D1608311

Thoracic Radiology

SERIES EDITOR

James H. Thrall, MD
Radiologist-in-Chief
Department of Radiology
Massachusetts General Hospital
Juan M. Taveras Professor of Radiology
Harvard Medical School
Boston, Massachusetts

OTHER VOLUMES IN
THE REQUISITES IN RADIOLOGY SERIES

THE REQUISITES

Thoracic Radiology

Second Edition

Theresa C. McLoud, MD
Professor of Radiology
Harvard Medical School
Associate Radiologist-in-Chief
Director of Education
Thoracic Radiologist
Massachusetts General Hospital
Boston, Massachusetts

Phillip M. Boiselle, MD
Associate Professor of Radiology
Harvard Medical School
Associate Radiologist-in-Chief of Administrative Affairs
Director, Thoracic Imaging Section
Beth Israel Deaconess Medical Center
Boston, Massachusetts

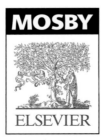

MOSBY

ELSEVIER

1600 John F. Kennedy Blvd.
Ste 1800
Philadelphia, PA 19103-2899

Thoracic Radiology : The Requisites   ISBN: 9780323027908
Copyright © 2010, 1998 by Mosby, Inc., an affiliate of Elsevier Inc.

All rights reserved. No part of this publication may be reproduced or transmitted in any form or by any means, electronic or mechanical, including photocopying, recording, or any information storage and retrieval system, without permission in writing from the publisher. Permissions may be sought directly from Elsevier's Rights Department: phone: (+1) 215 239 3804 (US) or (+44) 1865 843830 (UK); fax: (+44) 1865 853333; e-mail: healthpermissions@elsevier.com. You may also complete your request on-line via the Elsevier website at http://www.elsevier.com/permissions.

Notice

Knowledge and best practice in this field are constantly changing. As new research and experience broaden our knowledge, changes in practice, treatment and drug therapy may become necessary or appropriate. Readers are advised to check the most current information provided (i) on procedures featured or (ii) by the manufacturer of each product to be administered, to verify the recommended dose or formula, the method and duration of administration, and contraindications. It is the responsibility of the practitioner, relying on their own experience and knowledge of the patient, to make diagnoses, to determine dosages and the best treatment for each individual patient, and to take all appropriate safety precautions. To the fullest extent of the law, neither the Publisher nor the Editors assumes any liability for any injury and/or damage to persons or property arising out of or related to any use of the material contained in this book.

The Publisher

Library of Congress Cataloging-in-Publication Data

McLoud, Theresa C.
  Thoracic radiology : the requisites / Theresa McLoud, Phillip Boiselle. – 2nd ed.
     p. ; cm.–(Requisites series)
  ISBN 978-0-323-02790-8
  1. Chest–Imaging. I. Boiselle, Phillip M. II. Title. III. Series: Requisites series.
   [DNLM: 1. Thoracic Diseases–radiography. 2. Lung Diseases–radiography. 3. Radiography,
   Thoracic–methods. WF 975 M478t 2010]
  RC941.M356 2010
  617.5'407572–dc22

Acquisitions Editor: Rebecca Gaertner
Developmental Editor: Stacey Fisher
Publishing Services Manager: Hemamalini Rajendrababu
Project Manager: K. Anand Kumar
Design Direction: Steven Stave

Working together to grow
libraries in developing countries

www.elsevier.com | www.bookaid.org | www.sabre.org

ELSEVIER   BOOK AID International   Sabre Foundation

Printed in the United States of America

Last digit is the print number: 9 8 7 6 5 4 3 2 1

Dedication

"To my nephews, Malcolm and Paul"
                                    TCM

"To my wife, Ellen"

                                    PMB

List of Contributors

Suzanne Aquino, MD
Radiologist
Night Hawk Radiology Services
U.S. Corporate Office
Scottsdale, AZ

Jo-Anne O. Shepard, MD
Director of Thoracic Imaging
Radiologist
Department of Radiology
Massachusetts General Hospital
Boston, MA
Professor of Radiology
Harvard Medical School
Boston, MA

Beatrice Trotman-Dickenson, MD
Thoracic Radiologist
Brigham and Women's Hospital
Boston, MA
Instructor in Radiology
Harvard Medical School
Boston, MA

Conrad Wittram, MD
Radiologist
Night Hawk Radiology Services
U.S. Corporate Office
Scottsdale, AZ

Subba Digumarthy, MD
Assistant Radiologist
Thoracic Imaging Division
Massachusetts General Hospital
Boston, MA
Instructor in Radiology
Harvard Medical School
Boston, MA

Stephen Ledbetter, MD, MPH
Director of Emergency Radiology
Brigham and Women's Hospital
Boston, MA
Assistant Professor of Radiology
Harvard Medical School
Boston, MA

Foreword

THE REQUISITES series is designed to provide core material in major subspecialty areas of radiology for use by residents and fellows during their training and by practicing radiologists seeking to review or expand their knowledge. These books have also been found of value by non imaging specialists in their own respective areas of interest.

Thoracic Radiology: THE REQUISITES has been a particularly popular book in the requisites series. Thoracic imaging is part of the heart and soul of the specialty of radiology and encompasses a number of the most commonly performed procedures in our specialty. The subject is of interest to every radiologist.

Each book in the THE REQUISITES series presents special challenges in terms of its development. One of the challenges for thoracic radiology is that, taken together, imaging studies of the chest continue to represent the largest aggregate number of procedures performed in contemporary radiology practice. And, somehow, the "simple" chest x-ray is as complex and full of mystery as any of our more modern methods. Dr Theresa C. McLoud and her contributors have done a magnificent job of distilling the essential facts and concepts of thoracic radiology into a text that will serve the resident and practicing radiologist equally well.

As noted in the foreword to the first edition of *Thoracic Radiology: THE REQUISITES*, each volume in the series lends itself to a unique organizational structure. Dr McLoud is retaining the logical structure of the first volume. Technical and anatomical considerations are first presented followed by an exploration of the component parts of the chest including the lung, airways, pulmonary vasculature, mediastinum and pleura. Each chapter further subdivides the discussion by anatomy and disease category. This approach to organization maximizes the access by the reader to desired information and makes using the book extremely efficient for both an initial introduction and an in depth review.

Much of thoracic radiology is enduring but as with the rest of the specialty of radiology, there have been major changes and advances in both our understanding of disease and the technology that we apply to its diagnosis. Advances in CT from spiral scanning to progressively higher numbers of rows for multi-slice CT devices have revolutionized the application of CT. New approaches have been necessary for many conditions ranging from follow-up of pulmonary nodules to diagnosis of interstitial lung disease based on the superior resolution of today's imaging devices. CT has also displaced radionuclide imaging in many settings for the diagnosis of pulmonary embolism which was not nearly as important or well understood at the time of the previous edition of *Thoracic Radiology: THE REQUSITES*.

Since the first edition, positron emission tomography (PET) and PET/CT have become extraordinarily important in the practice of thoracic radiology. New insights into lung cancer have come from their application among other diseases. Magnetic resonance imaging has also begun to be applied more to diseases of the thorax although this modality still lags CT by a substantial margin. Dr McLoud and her co-authors have done a comprehensive job in including these and many other new directions into their book.

In a real sense, those entering training in radiology have a greater challenge than those entering many other disciplines. A surgical or medical house officer might find himself or herself performing a physical examination during their first days in their respective programs, something they learned in medical school. However, in radiology the knowledge base from medical school is only preparatory to the opportunity to begin learning radiology. Thus, THE REQUISITES series is specifically designed to help radiologists in training navigate from a very limited knowledge of imaging to a sufficient knowledge to begin engaging in clinical practice in a short period of time.

I believe residents in radiology will find *Thoracic Radiology: THE REQUISITES* to be an excellent tool for learning the subject. The book is comprehensively updated and illustrated with the most recent applications. In keeping with the philosophy of the series, the book can be reasonably read and reread during successive thoracic radiology rotations in a residency program. For practicing physicians, *Thoracic Radiology: THE REQUISITES* should be attractive as a concise and useful way to build or refresh their knowledge of thoracic imaging.

I congratulate Dr Theresa C. McLoud and her contributors for another outstanding edition of *Thoracic Radiology: THE REQUISITES*.

James H. Thrall, MD
Radiologist-in-Chief
Department of Radiology
Massachusetts General Hospital
Juan M. Taveras Professor of Radiology
Harvard Medical School
Boston, Massachusetts

Preface

The second edition of the THE REQUISITES in Radiology series similar to the original is designed to provide standard textbooks in each of the subspecialties of radiology, primarily for use by radiology residents throughout their years of training. This particular book in thoracic radiology is also designed to meet the educational needs of those training in pulmonary medicine, thoracic surgery, and critical care. This book defines the basic knowledge that radiology students need to master. It attempts to integrate a number of imaging modalities that are essential in the diagnostic imaging approach to clinical problems. These include standard chest radiography, computed tomography, magnetic resonance imaging and FDG positron emission tomography.

The book begins with chapters dealing with technical factors and the anatomy of the thorax. This is followed by an extensive review of important radiographic signs used in the diagnosis of chest disease. The approach is integrated, emphasizing signs on standard radiographs as well as cross-sectional imaging including CT, MRI and also FDG/PET imaging. The remainder of the text is devoted to specific disease processes with particular emphasis on anatomic areas such as the lung, the airways, the mediastinum, and pulmonary vasculature. The final chapter provides a brief summary of the important interventional techniques used by the radiologist in the diagnosis of thoracic disease. New additions to the second edition include updated imaging techniques including CT angiography, MDCT with multiplanar and 3D reconstructions, advanced CT methods for assessing emphysema including CT densitometry, advanced MR methods as well as FDG/PET applications in staging and evaluating malignancies. In addition to technical advances there is new subject matter which is addressed in this edition including an update on infections in HIV/AIDS, expanded information regarding CTA for diagnosis of acute and chronic pulmonary embolism, the new classification of idiopathic interstitial pneumonias and the new interventional technique of radiofrequency ablation of lung tumors.

Each of the chapters is extensively supplemented with tables and boxes that provide summaries of information presented in the text, including clinical features of disease processes, pathology, and radiographic signs. The intent of such a format is to allow the radiology resident to correlate clinical findings, pathophysiology, and radiographic observations in important disease processes.

Emphasis is placed on fairly common thoracic diseases, although uncommon diseases are addressed briefly, particularly if the imaging features are diagnostic. Tables of differential diagnosis are provided as appropriate.

The standard chest radiograph still remains the most frequently ordered imaging study. The number of disease processes affecting the thorax is legion, and it has been challenging to encompass all the necessary material in simple and direct form. However, the aim of this book is to provide a curriculum of the most important requisites in thoracic radiology, which will be beneficial to residents at any level of training, to fellows in allied clinical fields, and to physicians in practice. Hopefully, the second edition will continue to serve as a valuable learning tool for all of its readers.

Theresa C. McLoud, MD

Acknowledgements

I am indebted to several individuals who have contributed directly or indirectly to Thoracic Radiology: THE REQUISITES.

First of all, Dr James H. Thrall, Radiologist-in-Chief at Massachusetts General Hospital (MGH), Series Editor for THE REQUISITES, provided me with the encouragement to see the second edition of this project through to completion. This edition has been particularly enhanced by the contributions of Dr Phillip Boiselle from the Beth Israel Deaconess Medical Center and Harvard Medical School in Boston, who is now a co-author of this textbook.

A number of my present and previous colleagues at the Department of Radiology at MGH have also contributed original chapters and/or revisions. I am indebted to Dr Jo-Anne O. Shepard and Dr Subba Digumarthy, Dr Suzanne Aquino, as well as Dr Beatrice Trotman-Dickenson and Dr Stephen Ledbetter, currently radiologists at the Brigham and Women's Hospital in Boston, Harvard Medical School. Together we have attempted to craft an up-to-date textbook that reflects not only a large body of factual material about thoracic diseases, but that also offers our own approach to radiographic interpretation and diagnostic investigation.

I also wish to acknowledge all of my clinical colleagues in pulmonary medicine, critical care, and thoracic surgery who over the years have provided both the inspiration and the education in clinical decision-making that have helped to make this book possible. It is only appropriate to recognize the outstanding mentors who have helped to foster and support my career as a thoracic radiologist. Foremost is Dr Robert Fraser under whose tutelage I trained and with whose textbook mine, of course, will never be able to compete. Dr Juan Taveras provided me with the opportunity to flourish as a junior staff member and eventually as a division head at MGH. Finally, I wish to acknowledge Dr Edward Gaensler, a thoracic surgeon, pulmonologist, and clinical researcher extraordinaire, who helped to develop my interest in infiltrative and occupational lung disease.

Finally, this book could not have been possible without the dedication of many people involved in all stages of book preparation. Melanie Miller, Staff Assistant at MGH, provided secretarial assistance with the revised manuscripts. I also wish to thank and recognize all the professionals with whom I have worked at Elsevier. Their support and encouragement over the past few years have made this publication possible.

T.C.M.

Table of Contents

CHAPTER *1*

Thoracic Radiology: Imaging Methods, Radiographic Signs, and Diagnosis of Chest Disease

Theresa C. McLoud and Suzanne L. Aquino

■ EXAMINATION TECHNIQUES AND INDICATIONS

Chest Radiography

The plain chest radiograph is the most commonly performed imaging procedure in most radiology practices, constituting between 30% and 50% of studies. The standard routine chest radiograph consists of an erect radiograph made in the posteroanterior projection and a left lateral radiograph, both obtained at full inspiration.

The target film distance is 6 feet. Chest radiographs should be exposed using a high kilovoltage peak (kvp) technique, usually in the range of 100 to 140 kvp (Fig. 1-1). With this technique, a grid or air gap is required to reduce scatter radiation. The main advantage of this technique is that the bony structures appear less dense, permitting better visualization of the underlying parenchyma and the mediastinum. The only drawbacks are the decreased detectability of calcified lesions and loss of bony detail.

Additional views of the chest may be required in special instances (Table 1-1). Shallow oblique radiographs (15 degrees) may be useful in confirming the presence of a suspected nodule. Forty-five-degree oblique radiographs are recommended for the detection of asbestos-related pleural plaques. Apical lordotic views (Fig. 1-2) project the clavicles above the chest, improving visualization of the apices and the middle lobe, particularly in cases of middle lobe atelectasis. Expiration chest radiographs can be used to detect air trapping or to confirm small pneumothoraces. Lateral decubitus radiographs are commonly used to determine the presence or mobility of pleural effusion. These views can also be obtained to detect small pneumothoraces, particularly in patients who are confined to bed and unable to sit or stand erect. Bedside portable examinations may account for up to 50% of chest radiographs obtained for hospital patients.

The diagnostic quality of these images is usually limited because of the increased exposure time needed, which results in respiratory motion. Because the target film distance is considerably less than 6 feet, magnification occurs,

particularly of the heart and anterior structures. Many very ill patients, including patients in intensive care units, must be radiographed at the bedside, resulting in radiographs with limited diagnostic information.

During the past decade, rapid advances in electronics and computer technology have created new possibilities for x-ray imaging, including specific receptor systems independent of film that permit image information to be recorded in digital form and displayed on picture archiving and communication system (PACS) workstations. These systems include photostimulable phosphor computed radiography (PPCR) systems and selenium-based digital chest systems. A new generation of direct readout x-ray detectors based on thin film transistor arrays has emerged, offering unsurpassed image quality from a compact digital detector.

Storage PPCR systems employ a reusable imaging plate in place of the traditional screen film detector. These were first introduced in the middle to late 1980s and have been used for bedside radiography. The linear response of photostimulable phosphors over an extremely wide range of radiation exposures makes their application particularly good for portable radiography. A generation of digital x-ray systems based on flat panel detectors has emerged that provides good image quality and very rapid direct access to digital images. Most of these systems use large-area, thin-film transistor arrays. They offer compact packaging and direct connection to digital imaging networks. Image quality from digital acquisition systems is equivalent or better than standard film radiography.

Fluoroscopy

Fluoroscopy has become rather obsolete with the widespread application of computed tomography (CT) (Table 1-2). Fluoroscopy is mainly restricted to the evaluation of diaphragmatic motion. The patient is placed in an oblique position so that both hemidiaphragms can be visualized simultaneously. In patients with diaphragmatic paralysis, the affected hemidiaphragm moves up during a rapid inspiratory maneuver (e.g., a sniff).

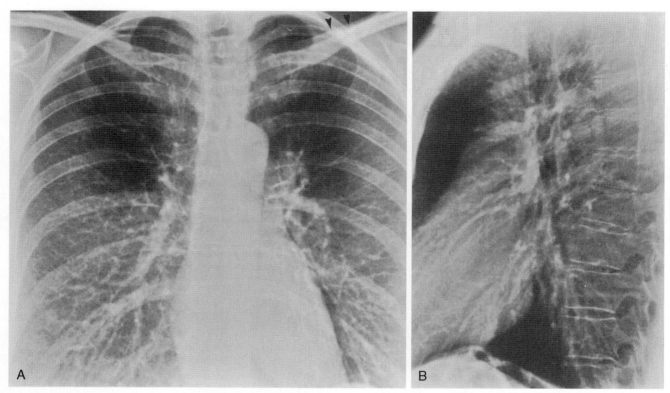

FIGURE 1-1. Standard posteroanterior and lateral chest radiographs obtained at 140 kvp, a 12:1 grid, and an automated phototimed exposure. Notice the visibility of retrocardiac vessels and mediastinal structures and the companion shadow of the left clavicle *(arrowheads)*.

TABLE 1-1 Indications for Nonstandard Chest Radiography

Projection	Indications
Oblique	Suspected nodule
	Plaques
Lordotic	Apical and middle lobe disease
Expiration	Air trapping
	Pneumothorax
Lateral decubitus	Pleural effusion
	Pneumothorax

Computed Tomography

Computed tomography typically is used as a diagnostic study, usually after a standard chest radiograph is obtained or when the chest radiograph result is considered to be abnormal (Box 1-1). Indications for CT include staging of lung carcinoma; a solitary pulmonary nodule, mass, or opacity; diffuse infiltrative lung disease; widened mediastinum, a mediastinal mass, or other abnormality of the mediastinum; an abnormal hilum; pleural abnormalities or the need to differentiate pleural from parenchymal abnormalities; chest wall lesions; trauma; and diagnosis of pulmonary embolism. CT may also be used for the detection of occult disease. Indications include detection of metastatic disease in tumors with a propensity for metastases to the lungs; hemoptysis or suspected bronchiectasis; evaluation of the thymus in patients who have myasthenia gravis; evaluation of patients with endocrine abnormalities that are associated with a suspected lung tumor or parathyroid adenoma; search for an unknown source of infection, especially in the immunocompromised population; evaluation of the pulmonary parenchyma in patients with normal chest radiographs and suspected diffuse infiltrative lung disease or emphysema; and suspicion of aortic dissection and other vascular abnormalities.

CT scans should be performed during deep inspiration at total lung capacity. For routine helical CT of the chest, contiguous 2.5- to 3-mm sections are recommended. High-resolution CT (HRCT) using thinner 1- to 1.25-mm sections can be used to study the fine details of the pulmonary parenchyma. A short scan time of 0.8 to 1 second is necessary to reduce the effect of motion. On routine studies, the field of view should be adjusted to the size of the thorax, but smaller fields of view may be selected for smaller anatomic parts that require study.

The routine approach is to obtain at least three window settings, used for the lung parenchyma, the mediastinum, and the bony structures. Suggested settings for the mediastinum are window level of +30 to +50 and window width of +350, and settings for the lung are a window width of +1500 and a window level of 2500 to 2700. The algorithm of reconstruction may be modified for the mediastinum or lung. For the mediastinum, a smoothing or standard algorithm is recommended. This is also sufficient for routine studies of the lung. However, HRCT requires an algorithm with high spatial resolution that corresponds to the bone algorithm on most scanners.

With thorough knowledge of mediastinal and hilar anatomy, contrast material may not be required for routine

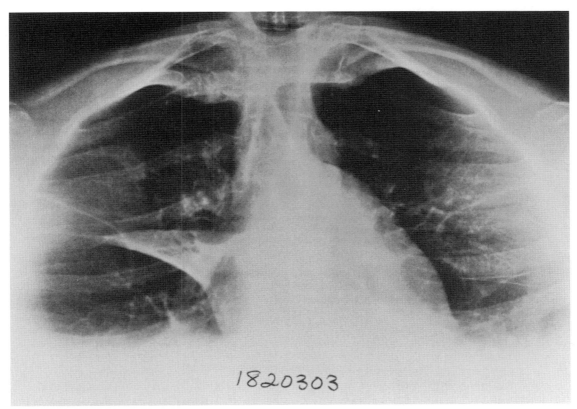

FIGURE 1-2. In an apical lordotic view, the clavicles are projected above the apices of the lungs. There is excellent demonstration of right middle lobe collapse.

TABLE 1-2 Indications for Chest Fluoroscopy

Technique	Indications
Fluoroscopy	Diaphragmatic movement
	Major airways, trachea

CT of the thorax, especially with a thinner slice thickness of 2.5 mm or less. However, contrast enhancement may be necessary for the evaluation of known or suspected vascular abnormalities (e.g., aortic aneurysm or dissection, pulmonary embolism), for evaluation of an abnormal hilum, or for abnormalities of the pleura. Approximately 100 to 150 mL at an injection rate of 2-4 mL/sec using an agent with 30% to 40% concentration of iodine is recommended. In hemodynamically normal individuals, the transit time of contrast from an antecubital vein to the right heart is about 3 seconds, 6 seconds to the pulmonary arteries, 9 seconds to the left heart, and 12 to 15 seconds to the major arteries. Although transit times vary among patients, we recommend as a routine a delay of at least 25 seconds between the onset of the injection and the first image. A power contrast injector should be used. Bolus tracking techniques allow for improved contrast opacification.

Improvement in scanner technology has led to the introduction of spiral or helical volumetric CT (Box 1-2). These CT scanners acquire data continuously and as the patient is transported through the scanner during a single breath

Box 1-1. Common Indications for Computed Tomography

ABNORMAL CHEST RADIOGRAPH
Staging lung carcinoma
Solitary nodule, mass, opacity
Infiltrative (interstitial) lung disease
Emphysema
Large and small airway disease
Mediastinum
  Widening
  Mass
  Other abnormality
Pleural abnormalities
Chest wall lesions

OCCULT DISEASE: NORMAL CHEST RADIOGRAPH
Metastases
Hemoptysis
Suspected bronchiectasis
Myasthenia gravis (thymus)
Endocrine abnormalities (suspected lung tumor or mediastinal parathyroid adenoma)
Unknown source of infection (immunocompromised host)
Suspected infiltrative (interstitial) lung disease
Suspected aortic dissection and other vascular abnormalities
Diagnosis of pulmonary embolism

Box 1-2. Indications for Helical and MDCT Computed Tomography

Routine assessment
Solitary pulmonary nodule
Metastatic disease
Airways
Vascular lesions
Peridiaphragmatic lesions
Pulmonary embolism

hold (Fig. 1-3). Multidetector helical CT (MDCT) revolutionized thoracic imaging by providing near-isocubic volumetric scanning. Initial multidetector imaging involved four slice detectors that are still popular today. However, this technology has expanded to 16- and 64-slice detectors as well as dual source scanners allowing even shorter scan times. With the newer technology, a patient's entire thorax is scanned in less than 10 seconds. MDCT slice acquisition provides a thinner slice thickness of an entire original dataset, with the elimination of interscan gaps and minimal respiratory motion. Capabilities include multiplanar imaging with little or no stair-stepping artifact on coronal, sagittal, and three-dimensional images. The greatest impact of MDCT in imaging the thorax involves reconstruction of the vasculature system and airways, and it provides comprehensive imaging of trauma patients (Fig. 1-4). Pulmonary embolism studies are obtained in shorter imaging sessions, improving on motion artifact and resolution of smaller subsegmental vessels.

Positron Emission Tomography

Increased metabolism of neoplastic cells can be detected by 2-[^{18}F]fluoro-2-deoxy-D-glucose (FDG) positron emission tomography (PET) imaging, and FDG-PET is there-fore useful in the detection of malignancy in pulmonary nodules, masses, and lymph nodes. PET is routinely used for the evaluation of a single pulmonary nodule equal to or greater than 1 cm in diameter and for staging and restaging of neoplasms, such as lung carcinoma, breast cancer, lymphoma, and melanoma, which commonly involve the thorax. A false-negative result for a pulmonary nodule may occur if the nodule is less than 1 cm. Tumors of relatively low metabolic activity, such as carcinoid tumor and bronchioloalveolar cell carcinoma, also may produce false-negative results. Because FDG-PET images the rate of glycolysis in tissues within the body, false-positive results can be seen in cases of infection and inflammation. False-negative results have been obtained for patients with focal infections such as mycobacterial disease and organizing pneumonia.

The implementation of FDG-PET has significantly improved the radiologic staging of lung cancer (Fig. 1-5). The characterization of lymph node disease by CT is limited by the use of size criteria to detect abnormal nodes. Lymph nodes are interpreted as abnormal if their short-axis diameter exceeds 1 cm. Because of reliance on size criteria, enlarged lymph nodes due to inflammatory or infectious disease are frequently misinterpreted as neoplastic. Early metastases in small nodes are not detected by CT. FDG-PET improves the specificity of lymph node disease detection by better identifying tumor involvement based on increased metabolic activity rather than anatomic enlargement. However, PET also has limitations when it comes to lymph node size. Detection of metastatic foci may also be limited by PET because of camera resolution. Lymph nodes with metastases that measure 5 mm in diameter or less may go undetected. False-positive results can be obtained in cases of granulomatous disease or silicosis. In the staging of lung cancer, mediastinoscopy should be performed on any patient with positive lymph nodes on FDG-PET to avoid erroneously overstaging a patient who has "hot" reactive nodes.

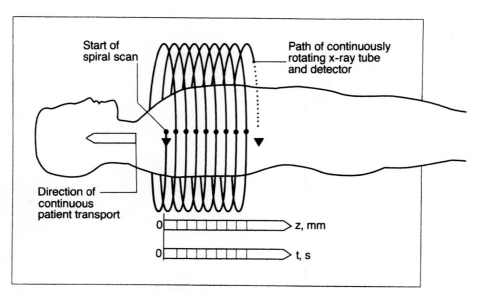

FIGURE 1-3. Helical CT scan principle. (From Kalender WA, Seissler W, Klotz E, Vock P: Spiral volumetric CT with single-breath-hold technique, continuous transport, and continuous scanner rotation. Radiology 176:181–183, 1990).

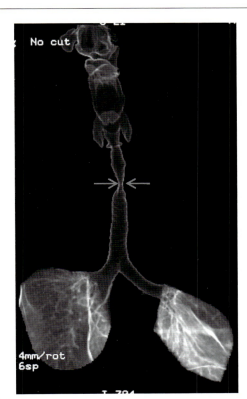

FIGURE 1-4. Three-dimensional external volume rendering shows subtle tracheal stenosis *(arrow)*.

Because of its relatively low spatial resolution, FDG-PET imaging should be interpreted with cross-sectional imaging such as a CT. Studies have shown that interpretation of PET improves when CT images are also available. The added application of fusion imaging of PET and CT by computer registration or dual PET/CT scanning has lead to even better radiologic sensitivity and specificity for detecting lymph node metastases and recurrent tumor. With dual PET/CT imaging, the CT scan is used for attenuation correction, thereby providing the high spatial resolution needed to better localize areas of increased FDG uptake on PET.

Magnetic Resonance Imaging

Magnetic resonance imaging (MRI) has not had extensive application in imaging the thorax, mainly because of problems due to motion artifacts caused by cardiac and respiratory movements. The normal lung does not produce an MR signal because of magnetic susceptibility effects. However, MRI does provide excellent images of the mediastinum and the chest wall, and it does permit direct imaging in the coronal, sagittal, and axial planes. General indications for MRI in the chest include evaluation of the mediastinum or vascular structures in patients in whom contrast media is contraindicated; diagnosis of aortic dissection and congenital abnormalities of the aorta; evaluation of superior sulcus tumors; imaging of chest wall lesions and brachial plexus abnormalities; staging of lung carcinoma with particular reference to direct chest wall and mediastinal invasion; and evaluation of posterior mediastinal masses (Box 1-3).

Some general recommendations can be made in regard to technique. Techniques can be varied according to the clinical indication. Typically, a body coil is used, and images are obtained in the axial plane using two different spin-echo sequences. With high field-strength magnets, electrocardiographic (ECG) gating should be employed. T1-weighted, multislice, single-echo (i.e., echo time [TE] values of 15 to 30 msec) sequences are always obtained, and a T2-weighted sequence with two echoes (i.e., TE of 60 to 100 msec) is obtained in most instances. T1-weighted images give information concerning diagnosis of masses and provide the best information about vascular anatomy. The T2-weighted images may render fluid collections distinguishable from solid masses and may help separate tumor from fibrosis (Fig. 1-6). Gadolinium contrast administration is often helpful in distinguishing benign from malignant conditions.

In addition to ECG gating, several other techniques can be used to limit or correct motion artifacts. Respiratory compensation and presaturation (i.e., destroying the magnetization of incoming blood by repeatedly imposing radiofrequency pulses to the areas adjacent to the image volume) to eliminate the artifacts related to blood motion are frequently used. Rapid scanning techniques (i.e., gradi-

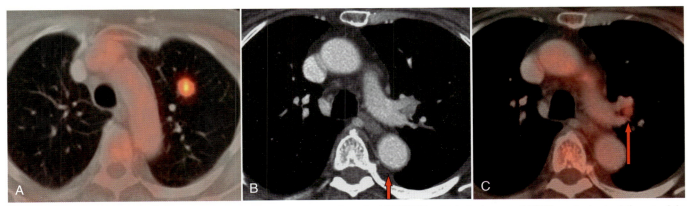

FIGURE 1-5. Dual FDG-PET/CT scan of lung cancer. **A,** Fusion image from dual PET/CT scan shows increased FDG uptake in the left upper lobe nodule. **B,** Subcentimeter hilar lymph node can be seen on the CT scan *(arrow)*. Because its size is less than 1 cm, this lymph node is not normally identified on CT. **C,** Fusion image from a dual PET/CT scan demonstrates increased FDG uptake in this node *(arrow)*. On surgical resection, the lymph node was found to contain metastatic adenocarcinoma.

Box 1-3. **Indications for Magnetic Resonance**

Contraindication to contrast medium; mediastinal or
vascular abnormality
Superior sulcus carcinoma
Chest wall and brachial plexus lesions
Posterior mediastinal masses
Mediastinal cysts

ent recalled acquisition of the steady-state [GRASS] or fast low-angle shot [FLASH]) that allow for acquisition of single or multiple images during a single breath hold have been developed. These techniques use decreased flip angles, gradient refocused echoes, and short repetition time (TR) and TE values.

Because MRI is often used as a problem-solving procedure, it needs to be correlated carefully with CT scans. For this reason, images are usually obtained in the transaxial plane. However, it is possible to have direct MRI in the sagittal and coronal planes. The benefits of imaging in the sagittal and coronal planes are that they better elucidate structures oriented longitudinally, and they reduce the chance of misinterpretation of findings due to volume averaging.

Fast imaging techniques, sometimes referred to as cine MRI, are available for imaging vascular structures and diagnosing vascular abnormalities. They are discussed in more detail by Miller in *Cardiac Radiology: The Requisites*, which is part of a series dealing with vascular diseases and cardiac imaging.

◼ ANATOMY

Airways

Trachea and Main Bronchi
The trachea is a midline structure that usually is 6 to 9 cm long. The wall contains horseshoe-shaped cartilage rings at regular intervals, but the posterior wall is membranous. The upper limits for coronal and sagittal diam-

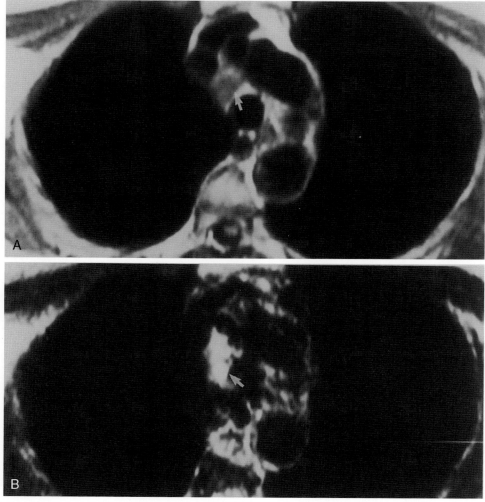

FIGURE 1-6. MRI of a bronchogenic cyst. **A,** T1-weighted image shows low signal intensity of the right paratracheal mass. The low signal intensity results from the water content of the cyst. **B,** On the T2-weighted image, the cyst has greater signal intensity than fat or muscle because of the long T2 value of water.

eters are 25 and 27 mm for men and 21 and 23 mm for women. The lower limit of normal in both dimensions is 13 mm in men and 10 mm in women. The trachea divides into two major bronchi at the carina. The carinal angle usually is about 60 degrees, but a wide range of 40 to 75 degrees can be seen in normal adults. The right main bronchus has a more vertical course than the left, and its length is considerably shorter. The air columns of the trachea, both major bronchi, and the intermediate bronchus are usually visible on well-exposed standard radiographs of the chest in the frontal projection (Figs. 1-7 and 1-8). The right lateral and posterior walls of the trachea are identifiable on posteroanterior and lateral chest radiographs as vertically oriented linear opacities, called the *right paratracheal* and *posterior tracheal stripes*. They are described in more detail in the "Mediastinum" section.

Lobar Bronchi and Bronchopulmonary Segments

Table 1-3 summarizes the bronchopulmonary segments of the right and left lung.

Right Side

The bronchus to the right upper lobe (Fig. 1-9) arises from the lateral aspect of the mainstem bronchus, approximately 2.5 cm from the carina. It then divides into three branches—the anterior, posterior, and apical—each supplying a segment of the right upper lobe. The intermediate bronchus continues distally for 3 to 4 cm from the takeoff of the right upper lobe bronchus and bifurcates to become the bronchi to the middle and lower lobes. The middle lobe bronchus arises from the anterolateral wall of the intermediate bronchus almost opposite the origin of the superior segmental bronchus of the lower lobe. It then bifurcates into lateral and medial segments.

The superior segmental bronchus is the first segment originating in the lower lobe. It arises from the posterior aspect of the lower lobe bronchus immediately beyond its origin and directly posterior to the takeoff of the middle lobe bronchus. Four basal segments subsequently arise from the root bronchus of the right lower lobe: anterior, lateral, posterior, and medial segments. This is the order of the basal bronchi from the lateral to the medial aspect of the hemithorax on a standard posteroanterior radiograph.

Left Side

The left upper lobe bronchus (Fig. 1-10) arises from the left main bronchus and then bifurcates or trifurcates. The upper division is the main left upper lobe bronchus and the lower division is the lingular bronchus. The upper division almost immediately divides into two segmental branches, the apical posterior and anterior. The lingular bronchus is analogous to the middle lobe bronchus of the right lung. The lingular bronchus then bifurcates into superior and inferior divisions or segments.

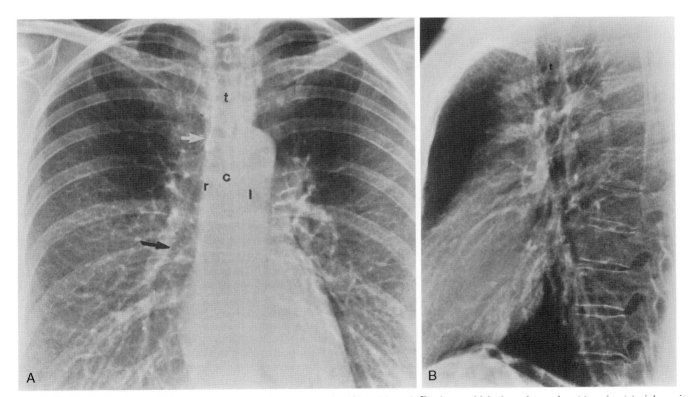

FIGURE 1-7. Tracheal and bronchial anatomy on standard posteroanterior (**A**) and lateral (**B**) views, which show the trachea (t), carina (c), right main bronchus (r), left main bronchus (l), right paratracheal stripe *(arrowhead)*, right intermediate bronchus *(large black arrow)*, and posterior paratracheal stripe *(arrowhead* in B).

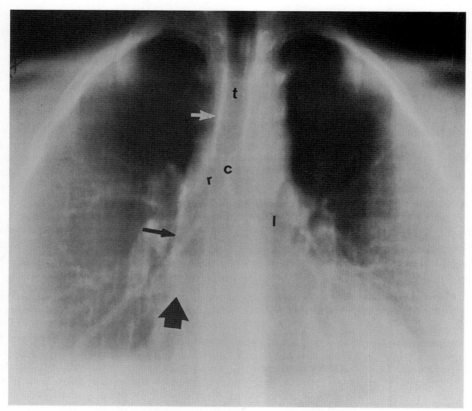

FIGURE 1-8. Anteroposterior tomogram shows the anatomy of the tracheobronchial tree, including the venous confluence *(black arrows)*, trachea (t), carina (c), right main bronchus (r), and left main bronchus (l). White arrow is the right paratracheal stripe, and the black arrow is the right intermediate bronchus, and the large arrow head is the venous confluence.

TABLE 1-3 Bronchopulmonary Segments

Right Lung Segments	Left Lung Segments
Upper Lobe	Upper Lobe
1. Apical	1 and 2. Apical posterior
2. Anterior	3. Anterior
3. Posterior	4. Superior lingula
Middle Lobe	5. Inferior lingula
4. Lateral	Lower Lobe
5. Medial	6. Superior
Lower Lobe	7 and 8. Anteromedial basal
6. Superior	9. Lateral basal
7. Medial basal	10. Posterior basal
8. Anterior basal	
9. Lateral basal	
10. Posterior basal	

The divisions of the left lower lobe bronchus are in name and anatomic distribution identical to the right lower lobe bronchus, except that there are usually three basal bronchi: anteromedial, lateral, and posterior. The distribution from lateral to medial on the frontal radiograph is anteromedial, lateral, and posterior. The lingular bronchus, like its corollary on the other side, the middle lobe bronchus, usually comes off directly anterior to the takeoff of the superior segmental bronchus of the lower lobe.

Pulmonary Vessels

The main pulmonary artery originates in the mediastinum at the pulmonic valve and passes upward, backward, and to the left before bifurcating within the pericardium into the short left and long right pulmonary arteries (Figs. 1-11 and 1-12). The right pulmonary artery courses to the right behind the ascending aorta before dividing behind the superior vena cava and in front of the right main bronchus into a right upper branch (i.e., truncus anterior) and the descending or interlobar branch. The interlobar artery subsequently divides into segmental arteries to the right middle and right lower lobes. The higher left pulmonary artery passes over the left main bronchus. It may give off a separate branch to the left upper lobe or, more commonly, continues directly into a vertical left interlobar or descending pulmonary artery from which the segmental arteries to the left upper and lower lobes arise directly. The left descending or interlobar artery lies posterior to the lower lobe bronchus.

The upper limit of normal diameters for the pulmonary arteries have been determined in normal subjects on the basis of CT scans: main pulmonary artery, 28.6 mm; left pulmonary artery, 28 mm; and proximal right pulmonary artery, 24.3 mm. The right interlobar artery can often be measured on standard radiographs, with the intermediate

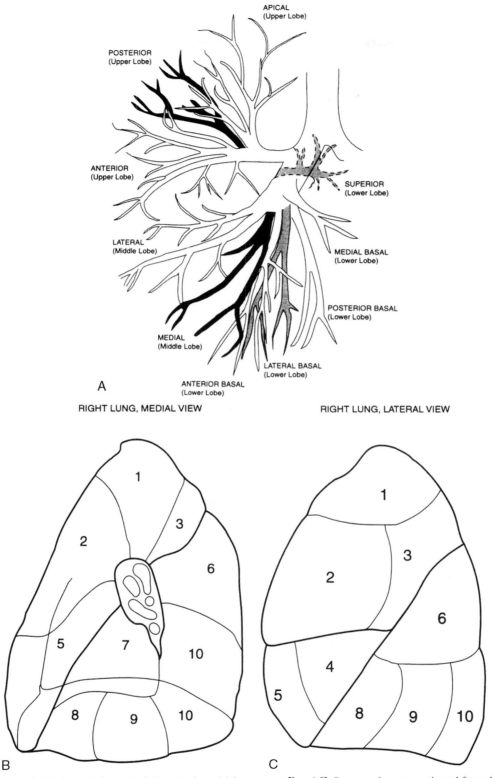

FIGURE 1-9. **A**, Anatomy of right bronchial tree, including the bronchial segments. **B** and **C**, Segmental anatomy viewed from the medial and lateral surfaces of the right lung.

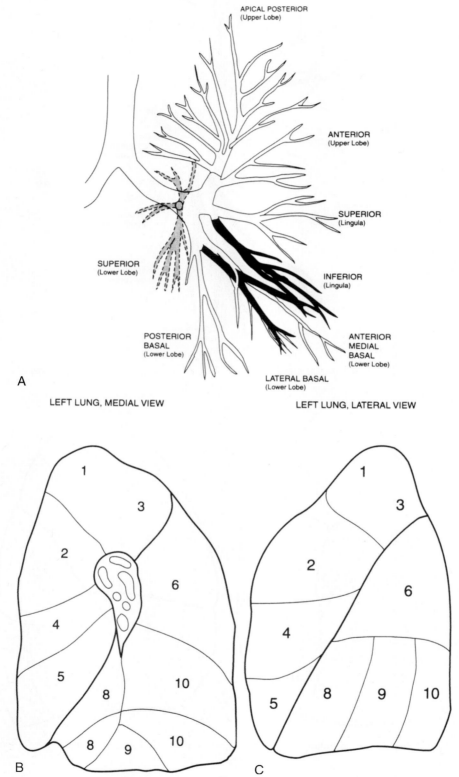

LEFT BRONCHIAL SEGMENTS

APICAL POSTERIOR
(Upper Lobe)

ANTERIOR
(Upper Lobe)

SUPERIOR
(Lingula)

INFERIOR
(Lingula)

SUPERIOR
(Lower Lobe)

POSTERIOR
BASAL
(Lower Lobe)

ANTERIOR
MEDIAL
BASAL
(Lower Lobe)

LATERAL BASAL
(Lower Lobe)

A

LEFT LUNG, MEDIAL VIEW

LEFT LUNG, LATERAL VIEW

B

C

FIGURE 1-10. A, Anatomy of the left bronchial tree, including the bronchial segments. B and C, Segmental anatomy viewed from the medial and lateral surfaces of the left lung.

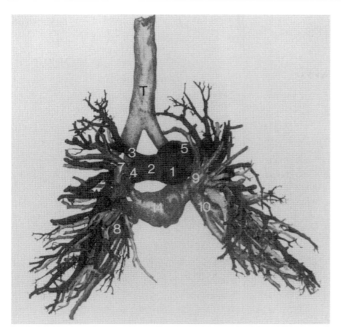

FIGURE 1-11. Central pulmonary vasculature: main pulmonary artery (1), right pulmonary artery (2), truncus anterior (3), right interlobar artery (4), left pulmonary artery (5), right superior pulmonary vein (7), right inferior pulmonary vein (8), left superior pulmonary vein (9), inferior pulmonary veins (10), and left atrium (14). (From Genereux GP: Conventional tomographic hilar anatomy emphasizing the pulmonary veins. Am J Roentgenol 141:1241–1257, 1983.)

bronchus serving as the medial border. The mean diameter is approximately 13 mm for men and approximately 12.5 mm for women. Another method for estimating changes in arterial caliber is the artery-to-bronchus index. Normally, the ratio of pulmonary artery to bronchus size at any point distal to the takeoff of the upper lobe bronchi is approximately 1.3:1 to 1.4:1. On CT scans, the more peripheral arteries can be visualized in the bronchovascular bundles, and the arterial bronchial index is approximately 1:1.

The right superior pulmonary vein drains the segmental veins of the right upper lobe and descends medially into the mediastinum to the upper and posterior aspect of the left atrium. After passing under the middle lobe bronchus, the middle lobe vein usually joins the left atrium at the base of the superior pulmonary venous confluence. The left superior pulmonary vein drains the left upper lobe and lingula and courses in an oblique fashion medially into the mediastinum to join the superior part of the left atrium. In the lower lobes, the right and left inferior pulmonary veins have a horizontal rather than an oblique course and drain into the left atrium medially. They form inferior pulmonary venous confluences.

Pulmonary Hila

The pulmonary hila, or roots, of the lungs contain bronchi, pulmonary and systemic arteries and veins, autonomic nerves, lymph vessels, and lymph nodes.

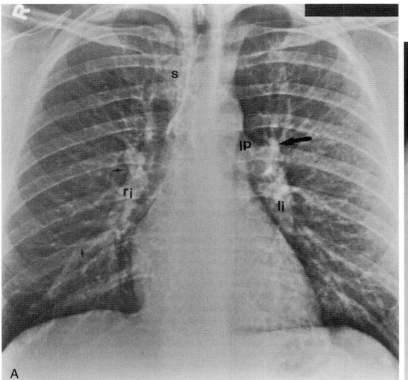

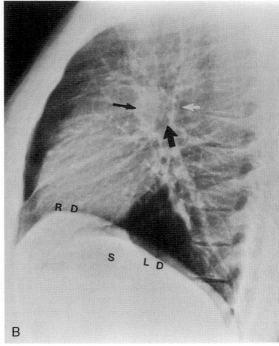

FIGURE 1-12. Central pulmonary vasculature. **A,** Left pulmonary artery (lp), left interlobar artery (li), right interlobar artery (ri), and sternum (s). *Small black arrows* on right indicate the right superior pulmonary vein that forms the upper border of the right hilum and a V configuration with the right interlobar artery. *Lower black arrow* on the right points to the horizontal course of the inferior pulmonary vein. *White arrow* on the left indicates the left superior pulmonary vein. **B,** Lateral view. Anterior portion of the hilar structures is made up mostly by the right pulmonary artery *(upper black arrow)*. The left pulmonary artery *(white arrow)* is seen as a longitudinal structure arching over and passing posterior to the left upper lobe bronchus *(lower black arrow)*. LD, left hemidiaphragm; RD, right hemidiaphragm; S, stomach bubble.

Standard Posteroanterior and Lateral Chest Radiography

The hila can be conveniently divided into upper and lower zones, and specific anatomic structures can be identified in each area (see Fig. 1-12). The upper part of the right hilum consists of the right superior pulmonary vein and the truncus anterior branch of the right pulmonary artery. A short segment of the upper lobe bronchus and the end-on anterior segmental artery and bronchus can often be identified. The lower portion of the right hilum is formed by the interlobar artery, which descends in a vertical manner and lies lateral to the intermediate bronchus. The horizontally oriented inferior pulmonary vein lies postero-inferior to the hilum. On the left side, the upper part of the left hilum is formed by the distal left pulmonary artery and the left superior pulmonary vein. The proximal left pulmonary artery is almost always higher than the highest point of the right interlobar artery, with the left hilum therefore being higher than the right. The lower portion of the left hilum is formed by the distal interlobar or descending artery and more caudally by the left inferior pulmonary vein. The air columns of the lingular and left lower lobe bronchus may be identified.

Occasionally, the venous confluences may be extremely prominent and produce vascular pseudotumors. This is particularly common in the right retrocardiac area when the inferior right venous confluence is prominent (see Fig. 1-8).

Understanding hilar anatomy on the lateral projection is critical (Fig. 1-13). The tracheal air column is always clearly visible and ends caudally in a rounded radiolucency that represents the distal mainstem or proximal left upper lobe bronchus seen end on. The right pulmonary artery is projected as a circular opacity anterior to this bronchus. The left pulmonary artery is tubular in configuration and arches over the left mainstem or left upper lobe bronchus. The right upper lobe bronchus can be identified approximately 1 cm above the left upper lobe bronchus. Between the right and left upper lobe bronchi, which are seen end on, is a thin, vertical, white line representing the posterior wall of the bronchus intermedius that courses inferiorly. It separates the lumen of the bronchus intermedius from the aerated right lung and the azygoesophageal recess posteriorly. The area beneath the left mainstem bronchus is sometimes referred to as the *inferior hilar window*. It should be clear and radiolucent. An opacity, particularly a rounded opacity, in this area suggests the presence of hilar or subcarinal adenopathy. Abnormalities of the hilum on standard radiographs may be increased opacity or changes in size, shape, or lobulation.

Computed Tomography

The pulmonary hila are probably best evaluated with CT. They can be visualized with or without the use of intravenous contrast medium. However, dense opacification of the pulmonary or the hilar vessels simplifies interpretation. The bronchial tree is best assessed at wide windows (i.e., 1500 to 2000 Hounsfield units [HU]). Visualization of hilar structures is also improved by thin (2-3 mm) sections. The anatomy of the hila is illustrated in Figure 1-14, and mediastinal anatomy is shown later (see Figs. 1-23 and 1-24).

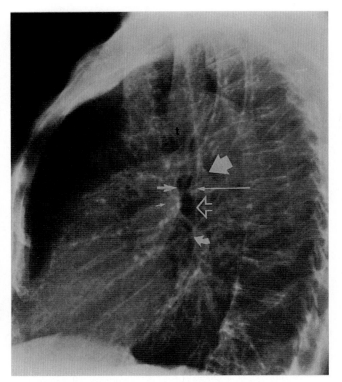

FIGURE 1-13. Hilar anatomy in the lateral view shows the trachea (t), right upper lobe bronchus *(large white arrow)*, left upper lobe bronchus *(white open arrowhead)*, right pulmonary artery *(small white arrow)*, left pulmonary artery *(large white arrowhead)*, posterior wall right intermediate bronchus *(long white arrow)*, and inferior hilar window *(curved white arrow)*.

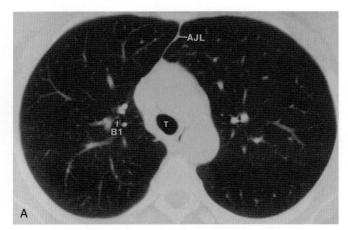

FIGURE 1-14. CT hilar anatomy. Sequential CT sections demonstrate anatomy of the major airways and central pulmonary vessels. ABSB, anterior basal segmental bronchus; AJL, anterior junction line; B1, apical segmental bronchus upper lobe; B2, anterior segmental bronchus upper lobe; B3, posterior segmental bronchus upper lobe; B6, superior segmental bronchus-right lower lobe and left lower lobe; BI, bronchus intermedius; LB, lingular bronchus; LBSB, lateral basal segmental bronchus; LDPA, left descending (interlobar) pulmonary artery; LLB, left lower lobe bronchus; LLLB, left lower lobe bronchus; LMB, left main bronchus; LULB, left upper lobe bronchus; MBSB, medial basal segmental bronchus; PBSB, posterior basal segmental bronchus; RIA, right interlobar artery; RLLB, right lower lobe bronchus; RMB, right main bronchus; RMLB, right middle lobe bronchus; RULB, right upper lobe bronchus; T, trachea.

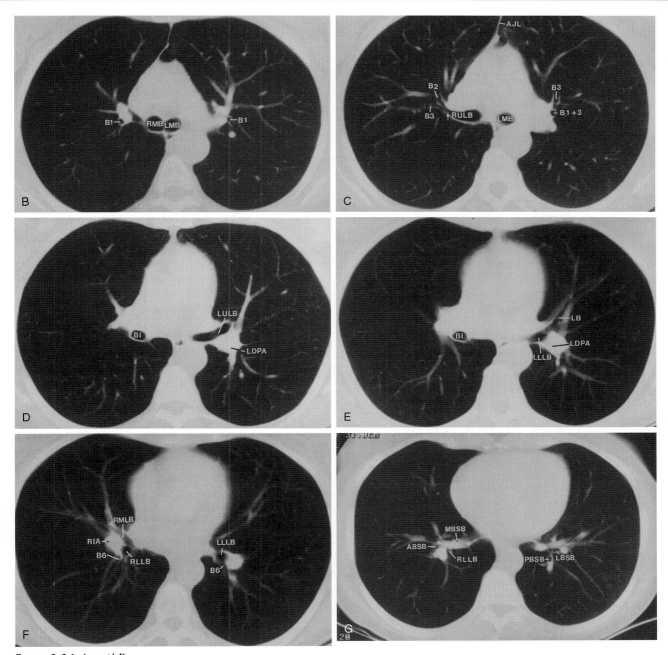

FIGURE 1-14. (cont'd)

Magnetic Resonance Imaging

MRI has several advantages in imaging the hila. Contrast is not required because flowing blood within hilar vessels generates no signal and can be easily differentiated from the lymph nodes and masses in the hila. The anatomy is identical to that described on CT in the axial plane. MRI also has the advantage of direct imaging in the coronal and sagittal planes.

The spatial resolution of MRI is less than that of CT, and on T1-weighted, spin-echo images, signal may be generated from soft tissues in the normal hilum that can be confused with enlarged nodes or masses. This signal is most likely caused by focal hilar fat and normal-sized lymph nodes. For these reasons, CT with contrast is the preferred method for evaluating the hila. However, MRI may be useful, particularly in patients who cannot tolerate intravenous contrast.

Pulmonary Parenchyma

Pulmonary Acinus

The pulmonary acinus is often considered an anatomic and functional unit of the lung parenchyma (Fig. 1-15). It refers to the gas-exchanging unit of the lung and is defined

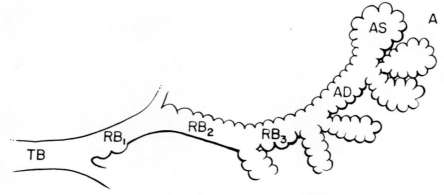

FIGURE 1-15. The pulmonary acinus. AD, alveolar duct; AS, alveolar sac; RB, respiratory bronchiole; TB, terminal bronchiole. From Thurlbeck WM: The Lung. In Sommers SC [ed]: Pathology Annual. New York, Appleton Communications, 1968.)

as that portion of the lung distal to the terminal bronchiole (i.e., the last purely conducting airway), which is composed of the respiratory bronchioles, alveolar ducts, alveolar sacs, and alveoli. There has been considerable debate about whether the acinus is radiologically visible. Experimentally, the acinus can be filled with bronchographic contrast medium, and the radiographic opacities that are produced are nodular opacities with a rosette appearance and a diameter of approximately 6 to 10 mm. However, it is debatable whether such "acinar shadows" can be identified with confidence in disease processes creating opacification in the lungs in living patients.

Secondary Lobule

The secondary lobule is defined as the smallest discrete portion of the lung that is surrounded by connective tissue septa (Fig. 1-16). It is composed of three to five terminal bronchioles with their accompanying airways and parenchyma.

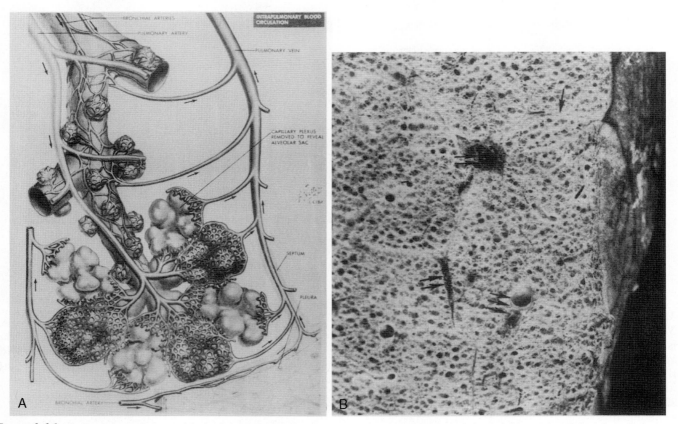

FIGURE 1-16. A, Secondary pulmonary lobule. Schematic drawing shows the pulmonary arteriole and airway in the center of the lobule. Pulmonary veins lie in the interlobular septum. **B,** Photograph of cut surface of inflated fixed lung. The margin of the secondary pulmonary lobule is formed by the interlobular septum, which is continuous with the pleural surface *(single arrow)*. The pulmonary arteriole and airway are seen in the center of the lobule *(three arrows)*, the pulmonary veins in the septa *(two arrows)*. (**A,** From Netter FH: Atlas of Human Anatomy. Basel, Novartis, 1989; **B,** from Groskin SA: Heitzman's the Lung: Radiologic Pathologic Correlations, 3rd ed. St. Louis, Mosby, 1993.)

The shape is usually polyhedral, and it usually is 1 to 2.5 cm in diameter. The secondary lobule has been recognized by some investigators as the radiographically visible basic structural unit of the lung. It is certainly the unit of the lung that is readily identified on HRCT. However, the distribution of lobules is not uniform throughout the lung, and the septa are better developed and more numerous in the lateral and anterior surfaces of the lower lobes. The secondary pulmonary lobule consists of core structures, which are the bronchus and accompanying pulmonary artery, and peripheral structures within the interlobular septa, which are the pulmonary veins and lymphatics.

In diffuse infiltrative (interstitial) lung diseases (see Chapter 7), the lobular architecture can often be readily identified on HRCT, and the relationship of the disease process to the center or the periphery of the lobule may be helpful in the diagnosis. However, lobular architecture is impossible to appreciate on standard chest radiographs.

Pleura

The pleurae consist of the parietal and visceral layers. The pleura is not of sufficient thickness to be visible on standard chest radiography. The pleura becomes visible when it is thickened, particularly over the lateral surfaces of the lungs and over the convexity, but such thickening cannot be appreciated along the mediastinal or diaphragmatic surfaces.

Interlobar Fissures

Between the lobes, contiguous layers of visceral pleura, called the *interlobar fissures*, separate individual lobes and can be visualized on standard chest radiographs (Fig. 1-17) and on CT. The fissures may or may not be complete, and incomplete fissures allow collateral air drift or spread of disease from one lobe to the other. The major or oblique fissures separate the upper and, on the right, the middle lobe from the lower lobes. They extend from

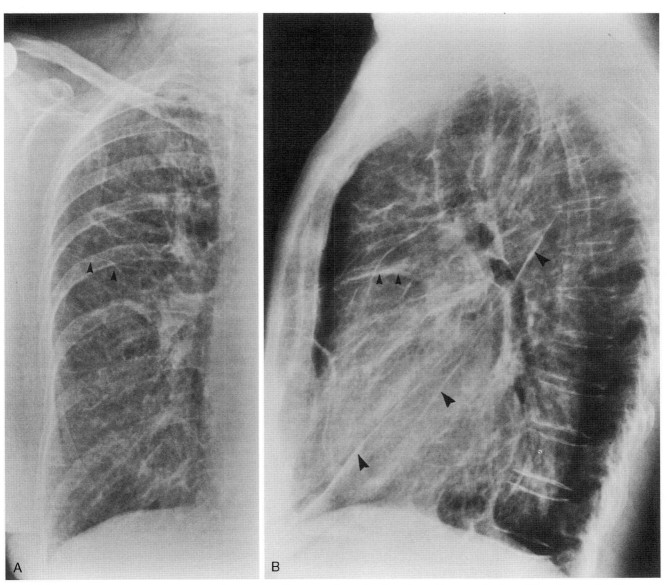

FIGURE 1-17. Interlobar fissures. Posteroanterior (**A**) and lateral (**B**) chest radiographs of a patient with congestive heart failure show a minor fissure *(small arrowheads)* and major fissures *(large arrowheads)*.

about the level of the fifth thoracic vertebra obliquely downward and forward, roughly paralleling the sixth rib to the diaphragm a few centimeters behind the anterior costophrenic angle. The minor or horizontal fissure separates the anterior segment of the right upper lobe from the middle lobe and lies in a horizontal plane at about the level of the fourth rib anteriorly. On a lateral chest radiograph, the posterior extent of the minor fissure is sometimes projected behind the hilum and the right major fissure due to the undulating course of the fissures. The position of the interlobar fissures is critical in the diagnosis of pulmonary volume changes such as lobar collapse. It is uncommon to see the normal major fissure on a frontal projection, and if it is visualized, it usually indicates thickening or fluid within the fissure or an abnormal position of the fissure due to volume loss and atelectasis.

The pleural fissures can usually be identified on CT (Figs. 1-18 and 1-19). On thick-section scans, they usually appear as lucent bands that are devoid of vessels and only occasionally as thin lines. However, on thinner-section CT, the fissures usually appear as thin lines or dense bands. On conventional thick-section CT, the minor fissure, because it is tangential to the CT scan, appears as a lucent area relatively devoid of vessels (Fig. 1-20).

Accessory Fissures

Accessory pleural fissures may occur between segments. Such fissures are more frequently incomplete and vary in the degree of development. The common accessory fissures include the azygos fissure, the inferior accessory fissure, the superior accessory fissure, and the left minor fissure (Box 1-4).

The azygos fissure (Fig. 1-21) is created by the downward invagination of the azygos vein through the apical portion of the right upper lobe. It creates a curvilinear opacity that extends obliquely from the upper portion of the right lung, and it terminates in a teardrop shadow caused by the vein itself above the right hilum. It contains four pleural layers. This fissure is visible in approximately 0.4% of chest radiographs. The portion of the lung lying medial to the fissure is often referred to as the *azygos lobe*.

The inferior accessory fissure separates the medial basal segment from the remainder of the lower lobe. It can often be identified on conventional posteroanterior chest radiographs. The fissure extends superiorly and slightly medially from the inner third of the right or left hemidiaphragm. It is seen on either side in approximately 8% of posteroanterior chest radiographs and in up to 16% of CT scans.

The superior accessory fissure separates the superior segment from the basal segments of the lower lobes. It lies in a horizontal plane at about the same level as the minor fissure, with which it may be confused on the posteroanterior chest radiograph, although it can be clearly identified on the lateral view.

The left minor fissure separates the lingula from the remainder of the left upper lobe. It is usually incomplete and may be identified in 1% to 2% of posteroanterior chest radiographs and more frequently on CT.

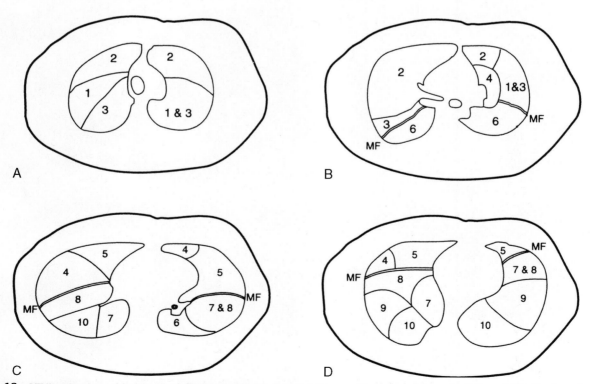

FIGURE 1-18. CT line drawings of four levels (**A-D**) from cephalad to caudad illustrate the course of the major fissures (MF). The bronchopulmonary segments are numbered. (Modified from Freundlich IM: Anatomy. In Freundlich IM, Bragg DG [eds]: A Radiologic Approach to Diseases of the Chest, 2nd ed. Baltimore, Williams & Wilkins, 1992.)

Inferior Pulmonary Ligament

The inferior pulmonary ligaments bilaterally are reflections of the parietal pleura that extend from just below the inferior margins of the pulmonary hila inferiorly and to the diaphragm posteriorly. They can be visualized in normal individuals on CT (Fig. 1-22). They usually appear as broad bands connected to the mediastinum extending from around the region of the esophagus to the diaphragm. The right inferior pulmonary ligament usually lies adjacent to the esophagus and posterior to the inferior vena cava. The ligaments should be distinguished from the phrenic nerves, which are nearby. The left phrenic nerve is usually identified lying adjacent to the pericardium, whereas the right phrenic nerve is only occasionally visualized.

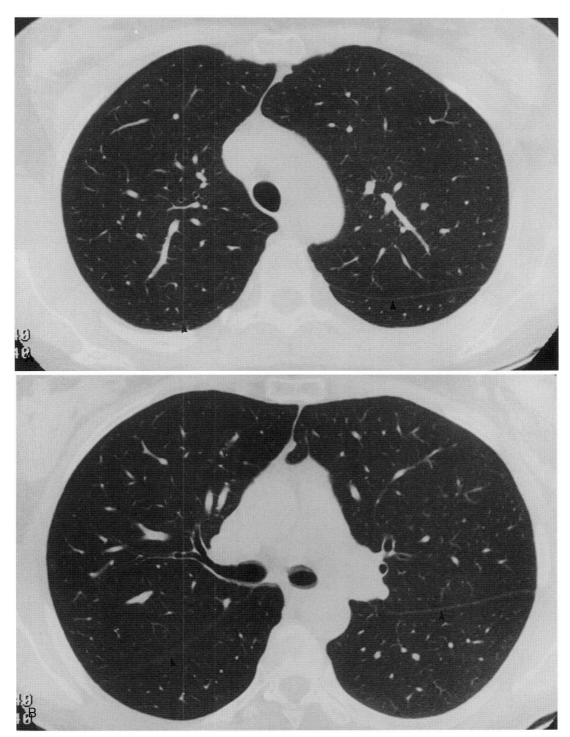

FIGURE 1-19. Comparable CT sections show the major fissures bilaterally. They appear as lines because of the thinness (1.5 mm) of the slices *(arrowheads).*

(Continued)

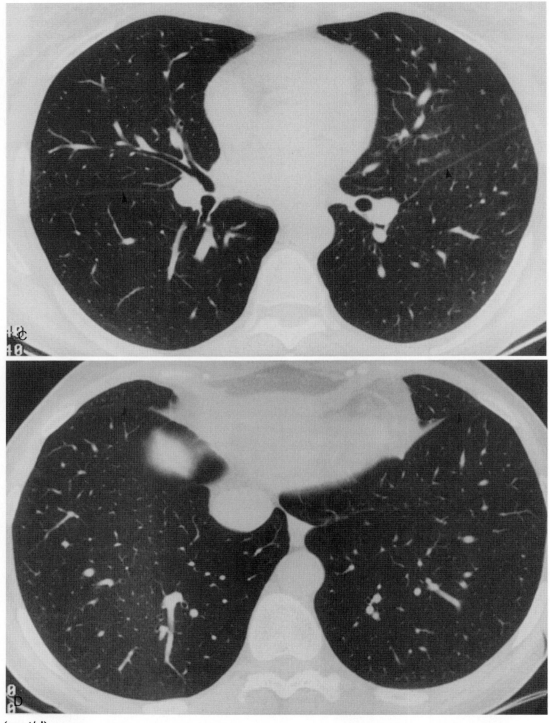

FIGURE 1-19. (cont'd)

MEDIASTINUM

The anatomy of the mediastinum on CT and MRI is shown in Figures 1-23 and 1-24.

Lymph Nodes

A number of lymph node classifications exist, the most important being that of Rouvière (Table 1-4). The American Thoracic Society has developed a numbered map of mediastinal lymph nodes that is used in the staging of lung carcinoma (Fig. 1-25).

Normal-sized lymph nodes can be identified on CT, and there is a range in size of normal lymph nodes. Most normal nodes are 7 mm or less in diameter, but normal nodes up to 11 mm and occasionally 15 mm in diameter may be observed. For practical analysis, lymph nodes up to 1 cm in

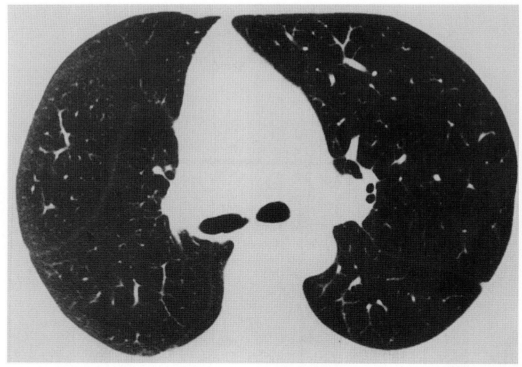

Figure 1-20. Minor fissure. Thin-section CT at the level of the carina demonstrates the minor fissure as a bandlike structure *(arrowheads).*

> **Box 1-4. Accessory Fissures**
>
> Azygos
> Superior accessory
> Inferior accessory
> Left minor

diameter should be considered to be within normal limits for size (see Fig. 1-23F). Normal lymph nodes on CT occasionally have low attenuation or fatty centers, a reliable indication that they are not involved with malignancy.

Anterior Mediastinal Lymph Nodes
Internal Mammary Nodes. The internal mammary nodes are parietal lymph nodes that communicate with lymphatics from the medial chest wall, including the breasts, pleurae, and diaphragm. They are located close to the anterior chest wall on either side of the sternum. They are usually not identified on standard radiographs unless they are markedly enlarged, but they are easy to identify on CT adjacent to the internal mammary vessels (see Fig. 1-23G).
Prevascular Nodes. Prevascular nodes are located anterior to the great vessels. They usually occur on the left side. These nodes communicate with the internal mammary nodes. The lowest node of this group is often referred to as the *aorticopulmonary window* or *ductus node*, and it is situated just above the left pulmonary artery near the ligamentum arteriosum (see Fig. 1-23F). This group communicates with the left paratracheal nodes.

Anterior Diaphragmatic Lymph Nodes. These lymph nodes are also parietal lymph nodes that occur on the anterior surface of the diaphragm. These lymph nodes communicate with diaphragmatic lymphatics from the peritoneal surface and drain the diaphragm on the thoracic side, the anterior pleura, and the pericardium. They are readily identified on CT between the pericardium, diaphragm, and anterior chest wall. The most medial node is referred to as the *pericardiac node.*

Middle Mediastinal Lymph Nodes
Paratracheal Nodes. There are right and left paratracheal chains along the anterolateral walls of the trachea (see Fig. 1-23F). On the right side, they drain mainly the right upper lobe, but they may drain the right middle and lower lobes indirectly. The lowest node of this chain is called the *azygous node*. It is usually the largest, and it is located in the tracheobronchial angle. The left paratracheal nodes are fewer and smaller than on the right side. These lymph nodes may drain cephalad along the trachea or toward the lymph nodes of the aortopulmonary window.
Subcarinal Lymph Nodes. The subcarinal lymph nodes are visceral lymph nodes that lie below the tracheal bifurcation anteriorly or posteriorly. They extend along the inferior margins of the main bronchi (see Fig. 1-23I).

Posterior Mediastinal Lymph Nodes
The posterior mediastinal lymph nodes occur in the paraesophageal, para-aortic, and prevertebral nodal groups. Even when enlarged, they are difficult to see on the standard

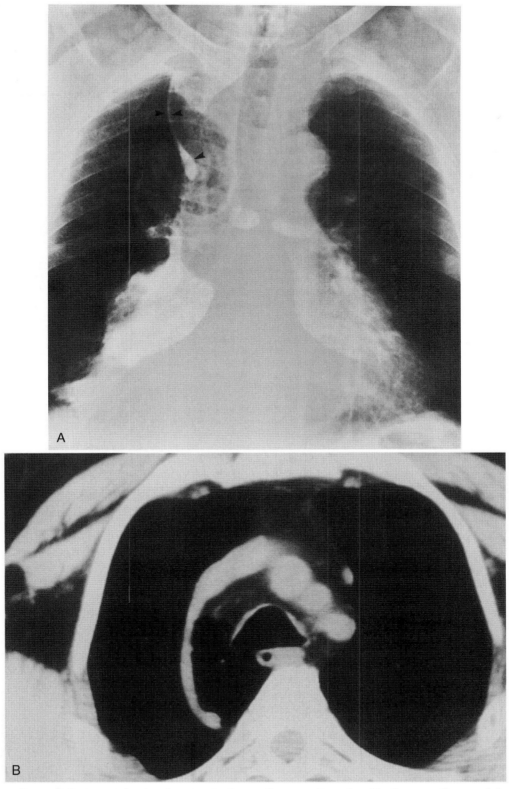

FIGURE 1-21. Azygos fissure. **A,** Posteroanterior view demonstrates the curvilinear opacity produced by the azygos fissure and the teardrop opacity of the azygos vein *(arrowheads).* The fissure is prominent because it contains fluid. **B,** CT appearance of the azygos fissure.

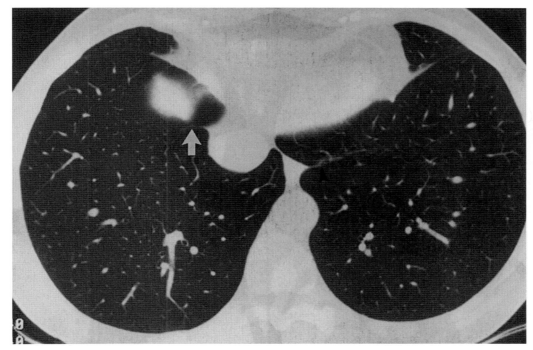

FIGURE 1-22. The left inferior pulmonary ligament can be seen as a band extending from and connected to the mediastinum just to the left of the esophagus *(arrowhead)*. The right phrenic nerve is seen adjacent to the inferior vena cava *(arrow)*.

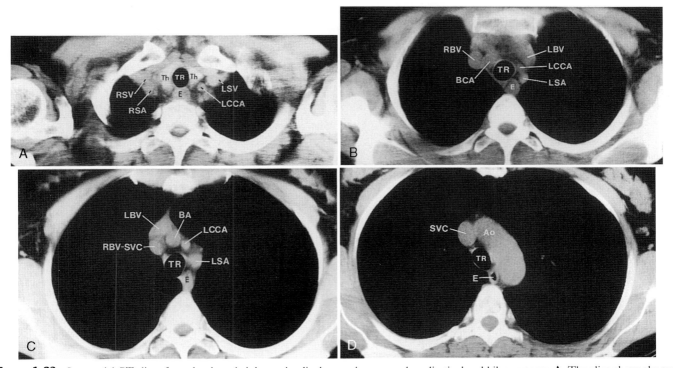

FIGURE 1-23. Sequential CT slices from the thoracic inlet to the diaphragm show normal mediastinal and hilar anatomy. **A,** The slice shows the trachea (TR), thyroid gland (Th), right subclavian vein (RSV), right subclavian artery (RSA), esophagus (E), left subclavian vein (LSV), and left common carotid artery (LCCA). **B,** The slice shows the right brachiocephalic vein (RBV), brachiocephalic artery (BCA), left brachiocephalic vein (LBV), and left subclavian artery (LSA). **C,** The slice shows the right brachiocephalic vein and superior vena cava junction (RBV-SVC). **D,** The slice shows the superior vena cava (SVC) and aorta (Ao).

(Continued)

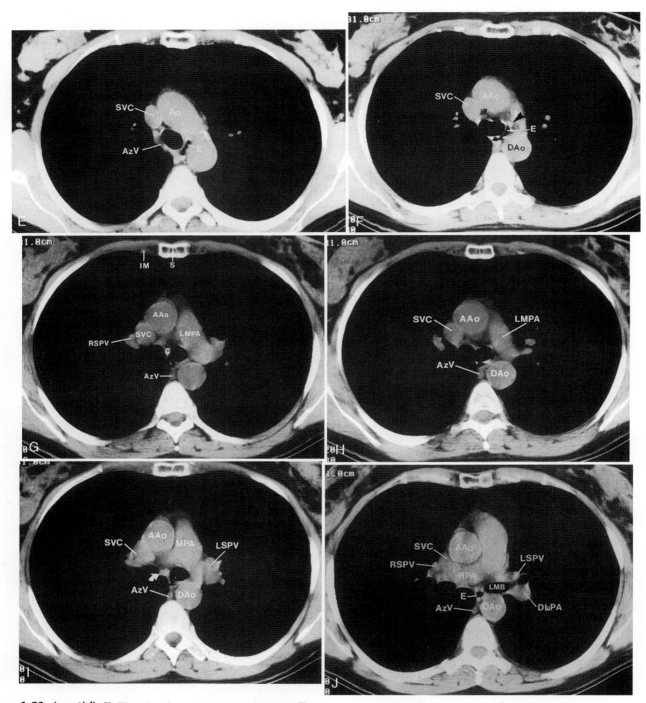

FIGURE 1-23. (cont'd) E, The slice shows the azygos vein (AzV). F, Slice shows the descending aorta (DAo). G, The slice shows the right superior pulmonary vein (RSPV), left main pulmonary artery (LMPA), internal mammary vessels (IM), sternum (S), tracheal carina (C), and main pulmonary artery (MPA). I, The slice shows the left superior pulmonary vein (LSPV). J, The slice shows the right pulmonary artery (RPA), descending (interlobar pulmonary artery) (DLPA), and left main bronchus (LMB).

chest radiograph. These nodes may communicate with the thoracic duct, inferior pulmonary ligament, subcarinal nodes, and intra-abdominal nodes. The intercostal nodes, which lie in the paravertebral fat by the rib heads, drain the pleura and, in the lower thorax, the posterior diaphragm. On CT, these nodes are usually not identified unless they are enlarged.

Hilar Nodes
Hilar nodes (i.e., tracheobronchial lymph nodes) are the nodes of the lung hila. They occur most frequently at the bifurcations of the bronchi and vessels. Illustrations of nodal enlargement in each of these locations can be found in Chapter 17.

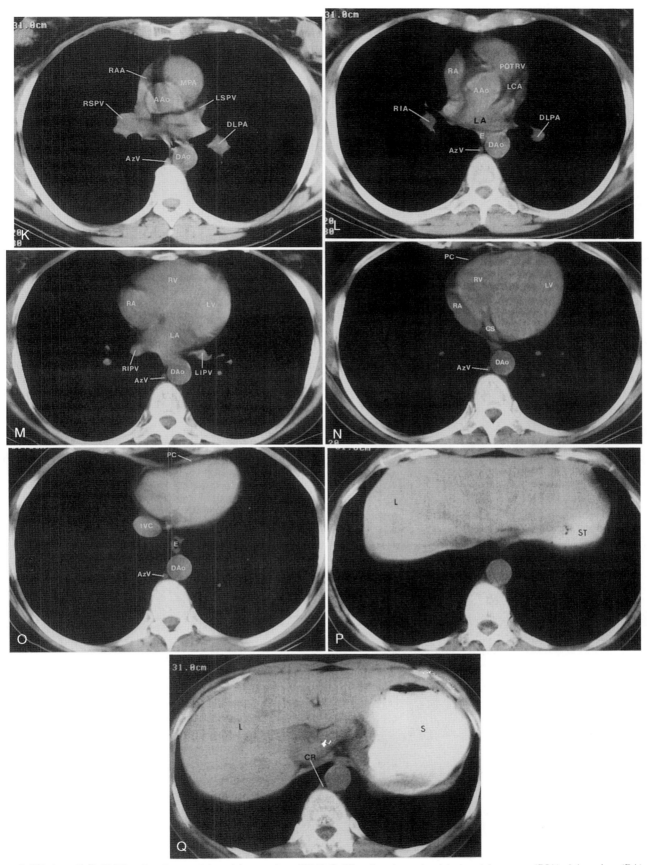

FIGURE 1-23. (cont'd) **K**, The slice shows a right atrial appendage (RAA). **L**, The slice shows the right interlobar artery (RIA), right atrium (RA), pulmonary outflow tract of the right ventricle (POTRV), and left coronary artery (LCA). **M**, The slice shows the left atrium (LA), right inferior pulmonary vein (RIPV), right ventricle (RV), left ventricle (LV), and left inferior pulmonary vein (LIPV). **N**, The slice shows the pericardium (PC) and coronary sinus (CS). **O**, The slice shows the inferior vena cava (IVC). **P**, The slice shows the liver (L) and stomach (ST). **Q**, The slice shows the crus of the diaphragm (CR), the liver (L), and the stomach (S). A normal-sized right paratracheal lymph node *(small black arrowhead)*, aorticopulmonary (anteroposterior window) lymph node *(large black arrowhead)*, and subcarinal lymph node *(curved white arrow)* can be seen.

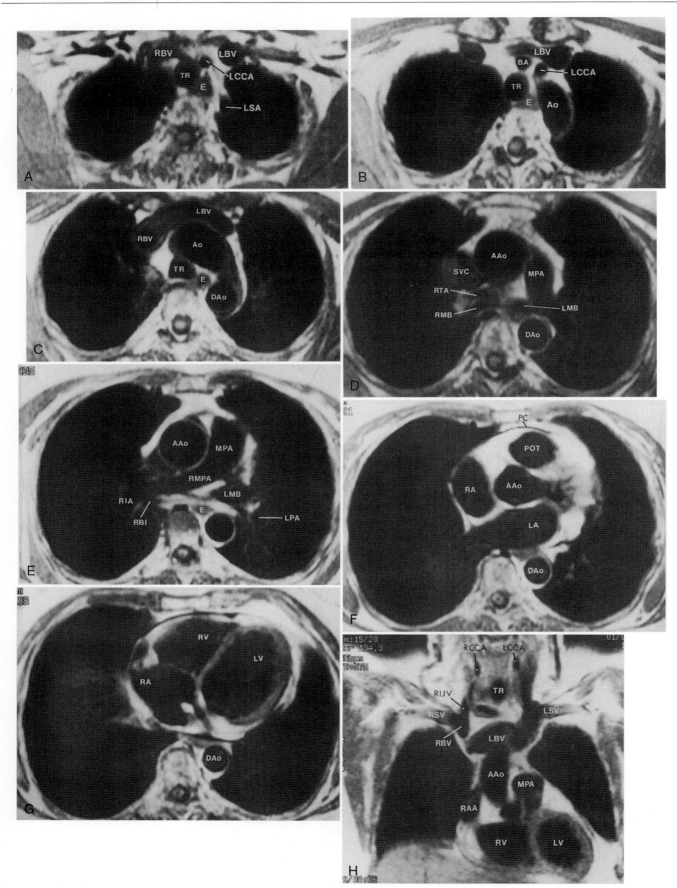

FIGURE 1-24. MRI of mediastinal and hilar anatomy. **A-G,** Sequential axial images from the thoracic inlet to the cardiac apex.

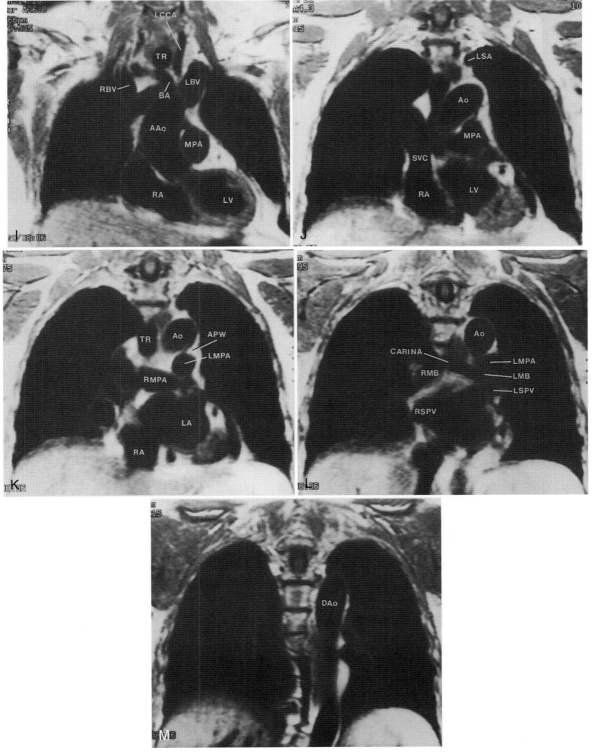

FIGURE 1-24. (cont'd) H-M, Coronal images proceeding from anterior to posterior.

(Continued)

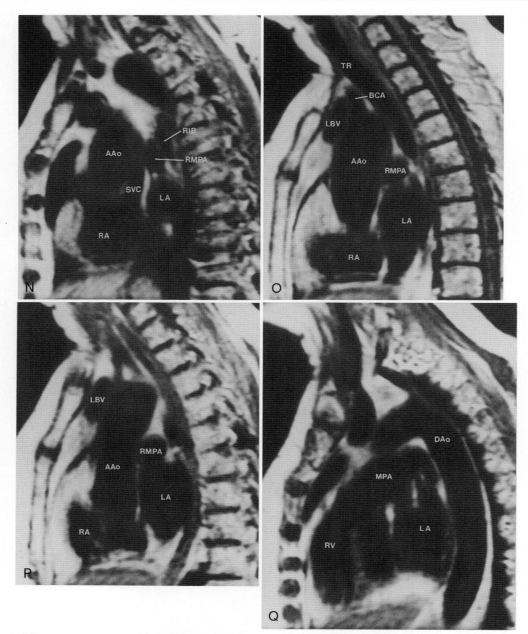

Figure 1-24 (cont'd) **N-Q,** Sagittal images from right to left. Ao, aorta; AAo, ascending aorta; APW, aorticopulmonary window; BA, brachial artery; BCA, brachiocephalic artery; DAo, descending aorta; E, esophagus; LA, left atrium; LBV, left brachiocephalic vein; LCCA, left common carotid artery; LMB, left main bronchus; LMPA, left main pulmonary artery; LSA, left subclavian artery; LSPV, left superior pulmonary vein; LV, left ventricle; MPA, main pulmonary artery; POT, pulmonary outflow tract; RA, right atrium; RBI, right bronchus intermedius; RBV, right brachiocephalic vein; RIA, right interlobar artery; RIB, right intermediate bronchus; RMB, right main bronchus; RMPA, right main pulmonary artery; RSPV, right superior pulmonary vein; RTA, right truncus anterior artery (right upper lobe branch); RV, right ventricle; SVC, superior vena cava; TR, trachea.

Other Mediastinal Anatomy

Other features of mediastinal anatomy are discussed in Chapters 15, 16, and 17.

Diaphragm

The diaphragm is a muscular tendinous sheath that separates the thoracic and abdominal cavities. It receives its blood supply from the phrenic and intercostal arteries and from branches of the internal mammary artery. Its nerve supply comes from the phrenic nerve. In most individuals, on standard posteroanterior radiographs, the right hemidiaphragm is approximately one half of an interspace above the left (see Fig. 1-12). The anterior portion of the left hemidiaphragm is obscured by the heart and lies above the stomach bubble. The diaphragm usually

TABLE **1-4** Lien and Lund's Modification of Rouvière's Classification System

Lymph Node Group	Drainage Area
Anterior Mediastinal Nodes	
Parietal group	Breasts, liver, anterior chest
Internal mammary nodes	and abdominal wall, diaphragm,
Superior diaphragmatic nodes	pleura, pericardium
Prevascular group	Thymus
Right anterior nodes	Heart
(prevenous)	Pericardium
Intermediate anterior nodes	Lungs, especially left upper
Left anterior nodes	lobe
(prearterial)	
Middle Mediastinal Nodes	
Paratracheal group	Lungs
Right lateral nodes	Trachea
Left lateral nodes	Bronchi
Pretracheal nodes	Esophagus
Retrotracheal nodes	Pericardium
Intertracheobronchial	
(subcarinal group)	
Tracheobronchial (pulmonary	
root) group	
Posterior Mediastinal Nodes	
Paraesophageal nodes	Esophagus, pericardium
Para-aortic nodes	Diaphragm, lower lung lobes
Paravertebral group	Posterior chest wall
Prevertebral nodes	Vertebrae
Lateral vertebral nodes	

From Lien HH, Lund G: Computed tomography of mediastinal nodes: anatomic review based on contrast enhanced nodes following foot lymphography. Acta Radiol Diagn 26:641–647, 1985.

has a smooth contour, but scalloping may occur; smooth arcuate elevations may be observed in about 5% of normal individuals.

Chest Wall

Certain soft tissue structures in the chest wall can be identified on standard radiographs. The pectoralis muscles form the anterior axillary fold. Calcification of the rib cartilages is a common and normal finding and one that increases with age. There is a difference in the pattern of calcification between men and women. Among men, the upper and lower borders of the cartilage become calcified first, whereas in women, the cartilage tends to calcify initially in a central location. Companion "shadows" can be seen outlining the clavicles and ribs (Fig. 1-26; see Fig. 1-1A). They are smooth soft tissue opacities that parallel these bones and measure 1 to 2 mm in diameter, particularly along the axillary portions of the lower ribs. They are caused by visualization in tangential projection of the parietal pleura and soft tissues immediately external to the pleura. They should not be confused with pleural thickening. Congenital anomalies of the ribs include supernumerary ribs (i.e., cervical ribs that arise from the seventh cervical vertebra). Intrathoracic ribs are rare congenital anomalies. They usually arise from a vertebral body and extend downward and laterally to end at or near the diaphragm. The normal thoracic spine is straight in frontal

projection and concave anteriorly in the lateral projection (see Fig. 1-1). The lateral and superior borders of the manubrium may be visible on standard posteroanterior chest radiographs (see Fig. 1-12A).

■ SIGNS OF DISEASE AND PATTERN RECOGNITION

Important radiographic signs of lung disease must be recognized when interpreting standard chest radiographs. Abnormalities on CT scans often parallel the changes observed on standard radiographs. However, the axial imaging of CT often provides more detailed information because it eliminates superimposition of abnormalities and provides more detailed and accurate anatomic localization, even to the level of the secondary pulmonary lobule. CT signs of disease are dealt with more specifically in each of the chapters discussing disease entities. Radiographic signs of pleural and mediastinal disease are also dealt with in their own chapters.

Alveolar Consolidation

It has been traditional to divide disease processes involving the pulmonary parenchyma into those that primarily involve the air spaces (i.e., the alveoli or distal acinus) and those that involve the interstitium. However, this approach to pattern recognition has many limitations, particularly poor correlation with histology. Many diffuse disease processes in the lung involve the alveoli and the interstitium, and it is almost impossible radiologically to differentiate nodules that are produced by disease in the interstitium from nodules that are caused by acinar or airspace filling. However, it is useful to consider homogeneous amorphous opacification, often with air bronchograms and ill-defined margins, as representing alveolar consolidation with airspace filling (Box 1-5). The term *alveolar consolidation* or *alveolar disease* is used in this textbook to describe these processes. The appearance may be caused by accumulation of edema, hemorrhage, or neoplastic elements within the alveolar spaces, and the interstitium also may be involved. Parenchymal consolidation is usually characterized radiographically by coalescent opacities that usually do not respect segmental boundaries (Fig. 1-27). The edge characteristics are ill defined and show poor margination. An example of this is the butterfly or bat wing appearance of acute pulmonary edema in left-sided congestive heart failure. Consolidation of the lung parenchyma often produces an air bronchogram (Fig. 1-28). The normally invisible air within the bronchial tree becomes apparent because of the surrounding consolidation. On standard radiographs, this sign usually is seen when the bronchus is not occluded, such as by lung carcinoma, although on CT, air bronchograms can definitely be observed even distal to a bronchial obstruction. Occasionally, minute radiolucencies may be seen within parenchymal consolidation. They may represent incompletely filled bronchioles and alveoli, an occurrence sometimes called an *air alveologram, pseudocavitation, or bubbly lucencies*. One of the important features of airspace consolidation is the absence of volume loss or atelectasis.

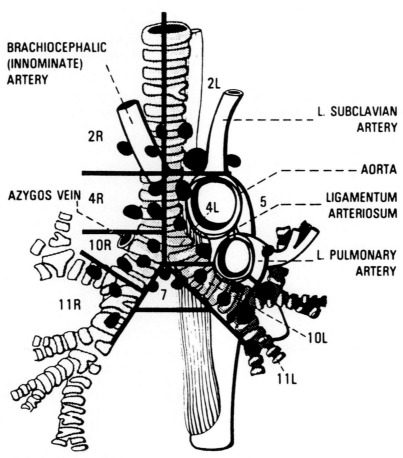

FIGURE 1-25. American Thoracic Society lymph node classification: 2R and 2L, high paratracheal; 4R and 4L, lower paratracheal; 5, aorticopulmonary; 7, subcarinal; 10R and 10L, tracheobronchial; 11R and 11L, bronchopulmonary (hilar) nodes.

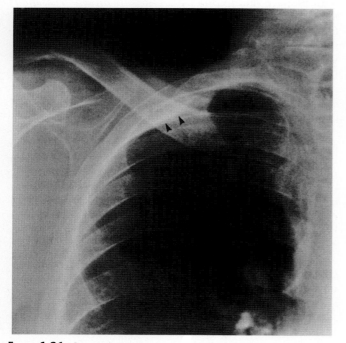

FIGURE 1-26. Companion shadow of the second rib on the right *(arrowheads).*

> *Box 1-5.* **Signs of Alveolar Disease**
>
> Homogeneous amorphous opacification
> Ill-defined margins
> Air bronchograms
> Coalescence
> Absence of volume loss
> Ground-glass pattern on computed tomography

There are many causes of parenchymal consolidation. The process may be localized or diffuse. It may be helpful to consider that the parenchyma of the lung and the alveoli may be filled with water, pus, blood, cells, or protein. Box 1-6 lists some of the more common causes of alveolar consolidation.

Infiltrative (Interstitial) Lung Disease

Many of the diffuse diseases involving the lungs arise primarily in the interstitium, although they may eventually involve the alveoli. This group of diseases may be referred to as *infiltrative lung disease* rather than purely interstitial disease,

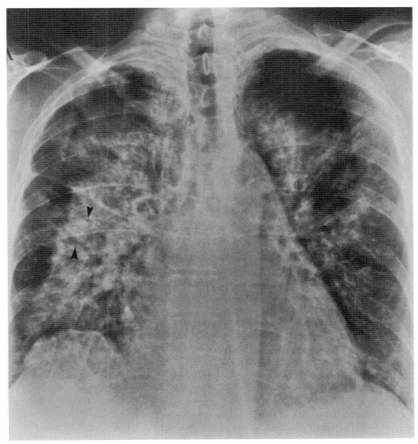

FIGURE 1-27. Alveolar disease causing pulmonary edema is characterized by diffuse, poorly marginated central opacities with air bronchograms *(arrowheads)* and a butterfly or bat wing appearance.

because both compartments are often involved. However, for the radiologist, it is useful to identify certain patterns that may occur in these diffuse diseases (Box 1-7). These patterns may be related to primary histologic involvement

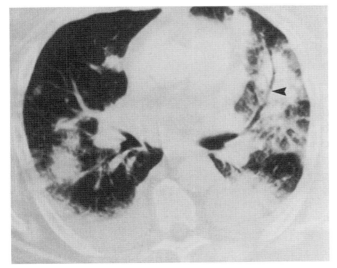

FIGURE 1-28. Bilateral pneumonia. Prominent air bronchograms can be seen in the left upper lobe *(arrowhead).*

of the interstitium. Examples of such diseases include sarcoidosis, lymphangitic carcinomatosis, and usual interstitial pneumonitis. A few of these infiltrative lung diseases primarily produce alveolar consolidation. They include chronic eosinophilic pneumonia and pulmonary alveolar proteinosis.

The interstitial space consists of two major anatomic compartments: the axial interstitial space and the parenchymal interstitial space. The former surrounds the bronchovascular bundles and occurs primarily in the central portions of the lung. The axial interstitium also extends out to the level of the terminal bronchioles. The parenchymal interstitial space is between the alveolar and capillary basement membranes in the peripheral portions of the lung (i.e., alveolar walls). Many interstitial or infiltrative lung diseases involve both compartments; interstitial pulmonary edema is a classic example (Fig. 1-29). The interlobular septa contain the veins and lymphatics. Thickening of the interlobular septa produces the classic short subpleural lines that lie perpendicular to the pleural space. The septal lines are also called *B lines of Kerley.*

Two major patterns of small opacities can be identified in interstitial lung disease: linear and nodular. The linear pattern may be fine, medium, or coarse. The nodular pattern consists of small, rounded opacities that are less than 1 cm in diameter (Fig. 1-30). Nodules 1 to 2 mm in diameter are sometimes to referred to as a *miliary* or *micronodular*

Box 1-6. Causes of Alveolar Disease

EDEMA
Hydrostatic
    Congestive heart failure
    Volume overload
    Renal failure
Capillary leak
    Acute respiratory distress syndrome

INFECTION

HEMORRHAGE AND VASCULITIS
Trauma, contusion
Overanticoagulation, hemorrhagic diathesis
Goodpasture's syndrome
Pulmonary and renal syndromes
Vasculitis
    Wegener's granulomatosis
Idiopathic pulmonary hemorrhage (hemosiderosis)

CHRONIC INFILTRATIVE (INTERSTITIAL) LUNG DISEASE
Organizing pneumonia
Pulmonary alveolar proteinosis
Eosinophilic pneumonias

NEOPLASM
Bronchioloalveolar carcinoma
Lymphoma

ASPIRATION
Lipoid pneumonia
Near-drowning
Gastric contents
Oropharyngeal material

Box 1-7. Interstitial (Infiltrative) Lung Disease

INTERSTITIUM
Compartments
Axial
Parenchymal

SIGNS OF INTERSTITIAL DISEASE
Patterns
Linear or reticular
    Fine
    Coarse
Nodular (less than 1 cm)
Reticulonodular
Ground glass (on CT)
Other Features
    Septal lines
    Honeycombing (fibrosis)

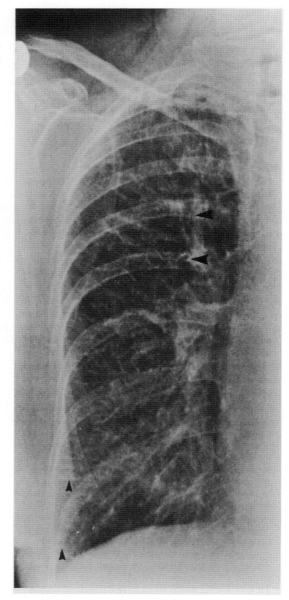

FIGURE 1-29. Interstitial edema. The axial interstitium is thickened by edema fluid, which is characterized by thickened bronchial walls *(large arrowheads)*. The interlobular septa are also thickened (i.e., Kerley B lines) by edema fluid. These short subpleural lines are best seen at the lung bases *(small arrowheads)*.

---

pattern, as seen in miliary tuberculosis. The two types of small opacities may combine to produce a reticulonodular pattern. A distinctive type of opacification may be identified in infiltrative lung disease on CT. This is referred to as *ground-glass opacification*, an amorphous increase in attenuation in the lung parenchyma through which the normal pulmonary vessels can be visualized (Fig. 1-31).

The latter characteristic differentiates ground-glass opacification from alveolar consolidation, which produces higher attenuation and usually obliterates the vessels within the lung parenchyma.

Linear or reticular opacities may be fine to coarse in nature, and the coarser reticular pattern usually correlates with more severe the underlying disease (Fig. 1-32). The linear or reticular pattern is most frequently seen in diseases that cause diffuse fibrosis in the lung. Severe fibrosis may result in *end-stage lung disease* (Fig. 1-33). This term refers to severe irreversible and chronic pathologic change. Typically, the lung consists of cystic spaces that result from the breakdown of alveolar walls or dilatation of terminal and respiratory bronchioles. These cystic spaces are thick

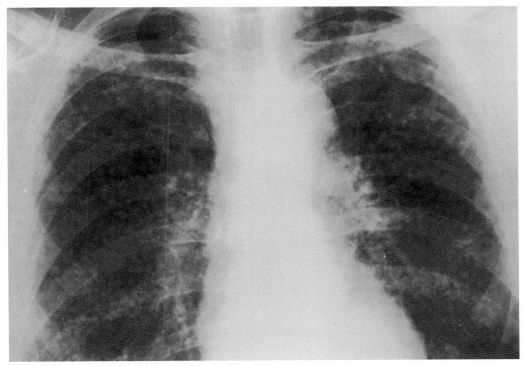

FIGURE 1-30. Nodular pattern of silicosis. Multiple, small, rounded opacities or nodules range in size from 2 to 4 mm in diameter.

walled and lined by fibrosis. Usually, the spaces are 1 cm or less in diameter, but they may be larger. Diseases that produce this honeycombing include idiopathic pulmonary fibrosis, fibrosis associated with other causes of usual interstitial pneumonia, asbestosis, and occasionally end-stage sarcoidosis.

Examples of diseases causing a diffuse nodular pattern include the pneumoconioses, such as silicosis and coal workers' pneumoconiosis, and the granulomatous diseases,

such as sarcoidosis and hematogenous dissemination of granulomatous infection (e.g., miliary tuberculosis). The CT and HRCT findings of small interstitial opacities are discussed in the chapter dealing with infiltrative lung diseases (see Chapter 7).

Atelectasis

Atelectasis is a decrease in the volume of a lung or a portion of the lung. Atelectasis may be referred to as *collapse*, although this definition is somewhat simplistic. Several types of atelectasis are related to the mechanism by which the loss in lung volume occurs (Box 1-8). The most common type is caused by central bronchial obstruction that usually leads to lobar or, less frequently, segmental collapse. When an obstruction occurs, gas is resorbed from the alveoli. This type of atelectasis is sometimes referred to as *resorption atelectasis*. The second major type is *passive atelectasis*, which is collapse caused by extrinsic pressure on the lung from air or fluid, or both, in the pleural space or at the edge of a local space-occupying lesion such as a mass in the lung. The third type, *cicatrization atelectasis*, occurs in areas of pulmonary fibrosis. Occasionally, atelectasis can be patchy and caused by widespread collapse of alveoli. This occurs in the postoperative situation or in the acute respiratory distress syndrome and has been called *adhesive atelectasis*.

Lobar Collapse

Collapse of a lobe may be complete or incomplete. The most common cause is obstruction of a central bronchus. The major or primary signs are opacification due to airlessness

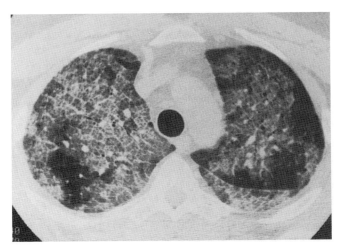

FIGURE 1-31. Ground-glass attenuation or pattern of pulmonary alveolar proteinosis. CT demonstrates increased diffuse opacification in both lungs. Pulmonary vessels in these areas can still be visualized. No air bronchograms are found, as in true consolidation.

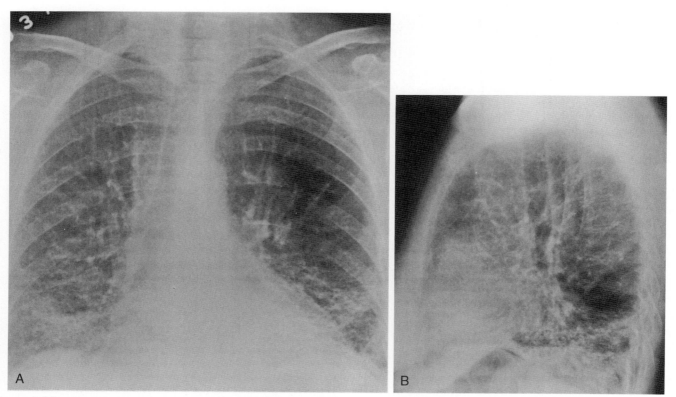

FIGURE 1-32. Linear pattern. Posteroanterior (**A**) and lateral (**B**) chest radiographs demonstrate fine to medium-coarse linear opacities at both lung bases. The patient has desquamative interstitial pneumonitis, a form of chronic interstitial pneumonia.

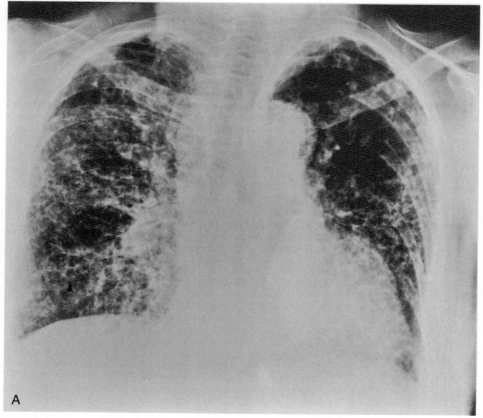

FIGURE 1-33. End-stage lung disease with honeycombing caused by rheumatoid lung with diffuse fibrosis. **A**, Posteroanterior chest radiograph shows multiple cystic spaces *(arrowhead)* that have thick walls and are less than 1 cm in diameter.

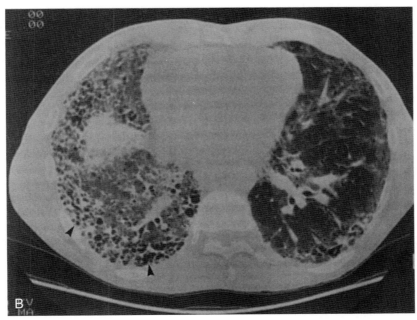

FIGURE 1-33. (cont'd) B, High-resolution CT demonstrates subpleural honeycomb spaces that are more marked on the right side *(arrowheads).*

Box 1-8. **Causes and Types of Atelectasis**

CENTRAL BRONCHIAL OBSTRUCTION (RESORPTION ATELECTASIS)
Endobronchial
Lung cancer
Other neoplasms
  Carcinoid
  Mucoepidermoid carcinoma
  Hamartoma
  Lipoma
  Metastases
    Breast
    Thyroid
    Melanoma
    Renal cell carcinoma
  Lymphoma
Foreign body
Mucoid impaction
Sarcoid
Misplaced endotracheal tube
Middle lobe syndrome, postinflammatory
Stricture
  Tuberculosis
  Trauma
Exobronchial
Lymphadenopathy
  Malignant
    Lung cancer
    Lymphoma
    Metastases
  Benign
    Sarcoid

Tuberculosis (particularly if nodes are calcified)
Histoplasmosis (particularly if nodes are calcified)
Enlarged left atrium
Mediastinal or adjacent mass

PASSIVE (COMPRESSION)
Pleura
  Pneumothorax
  Pleural effusion
  Rounded atelectasis
Lung (adjacent space-occupying lesion)
  Bulla
  Mass
Abdominal disease (e.g., ascites)

CICATRIZATION
Granulomatous infection
  Tuberculosis
  Fungal
Sarcoidosis
Pneumoconiosis
Interstitial Fibrosis

ADHESIVE
Adult acute respiratory distress syndrome
Postoperative (lower lobes)

OTHER TYPES
Subsegmental
Platelike
Discoid

Box 1-9. **Signs of Lobar Collapse**

Opacification of affected lobe
Displacement of fissures
Elevation of hemidiaphragm
Mediastinal displacement
    Heart
    Trachea
    Other mediastinal structures
Hilar displacement
Crowding of vessels
Compensatory overinflation of remaining lung

---

of the affected lobe and displacement of the interlobar fissures. The secondary signs include elevation of the hemidiaphragm; mediastinal displacement (e.g., heart, trachea, other mediastinal structures); hilar displacement; crowded vessels in the affected lobe if it is still partially aerated; and compensatory overinflation of the remaining lung (Box 1-9). If the obstruction of the lobar bronchus is caused by a large tumor mass, it may cause a bulge in the contour of the collapsed lobe (Fig. 1-34), and if the entire lobe is replaced by tumor, the lobe may appear lobular with undulation of the affected fissure. These signs also apply to CT features of lobar collapse. Additional CT features should be sought. Air bronchograms may be present, but if there is central endobronchial tumor causing the lobar collapse, the bronchus will be narrowed or occluded. The involved lobe usually becomes pie shaped rather than hemispherical in cross section, with the apex of the triangle situated at the origin of the affected bronchus. Loss of volume also produces a reduced zone of contact between the pleural surface of the lobe and the chest wall.

Right Upper Lobe Atelectasis

The right upper lobe collapses superiorly and medially, creating a wedge-shaped opacity in the right upper hemithorax (see Fig. 1-34). When collapsed completely, the right upper lobe progressively pancakes against the mediastinum. The minor fissure is displaced upward, and the major fissure is displaced anteriorly. If there is a large central mass causing lobar collapse, a convex bulge in the central medial portion of the minor fissure can be observed, which curves around the mass, the so-called reverse S sign of Golden (Fig. 1-35). On the lateral projection, the collapsed lobe may appear as an indistinctly defined triangular opacity with its apex at the hilum and its base at the parietal pleura at the apex of the hemithorax. On CT, the collapsed right upper lobe appears as a wedge of opacification extending along the mediastinum to the anterior chest wall (see Fig. 1-35). Hyperaeration of the middle and lower lobes occurs, and the vessels in those lobes typically are spread apart.

Left Upper Lobe Atelectasis

The major difference between collapse of the left and right upper lobes is the absence of the minor fissure on the left. With left upper lobe collapse, the major fissure is displaced forward roughly parallel to the anterior chest wall (Fig. 1-36). This fissure is well depicted on the lateral view, in which it can be seen to parallel the sternum. The opacity of the left upper lobe is anterior to the fissure extending from the apex of the lung to the diaphragm. On the posteroanterior view, the left upper lobe collapse does not appear as a wedge-shaped opacity like right upper lobe collapse. There is often a hazy opacification that obliterates the left heart border in the frontal projection (i.e., silhouette sign). The overinflated superior segment of the lower lobe occupies the far apex of the lung. There may be a para-aortic lucency on posteroanterior radiographs due to the hyperaeration of the left lower lobe. On CT, the left upper lobe usually retains more contact with the anterior and left lateral chest wall than the right upper lobe, which collapses against the mediastinum. Superiorly, the collapsed upper lobe has a wedge-shaped triangular configuration (Fig. 1-37). Hyperinflation of the lower lobe is somewhat greater than that seen in right upper lobe collapse. The left hilum commonly is elevated.

Middle Lobe Atelectasis

When the right middle lobe collapses, it often does not produce a discrete opacity on the posteroanterior projection (Fig. 1-38). The right middle lobe collapses medially toward the right heart border obliterating this border (i.e., silhouette sign). On the lateral projection, the right middle lobe is seen as a linear band or a wedge-shaped triangle, with displacement of the minor fissure inferiorly and the major fissure superiorly. Right middle lobe atelectasis may be seen to better advantage with a lordotic view. The lobe appears as a thin, triangular opacity, with the apex of the opacity directed away from the hilum and the base abutting the right cardiac border. Compensatory signs of middle lobe atelectasis are less marked than with other lobes because of the small volume of the middle lobe. On CT, the medial margin of the lobe abuts the right heart border, and the posterior margin of the lobe is displaced anteromedially (Fig. 1-39).

Although right middle lobe atelectasis may be caused by a central endobronchial tumor, this lobe appears to be susceptible to chronic collapse secondary to prior inflammatory episodes. This is sometimes called the *right middle lobe syndrome*. Typically, the middle lobe bronchus is patent but narrowed in this condition, and bronchiectasis is present peripherally in the collapsed lobe. The open bronchus and the absence of a mass can be identified on CT. Patients may be asymptomatic or may occasionally have recurrent pneumonias involving the lobe (see Fig. 1-39).

Lower Lobe Atelectasis

The pattern of lower lobe collapse is similar on both sides because of the equivalent anatomy bilaterally (Fig. 1-40). Both lower lobes collapse in a posterior medial and inferior direction. The upper part of the major fissure swings downward, and the lower half moves backward. The upper half of the fissure becomes evident on the posteroanterior projection, and the lower part of the fissure is displaced backward on the lateral projection. Eventually, as the collapse becomes complete, the lobe occupies a position in the posterior costophrenic gutter and medial costovertebral angle. Often, no discrete opacity can be seen on the lateral view except for a slight increase in opacification overlying the lower thoracic vertebra (normally, the vertebrae become relatively more radiolucent from above

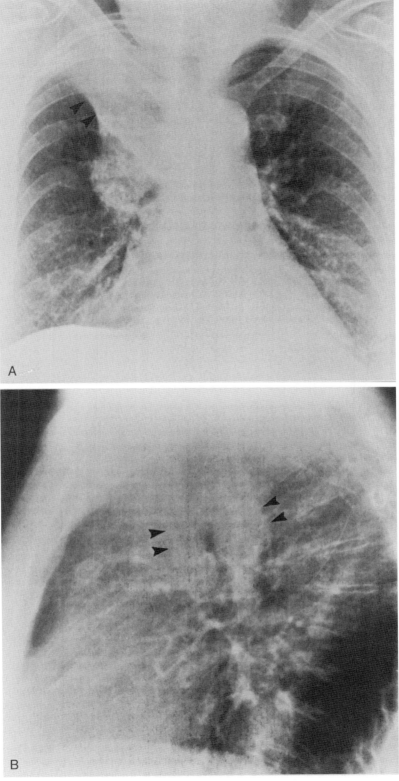

FIGURE 1-34. Right upper lobe atelectasis. **A,** Posteroanterior view demonstrates opacification of the right upper lobe and elevation of the minor fissure *(arrowheads).* There is a large mass in the right hilum (i.e., lung carcinoma) that is elevated slightly above the left hilum. **B,** The atelectasis is less visible on the lateral view. It appears as a wedge-shaped opacity in the center of the chest *(arrowheads).*

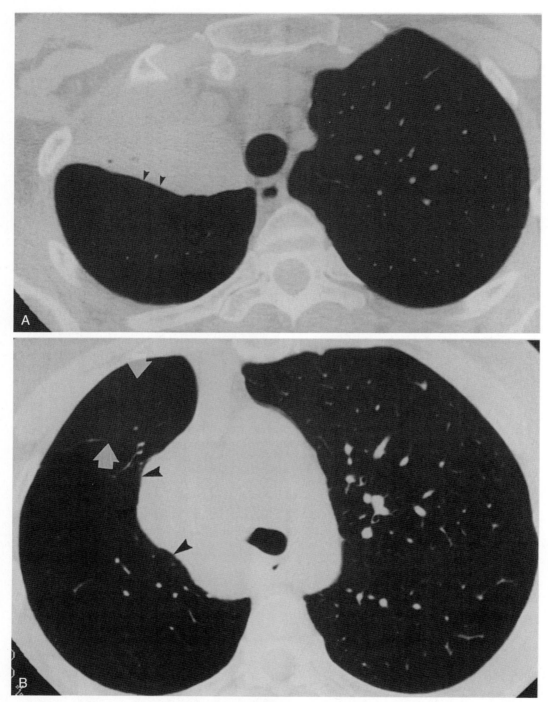

Figure 1-35. CT of right upper lobe atelectasis. The major fissure is displaced forward *(small black arrowheads)* and the minor fissure displaced around a central mass *(larger black arrowheads)*. The remaining right middle lobe *(large white arrowheads)* and right lower lobe *(posteriorly)* are hyperinflated, and their vessels spread apart.

downward) and loss of the contour of the posterior part of the hemidiaphragm. On a well-penetrated posteroanterior view, the collapsed lobe appears as a triangular opacity behind the heart and adjacent to the spine. The CT appearance can be induced from the previous description (Fig. 1-41). The right and left lower lobes collapse posteromedially against the posterior mediastinum and spine. The lateral contour of the collapse may be convex if a central tumor is present.

Combined Lobar Atelectasis
Combined right middle and lower lobe atelectasis can occur when a tumor obstructs the intermediate bronchus. The major and minor fissures in such an instance are displaced downward and backward, creating on the posteroanterior view an opacity that obliterates the right dome of the diaphragm. The upper surface of the opacity may be either concave or convex. This should not be confused with a medially loculated pleural effusion.

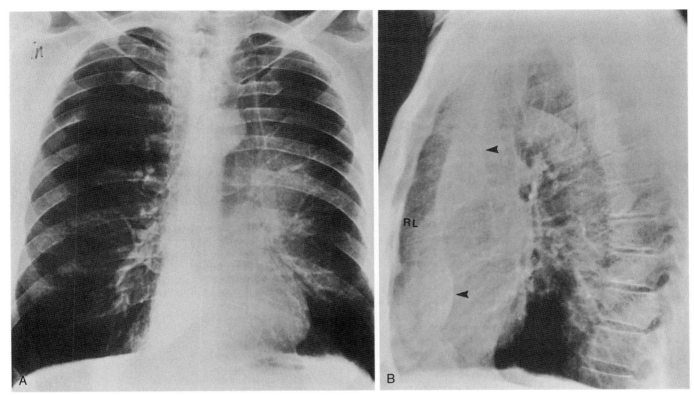

FIGURE 1-36. Left upper lobe collapse. **A,** Posteroanterior view shows hazy opacification in the left perihilar area with partial obliteration of the left heart border. The apex is aerated and occupied by the left lower lobe. **B,** The lateral view demonstrates forward displacement of the major fissure *(arrowheads)* parallel to the chest wall. The retrosternal lucency in front of the collapsed lobe is caused by herniation of the overinflated right lung (RL).

Combined right upper and right middle lobe atelectasis is unusual because the bronchi to these lobes are remote from each other. However, when this combination occurs, the appearance is identical to that of upper lobe atelectasis on the left.

Segmental and Subsegmental Atelectasis
It is unusual for a segment to undergo atelectasis because of channels that produce collateral air drift, even when a segmen-

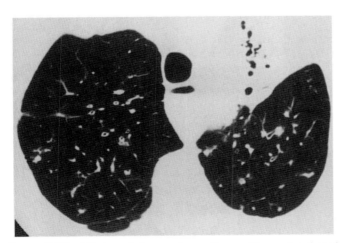

FIGURE 1-37. CT shows left upper lung collapse with a wedge-shaped configuration. The dilated bronchi in the collapsed lobe indicate bronchiectasis.

tal or subsegmental bronchus within a lobe is occluded. These forces tend to keep the segment aerated, and obstructive overinflation and air trapping occur rather than atelectasis.

Subsegmental, discoid, or *plate atelectasis* are terms used synonymously for linear opacities that are 1 to 3 mm thick and 4 to 10 cm long (Fig. 1-42). They are usually located in the lower lung zones and occur in a horizontal plane paralleling the diaphragm, although they occasionally may be oblique. These linear opacities are almost invariably associated with disease processes that diminish diaphragmatic excursion and are commonly seen after thoracic or abdominal surgery or in patients who are bedridden and who are kept in the supine position.

Total Collapse of the Lung
When an entire lung collapses the hemithorax on that side becomes completely opaque (Fig. 1-43). The mediastinum is shifted to the affected side. Elevation of the hemidiaphragm can be recognized only indirectly on the left side by the high position of the stomach bubble. The opposite lung overinflates and moves across the midline, particularly anteriorly behind the sternum, creating a large retrosternal air space on the lateral view. The appearance differs from that of a massive pleural effusion, which causes similar opacification of a hemithorax. In this condition, an increased retrosternal clear space is not observed, and there is a shift of the mediastinum to the opposite side. On the lateral view, a hazy opacification or uniform filter effect is observed.

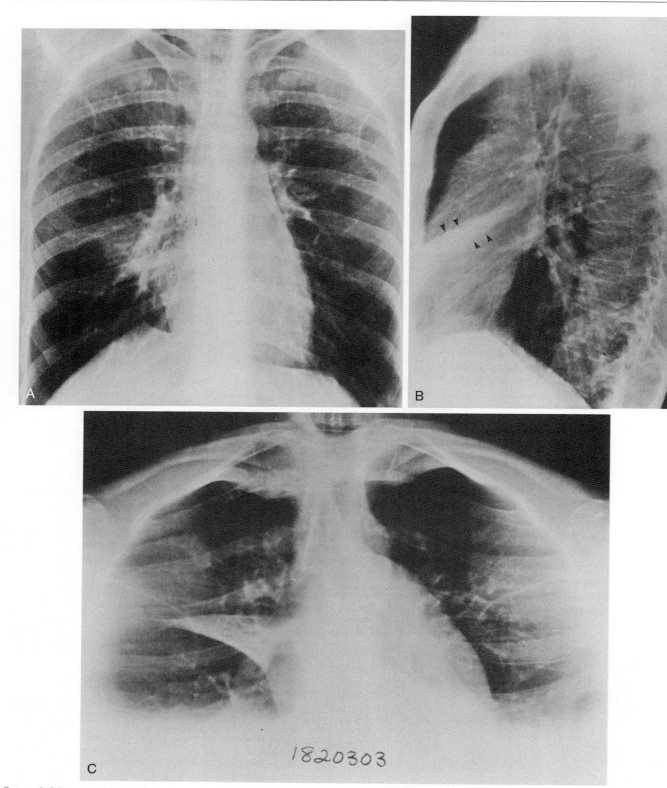

FIGURE 1-38. Right middle lobe atelectasis. **A,** Posteroanterior view shows a loss of definition of the right heart border (i.e., silhouette sign). There are no signs of volume loss. **B,** The lateral view demonstrates a wedge-shaped triangle bordered by the minor fissure above and major fissure below *(arrowheads)*. **C,** Collapse is evident on the lordotic view the middle lobe.

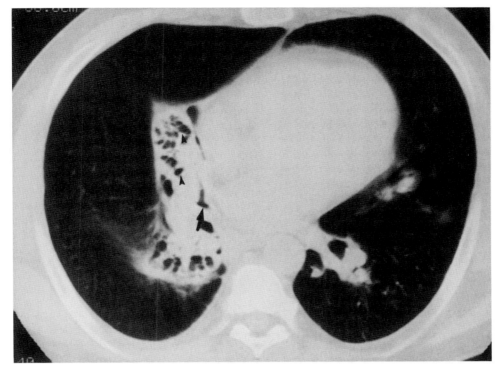

FIGURE 1-39. CT shows right middle lobe atelectasis. The lobe is collapsed medially along the right heart border. The lobe was chronically collapsed due to bronchiectasis. Dilated air-filled bronchi are seen in the lobe *(arrowheads)*, and the origin of the middle lobe bronchus is patent *(arrow)*.

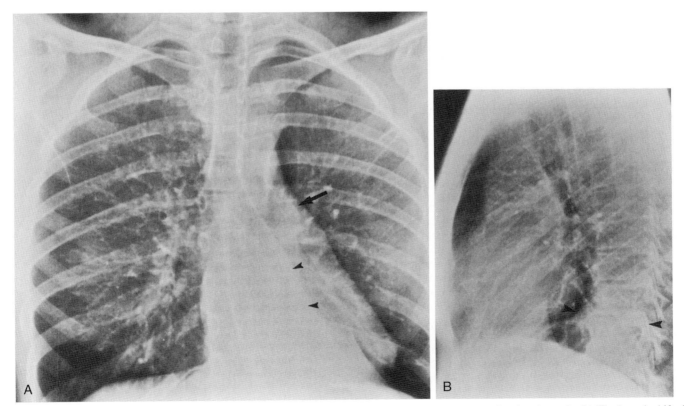

FIGURE 1-40. Left lower lobe atelectasis. **A,** A triangular opacity is seen behind the heart on the posteroanterior view *(arrowheads)*. The heart is shifted to the left, and the left ilium is depressed *(arrow)*. **B,** On the lateral view, there is loss of visualization of the left hemidiaphragm and increased opacity overlying the lower thoracic vertebrae *(arrowhead)* in the posterior costophrenic gutter.

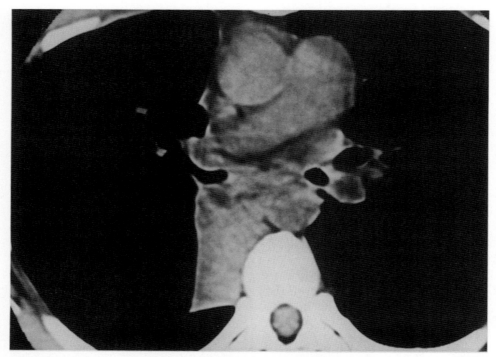

Figure 1-41. CT shows right lower lobe collapse. The lobe is collapsed posteriorly and medially along the posterior mediastinum and spine.

Postobstructive Pneumonitis and Drowned Lung

When a bronchus is obstructed, atelectasis is always accompanied by some fluid exudation or sequestration of blood in the obstructed lobe. Sometimes, the amount of fluid can become quite voluminous, resulting in a radiographic appearance with very little volume loss within the lobe despite the endobronchial obstruction. This appearance is sometimes referred to as *drowned lung* (Fig. 1-44). Infection may also occur distal to an obstructed bronchus, and the development of inflammatory exudate may result in little loss of volume of the affected lobe.

Passive Atelectasis

Passive atelectasis, also called *relaxation atelectasis*, refers to pulmonary collapse that occurs as a result of pneumothorax or hydrothorax (Fig. 1-45). If there are no pleural adhesions, the collapse of any portion of the lung is proportional to the amount of air or fluid in the adjacent pleural space. When a pneumothorax is large, the pulmonary collapse may be total; however, the opacity of the lung usually does not increase until it is approximately one tenth of its normal area at total lung capacity. More extensive discussion of pneumothorax and pleural effusion can be found in Chapter 18. *Compression atelectasis* is a similar phenomenon, and the term describes focal parenchymal collapse adjacent to a space-occupying mass within the thorax.

Rounded atelectasis (which is often an incidental finding on a chest radiograph) is a peripheral, focal type of atelectasis that is always associated with pleural thickening or, less commonly, with pleural effusion (Fig. 1-46). It appears as a sharply defined mass abutting the pleura, is 2 to 7 cm in diameter, and is usually located posteriorly in the lower lobes. Air bronchograms or focal collections of air (i.e., pseudocavitation) may be present within the atelectasis. The most distinctive finding is that vessels and bronchi located more centrally than the peripheral area of atelectasis are crowded together in a whorled pattern coursing like a comet tail toward the hilum. On CT, the finding is that of a rounded peripheral lung mass associated with pleural thickening. The comet tail appearance is easily visualized. Rounded atelectasis can be associated with any cause of pleural thickening but particularly with asbestos-related disease.

Cicatrization Atelectasis

Cicatrization atelectasis is a form of loss of volume that may be focal or diffuse. It is a form of collapse resulting from scarring and fibrosis. It is typically associated with old granulomatous infection, particularly tuberculosis. Endobronchial obstruction is absent, and bronchiectasis is a frequent feature. When an entire lobe is involved, the degree of volume loss is more marked than with other forms of lobar atelectasis (Fig. 1-47). More generalized fibrosis in the lungs may be associated with general loss of lung volume.

Adhesive, Nonobstructive, or Microscopic Atelectasis

Adhesive, nonobstructive, or microscopic forms of atelectasis usually are related to a number of forces and with decrease in the amount of surfactant. An example is diffuse microatelectasis associated with the acute respiratory distress syndrome.

Nodules and Masses

The definition of nodules and masses is somewhat arbitrary, but both are considered to be lesions that are roughly spherical. A nodule is usually less than 3 cm in diameter,

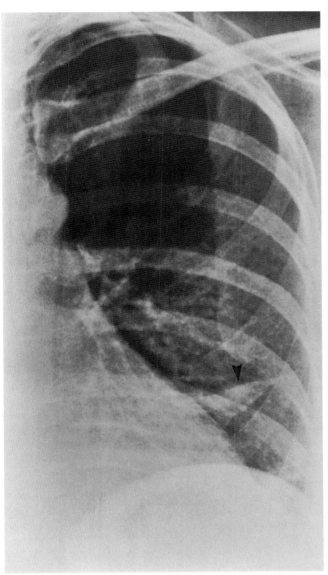

FIGURE 1-42. Platelike atelectasis. There is a broad band of increased opacity at the left base paralleling the left hemidiaphragm *(arrowhead).*

wall creates an obtuse angle with the chest wall, whereas an intraparenchymal lesion usually has an acute angle with the contiguous pleura. Extrapleural masses may have better defined margins than lung masses (Fig. 1-50).

Calcification and Ossification

Intrathoracic calcification is an important feature of pulmonary disease (Box 1-10). It is usually dystrophic (i.e., occurs in areas of necrosis). Less commonly, it is metastatic (i.e., related to hypercalcemia). Calcification may occur in focal lesions such as solitary pulmonary nodules (Fig. 1-51). The distribution and character of the calcification is important. This topic is discussed in more detail in Chapter 11. Occasionally, ossification can occur diffusely in the lung.

Diffuse pulmonary calcification can occur in a number of entities (Fig. 1-52). One is pulmonary alveolar microlithiasis, a hereditary disease in which calcified spherules occur within the alveoli. Other conditions with diffuse calcification include silicosis, end-stage mitral stenosis with hemosiderosis, and certain healed disseminated granulomatous or viral infections. Examples include tuberculosis, histoplasmosis, and varicella pneumonitis. The radiographic pattern consists of diffuse, round or punctate, calcific opacities. Interstitial ossification is rare but has been occasionally reported in cases of idiopathic pulmonary fibrosis and long-term busulfan therapy. The radiographic pattern is one of branching opacities distributed along the bronchovascular bundles.

Metastatic pulmonary calcification may occur with long-standing hypercalcemia. It is most common in patients with chronic renal disease who are maintained on dialysis and have secondary hyperparathyroidism. Metastatic calcification usually occurs in the apical and subapical lung zones, but it may be diffuse.

Cavities and Cysts

Abnormal air-filled spaces in the lung may develop in a variety of lung diseases, including infection, vascular embolic disorders, bronchiectasis, emphysema, pulmonary fibrosis, acute respiratory distress syndrome, lymphangioleiomyomatosis, and histiocytosis X (Box 1-11).

General Features

A pulmonary *cyst* is usually defined as a thin-walled (usually less than 3 mm), well-marginated, and circumscribed air- or fluid-containing lesion that is 1 cm or more in diameter (Fig. 1-53). A *cavity* is a lucency within a zone of pulmonary consolidation, a mass, or a nodule. It may or may not contain an air-fluid level, and it is surrounded by a wall of varied thickness but usually greater than 3 mm in diameter (Fig. 1-54). Pathologically, a cavity results from the expulsion of a necrotic part of the lesion into the bronchial tree. This may result in an air-fluid level that forms a straight line that is parallel to the bottom of the film (Fig. 1-55). An air-fluid level implies communication with the bronchial tree provided there has been no penetration of the chest wall. It usually also indicates liquefaction necrosis, as seen in pyogenic infection due to a lung abscess. Fluid-filled cysts cannot be distinguished on plain radiographs from solid masses. However, on CT, they may have

and a mass is greater than 3 cm in diameter. Nodules larger than 3 cm in diameter likely represent primary or secondary malignant disease in the lung. Further discussion of nodules and masses is available in Chapter 11, which specifically addresses the solitary pulmonary nodule. The smoothness of contour and edge characteristics of a nodular mass may be important. A smooth contour suggests benign disease, and nodularity or lobulation indicates malignancy, although these findings are relatively nonspecific and cannot be relied on to differentiate malignant from benign disease (Figs. 1-48 and 1-49). Nodules and masses may be associated with satellite lesions, which are small, often rounded opacities that lie close to the larger nodule or mass. They suggest an infectious cause, such as tuberculosis, rather than lung carcinoma. The relation of a mass or a nodule to the pleura or chest wall is important. A mass or nodule that arises within the extrapleural space in the chest

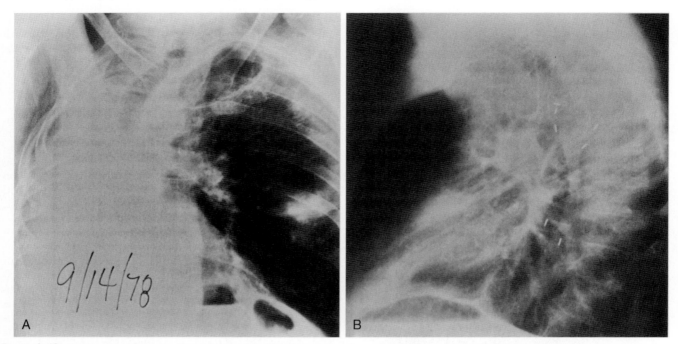

FIGURE 1-43. Right pneumonectomy. The appearance is equivalent to that of complete collapse of the right. **A,** The posteroanterior view shows a completely opaque right hemithorax with shift of the mediastinum toward that side. **B,** The lateral view demonstrates a large, retrosternal clear space and loss of visualization of the right hemidiaphragm (i.e., recurrent lung cancer in the left lung).

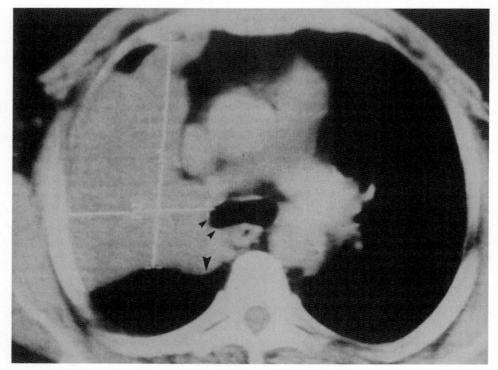

FIGURE 1-44. Postobstructive pneumonitis. There is atelectasis of the right upper lobe, and the bronchus is obstructed *(small arrowheads)*. There is no loss of volume and a lobulated contour of the fissure can be identified due to tumor *(large arrowhead)*.

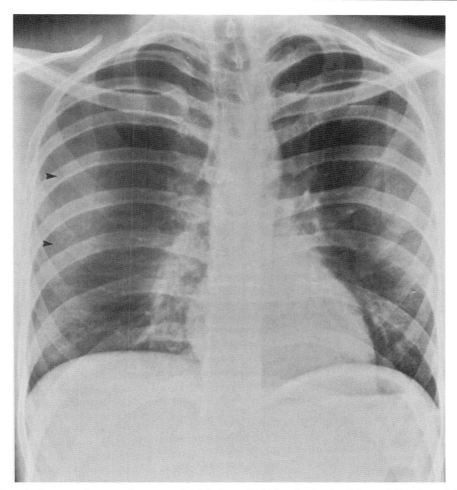

FIGURE 1-45. Passive atelectasis. A pneumothorax can be seen on the right *(arrowheads)*, but the density of the partially collapsed right lung has not changed.

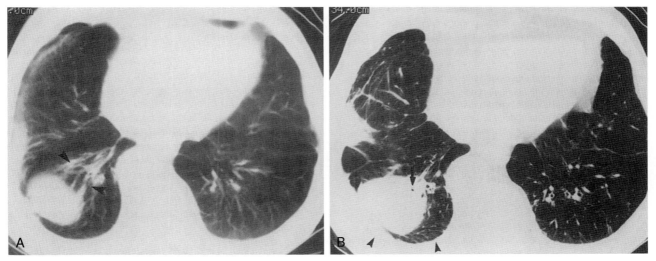

FIGURE 1-46. CT shows rounded atelectasis. A mass abutting the pleura is thickened *(small arrowheads)*. The pulmonary vessels are crowded together medial to the mass *(large arrowheads)*, producing a comet-tail appearance. Areas of pseudocavitation are present *(arrow)*.

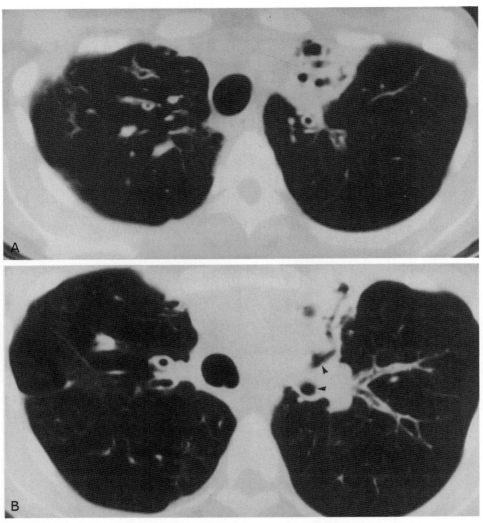

FIGURE 1-47. CT shows cicatrization atelectasis. **A,** There is atelectasis of the left upper lobe with bronchiectasis resulting from old tuberculosis. **B,** The upper lobe segmental bronchi are patent *(arrowheads).*

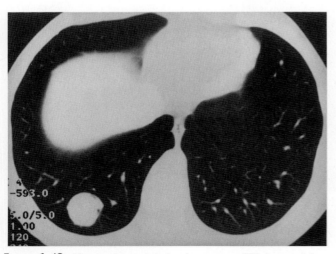

FIGURE 1-48. The benign nodule is a hamartoma. CT shows a 2.5-cm nodule with smooth borders in the right lower lobe.

low attenuation close to that of water (0 HU). However, cysts may contain fluid that is hemorrhagic or high in protein content, in which case they appear as soft tissue densities on CT. On MRI, cysts containing hemorrhagic or proteinaceous fluid usually appear bright on T1-weighted sequences and relatively heterogeneous on T2-weighted images, unlike *spring water* cysts, which have very low signal intensity on T1-weighted images and very bright signal intensity on T2-weighted images (see Fig. 1-6). Cysts will not enhance after administration of gadolinium contrast.

The thickness and irregularity of the wall of a cavity or abnormal space and the location and number of such spaces are important features in the differential diagnosis. For example, septic pulmonary infarcts associated with intravenous drug abuse are usually multiple, thick walled, and occur in the lower lung zones peripherally (Fig. 1-56). CT may be particularly helpful in characterizing abnormal spaces in the lung, particularly in regard to their number and internal architecture.

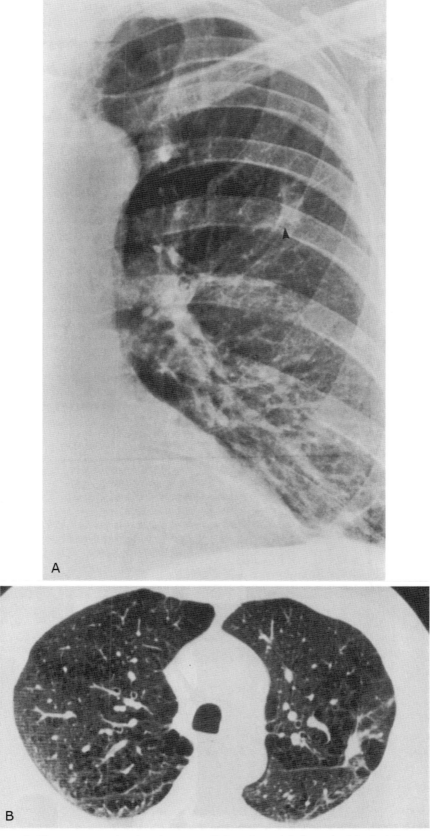

FIGURE 1-49. Lung carcinoma. **A,** The posteroanterior view shows a small, irregular nodule *(arrowhead)* in the left upper lobe. **B,** CT demonstrates that it has spiculated and irregular margins.

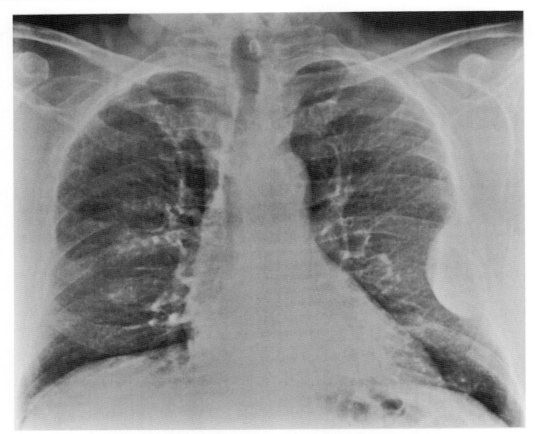

FIGURE 1-50. Extrapleural mass. The posteroanterior view shows a large, well-defined mass that has obtuse angles with the chest wall. The sixth anterior rib cannot be visualized because of destruction. The patient has metastatic renal cell carcinoma.

Box 1-10. Causes of Calcification

TYPES
Dystrophic
Metastatic

NODULES
Benign
   Tuberculosis
   Histoplasmosis
   Hamartoma
Malignant
Lung cancer
Metastases
   Osteogenic sarcoma (ossification)
   Chondrosarcoma
   Mucin-producing adenocarcinoma

DIFFUSE
Pulmonary alveolar microlithiasis
Silicosis
End-stage mitral stenosis (ossification)
Healed disseminated infections
   Varicella
   Tuberculosis
   Histoplasmosis
Secondary hyperparathyroidism (renal failure)
Idiopathic pulmonary fibrosis (usual interstitial
   pneumonia)

Congenital Cysts

Most congenital spaces in the lung are cysts. They are discussed in more detail in Chapter 2. Most arise from the primitive foregut. Examples include bronchogenic and esophageal duplication cysts (see Fig. 1-53) in the mediastinum, intrapulmonary abnormalities such as cystic adenomatoid malformation and pulmonary sequestration, and intrapulmonary bronchogenic cysts.

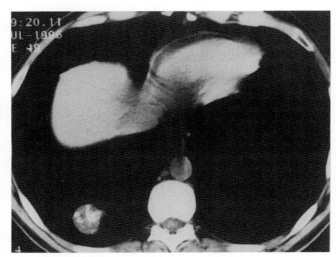

FIGURE 1-51. CT shows a calcified nodule that is a hamartoma.

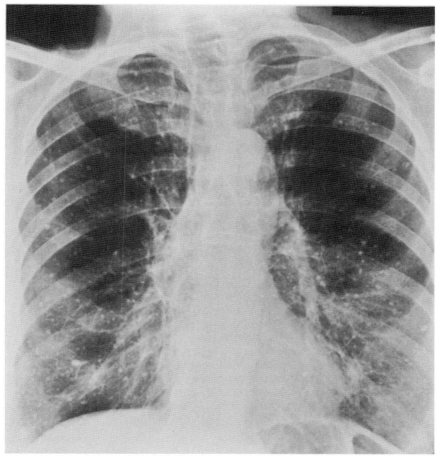

FIGURE 1-52. Diffuse pulmonary calcification in a patient with healed varicella pneumonia is characterized by multiple, small, dense nodules in both lungs.

Box 1-11. Cysts and Cavities

DEFINITION
Cyst
Thin wall (<3 mm)
Fluid- or air-filled
Air-fluid level (occasional)
Cavity
Thick wall (>3 mm)
Always contains air
Air-fluid level

TYPES
Congenital
Bronchogenic
Cystic adenomatoid malformation
Acquired
Infection
   Postinfectious pneumatocele
     Abscess
      Nonpyogenic
        Tuberculosis
        Fungal

Septic infarcts
Vasculitis and granulomatosis
   Wegener's granulomatosis
   Lymphomatoid granulomatosis
Rheumatoid nodules
Neoplasms
Primary lung carcinoma (squamous cell)
Metastatic
   Squamous cell
   Sarcomas
Trauma
Posttraumatic pneumatocele (laceration)
Emphysema
Bulla
Bronchiectasis
Diffuse infiltrative (interstitial) lung disease
Langerhans' histiocytosis
Lymphangioleiomyomatosis
Lymphocytic interstitial pneumonia
Honeycombing

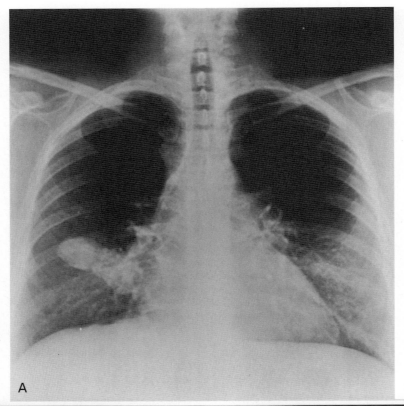

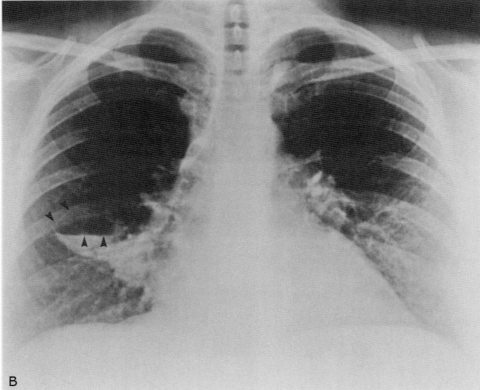

FIGURE 1-53. Bronchogenic cyst. **A,** The posteroanterior view shows an ovoid opacity that represents the fluid-filled cyst in the right lung. **B,** After a needle biopsy, an air-fluid level is seen, and a small, thin wall is delineated superiorly *(arrowheads)*.

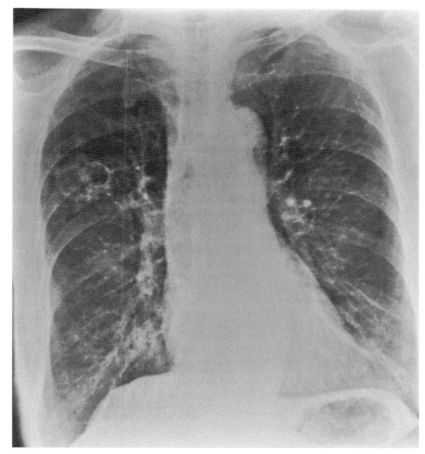

FIGURE 1-54. The thick-walled, multiloculated cavity in the right upper lobe resulted from tuberculosis.

Acquired Cysts and Cavities
Infection
Cavities may develop in pyogenic and nonpyogenic infections, and thin-walled cysts called *pneumatoceles* are a complication of some infections. Pneumatoceles are seen particularly in children who have had staphylococcal pneumonia, but they can also be identified in adult acquired immunodeficiency syndrome (AIDS) patients with *Pneumocystis jiroveci* (formerly called *Pneumocystis carinii*) pneumonia (Fig. 1-57). They are usually thin walled and do not contain air-fluid levels. Pneumothorax is an associated complication. The cysts eventually resolve in most patients.

Pyogenic abscesses develop as a result of liquefaction necrosis caused by bacteria. Lung abscesses are most frequently associated with aspiration and anaerobic pneumonia produced by mouth organisms. However, pyogenic abscesses can also be seen in staphylococcal, *Klebsiella*, and streptococcal pneumonia. If the abscess does not communicate with the bronchial tree, it will appear as a water or soft tissue density mass surrounded by pneumonia, but a solitary isolated mass occasionally is visualized. When bronchial communication occurs, an air-fluid level develops as the purulent material is drained through the bronchial tree (see Fig. 1-55). Because lung abscesses are roughly spherical, the air-fluid level has equal dimensions or lengths on views obtained 90 degrees to each other

(i.e. posteroanterior and lateral chest radiographs). In contrast, an empyema may contain an air-fluid level if there is a bronchopleural fistula. Air-fluid levels in the pleural space typically have different lengths on views obtained at 90 degrees to each other (i.e., posteroanterior and lateral views).

The classic examples of nonpyogenic cavitary lesions are the cavities associated with tuberculosis. They usually have thick but rather smooth walls (see Fig. 1-54). They are located in the apical and posterior segments of the upper lobes or the superior segments of the lower lobes. Similar cavities may occur in other granulomatous infections, particularly fungal infections. In immunocompromised patients, invasive fungi, particularly *Aspergillus*, may be associated with ischemic necrosis and the development of cavities with air crescents (Fig. 1-58). Echinococcal infection in the lung produces cystic lesions with thin walls. These cysts contain air, but three layers of the wall may be present. As the inner cyst wall collapses, the debris may float on the air-fluid level, producing a water-lily sign (see Chapter 3).

Vasculites and Granulomatoses
Cavities may be identified in a group of diseases often referred to as vasculites and granulomatoses. These diseases include Wegener's granulomatosis, lymphomatoid

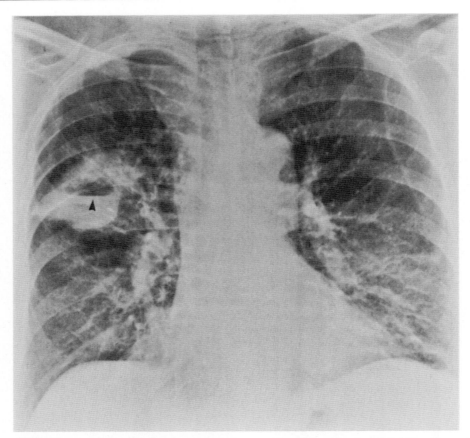

Figure 1-55. The posteroanterior view shows a lung abscess with a thick wall and an air-fluid level *(arrowhead)*.

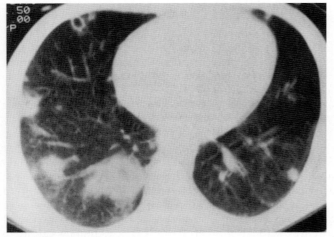

Figure 1-56. CT shows septic infarcts. Many nodules are peripheral, and some are cavitary in the lower lung zones.

granulomatosis, and other types of vasculitis. Necrobiotic nodules may be seen in rheumatoid lung disease. It is unusual for these cavities to contain air-fluid levels.

Neoplasms
A neoplasm in the lung may cavitate when it outgrows its blood supply. However, cavitation is most frequently identified with squamous cell carcinoma that is a primary tumor in the lung or metastatic. Such cavities are usually thick walled (Fig. 1-59). Metastatic neoplasms usually arise from squamous cell tumors of the head, neck, and cervix. It is not possible to radiologically differentiate cavitary neoplasms from other causes of cavitation.

Posttraumatic Pneumatoceles
Posttraumatic pneumatoceles result from penetrating or nonpenetrating trauma and from laceration of the lung parenchyma (Fig. 1-60). They are usually unilateral and peripheral in location at the site of injury. Traumatic lung cysts may be filled with blood initially. However, communication with the bronchus may occur, creating an air-fluid level. These pneumatoceles usually resolve in a few weeks, whereas hematomas may require months to resolve.

Pulmonary Infarcts
Pulmonary infarcts rarely undergo cavitation. However, if there is associated infection, usually as a result of septic emboli, cavitation may occur (Fig. 1-56). The classic features consist of ill-defined cavities at the bases of the lungs. Septic infarcts occur in intravenous drug abusers with tricuspid endocarditis or in patients with other causes of right-sided endocarditis, such as congenital valve anomalies or indwelling catheters.

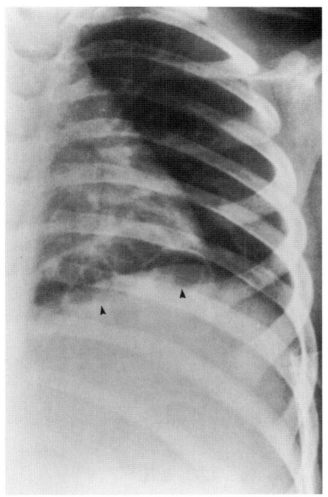

FIGURE 1-57. Pneumatoceles. Coned-down posteroanterior view shows multiple, thin-walled pneumatoceles above the left hemidiaphragm *(arrowheads)* in a child who had staphylococcal pneumonia.

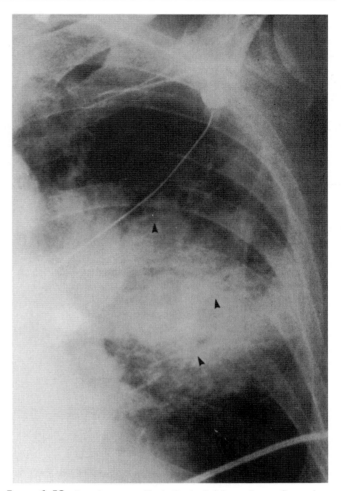

FIGURE 1-58. Invasive aspergillosis. In the left lung, the confluent, large nodules contain a rim of air (i.e., air crescent sign) *(arrowheads)*.

Blebs and Bullae

Bullae are air-containing spaces within the lung parenchyma that measure more than 1 cm in diameter when distended and have a wall thickness of less than 1 mm (Fig. 1-61). They result from obstruction to air flow and are associated usually with emphysema. A bleb is a gas-containing space within the visceral pleura of the lung. Radiologically, it appears as a sharply demarcated, thin-walled lucency that is contiguous with the pleura, usually at the lung apex. A bleb can be considered a bulla located in the visceral pleura outside the internal capsule of the lung.

Bronchiectasis

Cystic or saccular bronchiectasis may produce an appearance of multiple cystic spaces in the lung (Fig. 1-62). On standard radiographs, these cysts are usually associated with other signs of bronchiectasis, such as bronchial wall thickening seen en face or end on. If the bronchiectasis is diffuse, the lungs will be overinflated. These cystic structures are usually more marked in the medial third of the lung along the bronchovascular bundles.

Diffuse Infiltrative (Interstitial) Lung Disease

Several interstitial lung diseases may be associated with cyst formation in the lung. These may be thin-walled cysts resulting from bronchiolar obstruction, such as in lymphangioleiomyomatosis or Langerhans cell histiocytosis. *Honeycombing* refers to thick-walled cystic structures that are produced by dissolution of alveolar walls and fibrosis associated with architectural distortion. This appearance occurs as part of the end-stage lung disease discussed previously, which represents the final common pathway of diffuse fibrotic diseases.

Radiographically, honeycombing appears as closely approximated ring shadows that are usually less than 1 cm in diameter and with walls that are 2 to 3 mm thick. It is usually associated with a coarse reticular pattern in the lung (see Fig. 1-33). On HRCT, these spaces typically line up one on top of the other in the subpleural or peripheral zones of the lung and are associated with traction bronchiectasis and architectural distortion of the lung.

Intrathoracic Air Trapping

Intrathoracic air trapping produces changes in radiographic density that result in increased lucency in the lung. Air trapping is a relatively common condition. It may be

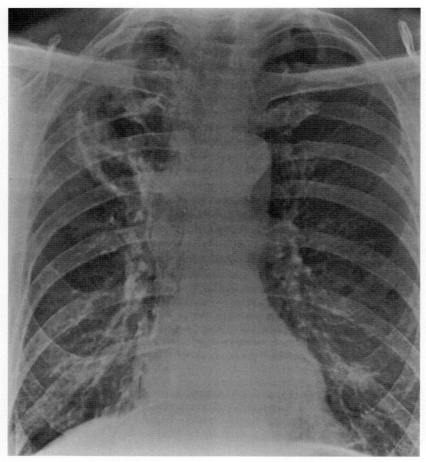

Figure 1-59. Cavitary squamous carcinoma in the right upper lobe.

localized or generalized, as in chronic obstructive pulmonary disease. Air trapping may be difficult to detect on routine chest radiographs, which are conventionally obtained at full inspiration (Fig. 1-63). Air trapping becomes apparent only on expiratory chest radiographs. It results in increased lucency of the affected lung or portion of the lung and in alteration of the lung volume. The overall size of the lung that air traps may be equal to, smaller than, or larger than the contralateral normal lung on the inspiration radiograph, but on expiration, the area containing trapped air maintains its size, whereas the normal lung becomes smaller. This results in signs of overexpansion of the portion of the lung that is trapping air. The signs include a shift of the mediastinum away from the involved side and failure of elevation of the ipsilateral hemidiaphragm. The area of trapping may appear relatively lucent when compared with the more normal lung. Air trapping may involve an entire lung, lobe, or segment, or it may be patchy and occur at the lobular level.

Causes of air trapping include obstruction of a central bronchus by endobronchial or exobronchial lesions such as tumors or foreign bodies. The airway or bronchus is usually of sufficient diameter to allow air to enter during inspiration. However, during expiration, when the bronchus decreases in caliber, air trapping occurs. Air trapping can occur distal to complete airway obstruction because of

collateral air drift through intra-alveolar connections (i.e., pores of Kohn) and intra-acinar connections (i.e., canals of Lambert), which permit air to pass from the normal portions of the lung to those distal to completely obstructed airways, keeping these obstructed areas inflated. Collateral air drift occurs when fissures are incomplete.

Areas of air trapping may appear more lucent on standard chest radiographs obtained at inspiration (i.e., total lung capacity) because the areas are relatively oligemic, with reduced pulmonary blood flow caused by alveolar hypoxia. Blood flow is then diverted to the more normal areas of the lung. Areas of air trapping must be distinguished from other causes of a radiolucent lung or lobe (Box 1-12). The other causes include technical factors, chest wall abnormalities, and pulmonary vascular disease. Technical factors that may produce unilateral hyperlucency include grid cut-off, misalignment of the x-ray beam, and anode heel effect. A few degrees of rotation of the patient may produce a difference in the relative density of the two hemithoraces. The most common chest wall abnormality associated with unilateral hyperlucency is mastectomy. However, rare congenital anomalies, such as absence of the pectoralis muscle or stroke, which produces unilateral atrophy of chest wall muscles, may be responsible. Several primary intravascular conditions, such as pulmonary emboli, may cause hyperlucency of the lung or a portion of the lung. However,

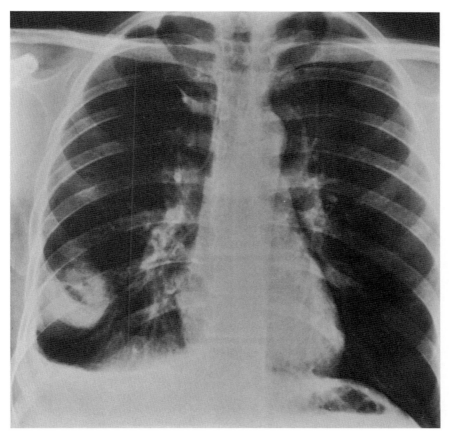

FIGURE 1-60. Lung laceration or posttraumatic pneumatocele. The posteroanterior view shows a partially air-containing, rounded opacity located peripherally and a small, right effusion. The patient was involved in a motor vehicle accident.

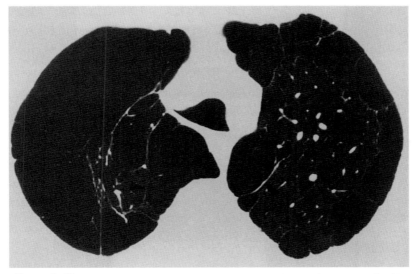

FIGURE 1-61. Multiple bullae with thin walls can be seen in both lungs *(arrowheads)*.

these disorders do not cause air trapping. Vascular causes of hyperlucency can be distinguished from air trapping by an expiration radiograph.

Expiratory chest radiographs are the simplest and easiest method for demonstrating air trapping. Expiration radiographs, however, are usually not sensitive in detecting generalized obstructive pulmonary disease such as emphysema. Limitation in the movement of the diaphragm can be appreciated only in the moderate to severe stages of the disease. For children or patients who

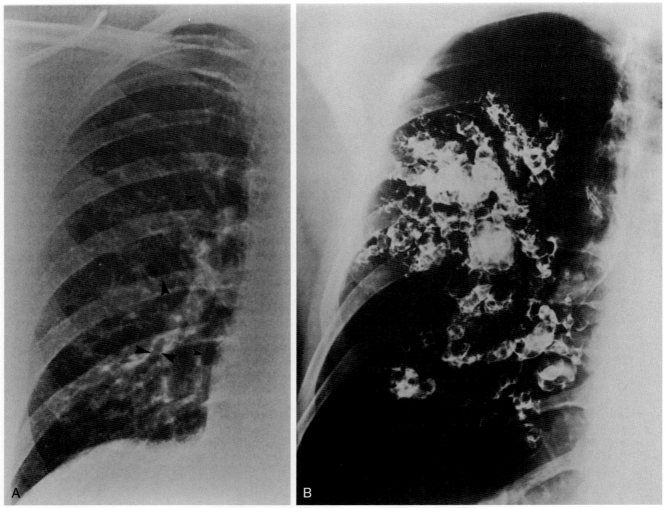

FIGURE 1-62. Bronchiectasis. **A,** The posteroanterior view shows multiple, central cystic structures with bronchial wall thickening *(arrowheads).* **B,** A bronchogram in which contrast is introduced into the bronchial tree shows markedly dilated saccular bronchi (i.e., cystic bronchiectasis).

are unable to cooperate, fluoroscopy of the chest may be helpful in demonstrating air trapping. Dynamic changes in volume with shift of mediastinal structures can be easily visualized.

There has been much interest in the use of CT for the identification of localized air trapping. Trapping occurs in diseases involving the small airways, such as bronchiolitis obliterans (Fig. 1-64). HRCT findings include areas of decreased lung opacity that are usually patchy in distribution, creating a *mosaic* pattern. The pulmonary vessels in the areas of decreased attenuation are decreased in caliber, and there may be associated central bronchiectasis. Expiration HRCT scans can confirm focal areas of suspected air trapping. Marked lung inhomogeneity is usually seen on the expiration scans as the normal lung increases in attenuation, and the areas of air trapping remain relatively radiolucent or of low attenuation. Further discussion of this topic can be found in Chapter 13.

Other Radiographic Signs of Disease

Localization of Disease

The anatomic localization of disease is usually easily determined on standard posteroanterior and lateral chest radiographs. A classic radiographic sign that helps in the localization of disease processes that have caused an increase in opacification is the silhouette sign (see Figs. 1-38 and 1-39). Normally, the mediastinal and diaphragmatic contours are visible because of their inherent contrast with the adjacent air-containing lung. When a lesion or opacity is situated in a portion of the lung adjacent to a mediastinal or diaphragmatic border, the border can no longer be seen. This sign is apparent only when structures have been adequately penetrated.

An example of the use of the silhouette sign is in differentiation of middle lobe and lingular disease from lower lobe disease. When disease processes involve the former lobes, the heart border is obliterated. Obliteration of the

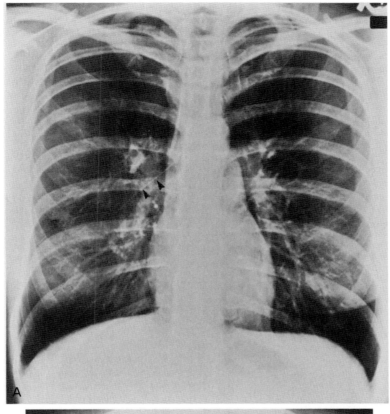

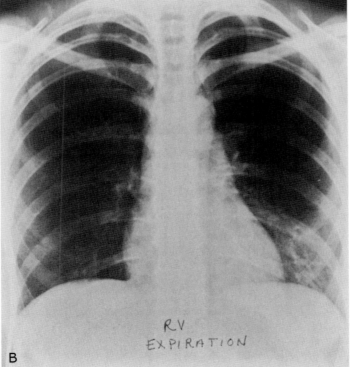

FIGURE 1-63. Air trapping in the right lower lobe. **A**, The posteroanterior view at inspiration shows a slightly smaller right lower lobe. The major fissure is depressed *(arrowheads)*. **B**, On expiration, the right lower lobe traps air. It is more lucent than the left base, and the right hemidiaphragm is lower than the left. The patient was diagnosed with bronchiolitis obliterans.

Box 1-12. **Unilateral Hyperlucency**

TECHNICAL FACTORS
Grid cutoff
Anode heel effect
Rotation

CHEST WALL
Mastectomy
Absent pectoralis muscle

PLEURA
Pneumothorax

LUNG
Vascular conditions
Congenital
   Absence of pulmonary artery
   Hypoplastic lung
      Congenital heart disease with abnormalities of
         pulmonary circulation

Acquired
   Pulmonary embolus
   Tumor invading pulmonary artery
   Inflammatory stenosis (fibrosing mediastinitis)

AIRWAYS OR PARENCHYMAL ABNORMALITIES (AIR TRAPPING)
Large airway obstruction
Foreign body
Tumor
Mucoid impaction
Small airways (bronchioles)
Bronchiolitis obliterans (Swyer-James)
Peripheral lung
Emphysema
   Bullae

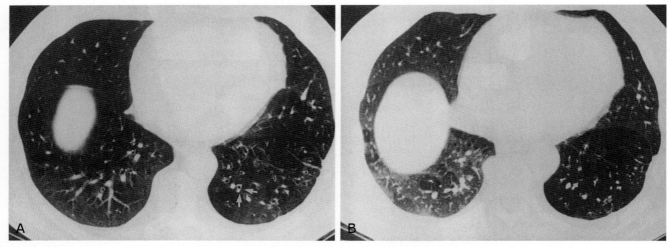

FIGURE 1-64. CT shows trapping. **A,** Inspiration scan shows patchy variation in attenuation, particularly in the left lower lobe where bronchiectasis is present *(arrows).* **B,** On expiration, CT shows air trapping in the left lower lobe, which remains lucent while most of the remainder of the lungs increases in attenuation. A pattern of mosaic perfusion is seen in the right lower lobe.

posterior part of the aortic arch (i.e., *aortic knob*) on the left side is caused by disease in the apical posterior segment of the left upper lobe. It may be difficult on standard posteroanterior chest radiographs to identify minor degrees of consolidation or atelectasis in the basal segments of the lower lobes. Lack of visibility of the posterior portion of the hemidiaphragm in the lateral projection is often an important clue to identifying such disease (see Fig. 1-40). Focal increase in opacity overlying the vertebral bodies may also be identified.

Distribution of Disease within the Lung
The distribution of disease in the lungs may be a clue to the diagnosis. Gravity is often an important factor. For example, aspiration pneumonia typically occurs in the posterior segments of the upper lobes and superior segments of the lower lobes when the patient is supine, and when the patient is erect, the basal segments of the lower lobes are involved.

Because there is much more blood flow to the base of the lungs than the apices in the erect position, certain processes related to the pulmonary circulation occur at the bases. For example, pulmonary infarction is much more common in the lower lobes, and metastatic lesions tend to occur at the bases.

Reactivation tuberculosis has an anatomic bias for the apices of the lung, particularly the apical and posterior segments of the upper lobes and superior segment of the lower lobes (see Fig. 1-54). These areas of the lung are characterized by higher oxygenation, with a high ventilation-to-perfusion ratio favoring the growth of mycobacteria.

Several diffuse lung diseases have an anatomic bias (see Fig. 1-32). For example, idiopathic pulmonary fibrosis and fibrosis associated with collagen vascular disease or asbestosis tend to occur predominantly in the lower lung zones, whereas upper lobe predilection is exhibited by diseases such as silicosis, sarcoidosis, and Langerhans cell histiocytosis.

▄▄▄ SUGGESTED READINGS

Aquino, S.L., Hayman, L.A., Loomis, S.L., Taber, K.H., 2003. The source and direction of thoracic lymphatics. Part I. The upper thorax. J. Comp. Assist. Tomogr. 27, 292–296.

Aquino, S.L., Hayman, L.A., Loomis, S.L., Taber, K.H., 2003. The source and direction of thoracic lymphatics. Part II. The lower thorax. J. Comput. Assist. Tomogr. 27, 479–484.

Blume, H., Jost, R.G., 1992. Chest imaging within the radiology department by means of photostimulable phosphor computed radiography: a review. J. Digit. Imaging. 5, 67–78.

Boyden, E.A., 1955. Segmental Anatomy of the Lungs. McGraw-Hill, New York.

Bragg, D.G., Freundlich, I.M., 1977. Cysts and cavities of the lung. In: Freundlich, I.M., Bragg, D.G. (Eds.), Radiologic Approach to Diseases of the Chest. second ed. Williams & Wilkins, Baltimore, pp. 119–130.

Doyle, T.C., Lawler, G.A., 1984. CT features of rounded atelectasis of the lung. AJR. Am. J. Roentgenol. 143, 225–228.

Felson, B., Felson, H., 1950. Localization of intrathoracic lesions by means of the postero-anterior roentgenogram: the silhouette sign. Radiology 55, 363–368.

Felson, B., 1967. The roentgen diagnosis of disseminated pulmonary alveolar diseases. Semin. Roentgenol. 2, 3–21.

Flaherty, R.A., Keegan, J.M., Sturtevant, H.N., 1960. Post-pneumonic pulmonary pneumatoceles. Radiology 74, 50–53.

Fleischner, F.G., 1967. Roentgenology of the pulmonary infarct. Semin. Roentgenol. 2, 61–66.

Fleischner, F.G., 1948. The visible bronchial tree: a roentgen sign in pneumonic and other pulmonary consolidations. Radiology 50, 184–190.

Floyd, C.E., Baker, J.A., Chotas, H.G., et al., 1995. Selenium-based digital radiography of the chest: radiologists' preference compared with film-screen radiographs. AJR. Am. J. Roentgenol. 165, 1353–1358.

Floyd, C.E., Warp, R.J., Dobbins, J.T., et al., 2001. Imaging characteristics of an amorphous silicon flat-panel detector for digital chest radiography. Radiology 218, 683–688.

Fraser, R.G., Fraser, R.S., Renner, J.W., et al., 1976. The roentgenologic diagnosis of chronic bronchitis: a reassessment with emphasis on parahilar bronchi seen end-on. Radiology 120, 1–8.

Fraser, R.G., Muller, N.L., Fraser, R.S., et al., 2001. Diagnosis of diseases of the chest. WB Saunders, Philadelphia.

Freundlich, I.M., 1997. Anatomy. In: Freundlich, I.M., Bragg, D.G. (Eds.), Radiologic Approach to Diseases of the Chest, second ed. Williams & Wilkins, Baltimore, pp. 31–48.

Freundlich, I.M., 1977. Pulmonary alveolar consolidation. In: Freundlich, I.M., Bragg, D.G. (Eds.), Radiologic Approach to Diseases of the Chest, second ed. Williams & Wilkins, Baltimore, pp. 89–100.

Freundlich, I.M., 1977. Pulmonary atelectasis. In: Freundlich, I.M., Bragg, D.G. (Eds.), Radiologic Approach to Diseases of the Chest, second ed. Williams & Wilkins, Baltimore, pp. 73–88.

Galvin, J.R., Gingrich, R.D., Hoffman, E., et al., 1994. Ultrafast computed tomography of the chest. Radiol. Clin. North. Am. 32, 775–793.

Gamsu, G., Thurlbeck, W.M., Macklem, P.T., et al., 1971. Roentgenographic appearance of the human pulmonary acinus. Invest. Radiol. 6, 171–176.

Genereux, G.P., 1984. CT of acute and chronic distal airspace (alveolar) disease. Semin. Roentgenol. 19, 211–217.

Genereux, G.P., 1975. The end-stage lung: pathogenesis, pathology, and radiology. Radiology 116, 279–284.

Glazer, G.M., Gross, B.H., Quint, L.E., et al., 1985. Normal mediastinal lymph nodes: number and size according to American Thoracic Society mapping. AJR. Am. J. Roentgenol. 144, 261–264.

Godwin, J.D., Vock, P., Osborne, D.R., 1983. CT of the pulmonary ligament. AJR. Am. J. Roentgenol. 141, 231–236.

Godwin, J.D., Webb, W.R., Savoca, C.J., et al., 1980. Review: multiple, thin-walled cystic lesions of the lung. AJR. Am. J. Roentgenol. 135, 593–604.

Greenspan, R.H., Curtis, A.M., 1977. Intrathoracic air trapping. In: Freundlich, I.M., Bragg, D.G. (Eds.), Radiologic Approach to Diseases of the Chest, second ed. Williams & Wilkins, Baltimore, pp. 195–210.

Groskin, S.A., 1993. In: Heitzman's the Lung: Radiologic Pathologic Correlations, third ed. Mosby–Year Book, St. Louis, pp. 43–105.

Gupta, N.C., Tamim, W.J., Graeber, G.C., et al., 2001. Mediastinal lymph node sampling following positron emission tomography with fluorodeoxyglucose imaging in lung cancer staging. Chest 120, 521–527.

Huang, R.M., Naidich, D.P., Lubat, E., et al., 1989. Septic pulmonary emboli: CT-radiologic correlation. AJR. Am. J. Roentgenol. 153, 41–45.

Jardin, M., Remy, J., 1986. Segmental bronchovascular anatomy of the lower lobes: CT analysis. AJR. Am. J. Roentgenol. 147, 457–468.

Kalender, W.A., 1994. Technical foundations of spiral CT. Semin. Ultrasound. CT. MRI. 15, 81–89.

Khoury, M.B., Godwin, J.D., Halvorsen Jr., R.A., et al., 1985. CT of obstructive lobar collapse. Invest. Radiol. 20, 708–711.

Kuhlman, J.E., Fishman, E.K., Teigen, C., 1990. Pulmonary septic emboli: diagnosis with CT. Radiology 174, 211–213.

Kuhlman, J.E., Hruban, R.H., Fishman, E.K., 1991. Wegener granulomatosis: CT features of parenchymal lung disease. J. Comput. Assist. Tomogr. 15, 948–952.

Kuhlman, J.E., Reyes, B.L., Hruban, R.H., et al., 1993. Abnormal air filled spaces in the lung. Radiographics 13, 47–75.

Lardinois, D., Weder, W., Hany, T.F., et al., 2003. Staging of non-small-cell lung cancer with integrated positron-emission tomography and computed tomography. N. Engl. J. Med. 348, 2500–2507.

Lien, H.H., Lund, G., 1985. Computed tomography of mediastinal lymph nodes: anatomic review based on contrast enhanced nodes following foot lymphography. Acta. Radiol. Diagn. 26, 641–647.

Lubert, M., Krause, G.R., 1951. Patterns of lobar collapse as observed radiographically. Radiology 56, 165–168.

McLoud, T.C., Carrington, C.B., Gaensler, E.A., 1983. Diffuse infiltrative lung disease: a new scheme for description. Radiology 149, 353–357.

McLoud, T.C., Meyer, J.E., 1985. Lymph node imaging of the thorax. In Clouse, M.E., Wallace, S. (Eds.), Golden's Diagnostic Radiology: Lymphatic Imaging: Lymphography, Computed Tomography and Scintigraphy, second ed. Waverly Press, Baltimore, pp. 451–471.

McLoud, T.C., 1981. Diffuse infiltrative disease. In: Putman, C.E. (Ed.), Pulmonary Diagnosis. Appleton Communications, Imaging, and Other Techniques, New York, pp. 125–153.

Moore, A.D.A., Godwin, J.D., Müller, N.L., et al., 1989. Pulmonary histiocytosis X: comparison of radiographic and CT findings. Radiology 172, 249–254.

Muller, N.L., 1991. Computed tomography in chronic interstitial lung disease. Radiol. Clin. North. Am. 29, 1085–1093.

Naidich, D.P., Khouri, N.F., Scott, W.W., et al., 1981. Computed tomography of the pulmonary hila: abnormal anatomy. J. Comput. Assist. Tomogr. 5, 468–472.

Naidich, D.P., Khouri, N.F., Scott, W.W., et al., 1981. Computed tomography of the pulmonary hila: normal anatomy. J. Comput. Assist. Tomgr. 5, 459–467.

Naidich, D.P., Webb, W.R., Zerhouni, E.A., et al., 1998. In: Computed tomography and magnetic resonance of the thorax, third ed. Lippincott Williams & Wilkins, New York, pp. 1–300.

Osborne, D., Vock, P., Godwin, J.D., Silverman, P.M., 1984. CT identification of bronchopulmonary segments: 50 normal subjects. AJR. Am. J. Roentgenol. 142, 47–52.

Pieterman, R.M., van Putten, J.W., Meuzelaar, J.J., et al., 2000. Preoperative staging of non-small-cell lung cancer with positron-emission tomography. N. Engl. J. Med. 343, 254–261.

Proto, A.V., Ball Jr., J.B., 1983. Computed tomography of the major and minor fissures. AJR. Am. J. Roentgenol. 140, 439–448.

Proto, A.V., Speckman, J.M., 1979. The left lateral radiograph of the chest. I. Med. Radiogr. Photogr. 55, 30–42.

Proto, A.V., Speckman, J.M., 1980. The left lateral radiograph of the chest. II. Med. Radiogr. Photogr. 56, 38–50.

Reed, J.C., Madewell, J.E., 1975. The air bronchogram in interstitial disease of the lungs: a radiological-pathological correlation. Radiology 116, 1–5.

Reich, S.B., Abouav, J., 1965. Interalveolar air drift. Radiology 85, 80–86.

Remy-Jardin, M., Giraud, F., Remy-Jardin, J., et al., 1993. Importance of ground-glass attenuation in chronic diffuse infiltrative lung disease. Radiology 189, 693–698.

Robbins, L.L., Hale, C.H., Merrill, O.E., 1945. Roentgen appearance of lobar and segmental collapse of the lung: technique of examination. Radiology 44, 474–1471.

Robbins, L.L., Hale, C.H., 1945. The roentgen appearance of lobar and segmental collapse of the lung. II. The normal chest as it pertains to collapse. Radiology 44, 543–548.

Robbins, L.L., Hale, C.H., 1945. The roentgen appearance of lobar and segmental collapse of the lung. III. Collapse of an entire lung or the major part thereof. Radiology 45, 23–26.

Robbins, L.L., Hale, C.H., 1945. The roentgen appearance of lobar and segmental collapse of the lung. IV. Collapse of the lower lobes. Radiology 45, 120–127.

Robbins, L.L., Hale, C.H., 1945. The roentgen appearance of lobar and segmental collapse of the lung. V. Collapse of the right middle lobe. Radiology 45, 260–266.

Robbins, L.L., Hale, C.H., 1945. The roentgen appearance of lobar and segmental collapse of the lung. VI. Collapse of the upper lobes. Radiology 45, 347–355.

Rost, R.C., Proto, A.V., 1983. Inferior pulmonary ligament: computed tomographic appearance. Radiology 14, 479–482.

Rouviere, H., 1938. Anatomy of the Human Lymphatic System. MI, Edwards Brothers, Ann Arbor.

Sandhu, J., Goodman, P.C., 1989. Pulmonary cysts associated with PCP in patients with AIDS. Radiology 173, 33–35.

Schneider, H.J., Felson, B., Gonzalez, L.L., 1980. Rounded atelectasis. AJR. Am. J. Roentgenol. 134, 225–229.

Sosman, M.C., Dodd, G.D., Jones, W.D., et al., 1957. The familial occurrence of pulmonary alveolar microlithiasis. AJR. Am. J. Roentgenol. 77, 947–952.

Swyer, P.R., James, G.C.W., 1953. A case of unilateral pulmonary emphysema. Thorax 8, 133–137.

Thurlbeck, W.M., Churg, A.M., 1995. In: Pathology of the Lung. Thieme Medical Publishers, New York. pp 589–737.

Thurlbeck, W.M., Muller, N.L., 1987. Emphysema: definition, imaging, and quantification. AJR. Am. J. Roentgenol. 163, 1017–1025.

Webb, W.R., Glazer, G., Gamsu, G., 1981. Computed tomography of the normal pulmonary hilum. J. Comput. Assist. Tomogr. 5, 476–484.

Webb, W.R., Jensen, B.G., Gamsu, G., et al., 1984. Coronal magnetic resonance imaging of the chest: normal and abnormal. Radiology 153, 729–735.

Webb, W.R., 1994. High resolution computed tomography of obstructive lung disease. Radiol. Clin. North. Am. 32, 745–757.

Webb, W.R., 1994. High resolution computed tomography of obstructive lung disease. Radiol. Clin. North. Am. 32, 745–757.

Woodring, J.H., Fried, M., Chuang, V.P., 1980. Solitary cavities of the lung: diagnostic implications of cavity wall thickness. AJR. Am. J. Roentgenol. 135, 1269–1274.

CHAPTER 2

Congenital Abnormalities of the Thorax

Theresa C. McLoud and Phillip M. Boiselle

Several congenital abnormalities of the thorax have been described, but most are rare. Classification of these anomalies is difficult because the embryologic basis often is not clearly understood. A classification based on thoracic anatomic structures uses the categories of trachea, bronchi, lung, and pulmonary vasculature. Congenital abnormalities involving the mediastinum are discussed in Chapter 15, and airway anomalies are discussed in Chapter 13.

The diagnosis usually can be established noninvasively by means of standard radiographs, ultrasound, computed tomography (CT), and magnetic resonance imaging (MRI). A comprehensive listing of congenital abnormalities of the chest is provided in Box 2-1. In this chapter, congenital abnormalities in adults are emphasized. Those more commonly identified in infancy are discussed in *Pediatric Radiology: The Requisites.*

TRACHEA

The most common anomalies of the trachea include congenital stenosis, tracheomalacia, congenital tracheobronchomegaly, aberrant tracheal bronchus, and tracheoesophageal fistula.

Congenital Tracheal Stenosis

The three patterns of congenital tracheal stenosis are diffuse or generalized hypoplasia; a funnel-like stenosis (i.e., carrot-shaped trachea), often associated with an anomalous origin of the left pulmonary artery (Fig. 2-1); and segmental stenosis. Diffuse or funnel-like stenosis may be associated with absence of the posterior membranous wall due to complete ringlike tracheal cartilages. Patients with complete tracheal rings usually present with respiratory distress in the first few weeks of life, and this condition is associated with a high mortality rate. Rarely, the diagnosis is delayed until adulthood.

Tracheomalacia

Tracheomalacia is abnormal collapsibility of the trachea, which is caused by softness or pliability of the tracheal cartilages. It may be primary, associated with a localized absence of the tracheal cartilage, or secondary, resulting from external compression, such as from an extrinsic mass. Tracheomalacia must be differentiated from excessive collapse, which is caused by abnormal expiratory pressures. For example, collapse of a long segment of the intrathoracic trachea may occur in late expiration in patients with asthma, chronic bronchitis, and bronchiolitis. Paired inspiratory and dynamic expiratory computed tomography (CT) using state-of-the-art multidetector-row CT scanners is excellent for evaluating tracheomalacia. The accuracy of this technique is comparable to that of bronchoscopy, the gold standard for diagnosing this condition. A greater than 50% collapse of the tracheal diameter is considered abnormal (Fig. 2-2), but healthy individuals may sometimes exceed this threshold.

Congenital Tracheobronchomegaly

Tracheobronchomegaly (i.e., Mounier-Kuhn syndrome) is characterized by loud, prolonged chronic cough with ineffective secretions and recurrent bronchitis or pneumonia. Imaging of the trachea demonstrates absence or atrophy of elastic fibers and thinning of muscle; airway dynamics are abnormal with dilation on inspiration and collapse on expiration. There are frequent saccular bulgings of the intercartilaginous membranes. The diagnosis can be established by chest radiography when the transverse diameter of the trachea is greater than 25 mm and the diameters of the right and left main bronchi are greater than 23 and 20 mm, respectively (Fig. 2-3). CT can confirm the increased diameter of the trachea. Frequently, there is bronchiectasis in the lung parenchyma.

Aberrant Tracheal Bronchus

Rarely, the right upper lobe bronchus or a segment of the right upper lobe bronchus may originate in the trachea (i.e., tracheal or pre-eparterial bronchus). This is usually of no clinical consequence. However, in a minority of affected patients, impaired drainage may result in recurrent infections (Fig. 2-4). After endotracheal intubation, the balloon may inadvertently obstruct such a bronchus, causing right upper lobe atelectasis.

Tracheoesophageal Fistula

Congenital tracheoesophageal fistula is invariably a pediatric disease. It occurs in newborns and is most frequently associated with esophageal atresia. However, about 3% of all tracheoesophageal fistulas occur with an otherwise normal esophagus, and patients may present in these instances in adult life. Roughly 75% show communication with the trachea, and the others communicate with the major bronchi (Fig. 2-5). Patients usually have a history of recurrent pneumonias. The chest roentgenogram

Box 2-1. **Congenital Abnormalities of the Thorax**

TRACHEA
Tracheomalacia
Tracheal stenosis
Tracheal abnormalities in skeletal dysplasia
  syndromes
Tracheobronchomegaly
Tracheopathia osteoplastica
Intratracheal masses (hemangioma)
Tracheoesophageal fistula
Tracheal diverticulum

BRONCHI
Bronchial isomerism syndromes
Tracheal accessory bronchus
Bridging bronchus
Bronchomalacia
Bronchial atresia
Bronchiectasis
Congenital lobar emphysema

LUNGS
Horseshoe lung
Agenesis of the lung
Hypoplasia of lung
Congenital pulmonary lymphangiectasia

Pulmonary blastoma or hamartomas
Sequestration
Scimitar syndrome
Congenital cystic adenomatoid malformation
Bronchogenic cyst
Cystic fibrosis

VASCULAR ABNORMALITIES
Arteries
Absence of main pulmonary artery
Proximal interruption of the pulmonary artery
Anomalous origin of left pulmonary artery from right
Pulmonary artery stenosis or coarctation
Congenital aneurysm of pulmonary arteries
Arteriovenous fistula

Veins
Hypogenetic lung (scimitar syndrome)
Pulmonary varix
Anomalous pulmonary venous drainage

Lymphatics
Lymphangiectasis
Lymphangiomatosis
Lymphangioleiomyomatosis

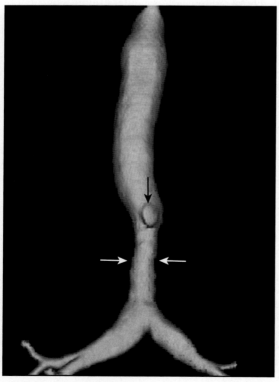

FIGURE 2-1. Congenital tracheal stenosis. External three-dimensional rendering of trachea demonstrates smooth stenosis *(white arrows)* of the lower trachea. Round protuberance *(black arrow)* above the level of stenosis represents a tracheal diverticulum viewed en face.

may show evidence of bronchiectasis. The diagnosis can be confirmed by a contrast esophagogram, which often can identify the fistula and show evidence of contrast material within the tracheobronchial tree and the lung.

■ BRONCHI

Bronchopulmonary Isomerism Syndrome

Bronchopulmonary isomerism has an identical pattern of bronchial branching and an equal number of lobes in each lung. The anomaly may be isolated or associated with other anomalies. The bilateral right lung type may be associated with asplenia, and the bilateral left lung type may be associated with polysplenia.

Bronchial Atresia

This anomaly consists of atresia of a lobar or segmental bronchus with obliteration of the lumen and preservation of distal structures. The most common site is the left upper lobe, particularly the apical posterior segment. The right middle and upper lobes are less common sites. Mucus secreted within the airways distal to the atretic segment cannot pass the stenosis and accumulates as a mucous plug or mucocele. Collateral air drift keeps the lobe or segment inflated, and it becomes hyperinflated as a result of expiratory air trapping. The chest radiograph shows an area of hyperlucency in the affected portion of the lung (Fig. 2-6). The mucocele appears as an ovoid or branching structure at the hilar level. CT demonstrates the mucoid impaction

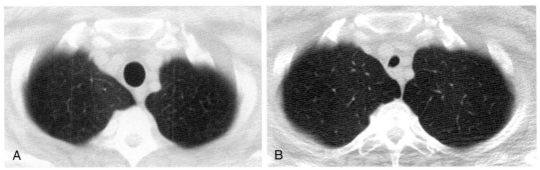

FIGURE 2-2. Tracheomalacia is shown on paired inspiratory and dynamic expiratory axial CT images. **A**, On inspiration, the trachea is of normal caliber. **B**, On expiration, excessive collapsibility of the trachea can be seen.

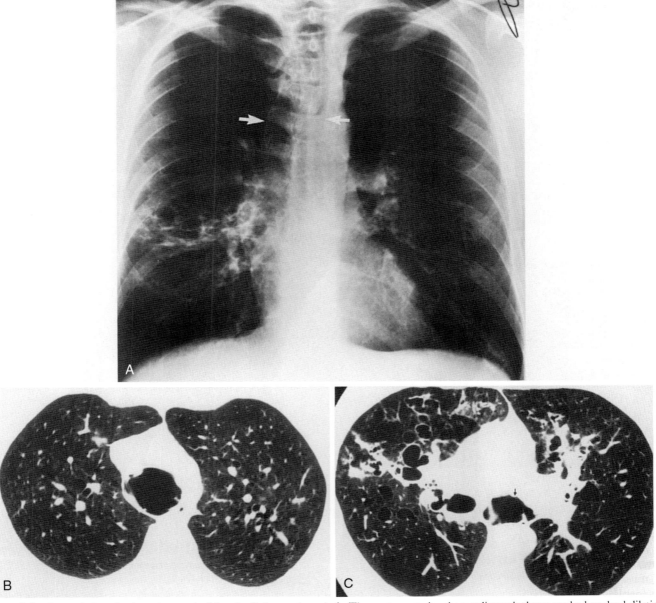

FIGURE 2-3. Congenital tracheobronchomegaly (Mounier-Kuhn syndrome). **A**, The posteroanterior chest radiograph shows marked tracheal dilation (43 mm) *(arrows)* and bronchiectasis in the right lung. **B**, CT confirms the large tracheal lumen. **C**, The dilation extends into the main bronchi, which exhibit saccular bulging of their walls *(arrow)*.

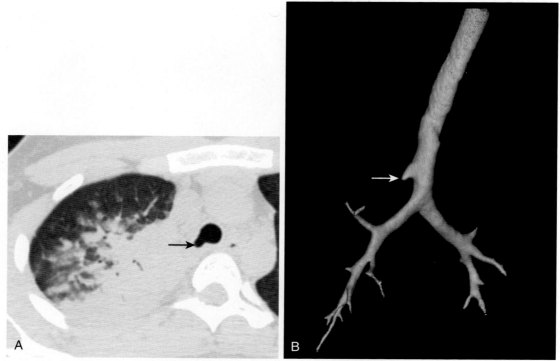

FIGURE 2-4. Tracheal bronchus. **A,** Axial CT shows the anomalous origin of the apical segment of the right upper lobe bronchus directly from the trachea, with an obstructed lumen *(arrow)* and postobstructive pneumonia. **B,** External three-dimensional rendering of the airways shows the anomalous origin of the right upper lobe apical segment bronchus *(arrow)* from the trachea.

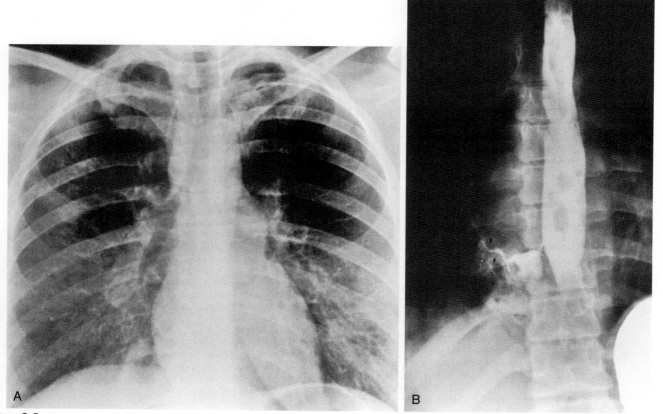

FIGURE 2-5. Congenital bronchoesophageal fistula in a 24-year-old woman with a history of repeated pneumonias since childhood. **A,** The posteroanterior chest radiograph shows patchy pneumonia in the right upper lobe and right base, with right hilar and paratracheal adenopathy caused by repeated infections. **B,** The barium esophagogram demonstrates a fistula between the lower esophagus and a branch of the right lower-lobe bronchus *(arrows).*

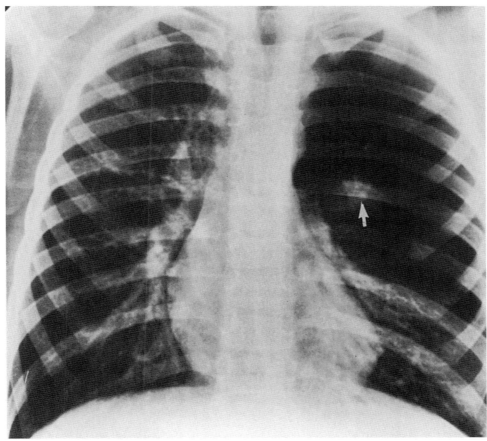

FIGURE 2-6. Bronchial atresia. The anteroposterior radiograph shows an overinflated left upper lobe with a slight mediastinal shift. The left perihilar opacity represents mucoid impaction distal to the atresia *(arrow)*.

at the site of obstruction, which is associated with lobar or segmental hyperinflation (Fig. 2-7). There may be an accompanying shift of the mediastinum and compression of the surrounding lung.

Congenital Bronchiectasis

Congenital bronchiectasis (i.e., Williams-Campbell syndrome) is rare, and its existence is controversial. It results from an intrinsic abnormality of cartilage. The cartilagi-

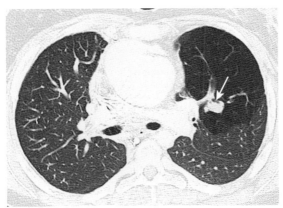

FIGURE 2-7. Bronchial atresia. Axial CT shows a site of mucoid impaction *(arrow)* distal to the atretic left upper lobe's apical posterior segmental bronchus and surrounding hyperlucency in the left upper lobe.

nous deficiency occurs within the fourth- to sixth-order bronchi and is manifested by cystic bronchiectasis and pulmonary hyperinflation (Fig. 2-8). Bronchiectasis, which is acquired and caused by chronic infection, may occur early in life as a result of other congenital, developmental, or genetic disorders. These conditions are listed in Box 2-2 (see Chapter 13).

■ LUNGS

Pulmonary Agenesis and Hypoplasia

Pulmonary agenesis is a condition with total absence of the lung parenchyma and the vessels and bronchi distal to the carina. Patients with pulmonary aplasia have a rudimentary bronchus, which ends in a blind pouch without lung tissue or pulmonary vasculature. A decrease in the number or size of airways, vessels, and alveoli characterizes pulmonary hypoplasia. The lesion may be primary, or it may result from several pathogenetic mechanisms that may occur during gestation. These conditions include decreased pulmonary vascular perfusion, oligohydramnios, or compression of the lung by a space-occupying mass within the pleural cavity (e.g., congenital diaphragmatic hernia).

Agenesis, aplasia, and hypoplasia more frequently involve the right lung. In agenesis, the radiograph shows complete absence of an aerated lung in one hemithorax,

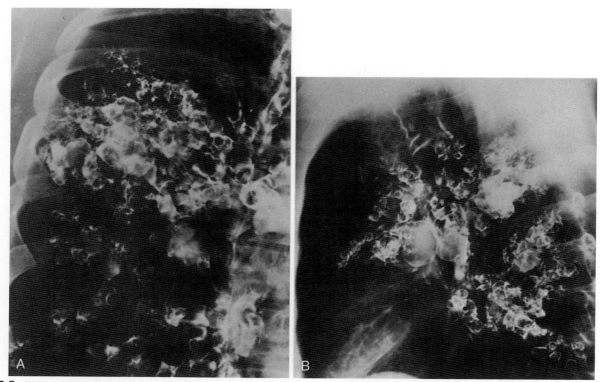

FIGURE 2-8. Williams-Campbell syndrome. The posteroanterior (**A**) and lateral (**B**) views of a bronchogram of the right lung shows diffuse cystic bronchiectasis involving all lobes.

Box 2-2. **Bronchiectasis Associated with Developmental or Congenital Disorders**

Congenital cystic bronchiectasis
Primary hypogammaglobulinemia
Yellow nail syndrome
Cystic fibrosis
Immotile-cilia syndrome (Kartagener's syndrome)

with pronounced reduction in the volume of that hemithorax and associated shift of the mediastinum to the affected side (Fig. 2-9). There is usually pronounced compensatory overinflation of the contralateral normal lung. Pulmonary hypoplasia has similar findings because of volume reduction; however, there is a small lung on the affected side. In some cases, it may be difficult on standard radiographs to distinguish severe pulmonary hypoplasia from aplasia or agenesis. In such instances, CT may help to identify the absence or

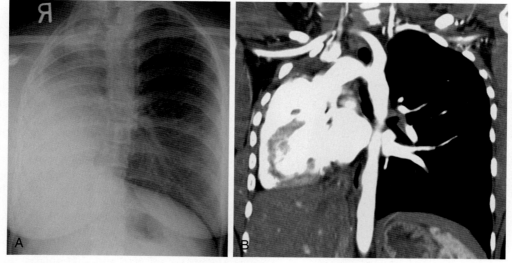

FIGURE 2-9. Pulmonary agenesis. **A,** PA radiograph of a 16 year-old girl shows complete absence of the right lung and pronounced mediastinal shift and overinflation of the left lung. **B,** Coronal multiplanar reformation of a CT angiogram demonstrates absence of the right lung and marked shift of mediastinal structures into the right hemithorax, which is reduced in size compared with the left. (Case courtesy of Edward Lee, MD, Children's Hospital, Boston, MA.)

presence of the ipsilateral pulmonary artery and bronchus or the presence of a rudimentary bronchus in pulmonary aplasia. CT also can demonstrate rudimentary pulmonary tissue in the base of the hemithorax in patients with severe pulmonary hypoplasia and show a patent bronchus and accompanying pulmonary artery (Fig. 2-10).

Pulmonary hypoplasia must be differentiated from other conditions that can produce a small lung with markedly reduced volume of the hemithorax, including total atelectasis of the lung, severe bronchiectasis with collapse, and advanced fibrothorax due to chronic pleural disease. CT is likely to be diagnostic in these cases.

Congenital Lobar Emphysema

The primary characteristic of congenital lobar emphysema is progressive overdistention of a lobe caused by an intrinsic bronchial obstruction due to a cartilage anomaly

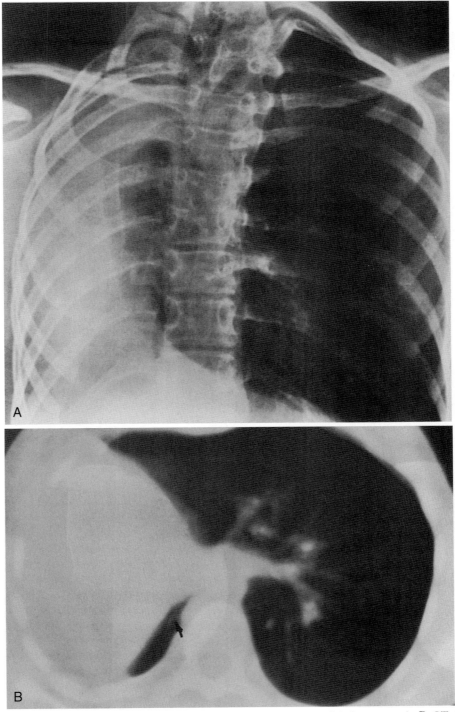

FIGURE 2-10. Severe pulmonary hypoplasia. **A,** The posteroanterior chest radiograph suggests right lung agenesis. **B,** CT demonstrates rudimentary lung tissue at the right base that contains pulmonary vessels *(arrow).*

or deficiency or because of compression by an extrinsic vascular structure or mass (i.e., bronchogenic cyst). In a few patients, the hyperinflated lobe may be caused by an abnormal increase in alveoli. The condition usually occurs in infants or young children. The left upper lobe is the most frequently affected, followed by the right middle lobe. The radiologic findings consist of overinflation of the affected lobe with various degrees of mediastinal shift (Fig. 2-11). Occasionally, the lobe may be opaque because of retained fetal lung fluid. The differential diagnosis includes a for-

eign body in an older infant; extraluminal compression of the bronchus by a bronchogenic cyst, teratoma, or other mass lesion; bronchial atresia with overinflation; and congenital lung cyst (Table 2-1).

Acute cases of respiratory distress require surgical resection, particularly in the neonatal period. However, the trend is toward supportive therapy because investigations show that these lesions may regress spontaneously without thoracotomy and lobar resection. A few cases are asymptomatic and may not be diagnosed until adult life.

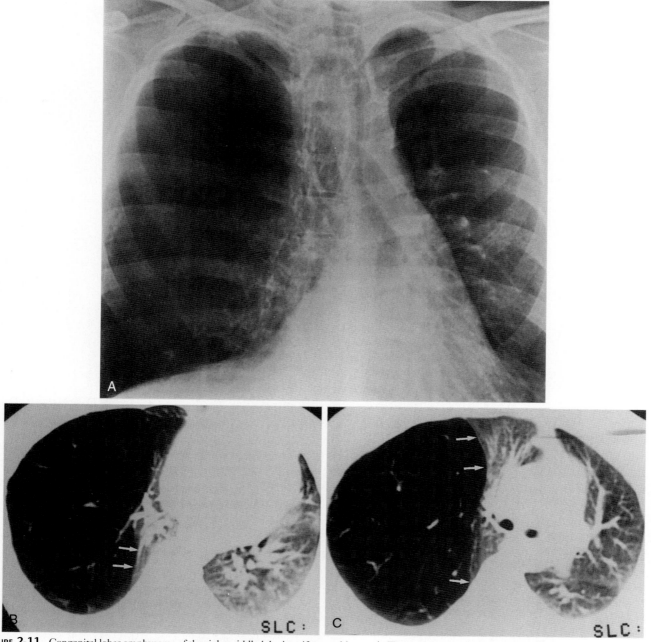

Figure 2-11. Congenital lobar emphysema of the right middle lobe in a 42-year-old man. **A,** The posteroanterior chest radiograph shows pronounced overinflation of the right lung and a mediastinal shift to the left. The vessels in the right lung are few and stretched, suggesting that the air-filled lung may represent only one lobe. **B** and **C,** CT demonstrates collapsed and compressed upper and lower lobes *(arrows)* and pronounced overinflation of the right middle lobe.

TABLE 2-1 Diagnosis of Cystic or Cystlike Developmental Lesions

Condition	Distinguishing Features
Congenital diaphragmatic hernia	Air-filled or contrast-filled bowel loops above diaphragm
Bronchogenic cyst	Usually mediastinal In lung, medial one third Usually opaque, occasionally has air-fluid level Marked displacement of lung and mediastinum not a feature
Congenital lobar emphysema	Left upper lobe, right middle lobe: no internal linear opacities Usually lucent Marked shift of mediastinum and compression of lung with mass effect If fluid-filled, may substitute cystic adenomatoid malformation type III
Cystic adenomatoid malformation	Lucent, air-filled, single or multiple cysts Mass effect Multiple internal linear opacities

Cystic Adenomatoid Malformation

Cystic adenomatoid malformation of the lung is a rare lesion that usually occurs in infancy with respiratory distress caused by a space-occupying effect that compromises lung tissue. Roughly 80% of patients are younger than 6 months, although 17% of cases are reported in older children.

There are three types. Type I, the most common, is characterized by single or multiple, large cysts of various sizes that are more than 2 cm in diameter. Type II consists of multiple, small cysts of more uniform size, not exceeding 2 cm in diameter, and type III consists of large, bulky, solid-appearing lesions that contain multiple, microscopic cysts.

The radiographic findings vary and correlate with the type of lesion. Chest radiographs of the type I lesion typically show unilateral, single or multiple air-filled cysts in the thorax of a neonate with respiratory distress (Fig. 2-12). The lesions may be very large and may occupy almost the entire lung, producing a mass effect with a shift of the mediastinum and compression of the remaining lung. A single, dominant cyst may be surrounded by smaller cysts. If fluid is present, air-fluid levels can be identified on horizontal beam images. Type II lesions may show evidence of multiple, small, uniform cysts. A type III lesion usually appears as a solid intrathoracic mass or consolidation rather than as a cystic or air-filled structure.

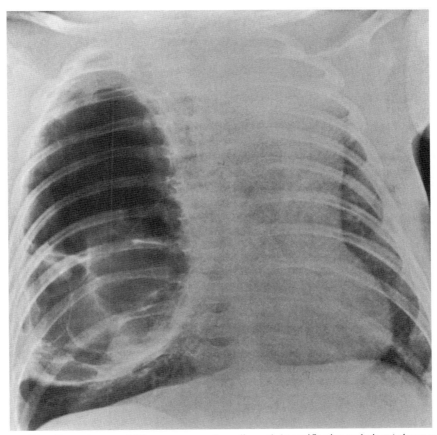

FIGURE 2-12. Cystic adenomatoid malformation type I. The posteroanterior radiograph (magnification technique) shows multiple, large, air-filled cysts in the right lung, with a shift of the mediastinum to the left and compression of the remaining right lung above the diaphragm.

The appearance on CT scanning is similar to the radiographic appearance, and CT may document the number of cysts. Although cystic adenomatoid malformation has been considered a unilateral disease, CT has found evidence of bilateral involvement. CT imaging may be helpful in differentiating congenital cystic adenomatoid malformation from other conditions. It can document the presence of air- or fluid-filled cysts, the extent of disease, and the degree of mass effect.

The definitive treatment is surgical excision. In neonates with severe respiratory distress, this lesion may constitute a surgical emergency.

Prognosis appears to be best for patients with type I lesions. If cysts are very large and interfere with normal pulmonary development, particularly if there is contralateral pulmonary hypoplasia, the prognosis is poor.

Pulmonary Sequestration

Pulmonary sequestration consists of aberrant lung tissue that has no normal connection with the bronchial tree or with the pulmonary arteries, or it is supplied by a systemic artery that usually arises from the aorta. It may be extralobar, contained within its own pleural envelope, or intralobar, contained within the substance of the lung (Table 2-2). It is generally agreed that extralobar sequestration is a congenital abnormality caused by failure of obliteration of one of the systemic arterial connections to the base of the developing fetal lung. Although somewhat controversial, there is growing consensus that intralobar sequestration may be an acquired anomaly resulting from recurrent infections that produce aberrant arterial vessels arising from the aorta.

The arterial blood supply to the sequestered pulmonary tissue usually arises from the descending thoracic aorta, although the origin may be from the upper abdominal aorta or one of its major branches. The venous drainage patterns of intralobar and extralobar sequestrations are different. Intralobar sequestration usually drains into a branch of the inferior pulmonary vein, creating a left-to-left shunt. Extralobar sequestration drains to the systemic veins, usually the azygos system.

Intralobar Sequestration

Intralobar sequestrations are more common than the extralobar variety, and they frequently manifest in adult life as an abnormality seen on a standard chest radiograph or as a cause of recurrent pneumonias. They almost invariably occur in the lower lobes in the area of the posterior basal segment. They affect the left side twice as frequently as the right.

The radiographic appearance may vary, but there are two major patterns. The patterns depend on the degree of aeration and the presence or absence of associated infection. The lesion may appear as a solid or water-density mass or area of consolidation, or it may appear as an air-containing, single or multicystic lesion (Figs. 2-13 and 2-14). The air gains entry into the sequestered lung from the surrounding pulmonary tissue by means of collateral ventilation. If there is an infection, an air-fluid level may be seen. CT and MRI may be useful in evaluation. With its ability to image directly in the coronal and sagittal planes, MRI has traditionally been superior to CT in identifying the systemic blood supply from the aorta. However, state-of-the-art CT scanners can provide high-quality multiplanar reformation and three-dimensional reconstructions that have enhanced the ability to display systemic blood supply to sequestrations. In these cases, the accuracy of CT is comparable to that of MRI (Fig. 2-15). CT also demonstrates the internal architecture of the sequestration and its cystic components when present. Failure to identify a systemic artery on these examinations, however, does not exclude the diagnosis. Angiography can demonstrate the anomalous systemic vessel (see Fig. 2-14). The ability of CT to simultaneously image the arterial supply, venous drainage, and internal architecture in a single examination makes it the imaging modality of choice for the diagnosis and preoperative assessment of pulmonary sequestration. MRI may be considered a secondary, problem-solving tool for inconclusive CT cases or as an alternative imaging test for patients with relative contraindications to iodinated contrast.

Extralobar Sequestration

Extralobar sequestration typically manifests in the newborn or early infancy. It most often occurs in the lower hemithorax between the lower lobe and the diaphragm, although it may occur within the substance of the diaphragm or in the mediastinum. Diagnosis can often be made without angiography by using CT and MRI, which may demonstrate the anomalous feeding and draining vessels.

On standard roentgenograms, the extralobar sequestration usually appears as a single, well-defined, homogeneous area of increased opacity in the lower thorax close to the posterior medial hemidiaphragm. It occasionally

TABLE 2-2 Pulmonary Sequestration

Characteristics	Intralobar Sequestration	Extralobar Sequestration
Clinical features	Affects adults Affects men and women equally Pneumonia or incidental finding	Affects infants Affects boys more than girls Asymptomatic or symptoms due to associated abnormalities
Location	60% occur in left side Posterior lower lobe	90% occur in left side Above or below diaphragm
Arterial supply	Large vessel from aorta	Single or multiple systemic arteries
Venous drainage	Pulmonary vein	Systemic (azygos, hemiazygos, vena cava)
Connection with foregut	Rare	Occasionally
Pleura	No separate pleural covering	Separate pleural covering

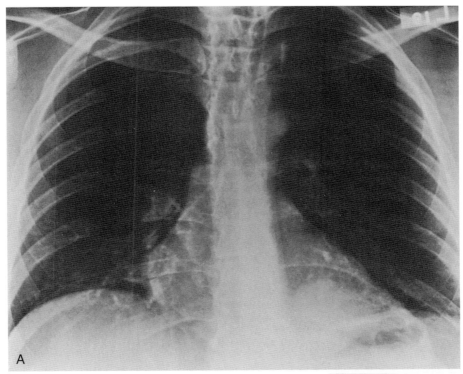

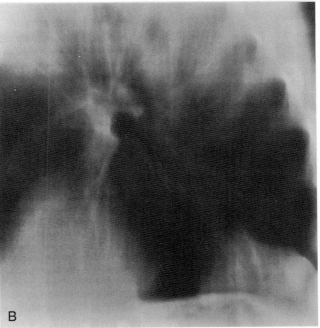

FIGURE 2-13. Intralobar sequestration. A, The posteroanterior radiograph shows a solid, masslike lesion in the left lower lobe abutting the diaphragm. B, The lateral tomogram confirms a well-defined mass posteriorly in the left lower lobe.

appears as a small "bump" on the hemidiaphragm or inferior paravertebral region. There are no air bronchograms. The lesion is usually well defined and does not blend with the surrounding lung parenchyma. It may also occur in the mediastinum and in the pericardium or upper thorax and rarely occur as a subdiaphragmatic mass. Occasionally, there may be communication with the stomach or esophagus, and an esophagogram is recommended to demonstrate the fistulous communication between the sequestration and the gastrointestinal tract.

Aortography depicts the anomalous systemic artery or arteries feeding the lesion. Demonstration of the venous drainage may require selective angiography of the anomalous feeding vessels.

Ultrasound may be useful in the diagnosis of pulmonary sequestration in neonates and infants with typical findings of a uniformly echogenic mass, occasionally with a hyperechoic rim. Duplex Doppler scanning and color Doppler flow imaging may be used to diagnose extralobar sequestration. Reports show aberrant arterial and venous structures

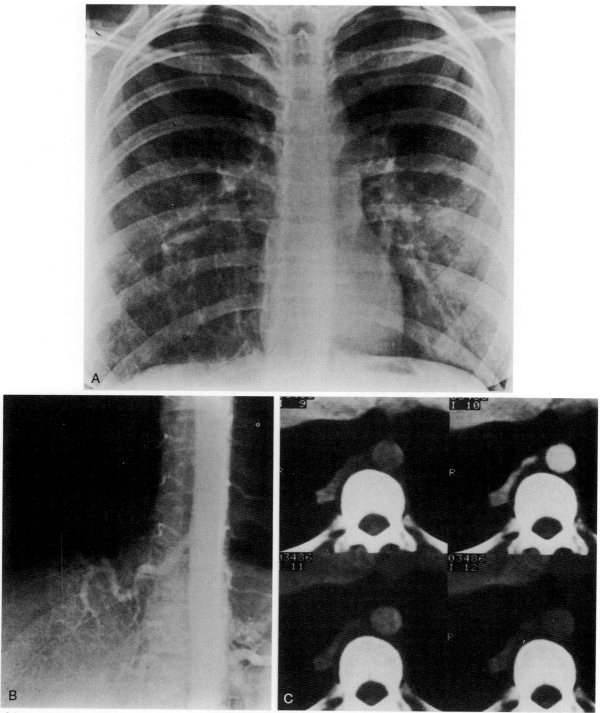

Figure 2-14. Air-filled intralobar sequestration. **A,** The posteroanterior radiograph shows the pulmonary vessels at the right base, which display an abnormal course. This suggests they may be draped around a space-occupying but air-filled lesion. The right hemidiaphragm is slightly depressed, and the heart is shifted slightly to the left. **B,** The aortogram demonstrates a large, single vessel arising from the distal aorta and supplying a portion of the right lower lobe. **C,** Contrast-enhanced CT confirms the vascular supply.

supplying and draining these lesions. Fetal MRI can provide additional diagnostic information to that of ultrasound in many cases and can aid in the diagnosis of sequestration by helping to identify the anomalous blood supply (Fig. 2-16). On CT images of the chest (Fig. 2-17), the lesions are usually homogenous, well-defined masses with soft tissue attenuation, sometimes with areas of emphysema in the adjacent normal lung. CT also may demonstrate cystic areas within the sequestration.

Bronchogenic Cyst

Bronchogenic cysts are bronchopulmonary foregut malformations resulting from an abnormality of budding or branching of the tracheobronchial tree during embryologic

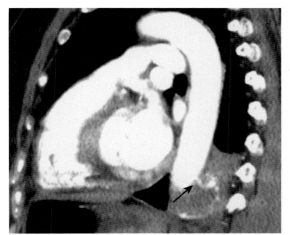

FIGURE 2-15. Systemic blood supply. Sagittal reformation of a CT angiogram shows a vessel *(arrow)* arising from the lower thoracic aorta to supply a mass in the posterior basal segment of the left lower lobe.

development. Bronchogenic cysts are lined by pseudostratified ciliated columnar epithelium, and they usually contain smooth muscle, mucous glands, and cartilage. They may occur in the mediastinum or, far less commonly, in the lung. They may be filled with clear or mucoid material. Mediastinal bronchogenic cysts are discussed in more detail in Chapter 16. The pulmonary variety typically occurs in the lower lobes, usually in the medial third of the lung. The cysts are sharply circumscribed, solitary, and typically round or oval, and on standard chest roentgenograms (Fig. 2-18), they appear to be of soft tissue or unit density. Most are not associated with symptoms, but intrapulmonary cysts may become infected, resulting in communication with the tracheobronchial tree. This may lead to the development of an air-fluid level or a surrounding consolidation in the lung parenchyma that obscures the wall of the cyst (Fig. 2-19).

CT can demonstrate a well-defined mass that may have various densities, depending on the nature of the fluid content.

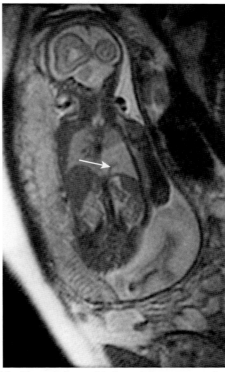

FIGURE 2-16. Prenatal diagnosis of extralobar sequestration using fetal MRI. Coronal, single-shot, fast spin-echo (SSFSE) MRI of the fetus demonstrates an anomalous systemic arterial supply *(arrow)* arising from the abdominal aorta and coursing above the diaphragm to supply a sequestration in the left lower lobe. (Case courtesy of Deborah Levine, MD, Beth Israel Deaconess Medical Center, Boston, MA.)

Roughly one half of the cysts have attenuation greater than that of muscle because of mucoid content or hemorrhage (see Chapter 16). On MRI, T1-weighted images the lesions have the typical appearance of cysts with long T1 and T2 values and will not enhance with contrast. Cysts that contain mucus may have high signal intensity on T1-weighted images.

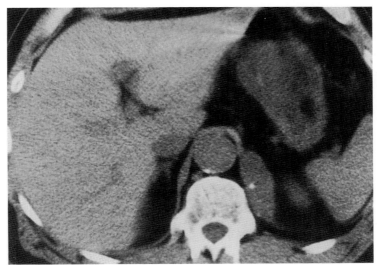

FIGURE 2-17. Extralobar sequestration. CT demonstrates a well-defined mass containing calcium and abutting the left diaphragmatic crus.

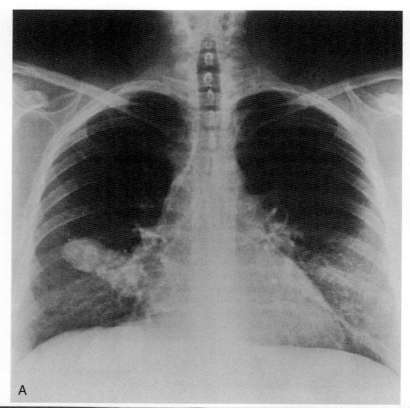

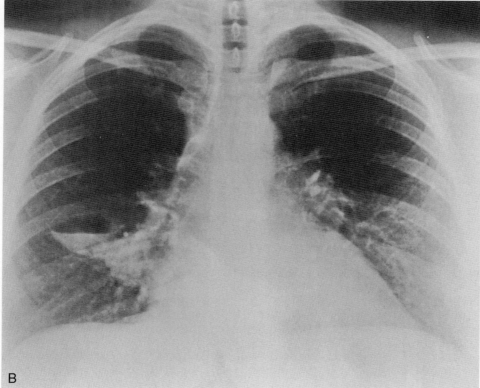

FIGURE 2-18. Bronchogenic cyst. **A,** The posteroanterior chest radiograph shows a well-defined, ovoid mass of soft tissue density in the medial third of the right lung. **B,** After needle aspiration biopsy, an air-fluid level can be seen, and the wall appears very thin, consistent with a cyst.

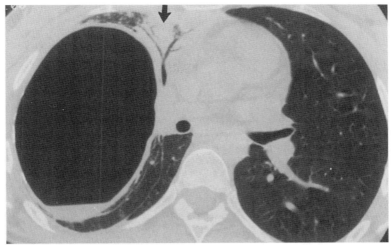

FIGURE 2-19. Infected bronchogenic cyst. CT demonstrates an air-fluid level in an infected bronchogenic cyst. There is evidence of pneumonia in the right middle lobe *(arrow)*.

■ PULMONARY VESSELS

Anomalies of the Pulmonary Arteries

Absence of the Main Pulmonary Artery and Proximal Interruption

Absence of the main pulmonary artery frequently consists of atresia of the artery's proximal portion or of its entire length. The right and left main pulmonary arteries persist and connect to the aorta by a ductus.

Congenital unilateral absence of a pulmonary artery usually occurs with cardiac lesions, but it may be an isolated finding when it occurs on the right side. Chest radiographic findings include evidence of a small lung as manifested by cardiac and mediastinal shift, absence of the pulmonary arterial shadow, elevation of the hemidiaphragm, and decrease in pulmonary vessels in the affected lung with oligemia (Fig. 2-20). There may be hyperinflation and herniation of the opposite lung across the midline. This entity must be distinguished from Swyer-James syndrome, which shares many of the radiographic features. This syndrome results from bronchiolitis and is always associated with air trapping, which can be documented by an expiration radiograph or CT. Absence of the pulmonary artery can be confirmed with CT scanning (see Fig. 2-20), which also reveals the small ipsilateral hemithorax and the enlarged intercostal vessels and transpleural collaterals that supply the affected lung. Although CT is the preferred method, MRI with either spin-echo or gradient-echo images also shows absence of the right pulmonary artery.

Anomalous Origin of the Left Pulmonary Artery from the Right

Anomalous origin of the left pulmonary artery from the right (i.e., pulmonary artery sling) is an uncommon anomaly in which the left pulmonary artery arises from the right

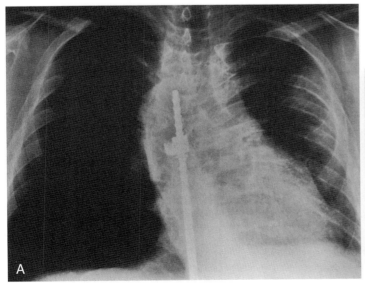

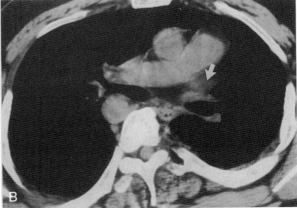

FIGURE 2-20. Congenital absence of the left pulmonary artery. **A,** The posteroanterior chest radiograph shows a small left lung, scoliosis, and a right aortic arch. **B,** CT demonstrates absence of the left pulmonary artery *(arrow)*.

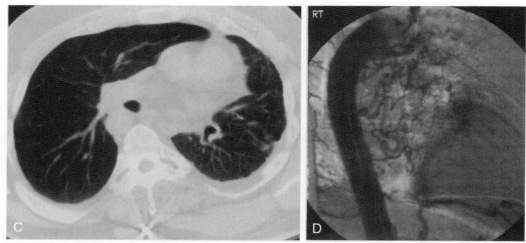

FIGURE 2-20. (cont'd) **C,** On the lung windows, the pulmonary vessels appear small, and there is a fine reticular pattern suggesting collateral systemic vascular supply. **D,** The aortogram shows a right arch with enlarged bronchial and intercostal arteries supplying the left lung. Later films demonstrated retrograde flow from these vessels into more peripheral pulmonary arteries.

and courses to the left between the esophagus and trachea in its course to the left hilum. It may produce compression of the right main bronchus and the trachea. It may occur as an isolated finding or be associated with congenital tracheal stenosis, particularly the type caused by complete or O-shaped cartilaginous rings, as described earlier. A barium swallow shows a focal impression on the anterior surface of the barium-filled esophagus in the region of the lower trachea. Diagnosis can be easily established with contrast-enhanced CT (Fig. 2-21) or MRI.

Pulmonary Artery Stenosis or Coarctation

Pulmonary artery stenosis is a rare anomaly characterized by single or multiple coarctations of the pulmonary arteries, commonly occurring with poststenotic dilation. The stenoses may occur anywhere in the pulmonary arterial

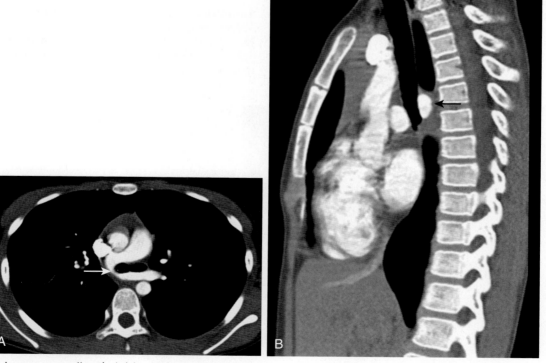

FIGURE 2-21. Pulmonary artery sling. **A,** Axial, contrast-enhanced CT shows the anomalous origin of the left pulmonary artery *(arrow)* arising from the distal right pulmonary artery and coursing to the left between the esophagus and the airway in its course to the left hilum. **B,** Sagittal reformation image shows the posterior course of the left pulmonary artery *(arrow),* which mildly compresses the posterior wall of the trachea. (Case courtesy of Edward Lee, MD, Children's Hospital, Boston, MA.)

tree. They may be short or long and unilateral or bilateral. This condition usually is associated with congenital cardiac or other anomalies.

The chest radiograph's appearance depends on the location and number of stenoses. The pulmonary vasculature may appear normal, diminished, or increased. If there is a stenosis of a main branch of the pulmonary artery, the affected lung distal to the stenosis may show radiographic changes of diffuse oligemia and signs of pulmonary arterial hypertension and cor pulmonale.

Congenital Aneurysms of the Pulmonary Arteries

Congenital aneurysms of the pulmonary artery are rare and are usually associated with other pulmonary abnormalities, such as arteriovenous fistulas or bronchopulmonary sequestration. When they occur in the central pulmonary arteries, they are usually associated with pulmonary valvular stenosis.

Anomalies of the Pulmonary Veins

Pulmonary Varix

A pulmonary varix is a rare localized enlargement of a segment of the pulmonary vein. It may be congenital or acquired. Acquired forms are caused by prolonged pulmonary venous hypertension, as seen in mitral stenosis. In the congenital variety, the varix occurs in a pulmonary vein that drains normally into the left atrium. Pulmonary varices occur more frequently on the right side and are usually not associated with symptoms, although there are rare cases of hemoptysis or dysphagia due to pressure on the esophagus.

On standard radiographic films, the varices appear as smooth, rounded or lobulated masses of unit density, frequently occurring in the lower lung zones. On the right, they may project behind the heart on the posteroanterior view, creating the impression of a solitary pulmonary nodule (Fig. 2-22). On the lateral view, they are localized posterior to the left atrium.

Dynamic enhanced CT or gradient-echo MRI can easily identify the vascular nature of the lesion and its course draining into the left atrium. Dynamic CT demonstrates opacification during the venous phase. The most important differential diagnosis is an arteriovenous fistula. Dynamic CT scanning should allow differentiation by demonstrating the absence of an enlarged arterial feeding vessel, enhancement during the venous phase, and drainage of the varix into the left atrium. Pulmonary angiography is seldom necessary for diagnosis.

Anomalous Pulmonary Venous Drainage

Anomalous pulmonary venous drainage is discussed in Chapter 9 of *Cardiac Radiology: The Requisites*.

Anomalies Involving Arteries and Veins

Pulmonary Arteriovenous Fistulas

Pulmonary arteriovenous fistulas are abnormal communications between the pulmonary arteries and the pulmonary veins, in which there is no capillary network that normally separates the arteries from the veins. There is a right-to-left shunt because blood passing through an arteriovenous fistula reaches the left atrium without being

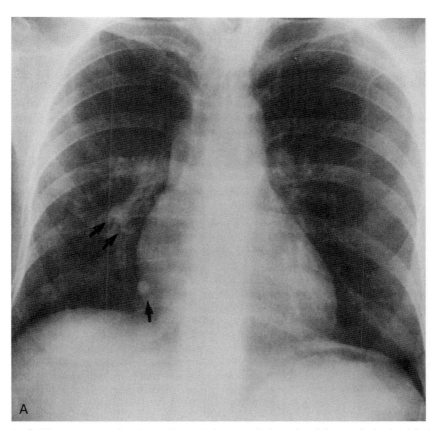

FIGURE 2-22. Pulmonary varix. **A,** The posteroanterior chest radiograph shows a tubular and nodular opacity in the right lower lung zone *(arrows).*

(Continued)

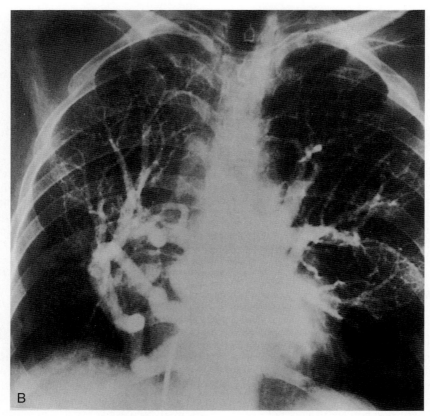

FIGURE 2-22. (cont'd) B, Venous phase of a pulmonary angiogram demonstrates a dilated, tortuous pulmonary vein draining into the left atrium.

oxygenated. Pulmonary arteriovenous malformations may be single or multiple. They are *simple* if there is a single feeding artery and a single draining vein; they are *complex* if there are two or more feeding arteries and two or more draining veins. Between 40% and 60% of patients with arteriovenous fistulas in the lungs have Osler-Weber-Rendu disease, characterized by cutaneous and mucosal telangiectasias and occasionally by arteriovenous fistulas in other organs.

Most patients are asymptomatic, but cyanosis, dyspnea, stroke, and brain abscess may occur as a result of the right-to-left shunt. Roughly 30% of the arteriovenous malformations in the lungs are multiple, and most occur in the lower lobes.

Standard chest radiographs show single or multiple, well-defined nodules, which are often lobulated. They typically occur in the medial third of the lung. The feeding artery and draining vein often can be identified. The artery appears as a dilated vessel originating in the hilum, and the vein drains into the left atrium (Fig. 2-23A).

Pulmonary angiography has historically been the method of choice for the identification of the size, number, and architecture of pulmonary venous malformations. Most patients receive pulmonary angiography because most of these lesions are treated with therapeutic embolization; however, it is not essential for diagnosis. The typical morphology of these lesions allows identification with CT with or without contrast injection (see Fig. 2-23B). Dynamic contrast-enhanced CT is recommended. Rarely, thrombosis may lead to a lack of contrast enhancement.

Multidetector-row CT with three-dimensional reconstruction is equivalent to angiography in the detection of small arteriovenous malformations and in the delineation of the angioarchitecture, which is important before therapeutic embolization.

Congenital Hypogenetic Lung Syndrome

Hypogenetic lung syndrome (i.e., scimitar or congenital pulmonary venolobar syndrome) encompasses a constellation of congenital anomalies of the thorax that often occur together. The anomaly consists of hypoplasia of the right lung and of the right pulmonary artery. There is usually partial anomalous pulmonary venous return and partial or complete arterial supply to the affected lung from systemic vessels. There may also be absence of the inferior vena cava and duplication of the diaphragm (i.e., accessory diaphragm). Dextroposition of the heart results from hypoplasia of the right lung. The most constant feature is anomalous venous drainage, with the entire right lung typically drained by a single vein that runs inferiorly parallel to the right border of the heart to join the inferior vena cava below the diaphragm. On the frontal radiograph, this vein appears like a Turkish sword or scimitar (Fig. 2-24A). Although the hypogenetic lung may occur occasionally on the left, the scimitar is almost exclusively right sided. Other standard radiographic findings include a small ipsilateral thorax with decreased pulmonary vascularity on the involved side. The heart and mediastinum are shifted toward the involved side, and the heart border may be indistinct. On the lateral radiograph (see

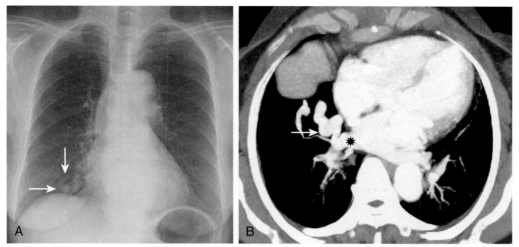

FIGURE 2-23. Pulmonary arteriovenous malformation. **A,** The posteroanterior radiograph shows a tubular, ringlike opacity inferolateral to the right hilum *(arrows)*. **B,** Curved, oblique, multiplanar reformation of an CT angiogram demonstrates a tangle of vessels in the right lung. The venous flow *(arrow)* drains to the inferior pulmonary vein *(asterisk)*.

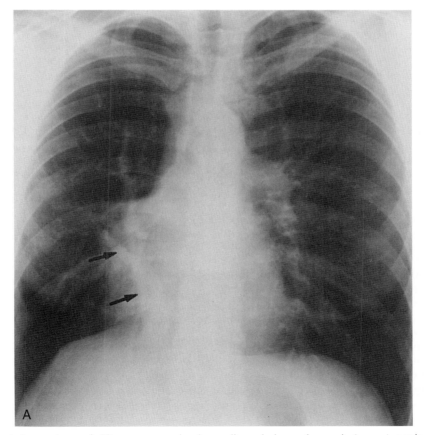

FIGURE 2-24. Venolobar or scimitar syndrome. **A,** The posteroanterior chest radiograph shows a large vein *(arrows)* coursing toward the diaphragm. The heart border is indistinct.

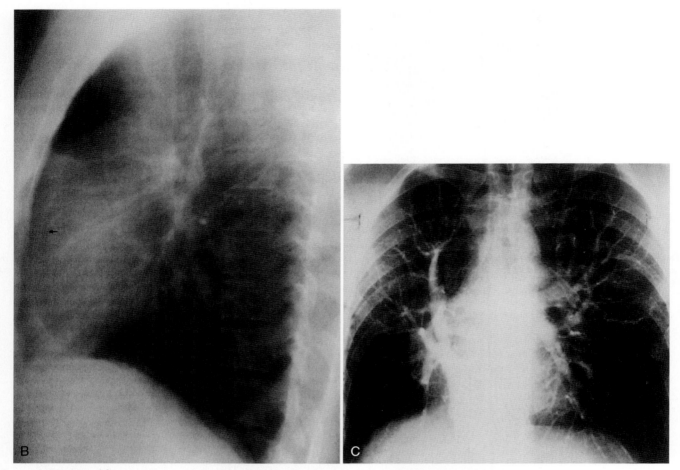

FIGURE 2-24. (cont'd) B, A retrosternal opacity can be seen on the lateral view *(arrow)*. C, The venous phase of a pulmonary angiogram confirms venous drainage of the right lung by means of a single, large vein, which drains into the inferior vena cava.

Fig. 2-24B), the cardiomediastinal shift produces a broad retrosternal band of opacity that may extend from the diaphragm to the apex of the involved hemithorax. This band is usually not an accessory diaphragm, which occurs in less than 10% of patients. It is a thin membrane fused anteriorly with the diaphragm that courses posterosuperiorly with the chest wall. It separates the right hemithorax into two parts, trapping part or all of the right middle or lower lobes below it. If the trapped lung is not aerated, it appears as a solid mass above the hemidiaphragm. If the lung is aerated, the accessory diaphragm appears as a fissure-like oblique line on the lateral radiograph. Aortography may be necessary to document the systemic arterial supply to the hypogenetic lung. CT may be useful in defining abnormalities of the central right pulmonary artery and delineating the anatomy and course of the anomalous pulmonary scimitar vein. It may show enlarged inferior pulmonary veins coalescing within the right lower lobe.

Congenital Anomalies of the Lymphatics

There are four major types of developmental lymphatic disorders that involve the thorax: pulmonary lymphangiectasis (see *Pediatric Radiology: The Requisites*), characterized by a congenital anomalous dilation of the pulmonary lymph vessels; localized lymphangioma, a cystic lesion occurring in the mediastinum; diffuse lymphangiomatosis, a proliferation of vascular spaces, mainly lymphatics, in which visceral and skeletal involvement are common; and lymphangioleiomyomatosis, a diffuse infiltrative lung disease characterized by haphazard proliferation of smooth muscle in the lungs and dilation of lymphatic spaces. Lymphangioma is discussed in Chapter 13, and lymphangioleiomyomatosis is discussed in Chapter 7.

▬ SUGGESTED READINGS

Ben-Menachem, Y., Kuroda, K., Kyger, E.R., et al., 1975. The various forms of pulmonary varices. AJR Am. J. Roentgenol. 125, 881–889.

Blickman, J., Parker, B., Bames, P. Pediatric Radiology: The Requisites, Ed 3. Mosby, 2009, Philadelphia.

Carpenter, B.L.M., Merten, D.F., 1991. Radiographic manifestations of congenital anomalies affecting the airway. Radiol. Clin. North. Am. 29, 219–240.

Davis, S.D., Umlas, S.L., 1992. Radiology of congenital abnormalities of the chest. Curr. Opin. Radiol. 4, 25–435.

Fraser, R.G., Paré, J.A.P., Paré, P.D., et al., 1989. Diagnosis of Diseases of the Chest. WB Saunders, Philadelphia, pp. 695–773.

Haddon, M.J., Bowen, A., 1991. Bronchopulmonary and neurenteric forms of foregut anomalies. Radiol. Clin. North. Am. 29, 241–254.

Kang, M., Khandelwal, N., Ojili, V., et al., 2006. Multidetector CT angiography in pulmonary sequestration. J. Comput. Assist. Tomogr. 30, 926–932.

Keslar, P., Newman, B., Oh, K.S., 1991. Radiographic manifestations of anomalies of the lung. Radiol. Clin. North. Am. 29, 255–270.

Landing, B.H., 1979. Congenital malformations and genetic disorders of the respiratory tract. Am. Rev. Respir. Dis. 120, 151–185.

Lee, K.S., Sun, M.R., Ernst, A., et al., 2007. Comparison of dynamic expiratory CT with bronchoscopy for diagnosing airway malacia: a pilot evaluation. Chest 131, 758–764.

Levine, D., Barnewolt, C.E., Mehta, T.S., et al., 2003. Fetal thoracic abnormalities: MR imaging. Radiology 228, 379–388.

Mata, J.M., Cáceres, J., Lucaya, J., García-Conesa, J.A., 1990. CT of congenital malformations of the lung. Radiographics 10, 651–674.

Miller, S.W. Cardiac Radiology: The Requisites ed 1. Mosby 1996, Philadelphia.

Morgan, P.W., Foley, D.W., Erickson, S.J., 1991. Proximal interruption of a main pulmonary artery with transpleural collateral vessels: CT and MR appearance. J. Comput. Assist. Tomogr. 15, 311–313.

Naidich, D.P., Webb, W.R., Müller, N.L., Vlahos, I and Krinsky, G.A., 2007, edn 4. Computed tomography and magnetic resonance of the thorax. Lippincott Williams & Wilkins.

Panicek, D.M., Heitzman, E.R., Randall, P.A., et al., 1987. The continuum of pulmonary developmental anomalies. Radiographics 7, 474–772.

Remy, J., Remy-Jardin, M., Wattinine, L., et al., 1992. Pulmonary arteriovenous malformations: evaluation with CT of the chest before and after treatment. Radiology 82, 809–816.

Rosado-de-Christenson, M.L., Frazier, A.A., Stocker, J.T., et al., 1993. Extralobar sequestration: radiologic-pathologic correlation. Radiographics 13, 425–441.

Scalzetti, E.M., Heitzman, E.R., Groskin, S.A., et al., 1991. Developmental lymphatic disorders of the thorax. Radiographics 11, 1069–1085.

White, R.I., Mitchell, S.E., Barth, K.H., et al., 1983. Angioarchitecture of pulmonary arteriovenous malformations: an important consideration before embolotherapy. Radiology 140, 681–686.

Woodring, J.H., Howard, R.S., Rehm, S.R., 1991. Congenital tracheobronchomegaly (Mounier-Kuhn syndrome): a report of 10 cases and review of the literature. J. Thorac. Imaging. 6, 1–10.

Woodring, J.H., Howard, T.A., Kanga, J.F., 1994. Congenital pulmonary venolobar syndrome revisited. Radiographics 14, 349–369.

Zylak, C.J., Eyler, W.R., Spizarny, D.L., Stone, C.H., 2002. Developmental lung anomalies in the adult: radiologic-pathologic correlation. Radiographics 22, S25–S43.

CHAPTER 3

Pulmonary Infections in the Normal Host

Theresa C. McLoud and Phillip M. Boiselle

Pneumonia ranks sixth among the causes of death in the United States and is the leading cause of death due to infection. The factors responsible for this high mortality rate include an increasing elderly population, immunocompromised hosts in greater numbers, new etiologic agents of pneumonia, antibiotic-resistant organisms, and unusual organisms acquired from international travel. The etiologic agent can reach the lungs by several routes. The most common is inhalation of airborne droplets, followed by aspiration of nasopharyngeal organisms, hematogenous spread to the lungs from other extrathoracic sources of infection, direct extension from a localized site of infection, and infection from penetrating wounds.

Clinical features are important in the determination of the etiologic agent of pneumonia (Table 3-1). Community-acquired pneumonias occurring in previously healthy individuals are caused by *Streptococcus pneumoniae* in 50% to 75% of cases and by *Mycoplasma pneumoniae*, viral organisms, or *Legionella pneumophila*. Nosocomial pneumonias (i.e., acquired in the hospital by patients who are already ill) typically are caused by gram-negative organisms or *Staphylococcus aureus*. Certain preexisting conditions are associated with pneumonias due to specific organisms. For example, patients with altered states of consciousness or those in coma are more likely to develop aspiration and subsequently develop infections due to mouth organisms (i.e., gram-negative organisms and anaerobes). *S. aureus* infection can occur after influenza pneumonia; in patients with chronic obstructive pulmonary disease (COPD), *Haemophilus influenzae* infection is common. *S. aureus* and *Pseudomonas aeruginosa* organisms are common superinfectants in patients with cystic fibrosis.

CLASSIFICATION

The pathologic classification of pneumonia is based on the anatomic localization of the disease process. Categories include lobar pneumonia, bronchopneumonia or lobular pneumonia, hematogenous bacterial infection, and acute interstitial pneumonia.

Lobar Pneumonia

Pathologic Features

Lobar pneumonia results when inhaled organisms reach the subpleural zone of the lung and produce alveolar wall injury with severe hemorrhagic edema. This is followed by a rapid multiplication of organisms and invasion of the infected edema fluid by polymorphonuclear leukocytes. Rapid spread occurs through the terminal airways and pores of Kohn, and consolidation of an entire lobe or segment may occur. This process is frequently aborted by administration of antibiotic therapy. The pattern commonly is seen in pneumonias due to *S. pneumoniae*. *Klebsiella pneumoniae*, *L. pneumophila*, and *M. pneumoniae* can also produce lobar consolidation.

Radiographic Features

This type of pneumonia produces a pattern of confluent opacification, often with air bronchograms (Fig. 3-1). The entire lobe may be involved, but more frequently because

TABLE 3-1 Clinical Clues to the Cause of Pneumonia

Clinical Circumstance	Likely Causative Organisms
Previously well, community-acquired	50% to 75% due to *Streptococcus pneumoniae* (pneumococcus), *Mycoplasma pneumoniae*, virus, or *Legionella pneumophila*
Hospital-acquired, otherwise ill	Gram-negative organisms, including *Pseudomonas aeruginosa*, *Klebsiella pneumoniae*, *Escherichia coli*, and *Enterobacter* species; *Staphylococcus aureus*; less commonly, *S. pneumoniae* and *Legionella*
Alcoholism	*S. pneumoniae* most common; gram-negative organisms, anaerobes, and *S. aureus* frequent causes
Diabetes mellitus	Suspect gram-negative organisms and *S. aureus*
Altered consciousness, coma	Gram-negative organisms and anaerobes
Drug addiction	If not an AIDS patient, suspect *Staphylococcus* and gram-negative organisms
After influenza	*S. aureus*
Chronic bronchitis with exacerbation	*Haemophilus influenzae* (common)
Cystic fibrosis	Mucoid, *P. aeruginosa*

From Woodring JH: Pulmonary bacterial and viral infections. In Freundlich IM, Bragg DG (eds): A radiologic approach to diseases of the chest. Baltimore, Williams & Wilkins, 1992.

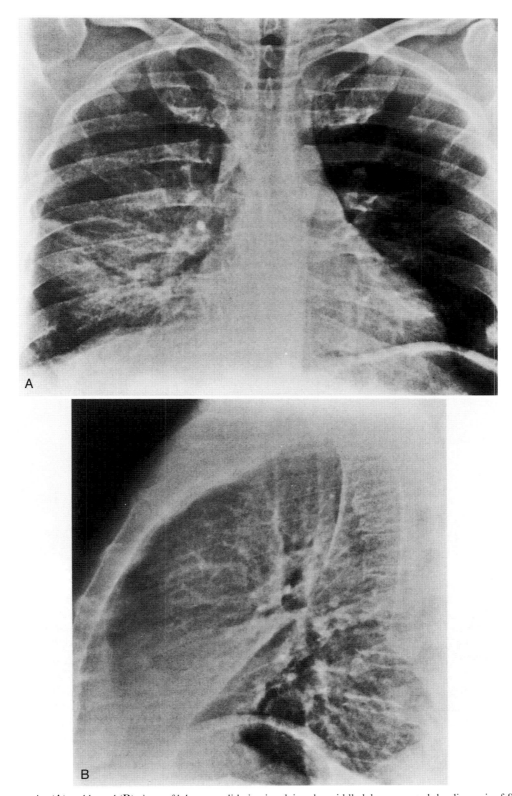

FIGURE 3-1. Posteroanterior (**A**) and lateral (**B**) views of lobar consolidation involving the middle lobe supported the diagnosis of *Streptococcus pneumoniae* (pneumococcus) infection.

of early use of antibiotics, the pneumonia involves only one or more segments within a lobe (i.e., sublobar form). A lobar pneumonia may result in expansion of the lobe due to voluminous edema, which is usually caused by infection with *K. pneumoniae* (Fig. 3-2). The enlargement of the lobe can be recognized radiographically by bulging of the interlobar fissures. Necrosis, cavitation, and development of a unique complication, pulmonary gangrene, may ensue.

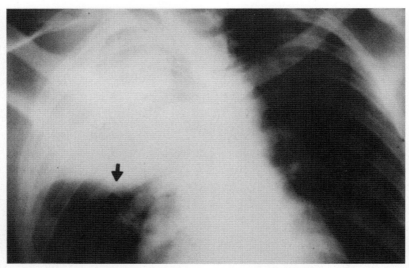

FIGURE 3-2. Anteroposterior view of a patient with *Klebsiella* pneumonia shows homogeneous opacity of the right upper lobe with slight bulging of the minor fissure *(arrow).*

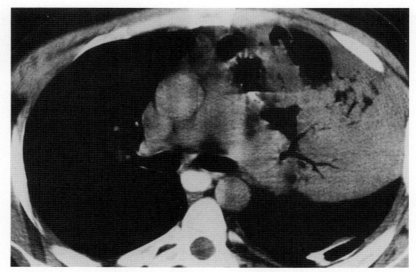

FIGURE 3-3. CT of a pneumococcal left upper lobar consolidation shows clearly defined air bronchograms and evidence of cavitation.

The computed tomography (CT) features of lobar pneumonia are similar to those seen on standard radiography (Fig. 3-3). There is usually evidence of confluent opacification with air bronchograms. The air bronchograms are often more easily visualized with CT examination. Table 3-2 summarizes the radiographic clues to the cause of pneumonia.

Bronchopneumonia

Pathologic Features
Bronchopneumonia (i.e., lobular pneumonia) results when organisms are deposited in the epithelium of peripheral airways (i.e., distal bronchi or bronchioles), resulting in epithelial ulcerations and formation of a peribronchiolar exudate. The inflammatory process spreads through the airway to involve the peribronchiolar alveoli, which become filled with edema and pus. Lobules may be affected in a patchy

pattern initially, and further spread results in involvement of contiguous pulmonary lobules. Eventually, a confluent bronchopneumonia may resemble lobar pneumonia. Offending organisms that produce this type of pathologic response include *S. aureus*, gram-negative organisms, anaerobic bacteria, and *L. pneumophila*.

Radiographic Features
The radiographic appearance of bronchopneumonia pneumonia is most frequently that of multiple, ill-defined nodular opacities that are patchy but that may eventually become confluent and produce consolidation with airspace opacification (Fig. 3-4). The opacification may be multifocal and involve several lobes, or it may be diffuse. As the disease progresses, segmental and lobar opacification develops, similar to the pattern of a lobar pneumonia. Early necrosis and cavitation can occur. The nodular opaci-

TABLE 3-2. Radiographic Clues to the Cause of Pneumonia

Radiographic Finding	Likely Causative Organisms
Round pneumonia	Suspect *Streptococcus pneumoniae* (pneumococcus)
Complete lobar consolidation	*S. pneumoniae, Klebsiella pneumoniae,* and other gram-negative bacilli; *Legionella pneumophila* and occasionally *Mycoplasma pneumoniae*
Lobar enlargement	*K. pneumoniae,* pneumococcus, *Staphylococcus aureus, Haemophilus influenzae*
Bilateral pneumonia (bronchopneumonia)	*S. pneumoniae* still common, but suspect others, including *S. aureus,* streptococci, gram-negative bacilli, anaerobes, *L. pneumophila,* virus, and aspiration syndromes
Interstitial pneumonia	Virus, *M. pneumoniae,* and occasionally *H. influenzae, S. pneumoniae,* and other bacteria
Septic emboli	Usually *S. aureus*; occasionally gram-negative bacilli, anaerobes, and streptococci
Empyema or bronchopleural fistula	*S. aureus,* gram-negative bacilli, anaerobes, and occasionally, pneumococcus; mixed bacterial infections common
Contiguous spread to chest wall	Actinomycosis; occasionally other bacteria or fungi
Cavitation	*S. aureus,* gram-negative bacilli, anaerobic bacteria, and streptococci; cavitation uncommon with *S. pneumoniae* or *L. pneumophila*
Pulmonary gangrene	*K. pneumoniae, Escherichia coli, H. influenzae, Mycobacterium tuberculosis, S. pneumoniae,* anaerobes, or fungi
Pneumatoceles	*S. aureus,* gram-negative bacilli, *H. influenzae, M. tuberculosis,* and measles; *S. pneumoniae* rare
Lymphadenopathy	*M. tuberculosis,* fungi, virus, *M. pneumoniae,* common bacterial lung abscess, and rarely plague, tularemia, and anthrax
Fulminant course with acute respiratory distress syndrome (ARDS)	Virus, *S. aureus,* streptococci, *M. tuberculosis,* and *L. pneumophila*

From Woodring JH: Pulmonary bacterial and viral infections. In Freundlich IM, Bragg DG (eds): A Radiologic Approach to Diseases of the Chest. Baltimore, Williams & Wilkins, 1992.

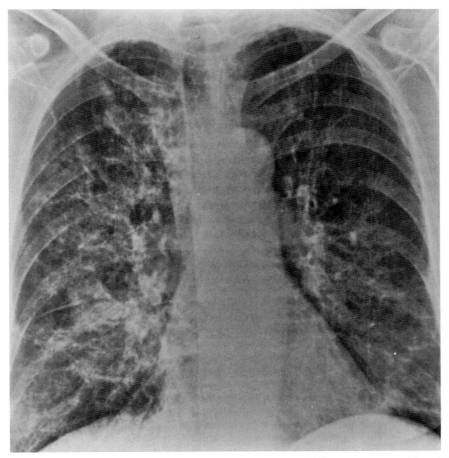

FIGURE 3-4. Bronchopneumonia. The posteroanterior view demonstrates bilateral, patchy, and inhomogeneous opacities, which have become confluent in some areas. The patient was diagnosed with viral influenza pneumonia.

ties of bronchopneumonia can be identified with facility on CT scans. The small nodules, usually less than 1 cm in diameter, represent peribronchiolar areas of consolidation or ground-glass opacity. They are called *acinar or airspace nodules*, but these nodules histologically are found in a peribronchiolar location. They are ill-defined and may be of homogenous soft tissue opacity and obscuring vessels, or they may be hazy and less dense so that adjacent vessels are clearly seen (i.e., ground-glass opacity). These nodules usually have a centrilobular location because of their proximity to small bronchioles.

Acute Interstitial Pneumonia

Pathologic Features
This type of pneumonia is usually produced by viral organisms, which result in edema and mononuclear cell infiltration around the bronchi and bronchiolar walls and extend into the interstitium of the alveolar walls.

Radiographic Features
Bronchopneumonia or an acute interstitial pneumonia may be seen with viral infections (Fig. 3-5). The early radiographic appearance is that of thickening of end-on bronchi and tram lines. However, this often evolves into a reticular pattern that may be seen extending outward from the hila.

Hematogenous Spread of Infection

Pathologic Features
Hematogenous spread to the lungs from bacterial infection may occur, although this is unusual. One of the most frequent manifestations is septic infarcts. They usually originate from right-sided tricuspid endocarditis or infected thrombi within major systemic veins. This phenomenon is seen in intravenous drug abusers and patients with long-standing indwelling central catheters.

Radiographic Features
Septic infarcts tend to be multiple and peripheral and to abut the pleural surface. They occur more frequently in the lower lobes. These nodules or wedge-shaped opacities may show evidence of cavitation (Fig. 3-6). CT often demonstrates a vessel connected to the area of infarction. On CT, the septic infarcts appear as wedge-shaped, peripheral opacities abutting the pleura. They may contain air bronchograms or rounded lucencies of air, sometimes referred to as *pseudocavitation*. True cavitation is common. Occasionally, septic bacterial infection may result in diffuse massive seeding of the lungs with a miliary pattern (i.e., very small nodular pattern), although this is much more common with hematogenous dissemination of granulomatous infections.

■ COMPLICATIONS OF PNEUMONIA

Box 3-1 outlines the complications of pneumonia.

Cavitation

Necrosis of lung parenchyma with cavitation (Fig. 3-7) may occur in pneumonia, particularly that produced by virulent

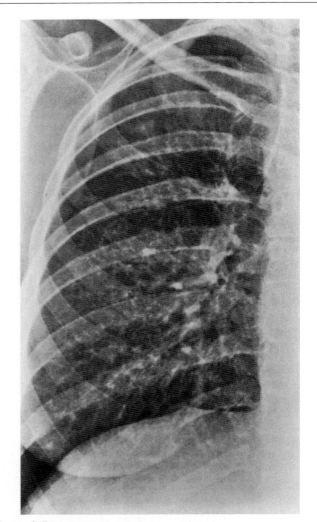

FIGURE 3-5. Acute interstitial pneumonia due to varicella (chickenpox). Coned-down view of the right lung demonstrates a fine reticulonodular pattern, which is more prominent centrally.

bacteria, including *S. aureus*, streptococci, gram-negative bacilli, and anaerobic bacteria. If the inflammatory process is localized, a lung abscess will form. It is usually rounded and focal, and it appears to be a mass (Fig. 3-8). With liquefaction of the central inflammatory process, a communication may develop with the bronchus; air enters the abscess, forming a cavity, which often contains an air-fluid level. The walls of the cavity may be smooth, but more often, they are thick and irregular.

Multiple, small cavities or microabscesses may develop in necrotizing pneumonia (Fig. 3-9). They are recognized as multiple areas of lucency within a consolidated lobe or segment. A similar appearance may be produced by consolidation superimposed on areas of preexisting emphysema. If the necrosis is extensive, arteritis and vascular thrombosis may occur in an area of intense inflammation, causing ischemic necrosis and death of a portion of lung. This is a particular complication of *Klebsiella* pneumonia and other pneumonias producing lobar enlargement. The radiographic features include multiple areas of cavitation, often with air-fluid levels. Portions of dead lung may slough and form intracavitary masses.

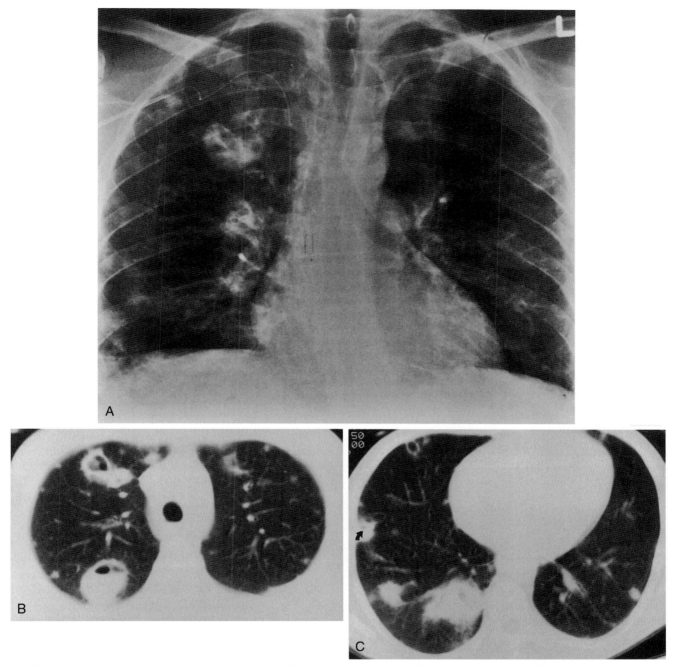

FIGURE 3-6. Septic infarcts in an intravenous drug abuser. **A,** The posteroanterior chest radiograph shows multiple, bilateral cavitary nodules. **B** and **C,** CT examination demonstrates that most of the infarcts are peripheral in location; some abut the pleura and occasionally are wedge shaped. True and pseudocavities *(curved arrow)* are present.

Pneumatocele Formation

Pneumatoceles are usually associated with pneumonia caused by virulent organisms; the classic offender is *S. aureus* (Fig. 3-10). They usually form subpleural collections of air, which result from alveolar rupture. Radiographically, they appear as single or multiple, cystic lesions with thin and smooth walls. They may show rapid change in size and location on serial radiographs.

Hilar and Mediastinal Adenopathy

Intrathoracic lymphadenopathy that can be recognized on standard radiographs is uncommon in most bacterial and viral infections; some notable exceptions include *Mycobacterium tuberculosis, Pasteurella tularensis,* and *Yersinia pestis.* Adenopathy may be associated with fungal infections or bacterial infections that are long-standing or virulent, as in lung abscesses. CT may show slightly enlarged

Box 3-1. Complications of Pneumonia

CAVITATION
Organisms
  Staphylococcus aureus
  Streptococci
  Gram-negative bacilli
  Anaerobes
Types
  Lung abscess (single, well-defined mass often with air-fluid level)
  Necrotizing pneumonia (small lucencies or cavities)
  Pulmonary gangrene (sloughed lung)

PNEUMATOCELES
S. aureus
Occur in children
Thin walls, multiple

ADENOPATHY
Common with granulomatous infections (tuberculosis, fungi)
Uncommon with most bacterial and viral infections

PLEURAL EFFUSIONS AND EMPYEMA
Common (40%)
Parapneumonic
Empyema (bronchopleural fistula)

OTHER COMPLICATIONS
Acute respiratory distress syndrome (ARDS)
Bronchiectasis
Slow resolution in the elderly
Recurrent pneumonias

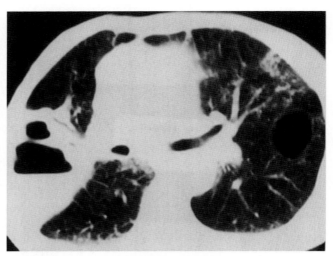

FIGURE 3-7. Cavitary pneumonia due to gram-negative organisms. CT shows two areas of cavitation with an air-fluid level in the more posterior area, indicating bronchial communication.

nodes (>1 cm) in patients with common bacterial infections that are not visible on standard radiography.

Pleural Effusions and Empyema

Pleural effusion is a common complication of pneumonia, occurring in about 40% of cases (Fig. 3-11). Most effusions are parapneumonic, but infection of the pleural space with empyema requiring drainage is an important but uncommon complication of some pneumonias. Empyemas can be recognized by the presence of gross pus within the pleural space, by a white blood cell count in the pleural fluid of greater than 15,000 cells/mm³, by the presence of bacteria within the pleural fluid, or by a pH less than 7.2. Chapter 18 provides more detail on the pleural complications of pneumonia.

Parenchymal necrosis in an underlying pneumonia may produce a fistula between the bronchus and the pleural space (i.e., bronchopleural fistula), and this results in an empyema with an air-fluid level. Further discussion of these entities can be found in Chapter 18.

Other Complications

Rapidly progressive and fulminant bacterial or viral pneumonia may result in the acute respiratory distress syndrome (ARDS). In the preantibiotic era, bronchiectasis was an extremely common complication of bacterial pneumonia,

but the incidence of bronchiectasis has declined with the advent of antibiotics. Most pneumonias clear within 2 or 3 weeks, but in elderly patients, resolution may take 3 to 4 months. Necrotizing pneumonias also tend to resolve slowly. Recurrent pneumonias are frequently found in patients with predisposing factors such as chronic obstructive lung disease, bronchiectasis, alcoholism, and diabetes. Although recurrent or persistent pneumonia in the same location raises the possibility of an obstructing endobronchial lesion due to lung carcinoma, cancer accounts for less than 5% of such cases.

▬ PNEUMONIAS CAUSED BY GRAM-POSITIVE BACTERIA

The most common gram-positive bacteria causing pneumonia include *S. pneumoniae* (pneumococcus), *S. aureus*, and *Streptococcus pyogenes*.

Streptococcus pneumoniae

S. pneumoniae (Box 3-2) is responsible for one third to one half of community-acquired pneumonias in adults. These infections occur more frequently in the winter and early spring. Pneumococcal pneumonia occurs in healthy people, but it is much more common in alcoholic, debilitated, and other immunocompromised individuals.

The radiographic features include consolidation that is usually unilateral, although it may be bilateral, and it typically affects the lower lobes (see Fig. 3-1). Although it is a lobar pneumonia, it is uncommon for the lobe to be completely consolidated. Cavitation is rare, and large pleural effusions are uncommon. When present, they suggest the development of empyema. Sometimes, especially in children, the pneumonia may have a rounded, masslike appearance (Fig. 3-12). This is called a *round pneumonia*; it results from centrifugal spread of the rapidly replicating bacteria by way of the pores of Kohn and canals of Lambert from a single primary focus in the lung.

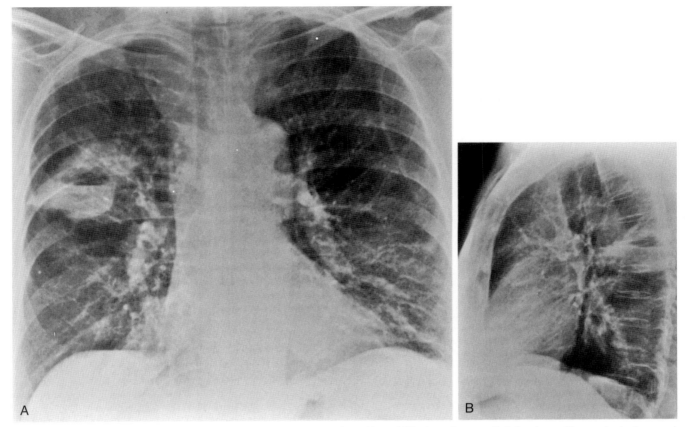

FIGURE 3-8. Primary lung abscess due to aspiration. The posteroanterior (**A**) and lateral (**B**) views show a well-defined, masslike opacity in the superior segment of the right lower lobe. There is cavitation with an air-fluid level and a thick wall.

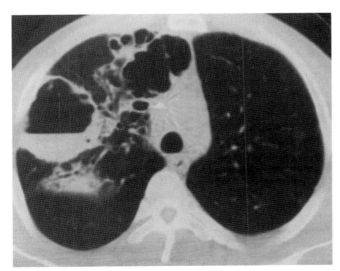

FIGURE 3-9. Microabscesses caused by *Pseudomonas* pneumonia in the right upper lobe. Multiple, thin-walled, multiloculated cavities can be seen with little surrounding parenchymal opacity.

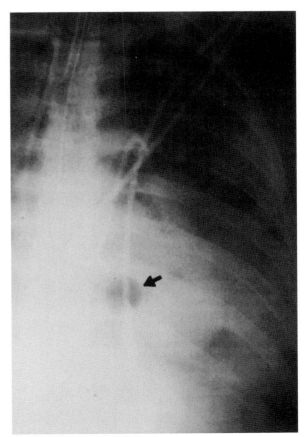

FIGURE 3-10. Pneumatocele. Coned-down (anteroposterior) view of the chest in a patient with fulminant staphylococcal pneumonia shows a rounded lucency in left lower lobe caused by a pneumatocele *(arrow)*.

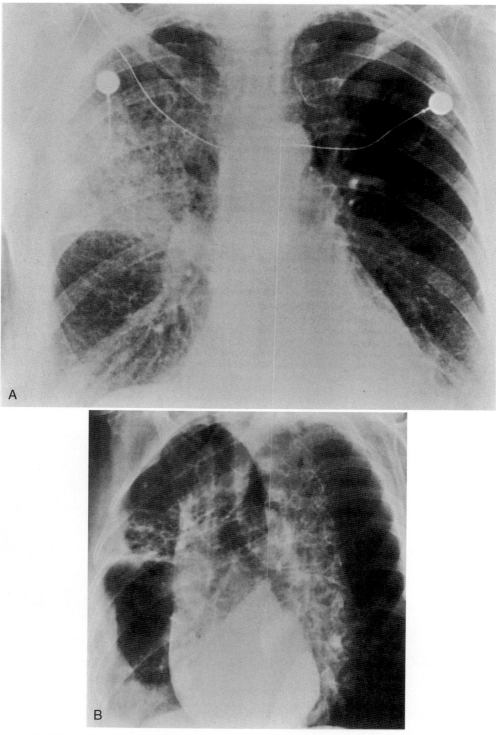

Figure 3-11. Parapneumonic effusion (pneumococcal pneumonia). **A,** The posteroanterior view shows a right upper lobe consolidation. **B,** An oblique view 2 days later demonstrates a right effusion.

Staphylococcus aureus

S. aureus (Box 3-3) is a gram-positive coccus, and the spherical organisms occur in pairs and clusters. This pneumonia rarely develops in healthy adults, but it is sometimes a complication of viral infections and is much more common in infants and children. In infants, unilateral or bilat- eral consolidation involving the lower lungs is the most frequent radiographic presentation. Pneumatoceles, thin-walled cysts filled with air or partially filled with fluid, may develop and occasionally rupture into the pleural space, resulting in pneumothorax. In adults, the disease is usually bilateral and is preceded by an atypical pneumonia such as

Box 3-2. Streptococcus pneumoniae

CHARACTERISTICS
Most common community-acquired pneumonia
More common among adults
Occurs in healthy and debilitated individuals

RADIOGRAPHIC FEATURES
Lower lobes
Consolidation
Lobar or sublobar
Round pneumonia in children

Box 3-3. Staphylococcus aureus

CHARACTERISTICS
Gram-positive coccus
Infants and children (more common)
Occurs after viral infection
Septic emboli
    Intravenous drug abusers
    Indwelling catheters

RADIOGRAPHIC FEATURES
Children
    Consolidation
    Lower lungs
    Pneumatoceles
Adults
    Bilateral
    Cavitation
    Empyema
Septic emboli (infarcts)
    Multiple
    Nodules or wedge-shaped opacities
    Peripheral, abut pleura
    Cavitation
    Seen on computed tomography
    Pseudocavitation or true cavitation
    Feeding vessel

influenza. Cavitation is a common feature, and the cavities may be multiple, thick walled, and irregular (Fig. 3-13). There is a high incidence of large pleural effusions, and empyema resulting from bronchopleural fistula is a common complication. Methicillin resistant staphylococcus aureus (MRSA) pneumonia usually occurs as a nosocomial infection in health care centers particularly in older, immunocompromised or intensive care unit patients.

Staphylococcal infection in the lungs may occur by way of the hematogenous route. This is usually the result of septic emboli, which arise in the central veins or as vegetations on cardiac valves, particularly in intravenous drug abusers and patients with indwelling intravenous catheters. The radiographic appearance is that of multiple nodular masses with or without cavitation, as previously described.

Streptococcus pyogenes

Streptococci (Box 3-4) are gram-positive cocci that occur in pairs and chains. The pneumonia occasionally occurs in epidemic proportions. This form of pneumonia is much less common than that caused by *Staphylococcus* or *S. pneumoniae* (pneumococcus).

The radiographic features include lower lobe consolidation, often occurring with a segmental distribution. Pleural effusions occur frequently, but localized empyema is unusual.

■ PNEUMONIAS CAUSED BY GRAM-NEGATIVE AEROBIC ORGANISMS

Pneumonias caused by gram-negative organisms usually are nosocomial pneumonias that affect hospitalized patients. These pneumonias tend to occur in patients maintained on artificial ventilators or in those who have intravenous catheters or a variety of other ancillary support systems. The incidence of gram-negative pneumonia acquired in the community is increasing, which may be related to the

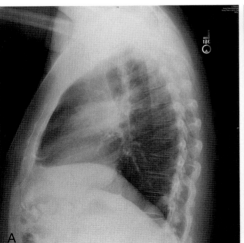
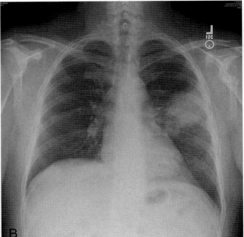
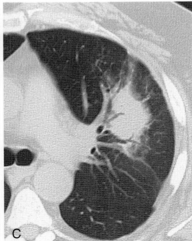

FIGURE 3-12. Rounded pneumonia. The lateral (**A**) and posteroanterior (**B**) chest radiographs and CT (**C**) of an adult patient shows an ill-defined, rounded opacity in the left upper lobe due to rounded pneumonia caused by pneumococcus. The opacity simulated a lung neoplasm radiographically, but it completely resolved after antibiotic therapy.

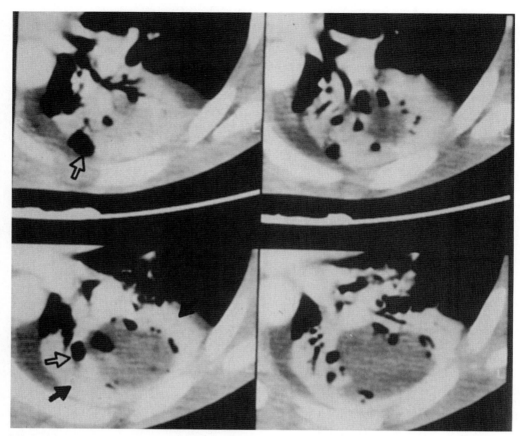

FIGURE 3-13. Staphylococcus aureus abscess. In the composite of four CT images of a patient with a left lower lobe staphylococcal abscess, notice the thick walls of the cavity *(closed arrows)* and the retained thick exudate in the center. Pockets of air in the peripheral regions of the cavity probably represent small pneumatoceles *(open arrows)*. (Courtesy of Dorothy L. McCauley, MD. New York University Medical Center, New York, NY.)

Box 3-4. **Streptococcus pyogenes**

CHARACTERISTICS
Gram-positive cocci
Uncommon but occasionally epidemic

RADIOGRAPHIC FEATURES
Consolidation
Segmental
Lower lobes
Effusion

Box 3-5. **Klebsiella pneumoniae**

CHARACTERISTICS
Middle-aged or elderly patients
Chronic lung disease and alcoholic patients

RADIOGRAPHIC FEATURES
Lobar consolidation
Bulging fissures
Cavitation
Pulmonary gangrene

---

overgrowth of resistant organisms because of widespread use of broad-spectrum antibiotics.

Klebsiella pneumoniae

Klebsiella pneumonia (Box 3-5) usually occurs in middle-aged or elderly patients, in those with underlying chronic lung disease, and in alcoholic individuals. Radiographic features consist of an upper lobe consolidation. Cavitation is common, and the lobar consolidation may lead to an expanded lobe with bulging interlobar fissures (see Fig. 3-2). If necrosis is extensive, pulmonary gangrene may develop.

Escherichia coli

E. coli pneumonia (Box 3-6) may be caused by direct extension from the gastrointestinal or genitourinary tract across the diaphragm or result from bacteremia. As is true of most of the gram-negative pneumonias, it is frequently characterized by the development of necrosis and multiple cavities. The lower lobes are more frequently involved.

Pseudomonas aeruginosa

P. aeruginosa pneumonia (Box 3-7) usually occurs in hospitalized patients, particularly those with debilitating disease (see Fig. 3-9). Organisms that affect the lungs often result from contamination of suction and tracheostomy devices. Radiographic features include a lower lobe predilection. However, the consolidation may spread rapidly to affect both lungs. Pleural effusions are uncommon. Multiple, irregular nodules may develop and are usually associated with bacteremia. These nodules may cavitate.

Haemophilus influenzae

H. influenzae pneumonia (Box 3-8) usually develops in patients with COPD. The appearance is typically that of a bronchopneumonia with homogeneous segmental opacities, usually in the lower lobes. Cavitation and pleural effusions are rare.

■ ASPIRATION PNEUMONITIS AND ANAEROBIC PNEUMONIA

Pulmonary aspiration (Box 3-9) is a common clinical problem. Many conditions predispose persons to aspiration, including reduced levels of consciousness, alcoholism, drug addiction, esophageal disease, periodontal and gingival disease, seizure disorders, and nasogastric tubes.

Box 3-6. Escherichia coli

CHARACTERISTICS
Direct extension from gastrointestinal or genitourinary tract
Results from bacteremia

RADIOGRAPHIC FEATURES
Necrosis, multiple cavities
Affects lower lobes

Box 3-7. Pseudomonas aeruginosa

CHARACTERISTICS
Hospitalized, debilitated patients
Tracheostomy tubes and suction devices

RADIOGRAPHIC FEATURES
Lower lobes, consolidation
Rapid spread to both lungs
Multiple, irregular nodules
Cavitation
Pleural effusions uncommon

Box 3-8. Haemophilus influenzae

CHARACTERISTICS
Chronic obstructive pulmonary disease (COPD)
Bronchopneumonia

RADIOGRAPHIC FEATURES
Homogeneous, segmental
Affects lower lobes

Box 3-9. Aspiration Pneumonitis and Anaerobic Pneumonia

CHARACTERISTICS
Common occurrence
Predisposing factors
 Reduced consciousness
 Alcoholism
 Drug addiction
 Seizures
 Esophageal disease
 Poor oral hygiene

CLINICAL SYNDROMES
Café coronary syndrome
 Obstruction of larynx or upper trachea
 Aphonia, respiratory distress, asphyxia
Bronchial obstruction
 Aspiration pneumonitis or pneumonia
  Mouth organisms
  Slow progression
 Aspiration of gastric acid
  Mendelson's syndrome

RADIOGRAPHIC FEATURES
Normal appearance
Opaque foreign body in airway
Air trapping if bronchus obstructed
 Inspiratory-expiration radiographs
 Fluoroscopy
Atelectasis
Aspiration pneumonia
 Superior segments of lower lobes
 Posterior segments of upper lobes
 Basilar segments of lower lobes
Primary lung abscess
 Focal walled-off area of anaerobic pneumonia
 Superior segments of lower lobes
 Thick-walled cavity
 Air-fluid level
 Rounded, masslike lesion may precede cavitation
Aspiration pneumonitis
 No infection
 Patchy basilar opacities
Mendelson's syndrome (aspiration of gastric acid)
 Chemical pneumonitis and acute lung injury
Diffuse consolidation resembling pulmonary edema

Aspiration of particulate matter or foreign bodies may produce different clinical syndromes, depending on the size of the aspirated material and the level of airway obstruction. Large food particles or foreign bodies may be aspirated into the larynx and upper trachea, resulting in the so-called café coronary syndrome, which is caused by acute upper airway obstruction. These patients exhibit respiratory distress and aphonia.

Results of chest radiographs are usually normal for patients who have aspirated foreign bodies. If the foreign body is opaque, it may be visible in the airways. Air trapping may occur if the foreign body causes airway obstruction of one of the major bronchi. This can be demonstrated by inspiratory and expiratory radiographs, decubitus views, or chest fluoroscopy. Occasionally, complete obstruction of the bronchus results in atelectasis and, if the foreign body is unrecognized, in the development of distal pneumonitis or bronchiectasis.

Ninety percent of aspiration pneumonias and lung abscesses are caused by anaerobic organisms. The pathogens include *Prevotella*, *Bacteroides*, *Fusobacterium*, and *Peptostreptococcus*. Because of the presence of oxygen in the lung, the progression of anaerobic infection is slow, beginning in the dependent lung zones. If the patient is in a supine position when the aspiration occurs, the superior segments of the lower lobes are most commonly affected, with the right side affected more frequently than the left (Fig. 3-14). Aspiration can also affect the posterior segments of both upper lobes. Chronic or recurrent aspiration, particularly in patients who are in the upright position, usually results in consolidation involving the basilar segments of the lower lobes. The middle lobe and lingula are uncommon sites for aspiration pneumonia. Aspiration is the most common cause of a primary lung abscess (see Fig. 3-8).

A *primary lung abscess* refers to a focal, walled-off area of anaerobic pneumonia with central liquefaction necrosis. It is most commonly identified in the superior segments of either lower lobe. Lung abscesses have a fairly thick wall and may or may not have an air-fluid level. A rounded, masslike lesion may precede the development of cavitation.

Occasionally, aspiration of nontoxic material that contains insufficient bacteria to produce an infection or insufficient volume to produce atelectasis may occur. The radiographic appearance usually consists of basilar patchy opacities resembling atelectasis, and these areas clear within several days. Mendelson's syndrome is a specific form of aspiration that results from the aspiration of gastric acid. This event produces a chemical pneumonitis and acute lung injury. The radiographic manifestations of gastric aspiration are similar to those of noncardiogenic pulmonary edema. The distribution is usually diffuse.

■ ATYPICAL PNEUMONIA SYNDROME

Atypical pneumonia syndrome (Box 3-10) describes pneumonias that do not respond to usual empiric antimicrobial therapy or do not have clinical features distinctive from the usual bacterial pathogens responsible for community-acquired pneumonias. Originally, these atypical pneumonias were thought to be caused by viruses. However, other treatable organisms have emerged as important causes of atypical pneumonia, including *M. pneumoniae*, *L. pneumophila*, and *Chlamydia*. These nonviral, atypical pneumonias are for the most part readily treatable with antibiotics.

Most patients with atypical pneumonia present with a nonspecific syndrome consisting of fever, usually without shaking chills, and nonproductive cough, headache, myalgias, and some degree of dyspnea. This contrasts with the classic presentation of bacterial pneumonia, which is characterized by abrupt onset with fever, shaking chills, and purulent sputum, often with chest pain. Patients with the latter signs and symptoms usually have a bacterial pneumonia attributable to pneumococci, group A streptococci, *Klebsiella*, *S. aureus*, or *H. influenzae*. Many of the atypical pneumonias are associated with extrapulmonary manifestations. For example, diarrhea is a prominent part of *Legionella* and *Mycoplasma* infection.

Mycoplasma pneumoniae

M. pneumoniae (Box 3-11) accounts for approximately 20% of all cases of pneumonia. It usually occurs during the winter months in enclosed populations, such as students in college dormitories. The incubation period is 2 to 3 weeks, and the onset is often insidious, with low-grade fever and nonproductive cough. Extrapulmonary manifestations may include otitis, nonexudative pharyngitis, and diarrhea.

The radiographic features are usually those of a fairly diffuse, interstitial, fine reticulonodular pattern. This may evolve to patchy airspace consolidation, particularly in the lower lobes (Fig. 3-15). Hilar adenopathy is seen in approximately 20% to 40% of patients. The radiographic appearance is very similar to that of many viral infections. The diagnosis is made by serologic evaluation.

Legionnaires' Disease

The first outbreak of Legionnaires' disease was recognized in Philadelphia at a Legionnaires' convention (Box 3-12).

Clinical Features
Clinical features include acute febrile illness without pneumonia; systemic disease with primarily pulmonary manifestations; a peak incidence in patients older than 60 years; a predisposition in smokers and those with alcoholic liver disease; high fever, shaking chills, and cough with small amounts of mucoid sputum; pleuritic chest pain; watery diarrhea in about one half of patients; and headache. The organism is spread by airborne transmission, usually through moist air exhaust or cooling towers.

Radiographic Features
The radiographic features of Legionnaires' disease often consist of segmental opacification and consolidation, particularly of an upper lobe. Rapid development of coalescence with complete consolidation of an involved lobe and rapid extension to adjacent lobes are common features (Fig. 3-16). Parenchymal changes are extensive, but pleural effusions are uncommon. The diagnosis of Legionnaires' disease is usually made by serology using indirect fluorescent antibody. Direct identification of the organism may

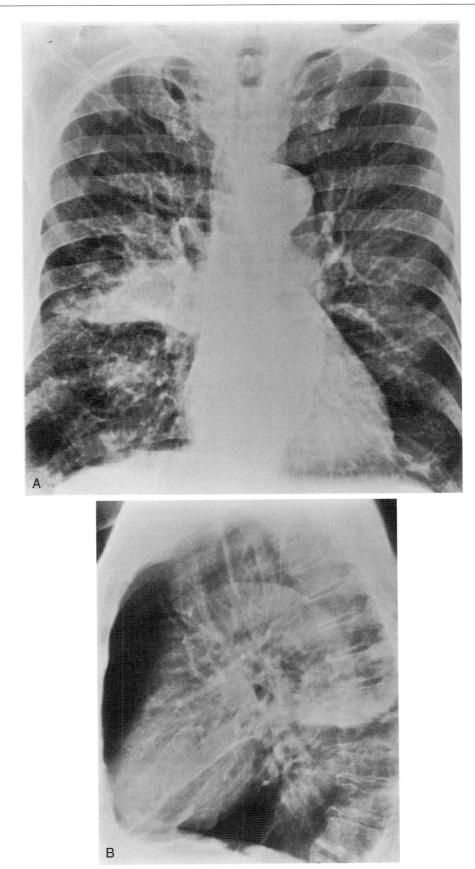

FIGURE 3-14. Aspiration pneumonia in a patient with a history of seizures. The posteroanterior (**A**) and lateral (**B**) chest radiographs demonstrate consolidation in the superior segment of the right lower lobe.

Box 3-10. Atypical Pneumonia Syndrome

ATYPICAL PNEUMONIA
Clinical Features
Nonproductive cough
Fever
Dyspnea
Headache, myalgias
Extrapulmonary manifestations
Organisms
Legionella
Mycoplasma
Chlamydia
Viruses

TYPICAL PNEUMONIA
Clinical Features
Abrupt onset
Fever with chills
Productive cough
Purulent sputum
Chest pain
Organisms
Streptococcus pneumoniae (pneumococcus)
Group A *Streptococcus*
Staphylococcus aureus
Haemophilus influenzae

Box 3-11. Mycoplasma pneumoniae

CHARACTERISTICS
Accounts for 20% of pneumonias
Occurs most often in winter
Affects enclosed populations

RADIOGRAPHIC FEATURES
Diffuse
Reticulonodular pattern evolves to patchy
   consolidation
Hilar adenopathy (20% to 40% of cases)
Similar to viral infections

---

be confirmed by direct fluorescent antibody (DFA) techniques using properly collected specimens.

Chlamydia

Chlamydia, a long recognized cause of pneumonia in neonates, is an increasingly frequent cause of community-acquired atypical pneumonia in adult patients (Box 3-13). It is caused by the TWAR agent *(Chlamydia pneumoniae)*. *Chlamydia* pneumonia may occur in compromised and noncompromised adults as an atypical pneumonia. The disease is characterized by fever and nonproductive cough. It is often preceded by pharyngitis.

Radiographic features may be similar to those of *Mycoplasma* pneumonia. However, more commonly there

is a localized area of consolidation in the middle or lower lobes, which may be patchy or homogeneous (Fig. 3-17).

Other Nonviral Atypical Pneumonias

Atypical nonviral pneumonias are rare. They include psittacosis; Q fever, a rickettsial disease; and tularemia.

Chlamydia psittaci is the etiologic agent of psittacosis, which may be transmitted by any avian species, and it is contracted by inhalation of infected aerosol material. The clue to the diagnosis is the history, which should include information about any contact with birds. Psittacosis usually mimics a standard bacterial pneumonia on chest radiography.

Coxiella burnetii is the etiologic agent of Q fever, which is a rickettsial disease. It is most common in the western and southwestern parts of the United States, and it can be transmitted by infected dust from animals. The radiographic features vary, but the most specific pattern simulates mycoplasma or viral pneumonia and usually consists of bilateral, diffuse reticulonodular opacities.

Tularemia, another animal-associated, atypical pneumonia, is transmitted by ticks in summer and rabbits in winter. There is an ulceroglandular form, which produces a skin papule that eventually ulcerates at the port of entry. Regional lymph nodes may become enlarged and eventually drain and ulcerate. In the typhoidal form, no portal of entry is apparent, but patients are characteristically extremely ill with gastrointestinal symptoms. Pneumonia may occur in patients with either of these presentations.

The most common radiographic feature is that of a localized and homogenous opacity, but lobar consolidation has also been reported. Occasionally, multiple lobes are involved. Bilateral hilar adenopathy may occur.

■ VIRAL PNEUMONIAS

Primary respiratory viruses (Box 3-14) include the parainfluenza and influenza group of viruses, respiratory syncytial virus (RSV), adenovirus, and picornavirus. The incidence of these infections varies with the age of the patient. For example, in children, RSV is responsible for up to 85% of epidemic lower respiratory tract infections and up to 60% of all pneumonias; in adults, the influenza and parainfluenza groups are responsible for most of the epidemic viral pneumonias. They usually occur during late winter. Adenovirus and picornavirus cause nonepidemic respiratory infections. Other viruses (e.g., cytomegalovirus) produce pneumonia as part of a systemic infection.

In all cases, the infection usually begins in the larger central airways. At this stage, the chest radiograph frequently appears normal. The radiologic correlates of severe inflammation and edema of the bronchial walls include coarse reticular opacities in the form of rings and parallel lines (i.e., tram tracks) due to bronchial wall thickening in the central perihilar lung zones. When the small airways are involved, bronchiolitis develops. Involvement of terminal bronchioles may lead to airway obstruction. This is more likely to occur in infants and young children because the cross-sectional area of the airways is small. Diffuse overinflation and air trapping can be visualized.

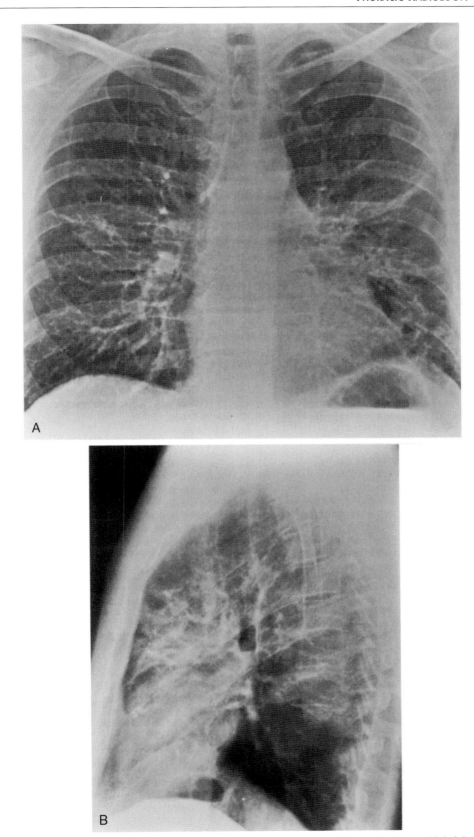

FIGURE 3-15. *Mycoplasma* pneumonia. **A** and **B**, Patchy, bilateral areas of inhomogeneous consolidation involve multiple lobes.

Box 3-12. Legionnaires' Disease

CHARACTERISTICS
Respiratory or systemic symptoms
Patients older than 60 years
Diarrhea common
Airborne spread through moist air exhaust or cooling towers
Diagnosis by serology with indirect fluorescent antibody

RADIOGRAPHIC FEATURES
Consolidation
Affects upper lobes
Rapid spread to other lobes

When the infection spreads to the alveoli, the disease is usually limited to the parenchyma around the terminal airways. The radiographic features in children and adults usually consist of a diffuse reticulonodular pattern, often with focal and patchy areas of consolidation (see Fig. 3-4). Multiple lobes are usually involved. CT may reveal the anatomic localization of the disease. The bronchiolitis and surrounding inflammation produces nodular opacities, which are located in the center of the lobules. Branching centrilobular opacities represent impaction of small airways, and their appearance has been referred to as the *tree-in-bud pattern* (Fig. 3-18). Other common CT findings of viral pneumonia include ground-glass attenuation with a lobular distribution and foci of segmental and subsegmental consolidation.

Influenza

Influenza is one of the most frequently reported contagious diseases. Symptoms include fever, nonproductive cough, weakness, and myalgias. Most patients who develop severe pneumonia have underlying disease or superinfection with bacterial organisms.

Radiographic features may reflect the complicating bacterial pneumonia. However, a diffuse reticulonodular pattern may be seen in infants and children with the disease.

Adenovirus

Adenovirus may occur in epidemic or pandemic proportions. When pneumonia develops, there may be destructive changes involving the peripheral airways, leading to chronic bronchitis, bronchiectasis, and bronchiolitis obliterans. Symptoms tend to persist after resolution of pneumonia. Radiographic features are very similar to pneumococcal pneumonia in pattern and distribution.

Respiratory Syncytial Virus

RSV, rarely reported in adults, is the most prevalent respiratory viral pathogen in the first 6 months of life. It usually produces focal and diffuse bronchiolitis. If radiographs are abnormal, they usually show increased lung volumes and air trapping, and linear interstitial opacities occasionally may be identified.

Varicella-Herpes Zoster

Varicella-herpes zoster (i.e., chickenpox) infection may be responsible for severe pneumonia in adults. The radiographic features are fairly characteristic. They consist of nodules ranging from 4 to 6 mm in diameter, with ill-defined margins diffusely distributed throughout both lungs (Fig. 3-19). Radiographic resolution usually occurs over many weeks. One of the interesting sequelae of chickenpox pneumonia is the development of diffuse, discrete pulmonary calcifications that can be identified on routine radiographs obtained after the infection (Fig. 3-20). Histoplasmosis should be considered in the differential diagnosis of this radiologic appearance.

Cytomegalovirus

Cytomegalovirus infection is discussed in Chapter 4.

Epstein-Barr Virus

The Epstein-Barr virus is the presumed etiologic agent for infectious mononucleosis. Although upper respiratory symptoms predominate, patients may develop a nonproductive cough. The chest radiograph is usually normal, but occasionally, pronounced hilar lymph node enlargement with an ill-defined, diffuse reticular pattern in the lungs may be seen.

◼ GRANULOMATOUS INFECTIONS

Mycobacterial Disease

Mycobacteria are aerobic, nonmotile, non–spore-forming rods that have in common the characteristics of staining bright red with carbol fuchsin and resistance to discoloration by strong acid solutions. The organisms are therefore referred to as acid-fast bacilli (AFB). There are several mycobacterial species, but the most important include *Mycobacterium leprae*, the cause of leprosy; *M. tuberculosis* and *Mycobacterium bovis*, responsible for tuberculosis; and the nontuberculous mycobacteria that are important etiologic agents in the development of pulmonary disease.

Tuberculosis
Characteristics

In the latter part of the 19th century, tuberculosis (Box 3-15) was a leading cause of death in the United States. The advent of drug therapy and improved public health measures led to a steady decline in the incidence of tuberculosis after World War II until 1985. For the next 7 years, a slow but steady increase in the incidence of tuberculosis was observed. This rise was primarily attributed to a large number of cases associated with acquired immunodeficiency syndrome (AIDS). Immigration into the United States of individuals from third world countries also might have contributed to the increased prevalence of tuberculosis.

Since 1993, the rate of tuberculosis has declined considerably. In 2006, the rate of tuberculosis in the United States was the lowest since the beginning of national record keeping in 1953. The tuberculosis rate is continuing to decline, but the rate of decline has recently slowed.

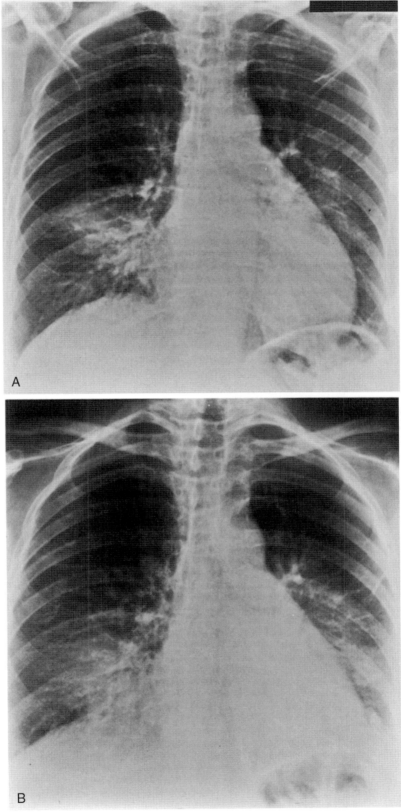

FIGURE 3-16. Legionnaires' disease. **A,** The posteroanterior chest radiograph shows consolidation involving the right middle lobe and left middle lung zones. **B,** Twenty-four hours later, the consolidation has become more extensive bilaterally.

Box 3-13. *Chlamydia* **Pneumonia**

CHARACTERISTICS
Chlamydia pneumoniae (TWAR agent)
Nonproductive cough
Preceding pharyngitis

RADIOGRAPHIC FEATURES
Localized consolidation in lower lobes
Patchy or homogeneous pattern

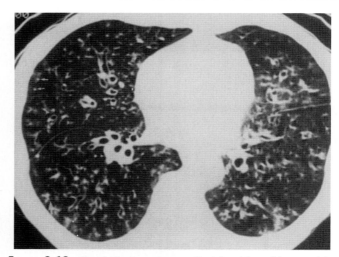

FIGURE 3-18. Tree-in-bud appearance. Peripheral branching opacities *(single arrow)* and centrilobular nodules 2 to 3 mm deep to the pleura *(double arrows)* can be identified. The appearance results from small airways filled with secretions and inflammatory debris.

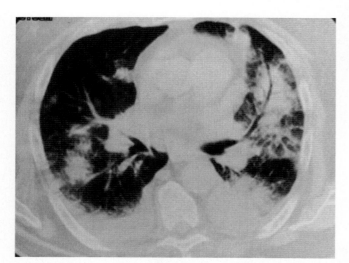

FIGURE 3-17. *Chlamydia* pneumonia. CT scan demonstrates bilateral, patchy areas of consolidation.

Box 3-14. **Viral Pneumonias**

CHARACTERISTICS
Viral organisms
    Influenza
    Parainfluenza
    Respiratory syncytial virus (RSV)
    Adenovirus
    Picornavirus

RADIOGRAPHIC FEATURES
Larger airways
    Normal radiograph
    Tram tracks and ring shadows
Small airways (bronchiolitis)
    Normal appearance
    Overinflation and air trapping
    Tree in bud opacities - CT
Alveoli
    Diffuse reticulonodular opacities
    Focal patchy consolidation
    Ground glass opacities - CT

From 1993 to 1997, there was also a decrease in the percentage of multidrug-resistant tuberculosis cases among persons with no prior history of tuberculosis, with a reduction from 2.4% to 1.1%. Since 1997, the rate has remained steady at approximately 1%.

In the United States, tuberculosis case rates vary considerably among different racial and ethnic populations and are lowest among whites. For example, compared with whites, the case rates are nearly 25 times higher for Asians and 10 times higher for blacks and Hispanics. The rate of tuberculosis among foreign-born persons in the United States is nearly 10 times higher than that of persons born in the United States. Other susceptible populations include the aged and the immunocompromised, particularly patients with AIDS.

Pathology and Pathogenesis

Infection with tuberculosis occurs as the result of inhalation of airborne droplets containing the tubercle bacilli. The initial infection, referred to as *primary tuberculosis*, is most common in the lower lobes. The bacteria are ingested by macrophages and initially spread to local lymph nodes at this stage, and they then may disseminate throughout the body. The infection is usually contained if the host is immunocompetent. However, walled-off tubercle bacilli representing a dormant focus of tuberculosis may activate under appropriate conditions. This may occur in the second type of tuberculosis, referred to as *reactivation or postprimary tuberculosis.*

Reactivation or post primary tuberculosis can occur any time after the primary infection, but the highest rate of reactivation occurs during the first and second years after the initial infection. Reactivation tuberculosis usually involves the lung apex, but a dormant focus of tuberculosis may become active in other organs, such as the bones, kidney, or brain. Clinically active disease may develop at the time of primary tuberculous infection (i.e., primary progressive tuberculosis) or when dissemination occurs (i.e., miliary tuberculosis). Clinical reactivation disease results when there is an ineffective T-cell immune reaction. The typical pathologic feature of tuberculosis is the caseating granuloma.

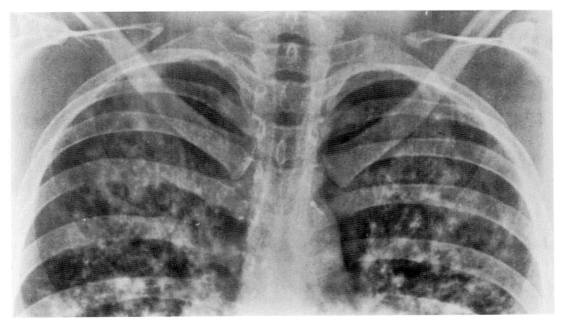

FIGURE 3-19. Varicella (chickenpox) pneumonia. Coned-down view of the upper lobes shows multiple, ill-defined nodules in both upper lobes.

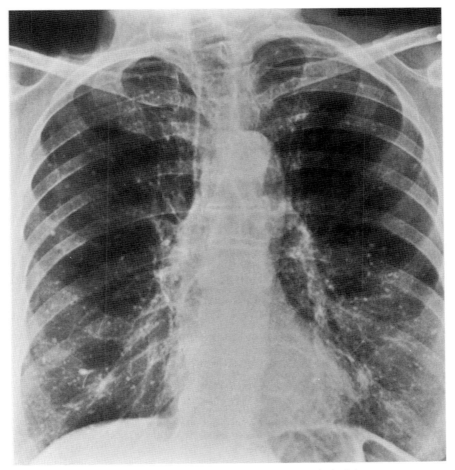

FIGURE 3-20. Healed varicella pneumonia. Multiple 1- to 3-mm calcified nodules can be seen in both lungs.

Box 3-15. Tuberculosis Clinical Features

EPIDEMIOLOGY
Increased incidence since 1985 due to AIDS, immigrants
Susceptible populations
    Human immunodeficiency virus positive
    Diabetes
    After gastrectomy
    Homeless
    Elderly in nursing homes
    Immigrants from endemic areas

PATHOGENESIS
Exposure to airborne droplets

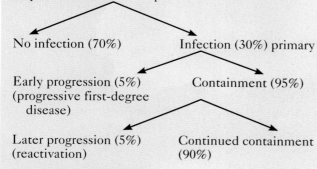

No infection (70%)   Infection (30%) primary

Early progression (5%)   Containment (95%)
(progressive first-degree disease)

Later progression (5%)   Continued containment (90%)
(reactivation)

CLINICAL FINDINGS
Primary
    Asymptomatic
    Symptomatic pneumonia
Reactivation
    Chronic cough
    Weight loss
    Hemoptysis
Positive skin test for 95%
Diagnosis by culture of organism

Clinical Findings

Patients with primary tuberculosis are usually asymptomatic but occasionally may have a symptomatic pneumonia. Patients with acute or chronic reactivation tuberculosis usually present with a chronic cough, weight loss, and occasionally with hemoptysis and dyspnea. The symptoms are often insidious. Ninety-five percent of patients with active tuberculosis have a positive tuberculin skin test result. The diagnosis must be made on the basis of culture of the organism, although the presence of AFB on the smear from the sputum is strong presumptive evidence of tuberculosis.

Classification of tuberculosis into primary or reactivation phases is based on the radiographic appearance. In third world countries and in the United States during 19th and early 20th centuries, primary tuberculosis was a disease of children, and reactivation tuberculosis was typically a disease of young adults. However, a significant change in the pattern of adult tuberculosis has occurred in the past several decades. Because of diminished exposure of children to tuberculosis, the disease often occurs in the primary form in adults. This has resulted in atypical radiographic manifestations of tuberculosis in adults, attributable to primary infection rather than reactivation of the disease.

Radiographic Features
Primary Tuberculosis

The radiographic features of primary tuberculosis are summarized in Box 3-16. Primary tuberculous pneumonia can occur in any lobe of the lung but is more common at the lung bases (Fig. 3-21). In more than one half of cases, the disease occurs in the lower lobes. Any chronic consolidation, particularly in the bases of the lungs, may suggest tuberculosis. Cavitation, although rare in primary tuberculosis, is more frequently reported in adults than in children with the primary form of disease.

Mediastinal and hilar adenopathy is another feature of primary tuberculosis (Fig. 3-22). It may occur alone or in association with consolidation in the lung. It tends to be particularly predominant in children. CT may be helpful in identifying and localizing adenopathy. On CT scans, tuberculous adenopathy has a predilection for the right paratracheal, right tracheobronchial, and subcarinal regions. Occasionally, atelectasis may result from extrinsic obstruction of a bronchus by enlarged lymph nodes. On CT scans obtained with intravenously administered contrast material, these nodes often demonstrate low-attenuation necrotic centers.

Pleural effusion due to tuberculous pleurisy, also a feature of primary infection, develops when subpleural foci of tuberculosis rupture into the pleural space. Patients present 3 to 7 months after the initial exposure. Organisms are rarely found in the fluid, and the diagnosis must be confirmed with a pleural biopsy.

Box 3-16. Tuberculosis: Radiographic Features

PRIMARY TUBERCULOSIS
Tuberculous pneumonia
    Basilar consolidation
    Cavitation rare
Mediastinal and hilar adenopathy
    Children
    Right side
    CT shows rim enhancement
Pleuritis
Ghon lesion and Rhanke complex
Calcification
Healed lesions

REACTIVATION TUBERCULOSIS
Apical and posterior segments, upper lobes, and superior segments, lower lobes
Patchy areas of consolidation
Cavitation
Bronchogenic spread, tree in bud opacities on CT
Chronic pattern
    Fibronodular
    Fibrocalcific
    Volume loss
    Bronchiectasis

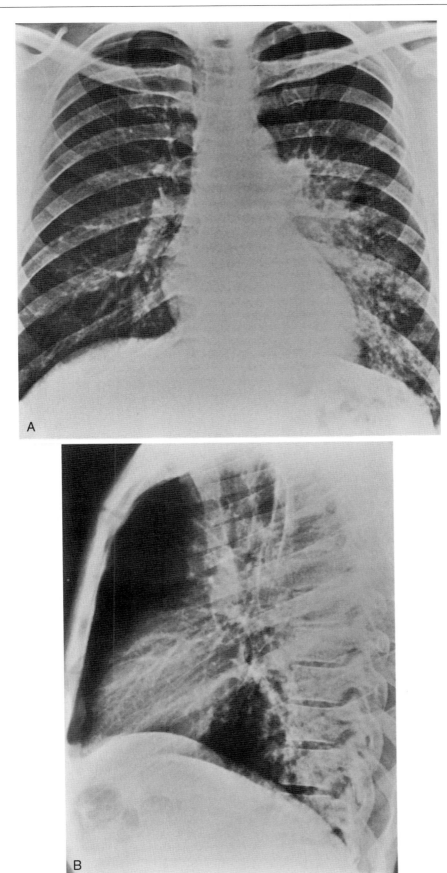

FIGURE 3-21. Posteroanterior (**A**) and lateral (**B**) views show primary tuberculous pneumonia. A patchy consolidation can be seen in the left lower lobe.

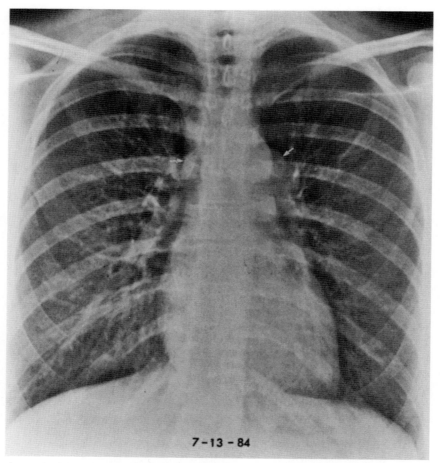

FIGURE 3-22. Mediastinal adenopathy in primary tuberculosis. A young, black woman presented with cervical adenopathy. The posteroanterior chest radiograph shows enlargement of the right paratracheal and left aorticopulmonary window nodes *(arrows)*.

The *Ghon lesion* (Fig. 3-23) is a manifestation of primary tuberculosis, which usually occurs in childhood and is self-limited. The host defense mechanisms handle the initial infection, and the area of consolidation in the lung slowly regresses to a well-circumscribed nodule. This nodule then shrinks and may disappear completely or remain as a solitary, calcified granuloma. The adenopathy regresses and may also exhibit calcification (i.e., Rhanke complex).

Reactivation Tuberculosis
Reactivation tuberculosis usually occurs in the apical and posterior segments of the upper lobes and in the superior segment of the lower lobes. It is characterized by chronic, patchy areas of consolidation (Fig. 3-24). Cavitation is a hallmark of reactivation tuberculosis (Fig. 3-25). Cavities result when areas of caseation necrosis erode into the bronchial tree, expelling liquefied debris. CT is more sensitive than plain radiography in the detection of small cavities (Fig. 3-26). They may have thick or thin walls, which can be smooth or irregular. Bronchogenic spread of tuberculosis occurs when a cavity erodes into an adjacent airway and organisms spread endobronchially to other parts of the lung.

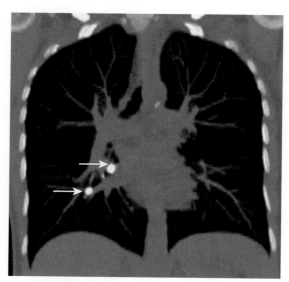

FIGURE 3-23. Ghon lesion and Rhanke complex. Coronal reformation chest CT image (bone windows) of a patient previously exposed to *Mycobacterium tuberculosis* shows a calcified right lower lobe nodule *(arrow)*, together with a calcified right hilar node (i.e., Rhanke complex) *(arrow)*.

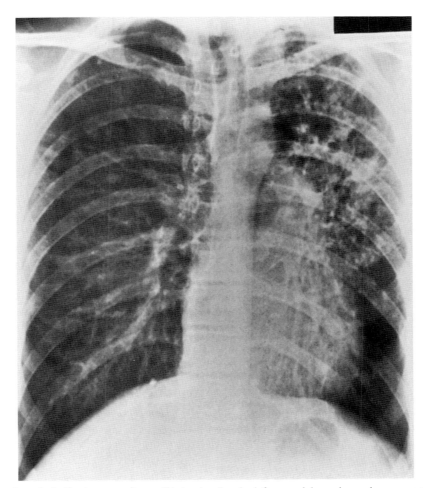

FIGURE 3-24. Reactivation tuberculosis. Patchy areas of consolidation involve the left upper lobe and superior segment of the left lower lobe. There is also evidence of some volume loss with a shift of the trachea to the left, a common finding with *Mycobacterium tuberculosis* infection, even in the early stages of disease. Nodular lesions can be identified in the right upper lobe.

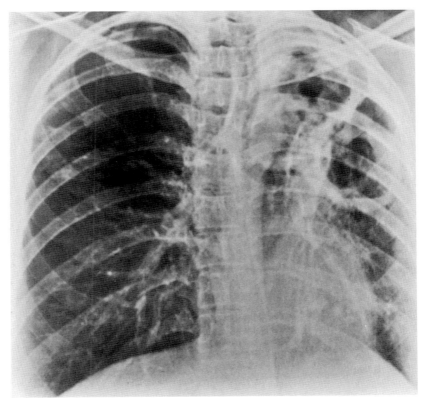

FIGURE 3-25. Cavitary tuberculosis. The posteroanterior chest radiograph shows multiple cavities in the left upper lobe. A thick-walled cavity can be seen lateral to the left hilum. There is pronounced volume loss in the left upper lobe and apical pleural thickening.

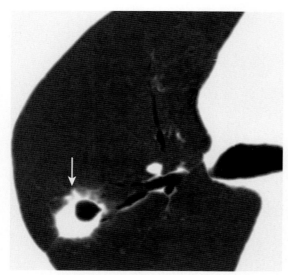

FIGURE 3-26. Cavitary tuberculosis. Minimal intensity projection CT image of a patient with reactivation tuberculosis shows a thick-walled cavity *(arrow)* in the posterior segment of the right upper lobe.

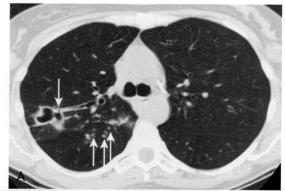

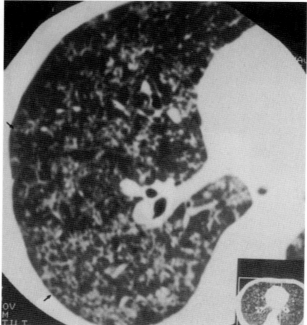

FIGURE 3-27. Bronchogenic spread of tuberculosis. **A,** CT shows a cavitary nodule communicating with the right upper lobe posterior segment bronchus *(single arrow)*, with associated centrilobular nodular opacities in the superior segment of the right lower lobe *(three arrows)*. **B,** CT of another patient shows a typical tree-in-bud pattern. Centrilobular nodules and branching opacities can be identified close to the pleural surface *(arrows)*.

The typical radiographic features (Fig. 3-27) consist of ill-defined nodules that usually are 5 to 6 mm in diameter. They are numerous and often bilateral. On CT, the pattern of bronchogenic spread can easily be recognized by a tree-in-bud pattern. This consists of centrilobular, branching, linear opacities with or without the presence of centrilobular nodules within 3 to 5 mm of the pleural surface or interlobular septa. This pattern is best appreciated on high-resolution CT (HRCT). It is not specific for bronchogenic spread of tuberculosis and may occur in other inflammatory diseases involving the peripheral airways.

The chronic lesion of reactivation tuberculosis usually consists of fibronodular opacities in the upper lobes, often with the presence of calcification (Fig. 3-28). It is usually associated with volume loss and retraction of the hila. Another feature of chronic reactivation tuberculosis is bronchiectasis. Tuberculosis should be considered in the differential diagnosis of upper lobe bronchiectasis. The activity of tuberculous disease cannot be determined by radiographs; it is confirmed only by positive cultures. However, tuberculosis is considered radiographically stable if there has been no change over 6 months.

Other Radiographic Features of Tuberculosis
Unusual patterns of tuberculosis (Box 3-17) may occur in the patient who has altered host resistance to the primary infection. *Miliary tuberculosis* is a term used to describe diffuse hematogenous dissemination of tuberculosis that has progressed when the host defense system is overwhelmed by massive hematogenous dissemination of organisms. It may occur at any time after the primary infection. The radiographic appearance (Fig. 3-29) is that of multiple, tiny nodules in the interstitium of the lung that are approximately 1 to 2 mm in diameter. CT may allow earlier detection than standard radiography (Fig. 3-30). Miliary disease takes up to 6 weeks to become apparent on plain radiographs.

Pneumothorax occasionally results from tuberculosis. Tuberculosis may also cause ulceration of the bronchi, and advanced endobronchial tuberculosis may produce lobar atelectasis and strongly simulate a primary carcinoma of the lung. A localized nodular focus of tuberculosis, referred to as a *tuberculoma* (Fig. 3-31), occurs in any portion of the lung and may result from primary or reactivation tuberculosis. It is usually solitary, spherical, and smooth. It may contain a central calcification, but tuberculomas occasionally may be multiple and simulate metastatic disease.

Tuberculous empyema and *bronchopleural fistula* may result from a tuberculous pleural effusion. Such effusions can become loculated and remain dormant for years.

Radiographic patterns of tuberculous disease in patients with acquired immune deficiency syndrome (AIDS) may vary. They are described in Chapter 4.

THORACIC RADIOLOGY: THE REQUISITES

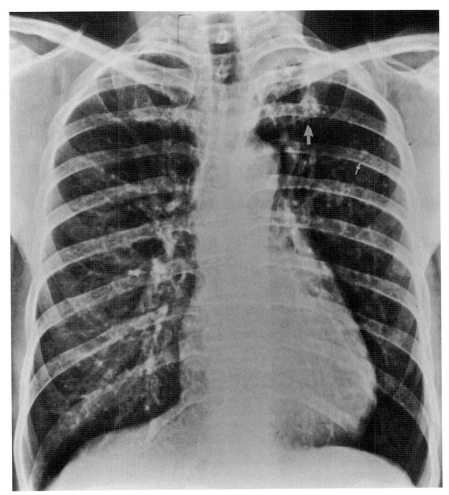

FIGURE 3-28. Fibrocalcific tuberculosis. The posteroanterior chest radiograph demonstrates the features of chronic, healed tuberculosis. Apical pleural thickening and multiple, calcified nodular and irregular opacities can be seen in the left upper lobe *(arrows)*. Volume loss is not a prominent feature in this case. Although such an appearance suggests inactive disease, serial radiographs are necessary to determine stability. Viable organisms may be present, and the development of clinically active disease may rarely occur.

Box 3-17. Tuberculosis: Other Radiographic Features

Miliary tuberculosis
  Hematogenous dissemination
  Diffuse, 1- to 2-mm nodules
Pneumothorax
Endobronchial tuberculosis
  Lobar or segmental atelectasis
Tuberculoma
  Single or multiple
  Nodules larger than 1 cm
Tuberculous empyema
Bronchopleural fistula

Nontuberculous Mycobacterial Infections
Characteristics

Some nontuberculous mycobacteria (Box 3-18) are pathogenic in humans. The most important of these organisms are *Mycobacterium avium-intracellulare*, often referred to as the MAC complex, and *Mycobacterium kansasii*. These

organisms often exhibit common features. They are usually found in the soil and water. Bronchopulmonary disease is caused by inhalation of the organisms, but no human-to-human transmission occurs. Unlike tuberculosis, nontuberculous mycobacterial infections do not manifest separate patterns of primary or reactivation disease.

Certain geographic areas have a preponderance of these forms of nontuberculous mycobacterial disease. For example, *M. kansasii* is more prevalent in the western and southern United States, and MAC is found more often in the southeastern United States.

The three major clinical presentations depend to some degree on the immune status of the host (Chapter 4 describes MAC disease in AIDS patients). In human immunodeficiency virus (HIV)–negative hosts, MAC typically affects male patients who are heavy smokers with underlying COPD. Similar infections may occur in patients with silicosis or bronchiectasis. The radiographic features of *M. kansasii* and MAC in this group of patients are indistinguishable from tuberculosis. However, MAC lung disease may develop in older women who are considered immunologically competent and who do not have a background of

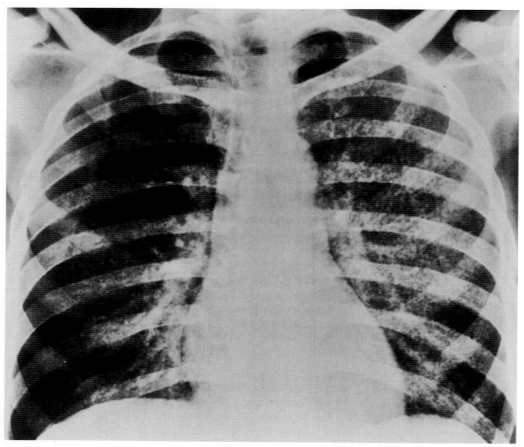

FIGURE 3-29. Miliary tuberculosis. The posteroanterior chest radiograph demonstrates innumerable tiny, 1- to 2-mm nodules in both lungs.

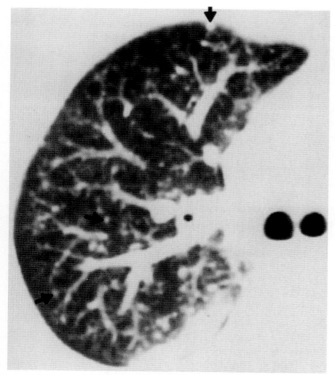

FIGURE 3-30. CT findings for miliary tuberculosis. In contrast to bronchogenic spread, the nodules are diffuse and uniformly distributed *(arrows)*.

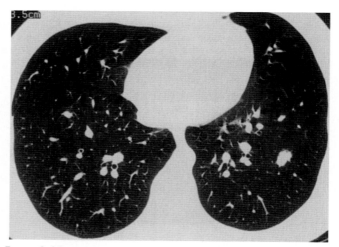

FIGURE 3-31. Tuberculoma. CT shows a somewhat lobulated nodule in the left lower lobe. There was no evidence of calcification or other manifestations of tuberculosis in the lungs.

COPD. This disease is usually noncavitary. Many women with this form of nontuberculous mycobacterial infection share similar clinical characteristics and bodily features, including scoliosis and pectus excavatum. It is uncertain whether these skeletal features predispose patients to infection due to poor tracheobronchial secretion drainage and ineffective mucociliary clearance or they are associated

Box 3-18. Nontuberculous Mycobacterial Infections

CHARACTERISTICS
Organisms
  Mycobacterium avium-intracellulare complex
    (MAC)
  Mycobacterium kansasii
  Found in soil and water
No human-to-human transmission
Human immunodeficiency virus–negative patients
  Men with chronic obstructive pulmonary disease
    (COPD)
  Immunologically competent older women without
    COPD
  Silicosis
  Bronchiectasis
RADIOGRAPHIC FEATURES
Classic form
  Almost identical to tuberculosis
  Frequent cavitation
  Slowly progressive
MAC in older women
  Bronchiectasis (CT finding)
  Focal nodules (CT finding)
  No cavitation (CT finding)

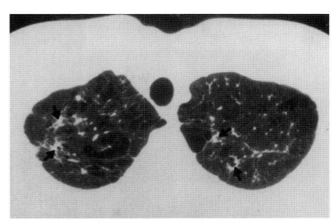

FIGURE 3-32. Atypical mycobacterial infection. Chest CT of a patient with emphysema shows the appearance of classic atypical mycobacterial infection. Biapical fibronodular opacities *(arrows)* are accompanied by architectural distortion resembling the appearance of reactivation tuberculosis.

with markers for specific genotypes that affect body morphotype and susceptibility to infection.

Because nontuberculous mycobacteria are common contaminants, the identification of invasive disease caused by these infections should be made only when defined clinical, radiographic, and microbiologic criteria have been met as defined by the American Thoracic Society (ATS) and Infectious Disease Society of America (IDSA) guidelines. Radiologic criteria include the presence of nodular or cavitary opacities on the chest radiograph or an HRCT scan that shows multifocal bronchiectasis with multiple small nodules. Establishing a diagnosis of nontuberculous mycobacteria does not necessitate the need for treatment in all cases: rather, the decision to institute multidrug therapy should be based on an assessment of the relative risks and benefits of therapy on an individual patient basis.

Radiographic Features

The classic form of atypical mycobacterial infection produces features almost identical to those of reactivation tuberculosis (Fig. 3-32). Involvement occurs in the apical and posterior segments of the upper lobes and superior segment of the lower lobes. Cavitation is common, and multiple cavities may be observed. The disease tends to be slowly progressive.

MAC lung disease occurring in older women who are usually nonsmokers without evidence of COPD is noncavitary and is associated with bronchiectasis. The classic radiographic features are best appreciated on CT (Fig. 3-33). The findings are those of cylindrical bronchiectasis associated with multiple, small, focal lung

nodules that are approximately 5 mm in diameter. Any lobe may be involved, but disease in the lingula and middle lobe has the highest prevalence. Occasionally, airspace disease may be delineated. Evidence indicates that patients with these findings are truly infected and not colonized with MAC and that the MAC infection causes the bronchiectasis rather than colonizing preexisting disease.

Fungal Diseases of the Lung

The wide variety of fungi that may produce lung disease can be divided into two groups. Some are truly pathogenic and can produce pulmonary infection in normal hosts. They include *Histoplasma, Coccidioides, Blastomyces,* and *Cryptococcus.* A second group of fungi are secondary invaders or opportunistic organisms, which produce disease in immunosuppressed patients. This group includes *Aspergillus, Candida, Cryptococcus,* and *Mucor.* The latter group is discussed in Chapter 4.

Histoplasmosis
Characteristics
Histoplasma capsulatum (Box 3-19) is a dimorphous fungus that gains entry to the lung by inhalation. Distribution is worldwide, and in the United States, it occurs along river valleys, particularly the Ohio, Mississippi, and St. Lawrence. The organism exists in the soil, particularly when it is contaminated by the excrement of birds (e.g., pigeons) or bats. Many epidemics may occur when there is heavy exposure due to demolition or construction in areas containing these droppings, such as bat caves, chicken houses, or attics of old buildings. In endemic areas, up to 80% of the population may be infected, but most individuals are asymptomatic. Inhalation of spores results in a localized infection of the lung, which then migrates to mediastinal and hilar lymph nodes and eventually migrates to the spleen and liver. The organisms usually are destroyed, and there is no residual of the initial infection, although a scar or calcification may occur. If individual foci of infection and

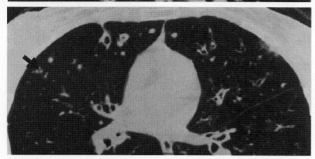
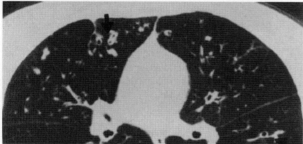

FIGURE **3-33.** *Mycobacterial avium* complex infection. Three selected images from a chest CT study of an elderly woman show scattered nodules and peripheral areas of bronchiectasis with mucous plugging *(arrows)*.

Box 3-19. Histoplasmosis

CHARACTERISTICS
Dimorphic fungus
River valleys in the United States
Soil containing excrement of birds or bats

ENDEMIC AREAS
80% of population infected
Most asymptomatic

PATHOGENESIS AND PATHOLOGY
Inhalation of spores
↓
Localized lung infection
↓
Hilar and mediastinal nodes
↓
Dissemination to liver and spleen
↙ ↘
Containment Chronic cavitary lung infection

RADIOGRAPHIC FEATURES
Acute phase
    Consolidation (segmental or sublobar)
    Ipsilateral mediastinal or hilar adenopathy
Epidemic form
    Multiple nodules
    May or may not have adenopathy
    Healed phase (calcification)
Solitary histoplasmoma
    Up to 4 cm
    Central nidus of calcium
Chronic cavitary form (simulates tuberculosis)
Additional features
Splenic calcification
Adenopathy (eventually calcifies)
Broncholith
Fibrosing mediastinitis
Disseminated (miliary pattern)

necrosis persist, they may enlarge, resulting in a chronic cavitary lesion indistinguishable from that of tuberculosis. Pathologically, well-defined granulomas may be found during the acute phase of disease in the lung, in the mediastinum, and in the various organs to which the organism disseminates. When healed, these granulomas are small and densely calcified.

Outbreaks of histoplasmosis are usually associated with constitutional symptoms and nonproductive cough. Many cases never come to medical attention.

Radiographic Features
The radiographic manifestations of histoplasmosis vary. The acute phase of the disease is characterized by single or multiple areas of consolidation, which are usually segmental or sublobar in distribution. These areas may be accompanied by ipsilateral hilar or mediastinal adenopathy, and occasionally, adenopathy alone may be the only finding. In the epidemic form of the disease, multiple, discrete nodules may be seen throughout both lungs; nodules may occur alone or be associated with hilar adenopathy (Fig. 3-34). They are usually 1 to 5 mm in diameter, discrete, and poorly marginated. With healing, the nodules may remain visible as multiple, discrete, calcified lesions less than 1 cm in diameter with or without calcified hilar lymph nodes (Fig. 3-35). A

third radiographic pattern consists of a solitary granuloma or histoplasmoma, which is usually well defined and can range in size from several millimeters to 4 cm. It typically contains a central or target type of calcification. These lesions usually occur in the lower lobes, and they may have associated smaller, calcified satellite nodules.

Additional radiographic features may be identified in patients with *Histoplasma* infection. They include calcifications in the spleen, which often are best detected on CT. Mediastinal lymphadenopathy is common as a sole manifestation of histoplasmosis or accompanying pulmonary consolidation or nodules. Nodes frequently calcify as healing occurs. Calcified lymph nodes may lead to two complications: broncholiths and fibrosing mediastinitis. Calcified lymph nodes may over time erode into a bronchus, producing broncholithiasis and its resulting symptom complex. Patients may have unexplained chronic cough and hemoptysis. CT can best identify the

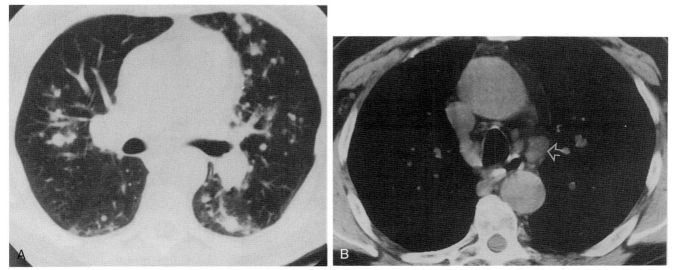

FIGURE 3-34. CT shows acute histoplasmosis. **A,** The lung windows demonstrate multiple, bilateral pulmonary nodules. **B,** On the mediastinal windows, there is adenopathy in the aorticopulmonary window *(arrow).*

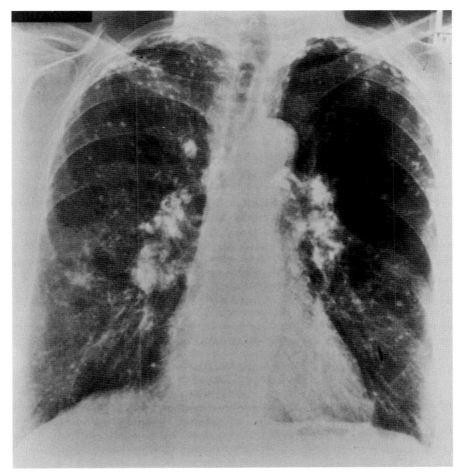

FIGURE 3-35. Healed histoplasmosis is characterized by multiple, small, calcified nodules in both lungs and by densely calcified hilar and mediastinal nodes.

intrabronchial calcification that may be associated with distal atelectasis of a segment or lobe (Fig. 3-36). The other complication, fibrosing mediastinitis, is discussed in Chapter 17. This condition is caused by the effect of large, calcified lymph nodes constricting and encasing important mediastinal structures, particularly the superior vena cava, with resultant superior vena caval syndrome; the trachea; right main bronchus; and central pulmonary arteries. Compression of pulmonary veins may lead to venous infarcts in the lungs.

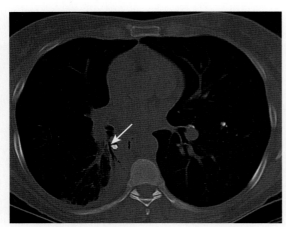

FIGURE 3-36. Broncholith. CT (bone window setting) demonstrates a small, rounded calcification *(arrow)* eroding into the superior segment right lower lobe bronchus and shows distal atelectasis. Notice the small, calcified granuloma in left lower lobe.

A rare chronic form of histoplasmosis can simulate tuberculosis. It usually consists of thin- or thick-walled cavities with patchy areas of consolidation, particularly involving the upper lobes with fibrosis and retraction. Disseminated histoplasmosis, which may occur in normal individuals, is much more common in immunosuppressed patients. Radiographically, the appearance is identical to that of miliary tuberculosis.

Coccidioidomycosis
Characteristics
Coccidioides immitis infection (Box 3-20) follows inhalation of infected spores in endemic areas such as desert areas of the southwestern United States and Central and South America. Clinical manifestations vary. Most individuals are asymptomatic, or they may experience a mild flulike illness of the lower respiratory system. Acute, severe disease may be associated with fever, cough, and pleuritic chest pain.

Pathology and Pathogenesis
With the initial inhalation of the spores, a local response or pneumonitis occurs. The immune system eventually destroys the organism, with resolution of the pneumonia. About 5% of individuals may have a chronic, often asymptomatic pulmonary lesion, such as a pulmonary nodule or cavity. Similar to tuberculosis, reactivation of the initial focus can occur. Dissemination of the organism to hilar and mediastinal nodes is common, and diffuse dissemination is rare but almost universally fatal.

Radiographic Features
The initial pneumonic form of the disease is characterized by an area of consolidation anywhere in the lung but most commonly in the lower lobes. It is usually sublobar, segmental, or patchy. It may be bilateral. Hilar and mediastinal lymph node involvement occurs in about 20% of cases, and rarely, it can be seen in the absence of the parenchymal consolidation. Most of these lesions resolve spontaneously without therapy.

Box 3-20. Coccidioidomycosis

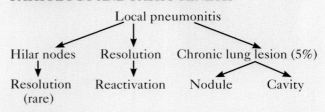

CHARACTERISTICS
Endemic areas
  Deserts
    Southwestern United States
Symptoms
  Flulike illness
  No symptoms

PATHOLOGY AND PATHOGENESIS

Local pneumonitis → Hilar nodes → Resolution (rare); Resolution → Reactivation; Chronic lung lesion (5%) → Nodule, Cavity

RADIOGRAPHIC FINDINGS
Pneumonic form
  Sublobar, segmental, patchy consolidation (lower lobes)
  Adenopathy (20%)
Chronic form
  Solitary or multiple nodules
  Thin-walled cavity (classic form found in 10% to 15%)
Disseminated pattern
  Nodules 5 mm to 1 cm
  Rare

The radiographic features of chronic coccidioidomycosis include solitary or multiple nodules. These tend to cavitate rapidly, and the cavities typically have very thin walls (Fig. 3-37). The thin-walled cavity is the classic lesion of coccidioidomycosis, but it occurs in only 10% to 15% of cases. Disseminated coccidioidomycosis is rare and is characterized radiographically by nodules ranging from 5 mm to 1 cm in diameter. A classic miliary pattern can also be observed.

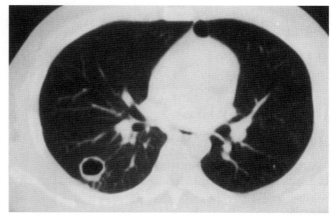

FIGURE 3-37. Coccidioidomycosis. CT demonstrates a relatively thin-walled cavity in the right lower lobe. The classic lesion of coccidioidomycosis has a paper-thin wall.

Box 3-21. North American Blastomycosis

CHARACTERISTICS
Dimorphic fungus
Wooded areas (hunters)

RADIOGRAPHIC FEATURES
Patchy segmental or nonsegmented consolidation
Solitary or multiple nodules
Disseminated (miliary pattern)

North American Blastomycosis
Characteristics
Blastomyces dermatitidis (Box 3-21) is a dimorphic fungus that grows in a mycelial form in the soil. Infection can occur by inoculation of the skin or by inhalation of organisms into the lungs. The organism is endemic in North America, occurring mostly in the same areas where histoplasmosis occurs but also in the southeastern United States. Blastomycosis is an infection associated with hunters because the organisms are prevalent in wooded areas.

Pathology and Pathogenesis
The organism is usually inhaled from the soil, and if the initial port of entry is the lung, a focal pneumonic process will occur. The disease can be self-limited, or a disseminated form can occur.

Radiographic Features
The radiographic findings are nonspecific but consist of areas of inhomogeneous consolidation in a segmental or nonsegmental distribution in any area of the lung. The next most common manifestation is that of solitary and multiple pulmonary nodules. The solitary nodules may simulate lung carcinoma. These nodules are 3 to 6 mm in diameter. A third pattern results from disseminated disease and consists of a diffuse nodular or micronodular pattern.

Cryptococcal Disease
Characteristics
Cryptococcus neoformans (Box 3-22) is an encapsulated, yeastlike fungus that exists in the soil and in the yeast form in humans. The soil may be contaminated by pigeon or chicken excreta. Seventy percent of individuals

Box 3-22. Cryptococcal Disease

CHARACTERISTICS
Spores in soil contaminated with pigeon and chicken
   excreta
Of patients with clinical disease, 70% are
   immunocompromised
Central nervous system involvement

RADIOGRAPHIC FINDINGS
Single or multiple nodules larger than 1 cm
Affects lower lobes

who have clinical disease are immunocompromised (see Chapter 4). The central nervous system is the most frequently affected site.

Radiographic Features
In the normal host, the most common finding is that of single or multiple pulmonary nodules that are approximately 1 to 5 cm in diameter and that usually occur in the lower lobes (Fig. 3-38). Cavitation, lymph node enlargement, and pleural effusion are uncommon. Adenopathy is rarely identified. Characteristically, the single or multiple nodules tend to abut the pleura.

Candidiasis
Characteristics
Candidiasis (Box 3-23) may be caused by a group of various organisms in the *Candida* genus, of which *Candida albicans* is the most important species. *C. albicans* lives in human and animal sources and may be a normal inhabitant of the

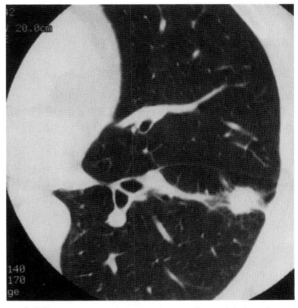

FIGURE 3-38. *Cryptococcus* infection in a patient with lymphoma. CT demonstrates an irregular nodule with a tag extending to the pleura.

Box 3-23. Candidiasis

CHARACTERISTICS
Candida albicans most common
Immunocompromised hosts
Exists in oropharynx

PATHOLOGY AND PATHOGENESIS
Mucous membranes and skin
Pulmonary features
   Aspirated organisms from oral cavity
   Results from fungemia

RADIOGRAPHIC FINDINGS
Multiple, patchy, bilateral areas of consolidation
Multiple nodules with or without cavitation

oral pharynx. As a result, short of an open lung biopsy, the true invasiveness or pathogenicity of this organism when recovered from the sputum is difficult to determine. It is an unusual infection found in immunocompromised individuals.

Pathology and Pathogenesis

The most common sites of infection are the mucous membranes and skin. Pulmonary candidiasis is unusual but may occur as a primary infection of the lungs, presumably resulting from aspiration of the organisms from the oral cavity. In most immunocompromised patients, pulmonary infection accompanies a diffuse, widespread fungemia.

Radiographic Features

The radiographic findings are usually nonspecific. Although most fungal diseases, particularly in immunocompromised hosts, are characterized by multiple nodules with cavitation, *Candida* pneumonia is more likely to produce areas of consolidation that are multiple and patchy and involve both lungs. Cavitation and hilar adenopathy are rare, and pleural effusion occurs in approximately 25% of cases.

Actinomycosis
Characteristics

Actinomyces (Box 3-24) is a rod-shaped bacterium rather than a fungus, but it is often considered a fungus because of its clinical presentation and radiographic findings. The organism is found in the mouth, and pulmonary infection usually occurs in people with extensive dental caries and poor oral hygiene. Involvement results from aspiration of these organisms.

There are three forms of actinomycosis: cervicofacial, gastrointestinal, and thoracic. The hallmark of the pulmonary disease is a focal abscess with extension to the chest wall, with secondary complications such as osteomyelitis, bronchopleural fistula, and pericarditis. The organism is an

---

Box 3-24. Actinomycosis

CHARACTERISTICS
Rod-shaped bacterium, anaerobe
Mouth organisms
Poor oral hygiene
Forms
   Cervicofacial
   Gastrointestinal
   Thoracic
      Focal abscess
      Invasion of chest wall

RADIOGRAPHIC FEATURES
Consolidation
Rounded abscess
Chest wall invasion (best seen on CT)
   Bone destruction
   Osteomyelitis and periostitis
   Pleural effusion

---

anaerobe, and anaerobic cultures must be obtained to confirm the diagnosis. Typical sulfur granules may be identified on pathologic specimens.

Radiographic Features

The radiographic features initially consist of an area of consolidation in the lung. This area may become rounded and suggest an abscess. Classic signs include extension of the disease process into the chest wall with bone destruction and osteomyelitis (Fig. 3-39). Chest wall invasion is best appreciated on CT. Pleural effusions are moderately common. Invasion of the ribs or vertebral bodies characteristically causes bone destruction and fairly extensive reactive periostitis.

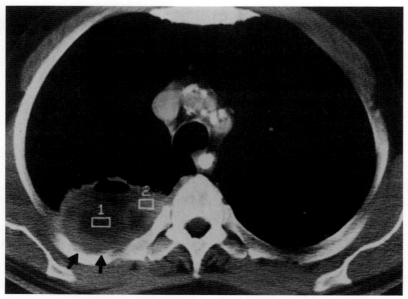

FIGURE 3-39. CT shows actinomycosis in a patient who developed a right upper lobe, posterior segment necrotic consolidation after dental extraction. Notice the erosion of the cortex of the overlying rib *(arrows)*.

Nocardiosis
Characteristics
Nocardia (Box 3-25) is a gram-positive organism, and although it is classified as a bacterium, it shares many features with fungal disease. It is weakly acid fast and can be confused with mycobacteria or *Legionella*. It is similar to *Actinomyces*, but the disease usually occurs in immunocompromised patients rather than in normal hosts (see Chapter 4).

Radiographic Features
Focal consolidation is the most common finding, although the disease can appear as single or multiple nodules with cavitation. Unlike aspergillosis, progression of disease usually is rather slow. Chest wall involvement may occur but is rare.

Aspergillosis
Aspergillus (Table 3-3) is a dimorphic fungus. The most common of the many species is *Aspergillus fumigatus*. *Aspergillus* grows widely in soil and water, in decaying vegetation, and in animal material.

Aspergillosis occurs in several different forms in the lung, including noninvasive (mycetoma) and semi-invasive aspergillosis, invasive aspergillosis, and allergic bronchopulmonary aspergillosis. The type of involvement depends on the immune status of the host. Infection is initiated by the inhalation route, and *Aspergillus* spores may exist in the mouth and airways of normal hosts. Immunocompetent or mildly immunosuppressed patients may acquire mycetomas or semi-invasive aspergillosis, whereas those who are severely immunosuppressed develop invasive aspergillosis. Allergic bronchopulmonary aspergillosis usually occurs in asthmatic patients.

Aspergilloma or Mycetoma: Noninvasive Aspergillosis
Characteristics
The most common radiographic form of aspergillosis is the mycetoma or fungus ball. The fungus ball consists of aspergillus hyphae, mucus, and cellular debris developing within a preexisting cyst, cavity, bulla, or area of bronchiectasis. It grows as a saprophytic organism and usually is noninvasive. A high prevalence of mycetoma has been found among patients with sarcoidosis or cystic fibrosis. Symptoms usually include hemoptysis, which may be life threatening.

Radiographic Features
The radiographic appearance of a fungus ball or mycetoma can be quite characteristic (Fig. 3-40). Typically, there is a solid, round opacity within a cavity or thin-walled cyst. Air may dissect into the solid mass, creating the appearance of an air crescent. In most cases, the fungus ball is mobile, and changes in position occur with changes in body posture. Extensive pleural thickening at the apex of the thorax frequently accompanies the development of a mycetoma. In making the differential diagnosis, necrotizing squamous cell carcinoma and an intrapulmonary abscess should be considered.

No treatment is necessary for asymptomatic individuals, but for those who develop severe hemoptysis, there

---

Box 3-25. Nocardiosis

CHARACTERISTICS
Gram-positive, acid-fast bacilli
Immunocompromised hosts

RADIOGRAPHIC FINDINGS
Single or multiple nodules with or without cavitation
Slow progression
Focal consolidation

TABLE 3-3 Aspergillosis

Aspergilloma or Mycetoma	Semi-invasive Aspergillosis	Invasive Aspergillosis	Allergic Bronchopulmonary Aspergillosis
Characteristics			
Fungus ball	Mildly immunosuppressed hosts	Immunocompromised hosts	Hypersensitivity reaction to *Aspergillus* in mucous plugs

Preexisting
  Cavity
  Bulla
  Bronchiectasis
	Focal consolidation→cavity→air crescent→thick-walled cavity→fungus ball	Granulocytopenia	Mucoid impaction

Saprophytic			Asthmatic patients
Sarcoidosis, cystic fibrosis			
Hemoptysis			
Radiographic Features			
Round opacity within cyst or cavity	Cavity ± fungus ball	Single or multiple nodules	Mucoid impaction Central branching opacities Central bronchiectasis
Air crescent	Air crescent	Cavitation	Lobar consolidation
Mobile	Pleural thickening	Air crescent	Chronic: upper lobe scarring and bronchiectasis
Plural thickening		Halo sign on CT	

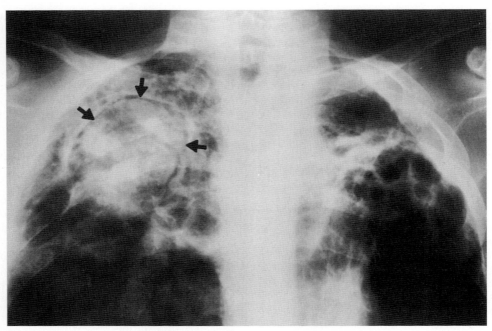

Figure 3-40. Fungus ball or mycetoma due to *Aspergillus*. Coned-down posteroanterior view shows the chest of a patient with biapical, fibrocavitary tuberculosis accompanied by volume loss. There is a mass in a large, right upper lobe cavity, with air dissecting into the cavity producing air crescents *(arrows)*.

are several therapeutic options. One is an interventional radiologic technique that consists of embolization of bronchial arteries that supply the cavity. Direct installation of amphotericin B in the form of a paste inserted through a percutaneous catheter into the cavity has been successful in some cases.

Semi-invasive Aspergillosis
Characteristics
Semi-invasive aspergillosis occurs in mildly immunosuppressed patients, such as those with alcoholism, chronic debilitating illness, or advanced malignancy. The lesion usually begins as a focal consolidation in the apex of one or both lungs that progresses over a period of months to become cavitary. It may form a crescent of air (i.e., air crescent sign) similar to that seen in a mycetoma. A thick-walled cavity, which later becomes thin walled and contains a fungus ball, is then formed.

Radiographic Features
The appearance may be identical to that of a mycetoma. It consists of a cavity with or without a fungus ball and air crescent, or it may be a localized area of consolidation. Extensive pleural thickening can be identified.

Invasive Aspergillosis
The features of invasive aspergillosis are described in Chapter 4, which discusses pulmonary infections in the immunocompromised patient.

Allergic Bronchopulmonary Aspergillosis
Characteristics
Allergic bronchopulmonary aspergillosis (see Chapter 13) occurs almost exclusively in asthmatic individuals. *Aspergillus* spores contained within mucous plugs in the tracheobronchial tree incite an allergic reaction. The syndrome consists of blood eosinophilia with positive precipitins and marked elevation of IgE antibodies. Large masses of mucus and *Aspergillus* hyphae can become trapped in the airways, producing mucoid impaction of the bronchi.

Radiographic Features
The most characteristic pattern is that of mucoid impaction of the bronchus. Central branching opacities, which sometimes are referred to as a finger-in-glove or V pattern, are identified. A more extensive description is provided in Chapter 13. Atelectasis distal to the areas of mucoid impaction usually does not occur because of collateral air drift. Air trapping may be identified, and lobar consolidation may be present. As the mucous plugs are expectorated, areas of central bronchiectasis can be identified, particularly on CT scans. Patients usually respond to steroids, but in the chronic form of the disease, scarring and upper lobe bronchiectasis are prominent features.

Mucormycosis
Mucormycosis, almost exclusively a disease in immunocompromised patients, is discussed in Chapter 4.

Pneumocystis jiroveci
Pneumocystis jiroveci (formerly called *Pneumocystis carinii*) is discussed in Chapter 4.

▬ PROTOZOAN AND OTHER PARASITIC INFECTIONS

In the United States, parasitic infection of the lung is rare. Pneumonia is caused by a hypersensitivity reaction to the organisms, or it results from systemic invasion of the lungs and pleura.

Toxoplasmosis

Toxoplasma gondii pulmonary involvement usually develops as part of a more generalized disease. The congenital variety is the most common, and it results from transmission of the organism from mother to fetus. It is associated with a consolidative and hemorrhagic pneumonia in neonates. In adults, toxoplasmosis, like pneumocystosis, occurs in patients who are immunocompromised. The radiographic appearance is that of fairly diffuse reticulonodular opacities.

Echinococcal Disease

Characteristics

Echinococcus granulosus (Box 3-26), the cause of most cases of human hydatid disease, occurs in two forms: pastoral and sylvatic, which differ in definitive and intermediate hosts and in geographic distribution. The pastoral variety is more common and occurs in sheep, cows, or pigs as the intermediate hosts, and in dogs as the definitive host. It is particularly common in sheep-raising areas. The sylvatic variety has as the definitive host the dog, wolf, or arctic fox.

Approximately 65% to 70% of *Echinococcus* cysts occur in the liver, and 15% to 30% occur in the lungs. The hydatid cyst is composed of two layers, an exocyst and an endocyst. Daughter cysts may be formed within the endocyst. Cysts may rupture in the lung parenchyma, with resulting intense inflammation. Rupture into the bronchus may result in severe hypotensive shock.

Radiographic Features

Echinococcal cysts are usually well-circumscribed, spherical or oval masses that may be single or multiple (Fig. 3-41).

Box 3-26. Echinococcus

CHARACTERISTICS
Pastoral form
  Sheep, cows, or pigs (intermediate hosts)
  Dogs (definitive host)
Sylvatic form
  Dog, wolf, arctic fox (definitive hosts)
Sites of involvement
  Liver (65% to 70%)
  Lung (15% to 30%)
Cystic structure
  Endocyst
  Exocyst
  Daughter cysts
Complications
  Rupture (local inflammation)
  Anaphylaxis

RADIOGRAPHIC FEATURES
Single or multiple lesions
Spherical lesions
Affects lower lobes
Meniscus or crescent sign
Air-fluid level (water lily sign)
No calcification

They are usually located in the lower lobes. If communication develops between the cysts and the bronchial tree, air may enter between the pericyst and exocyst, producing the appearance of a thin crescent of air around the periphery of the cyst, sometimes called the *meniscus* or *crescent sign*. Bronchial communication occurs directly into the endocyst. Occasionally, an air crescent sign and air-fluid level can be identified. The membrane of the cyst, which has ruptured into the bronchial tree, may float on the fluid within the cyst, giving rise to the classic water lily sign. CT can differentiate cystic from solid lesions and may identify the pathognomonic features in ruptured or complicated hydatid cysts, such as the presence of daughter cysts and endocyst membranes. Calcification of a pulmonary hydatid cyst is rare.

Amebiasis

Characteristics

Pulmonary amebiasis is rare and is usually a sequela of hepatic or gastrointestinal involvement. Amebiasis is caused by the protozoan *Entamoeba histolytica*. This organism causes dysentery and has a worldwide distribution. Pleuropulmonary complications usually occur when the liver is involved. Patients present with right upper quadrant and right-sided pleuritic chest pain.

Radiographic Features

The common radiographic features are right-sided pleural effusion with basal consolidation. Involvement of the lung may result from rupture of an amebic abscess in the liver. Occasionally, areas of consolidation in the right lower lobe may progress to abscess formation with cavitation.

Schistosomiasis

Characteristics

Schistosomiasis is a common disease in many areas of the world, including Central and South America, the Middle East, and the Far East. The intermediate host of this parasite is the snail. Humans contact the parasites in water. The parasites penetrate the skin, reach the circulation, and eventually grow in the mesenteric or pelvic venous plexus, where they mature into adult worms and lay eggs. Pulmonary symptoms may occur during the larval migration phase in the lungs due to a hypersensitivity reaction. A progressive diffuse endarteritis and thrombosis may result from impaction of ova in the pulmonary circulation, with the eventual development of pulmonary arterial hypertension.

Pathology and Pathogenesis

Pathologic changes in the lungs result from deposition of eggs or ova, which are released directly into the systemic venous blood or occasionally into the portal system, where eggs can reach the lungs through anastomotic channels as the liver becomes cirrhotic. The embolized ova become impacted in pulmonary arterioles and then extruded into the surrounding tissue. This causes an obliterative arteriolitis, which can result in increased pulmonary artery pressure. The ova may mature into adult worms in the lungs and can cause lung damage.

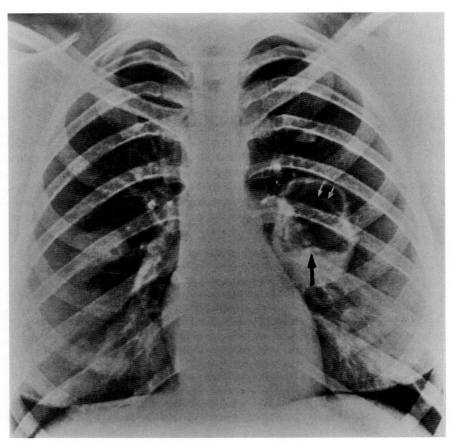

FIGURE 3-41. Echinococcal cysts. Both lungs contain multiple nodules, some of which are cavitated. A meniscus or crescent can be identified *(white arrows)* in the large cyst in the left lung, which also displays an air-fluid level and water lily sign *(black arrow).*

Radiographic Features

Pulmonary arterial hypertension is the most common finding in patients with pulmonary schistosomiasis (Fig. 3-42). The appearance consists of dilation of the central pulmonary arteries with rapid tapering. The passage of larva through the pulmonary capillaries can cause a transitory eosinophilic pneumonia, simulating Loeffler's syndrome. This is characterized by the presence of peripheral areas of consolidation.

Other Metazoan Infections

The lungs may be infected by a number of worms, causing ascariasis, strongyloidiasis, trichinosis, ancylostomiasis (i.e., hookworm disease), and filariasis (i.e., tropical eosinophilia). Most of these organisms produce hypersensitivity reactions in the lungs, similar to Loeffler's syndrome (see Chapter 9).

■ EMERGING VIRAL INFECTIONS

Outbreaks of several newly recognized viral infections, including avian influenza, severe acute respiratory syndrome–associated coronavirus, and hantavirus, have been associated with high mortality rates. These infections have presented challenges to clinicians, radiologists, scientists, and public health officials.

H5N1 Avian Influenza

Avian influenza is caused by the H5N1 subtype of the influenza A virus. Human transmission occurs through close contact with infected birds, usually from ingestion of infected poultry. The first documented case occurred in 1997 in Hong Kong. In 2003, the virus resurfaced in Vietnam. Approximately 180 people throughout Southeast Asia have been infected, with a nearly 50% mortality rate. Affected patients present with a rapidly progressive pneumonia that may lead to respiratory failure and ARDS.

Chest radiographs usually show abnormalities at the time of presentation. The most common finding is multifocal consolidation (Fig 3-43), which is bilateral in 80% of cases. Consolidation may infrequently be complicated by areas of cavitation. Bilateral pleural effusions occur in about one third of cases.

Severe Acute Respiratory Syndrome–Associated Coronavirus

Severe acute respiratory syndrome (SARS) is caused by the SARS-associated coronavirus. It results in a systemic infection that is manifested clinically as a progressive pneumonia. The first reported case in humans occurred in China in 2002. In 2003, SARS spread to Hong Kong and subsequently to Canada, Singapore, and Vietnam. Before the

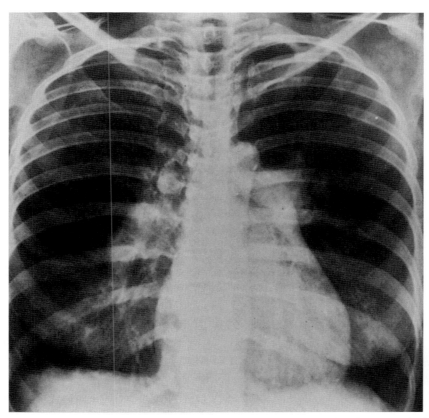

FIGURE 3-42. Pulmonary arterial hypertension in pulmonary schistosomiasis is characterized by dilation of the central pulmonary arteries. The patient was a 48-year-old Puerto Rican woman with proven schistosomiasis, cirrhosis, and portal hypertension.

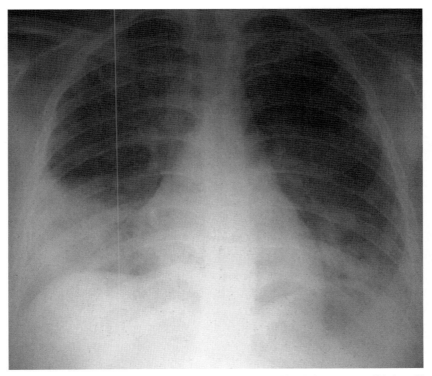

FIGURE 3-43. H5N1 avian influenza. The chest radiograph demonstrates bilateral, multifocal airspace consolidation. (From Ketai L, Paul NS, Wong KT: Radiology of severe acute respiratory syndrome [SARS]: the emerging pathologic-radiologic correlates of an emerging disease. J Thorac Imaging 21:276–283, 2006).

infection could be contained by vigorous public health measures, more than 8000 persons were infected, with a nearly 10% fatality rate. No additional human infections have been reported since 2003. After an initial incubation period of 2 to 10 days (mean, 6 days), affected patients typically present with headache, malaise, fever, and nonproductive cough.

Chest radiographs show abnormalities at the time of clinical presentation in about 80% of cases. The most common radiographic finding is poorly defined airspace consolidation. Although about one half of cases appear to have a focal distribution at the time of presentation, progression to multifocal involvement is common. Areas of consolidation have a predilection for the lower lobes and lung periphery. CT shows abnormalities at the time of clinical presentation, even when chest radiographs do not. The most common CT finding is ground-glass opacification (Fig 3-44), which is often accompanied by small foci of consolidation and interlobular and intralobular thickening. Severe SARS may progress to diffuse alveolar damage.

Overall, 20% of patients with SARS require mechanical ventilation, and 10% of patients do not survive the

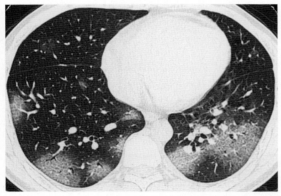

FIGURE 3-44. Severe acute respiratory syndrome (SARS). CT shows multifocal, peripheral foci of ground-glass attenuation with superimposed reticular opacities. (From Ketai L, Paul NS, Wong KT: Radiology of severe acute respiratory syndrome [SARS]: the emerging pathologic-radiologic correlates of an emerging disease. J Thorac Imaging 21:276–283, 2006).

infection. Survivors often have residual abnormalities seen on CT, reflecting interstitial fibrosis and small airways disease.

Hantavirus

Hantaviruses are carried by rodent vectors. Human infection occurs after inhalation of aerosolized rodent feces or urine. The Sin Nombre hantavirus (translated as "the nameless virus") was initially discovered in the southwestern United States in 1993 as a cause of pulmonary edema and respiratory failure accompanied by hematologic abnormalities. This clinical entity is referred to as the hantavirus pulmonary syndrome (HPS).

HPS is caused by endothelial damage to the lung. The initial interstitial edema manifests radiographically as Kerley lines, bronchial wall thickening, and subpleural edema. Although some patients recover fully from the initial stage of infection, many progress to diffuse alveolar edema, which is manifested by symmetric perihilar and basilar airspace consolidation (Fig 3-45). This phase of illness requires mechanical ventilation and is associated with a high mortality rate. As the disease progresses, it may be accompanied by myocardial depression, which worsens tissue hypoxia and contributes to the high mortality rate associated with this syndrome.

■ INFECTIONS RELATED TO BIOTERRORISM

The Centers for Disease Control and Prevention (CDC) lists several infectious agents as a category A threats, denoting the highest potential for public health impact. These agents include inhalational anthrax *(Bacillus anthracis)*, plague *(Y. pestis)*, smallpox (variola major), botulism *(Clostridium, botulinum)*, tularemia *(Francisella tularensis)*, and hemorrhagic fever (Ebola and Marburg filoviruses). Among these infections, anthrax has the unique distinction that imaging studies may allow prompt diagnosis and institution of life-saving therapy before organ damage is irreversible. For this reason, the discussion focuses on anthrax.

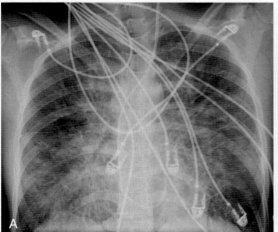
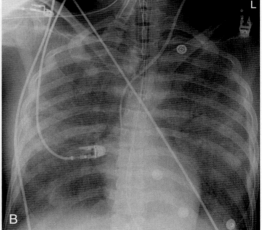

FIGURE 3-45. Hantavirus pulmonary syndrome. **A,** Portable chest radiograph shows bilateral central airspace opacities and diffuse Kerley lines due to combined alveolar and interstitial edema. **B,** Portable chest radiograph of same patient 1 day later shows progressive alveolar pulmonary edema and interval intubation. (Courtesy of Loren Ketai, MD, University of New Mexico, Albuquerque, NM.)

Anthrax

Anthrax has been used as a biologic weapon since World War II. The most recent episode occurred in 2001, when highly refined anthrax spores were placed in envelopes and mailed through the United States postal system. This act of bioterrorism resulted in 22 diagnosed cases of anthrax, which were evenly split between inhalational and cutaneous forms. Almost one half of those with the inhalational form died.

B. anthracis is a sporulating, gram-positive bacterium that may result in cutaneous, gastrointestinal, or pulmonary infection. The latter, which is also referred to as inhalational anthrax, is the deadliest form. The spores are 2 to 6 μm, an ideal size for deposition in the distal respiratory tract after inhalation. Once inhaled, the spores are ingested by macrophages. Surviving spores are transported to mediastinal lymph nodes, where they germinate for 2 to 30 days (mean, 1 week).

Radiologic findings have not been identified before germination. After germination, the organisms synthesize a toxin, resulting in the prodromal phase of the disease. This is manifested by flulike symptoms of fever, chills, fatigue, and cough. The prodromal phase lasts about 4 days and is rapidly followed by the second phase of the illness, which is characterized by stridor, respiratory failure, and shock. In many cases, death occurs despite antibiotic therapy.

Imaging findings for anthrax reflect hemorrhagic lymphadenitis and mediastinitis caused by the release of anthrax toxin within the mediastinum. In the prodromal phase of the illness, the chest radiograph typically demonstrates mediastinal widening and unilateral or bilateral hilar enlargement. These findings are frequently accompanied by pleural effusions. Although limited peribronchovascular airspace opacities may be present, extensive consolidation is uncommon. Imaging findings of mediastinal widening and pleural effusions are helpful for differentiating inhalational anthrax from a community-acquired respiratory infection.

CT may provide convincing evidence of inhalational anthrax before confirmatory laboratory tests have returned (Fig 3-46). Unenhanced CT may show high-attenuation (46 to 62 Hounsfield units) mediastinal and hilar lymph nodes,

which may rapidly enlarge over a period of days. These findings reflect the presence of hemorrhage and edema within lymph nodes. Because of this characteristic appearance, unenhanced CT is considered the imaging modality of choice for the diagnosis of inhalational anthrax.

After contrast administration, rim enhancement and central low attenuation of lymph nodes may be seen. Rapidly enlarging pleural effusions are commonly identified by CT, and they may contain dependently layering, high-attenuation fluid, reflecting serosanguineous exudates. Peribronchovascular thickening correlates with the presence of edema, hemorrhage, and necrosis of the airways and adjacent lymphatics. The constellation of these CT findings is almost pathognomonic for inhalational anthrax, but a variety of other causes of mediastinitis may produce similar findings in the appropriate clinical setting.

Inhalational anthrax is treated with an antibiotic regimen that includes ciprofloxacin or doxycycline combined with two other agents, usually rifampin and clindamycin. Early recognition of anthrax and prompt administration of antibiotics before the onset of fulminant illness can dramatically improve patient survival.

■ SUGGESTED READINGS

Aquino, S., Gamsu, G., Webb, W.R., et al., 1996. Tree-in-bud pattern: frequency and significance on thin section CT. J. Comput. Assist. Tomogr. 20, 594–599.

Berkmen, Y.M., 1980. Aspiration and inhalation pneumonias. Semin. Roentgenol. 15, 73–84.

Cantanzaro, A., 1980. Pulmonary coccidioidomycosis. Med. Clin. North. Am. 64, 461–465.

Centers for Disease Control, 2006. Reported Tuberculosis in the United States. Department of Health and Human Services, CDC, October 2007, Atlanta, U.S. Available at www.cdc.gov/tb/surv/surv2006/default.htm (accessed January 18, 2008).

Christensen, E.E., Dietz, G.W., Ahn, C.H., et al., 1979. Pulmonary manifestations of *Mycobacterium intracellulare*. AJR. Am. J. Roentgenol. 133, 59–66.

Comstock, G.W., 1982. Epidemiology of tuberculosis. Am. Rev. Respir. Dis. 125, 8–16.

Dalhoff, K., Maass, M., 1996. *Chlamydia pneumoniae* pneumonia in hospitalized patients. Chest 110, 351–356.

Davies, S.F., 1987. An overview of pulmonary fungal infections. Clin. Chest. Med. 8, 495–512.

Des Prez, R.M., Goodwin Jr., R.A., 1985. Mycobacterium tuberculosis. In: Mandell, G.L., Douglas Jr., R.G., Bennet, J. (Eds.), Principles and Practice of Infectious Diseases, second ed. Churchill Livingstone, New York, pp. 1383–1412.

Drutz, D.J., 1994. Coccidioidal pneumonia. In: Pennington, J.E. (Ed.), Respiratory Infections—Diagnosis and Management. third ed.. Raven Press, New York, pp. 569–597.

Edelstein, P.H., Meyer, R.D., 1994. *Legionella* pneumonias. In: Pennington, J.E. (Ed.), Respiratory Infections—Diagnosis and Management. third ed. Raven Press, New York, pp. 455–484.

Eisenstadt, J., Crane, L.R., 1994. Gram-negative bacillary pneumonias. In: Pennington, J.E. (Ed.), Respiratory Infections—Diagnosis and Management. third ed. Raven Press, New York, pp. 369–406.

Epstein, D.M., Kline, L.R., Albelda, S.M., et al., 1987. Tuberculous pleural effusions. Chest 91, 106–110.

Fairbank, J.T., Mamourian, A.C., Dietrich, P.A., et al., 1983. The chest radiograph in Legionnaires' disease: further observations. Radiology 147, 33–34.

Finegold, S.M., 1994. Aspiration pneumonia, lung abscess, and empyema. In: Pennington, J.E. (Ed.), Respiratory Infections—Diagnosis and Management. third ed. Raven Press, New York, pp. 311–322.

Flynn, M.W., Felson, B., 1970. The roentgen manifestations of thoracic actinomycosis. Am. J. Roentgenol. Radium. Ther. Nucl. Med. 110, 707–716.

Fraser, R.S., Muller, N.L., Colman, N.C., Paré, R.D., 1999. Fraser and Pare's Diagnosis of diseases of the chest. Fourth edition. Philadelphia, Elsevier.

Frasier, A.A., Franks, T.J., Galvin, J.R., 2006. Inhalational anthrax. J. Thorac. Imaging. 21, 252–258.

Gefter, W.B., Weingard, T.R., Epstein, D.M., et al., 1981. Semi-invasive pulmonary aspergillosis: a new look at the spectrum of aspergillus infections of the lung. Radiology 140, 313–321.

Gefter, W.B., 1992. The spectrum of pulmonary aspergillosis. J. Thorac. Imaging. 7, 56–74.

Genereux, G.P., Stilwell, G.A., 1980. The acute bacterial pneumonias. Semin. Roentgenol. 15, 9–16.

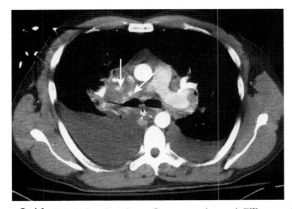

FIGURE 3-46. Inhalational anthrax. Contrast-enhanced CT scan of the chest shows diffuse widening of mediastinal and hilar regions due to a combination of widespread edema and enlarged lymph nodes. High-attenuation foci in the right paratracheal soft tissue *(arrows)* likely are caused by hemorrhagic foci in the lymph nodes. Notice the bilateral pleural effusions. (From Ketai L, Alrahji AA, Hart B, et al: Radiologic manifestations of potential bioterrorist agents of infection. AJR Am J Roentgenol 180:565–575, 2003.)

Goodwin Jr., R.A., DesPrez, R.M., 1985. *Histoplasma capsulatum*. In: Mandell, G.L., Douglas Jr., R.G., Bennett, J. (Eds.), Principles and Practice of Infectious Diseases, second ed. Churchill Livingstone, New York, pp. 1468–1479.

Greendyke, W.H., Resnick, D.L., Harvey, W.C., 1970. The varied roentgen manifestations of primary coccidioidomycosis. AJR. Am. J. Roentgenol. 109, 491–499.

Griffith, D.E., Aksamit, T., Brown-Elliott, B.A., et al., 2007. An official ATS/IDSA statement: diagnosis, treatment, and prevention of nontuberculous mycobacterial diseases. Am. J. Respir. Crit. Care. Med. 175, 367–416.

Halvorsen, R.A., Duncan, J.D., Merten, D.F., et al., 1984. Pulmonary blastomycosis: radiologic manifestations. Radiology 150, 1–5.

Hartman, T.E., Swensen, S.J., Williams, D.E., 1992. *Mycobacterium avium-intracellulare* complex: evaluation with CT. Radiology 187, 1–4.

Janower, M.L., Weiss, E.B., 1980. Mycoplasmal, viral, and rickettsial pneumonias. Semin. Roentgenol. 15, 25–34.

Kauffman, R.S., 1994. Viral pneumonia. In: Pennington, J.E. (Ed.), Respiratory Infections—Diagnosis and Management, third ed. Raven Press, New York, pp. 515–532.

Ketai, L.H., Paul, N.S., Wong, K.T., 2006. Radiology of severe acute respiratory syndrome (SARS): the emerging pathologic-radiologic correlates of an emerging disease. J. Thorac. Imaging. 21, 267–283.

Ketai, L.H., Tchoyoson Lim, C.C., 2007. Radiology of bacterial weapons—old and the new? Semin. Roentgenol. 42, 49–59.

Ketai, L.H., Williamson, M.R., Telepak, R.J., et al., 1994. Hantavirus pulmonary syndrome: radiologic findings in 16 patients. Radiology 191, 665–668.

Khoury, M.B., Goodwin, J.D., Ravin, C.E., et al., 1984. Thoracic cryptococcosis: immunologic competence and radiologic appearance. AJR. Am. J. Roentgenol. 142, 893–896.

Kim, E.A., Lee, K.S., Primack, S.L., et al., 2002. Viral pneumonia in adults: radiologic and pathologic findings. Radiographics 22, S137–S149.

Kroboth, F.J., Yu, V.L., Reddy, S.C., et al., 1983. Clinicoradiographic correlation with the extent of Legionnaire disease. AJR. Am. J. Roentgenol. 141, 263–268.

Kuhlman, J.E., Deutsch, J.H., Fishman, E.K., et al., 1990. CT features of thoracic mycobacterial disease. Radiographics 10, 413–431.

Kuhlman, J.E., Fishman, E.K., Teigin, C., 1990. Pulmonary septic emboli: changes with CT. Radiology 174, 211–213.

Landay, M.J., Christensen, E.E., Bynum, L.J., et al., 1980. Anaerobic pleural and pulmonary infections. AJR. Am. J. Roentgenol. 134, 233–240.

Luby, J.P., 1991. Pneumonia caused by *Mycoplasma pneumoniae* infection. Clin. Chest. Med. 12, 237–244.

Lynch, D.A., Simone, P.M., Fox, M.A., et al., 1995. CT features of pulmonary *Mycobacterium avium* complex infection. J. Comput. Assist. Tomogr. 19, 353–360.

Malo, J.L., Hawkins, R., Pepys, J., 1977. Studies in chronic allergic bronchopulmonary aspergillosis. I. Clinical and physiological findings. Thorax 32, 254–257.

Martinez, S., Restrepo, C.S., Carrillo, J.A., et al., 2006. Thoracic manifestations of tropical parasitic infections: a pictorial review. Radiographics 25, 135–155.

McGarry, T., Giosa, R., Rohman, M., et al., 1987. Pneumatocele formation in adult pneumonia. Chest 92, 717–720.

Miller, W.T., MacGregor, R.R., 1978. Tuberculosis: frequency of unusual radiographic findings. AJR Am J Roentgenol 130, 867–875.

Miller, W.T., 1988. Pulmonary infections. In: Taveras, J.M., Ferrucci, J.T. (Eds.), Radiology: Diagnosis–Imaging–Intervention, vol. 1. JB Lippincott, Philadelphia.

Miller, W.T., 1992. Granulomatous infections of the lung. In: Freundlich, I.M., Bragg, D.G. (Eds.), A Radiologic Approach to Diseases of the Chest. Williams & Wilkins, Baltimore.

Miller, W.T., Miller Jr., W.T., 1993. Tuberculosis in the normal host: radiological findings. Semin Roentgenol 23, 109–118.

Miller, W.T., 1994. Spectrum of pulmonary non-tuberculous mycobacterial infection. Radiology 191, 343–350.

Moore, E.H., 1993. Atypical mycobacterial infection in the lung: CT appearance. Radiology 187, 777–782.

Newman, G.E., Effman, E.L., Putman, C.E., 1982. Pulmonary aspiration complexes in adults. Curr Probl Diagn Radiol 11, 1–47.

Niederman, M.S., Mandell, L.A., Anzueto, A., et al., 2001. Guidelines for the management of adults with community-acquired pneumonia: diagnosis, assessment of severity, antimicrobial therapy, and prevention. Am J Respir Crit Care Med 163, 1730–1754.

Ort, S., Ryan, J.L., Barden, G., et al., 1983. Pneumococcal pneumonia in hospitalized patients' clinical and radiological presentations. JAMA 249, 214–218.

Patz, E.F., Goodman, P.C., 1992. Pulmonary cryptococcosis. J Thorac Imaging 7, 51–55.

Petty, T.L., 1982. Adult respiratory distress syndrome. Semin Respir Med 3, 219–224.

Putman, C.E., 1994. Infectious pneumonias—including aspiration states. In: Putman, C.E., Ravin, C.E. (Eds.), Textbook of Diagnostic Imaging, second ed. WB Saunders, Philadelphia, pp. 495–525.

Qureshi, N.R., Hien, T.T., Farrar, J., Gleeson, F.V., 2006. The radiologic manifestations of H5N1 avian influenza. J Thorac Imaging 21, 259–264.

Rohlfing, B.M., White, E.A., Webb, W.R., Goodman, P.C., 1978. Hilar and mediastinal adenopathy caused by bacterial abscess of the lung. Radiology 128, 289–293.

Ruben, F.L., Nguyen, M.L.T., 1991. Viral pneumonitis. Clin Chest Med 12, 223–235.

Rubin, S.A., Winer-Muram, H.T., 1992. Thoracic histoplasmosis. J Thorac Imaging 7, 39–50.

Sanders Jr., W.E., 1985. Other mycobacterium species. In: Mandell, G.L., Douglas Jr., R.G., Bennett, J.E. (Eds.), Principles and Practice of Infectious Diseases. second ed. Churchill Livingstone, New York, pp. 1413–1430.

Stead, W.W., 1981. Tuberculosis among elderly persons: an outbreak in a nursing home. Ann Intern Med 94, 606–610.

Washington, L., Palacio, D., 2007. Imaging of bacterial pulmonary infection in the immunocompetent patient. Semin Roentgenol 42, 122–145.

Wong, K.T., Antonio, G.E., Hui, D.S.C., 2003. Severe acute respiratory syndrome: radiographic appearance and pattern of progression in 138 patients. Radiology 228, 401–406.

Woodring, J.H., Rehm, S.R., Broderson, H., et al., 1985. Pulmonary aspiration of gastric contents. J KY Med Assoc 83, 299–306.

Woodring, J.H., Vandiviere, H.M., Fried, A.M., et al., 1986. Update: the radiographic features of pulmonary tuberculosis. AJR Am J Roentgenol 146, 497–506.

Woodring, J.H., 1992. Pulmonary bacterial and viral infections. In: Freundlich, I.M., Bragg, D.G. (Eds.), A Radiologic Approach to Diseases of the Chest. Williams & Wilkins, Baltimore.

CHAPTER 4

Pulmonary Diseases in the Immunocompromised Host with or without Acquired Immunodeficiency Syndrome

Theresa C. McLoud and Phillip M. Boiselle

▬ PULMONARY INFECTIONS IN THE IMMUNOCOMPROMISED PATIENT WITHOUT HUMAN IMMUNODEFICIENCY VIRUS INFECTION

The immunocompromised host is an individual with altered defense mechanisms or immunity. Immunocompromised hosts without human immunodeficiency virus (HIV) infection include patients with hematologic malignancies such as lymphoma and leukemia, recipients of organ transplants, patients treated aggressively with cytotoxic drugs for solid tumors, and those receiving high-dose corticosteroid therapy for collagen vascular disease and other disorders.

The lung is a frequent target of infection in the immunocompromised host, and mortality rates associated with pulmonary disease often are as high as 40% to 50%. Infection is the most frequent cause of the radiographic abnormality; however, conditions such as extension of malignancy (e.g., lymphoma, metastases), drug reactions, or other noninfectious processes may be diagnostic possibilities (Table 4-1). Unfortunately, noninvasive diagnostic methods such as sputum smears and cultures that are used for evaluation of pneumonia are less useful in the immunocompromised host. The clinician must therefore choose between using invasive techniques to determine the exact cause of the pneumonia or employing empirically chosen therapy. The former choice is not without hazard in debilitated patients; the latter is complicated by the broad range of possible causes and appropriate therapies.

The radiologist plays an important role, which involves detection of an abnormality on the chest radiograph, analysis of the radiographic features with regard to diagnosis and choice of an appropriate interventional technique, performance of percutaneous needle biopsy of focal lesions when appropriate, and monitoring response to therapy and the development of complications. Although the radiographic features in most opportunistic infections are relatively nonspecific, there is a general correlation between the type of radiographic pattern and the microorganism producing the pneumonia. Three major patterns are used for classification: lobar or segmental consolidation, nodules with rapid growth or cavitation, and diffuse lung disease.

Radiologic Patterns

Table 4-1 summarizes the radiographic patterns for HIV-negative immunocompromised patients with pulmonary disease.

Lobar or Segmental Consolidation: Bacterial Pneumonia
Causes
Bacteria are the most common infectious agents invading the lungs of immunocompromised hosts. Colonization of the oral pharynx by altered flora in the presence of reduced lung defense mechanisms leads to a preponderance of gram-negative bacillary pneumonias. Organisms include *Klebsiella*, *Enterobacter*, *Pseudomonas*, *Escherichia coli*, *Proteus*, and *Serratia*. Among gram-positive organisms, staphylococci are the most common.

The radiographic features include localized dense consolidation, which may be lobar or segmental. Cavitation is a common feature. Cavities may be solitary, but many small microabscesses often are identified. Patchy, multilobar pneumonia may also occur. Effusions are typically small, and empyemas are unusual. Occasionally, the chest roentgenogram may be normal, especially in the setting of neutropenia. Bacterial pneumonia can be diagnosed by isolation and culture of the organisms from sputum samples or by observing a clinical response to empirically chosen antibiotics.

The Legionnaires' disease bacterium *(Legionella pneumophila)* and Pittsburgh pneumonia agent are causes of

TABLE 4-1 Radiographic Patterns in HIV-Negative Immunocompromised Patients with Pulmonary Disease

Lobar or Segmental Consolidation	Nodules with Rapid Growth ± Cavitation	Diffuse Lung Disease

Causes
  Gram-negative bacteria
  Gram-positive bacteria
  Legionella pneumophila
	Causes
	  Fungi
	  Nocardia
	  Legionella (Pittsburgh agent)
	  Staphylococcus aureus (septic infarcts)
		Causes
		  Infection
		    Pneumocystis jiroveci
		    Viruses (cytomegalovirus)
		  Cytotoxic drug reactions
		  Lymphangitic spread of tumor
		  Radiation pneumonitis
		  Nonspecific interstitial pneumonitis

Radiographic features
  Lobar or segmental
  Frequent cavitation
	Aspergillus
	  Characteristics
	    Blood vessel invasion, infarction
	    Neutropenia
	  Radiographic features
	    Nodules
	    Cavitation
	    Air crescent sign
	    Halo sign on CT
		Pneumocystis jiroveci pneumonia
		  Characteristics
		    40% diffuse pneumonias in
		      immunocompromised hosts
		    Acute and fulminating
		  Radiographic findings
		    Central perihilar linear opacities
		      (diffuse consolidation)
		    CT findings (ground-glass
		      opacification)
		  Diagnosis
		    BAL

Diagnosis
  Sputum smear and culture
  Serology *(Legionella)*
	Mucormycosis
	  Diabetes, leukopenia
	  Blood vessel invasion
	  Radiographic appearance identical to *Aspergillus*
		Cytomegalovirus
		  Organ transplants
		  Diffuse nodular or linear pattern on
		    radiograph

Differential diagnosis
  Neoplasms (lymphoma)
	Diagnosis
	  Invasive procedure (TBB, TNB)	

	Differential diagnosis
	  Metastases
	  Lymphoma
	  Lymphoproliferative disease	

BAL, bronchoalveolar lavage; TBB, transbronchial biopsy; TNB, transthoracic needle biopsy.

acute bronchopneumonia in the immunocompromised host, particularly in renal transplant recipients. The clinical and radiographic appearance of *Legionella pneumophila* in these patients is usually identical to that seen in the normal host. Multilobar consolidation is common. However, the Pittsburgh agent (*Legionella micdadei*) typically produces circumscribed areas of pneumonia, creating a nodular appearance on the chest radiograph (Fig. 4-1).

Tuberculosis occurs with increased frequency in certain subgroups of immunosuppressed patients. However, in most reported series of pneumonias, the presence of mycobacterial disease in immunocompromised hosts is low. Tuberculosis, when it occurs in this setting, does carry a high fatality rate. The typical radiologic features of pulmonary tuberculosis consist of apical and posterior segmental disease in the upper lobes, with or without the development of cavitation. The differential diagnosis should include infection with atypical mycobacteria.

Differential Diagnosis

The differential diagnosis of lobar or segmental consolidation in the immunosuppressed patient is limited. Lymphoma involving the lung parenchyma may appear as a localized airspace or alveolar consolidation with prominent air bronchograms. This appearance may signal relapse after treatment, and hilar and mediastinal adenopathy may not be present.

Nodules with Rapid Growth or Cavitation: Fungal Pneumonias
Causes

Multiple nodules with rapid growth or cavitation are common features of fungal infection in the compromised host. This group includes pneumonias produced by *Nocardia*, although *Nocardia asteroides* is a higher transitional form of bacterium. The fungi most frequently isolated include the commensals, such as *Aspergillus, Candida, Mucor,* and true pathogenetic fungi, such as *Cryptococcus*. Fungal pneumonia characteristically develops in patients with hematologic malignancies who are neutropenic from cytotoxic drugs or who are receiving or have just completed a course of broad-spectrum antibiotics for fever of unknown cause.

Aspergillus pneumonia is the most common fungal pulmonary infection in immunosuppressed patients. *Aspergillus* causes an invasive necrotizing pneumonia resulting from invasion of blood vessels with accompanying pulmonary infarction. The roentgenographic features consist of multiple nodular areas of consolidation that often abut the pleural surfaces (Fig. 4-2). These areas frequently cavitate and may show crescentic radiolucencies around the parenchymal opacities (i.e., air crescent sign) that may mimic mycetoma. This sign also can be identified on CT studies (Fig. 4-3). Another characteristic finding is a pulmonary mass surrounded by a zone of lower attenuation with ground-glass opacification (i.e., halo sign), probably produced by adjacent hemorrhage. The diagnosis of *Aspergillus*

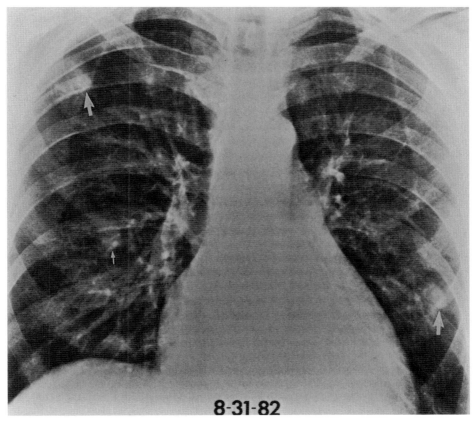

FIGURE 4-1. *Legionella micdadei* pneumonia. A posteroanterior chest radiograph shows multiple nodules in both lungs *(arrows).*

pneumonia usually requires invasive procedures, such as needle aspiration or open lung biopsy.

Pulmonary disease caused by *Mucor* is clinically and radiographically indistinguishable from that caused by *Aspergillus*. It is frequently seen in patients with lymphoproliferative disease, leukopenia, and diabetes, and it is detected in patients after antibiotic use. The organism likewise has a predilection for blood vessel invasion and pulmonary infarction (Fig. 4-4).

Primary candidal pneumonias are rare in immunosuppressed patients; the lung is more likely to be involved by disseminated fungemia. Invasive biopsy is usually required for diagnosis. The radiologic appearance is nonspecific, and there may be areas of airspace consolidation or nodular opacities.

Cryptococcal pneumonia, much less common than *Aspergillus* pneumonia, usually occurs in patients with defective cellular immunity rather than in neutropenic hosts.

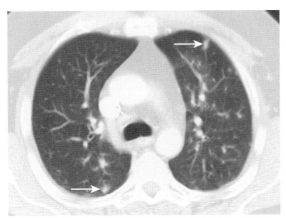

FIGURE 4-2. Invasive aspergillosis. There are multiple, bilateral nodules *(arrows)*, and blood vessels leading to the nodules can be identified in some instances.

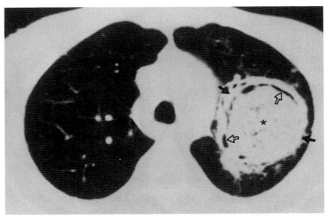

FIGURE 4-3. Invasive aspergillosis in an immunocompromised patient. CR shows a rim of air in the periphery; the air crescent *(open arrows)* separates the central amorphous infarcted lung *(asterisk)* from the rim of inflamed viable lung *(black arrows)*. This appearance is often seen as the patient's white cell count is recovering.

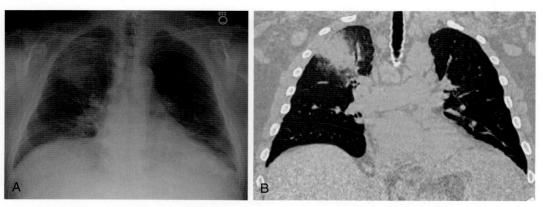

FIGURE 4-4. Mucormycosis. **A,** Standard posteroanterior chest radiograph demonstrates a wedge-shaped area of consolidation in the right upper lobe. **B,** Coronal reformation CT image (lung window setting) shows a halo of ground glass surrounding the right upper lobe consolidation.

Disseminated disease with central nervous system involvement is the rule, and neurologic symptoms may first call attention to the presence of cryptococcal disease. The radiographic manifestations consist of single or multiple nodules with or without cavitation. Well-defined lobar or segmental consolidation is uncommon. *Cryptococcus* may be isolated from the sputum or, more frequently, from the cerebrospinal fluid on lumbar puncture. In some cases, a lung biopsy is required.

Nocardia asteroides is an opportunistic bacterium that causes pneumonia in the compromised host with diseases or conditions in which cellular immunity is depressed. Antecedent corticosteroid therapy is a common history, but white blood cell counts are often normal. *Nocardia* usually does not cause a fulminant, rapidly progressive pulmonary infection. The usual radiologic appearance is that of single or multiple nodules with or without cavitation (Fig. 4-5). They may extend to the pleural surface with associated pleural effusion or chest-wall invasion. The diagnosis can occasionally be made on sputum smears or cultures, but invasive procedures are usually required.

Differential Diagnosis
The differential diagnosis for the radiographic appearance of multiple nodules in the immunocompromised host is rather limited. The appearance may be produced by metastatic disease or occasionally by lymphoma

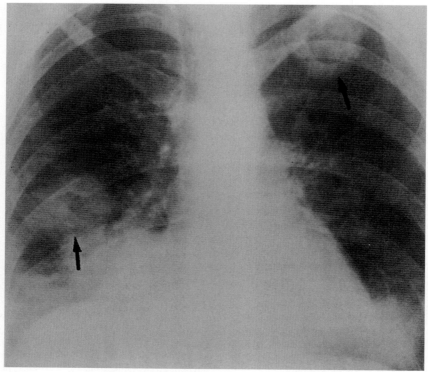

FIGURE 4-5. Nocardiosis in a patient on high-dose steroids. There are multiple nodules, and some are cavitated *(arrows)*.

involving the lung parenchyma. In both instances, rapid growth is usually not a feature. Transplant recipients who receive cyclosporine as a principal immunosuppressive agent may develop an unusual lymphoproliferative disorder in the lung (PTLD). It usually manifests 4 to 6 months after transplantation, although its appearance may be delayed as long as 2 years. The pulmonary manifestations include a solitary mass or multiple pulmonary nodules that are often associated with hilar adenopathy. Multiple organs are frequently involved. The radiographic abnormalities often regress after the reduction of immunosuppression.

Diffuse Lung Disease
Causes

A radiologic pattern of diffuse infiltration of the lungs in the immunocompromised host can be produced by a number of microorganisms, the most common of which are the fungus *Pneumocystis jiroveci* (formerly called *P. carinii*) and a variety of viral agents, including herpes zoster, cytomegalovirus (CMV), and respiratory syncytial virus (RSV). A diffuse interstitial pattern can be seen as a result of nonspecific interstitial pneumonitis, cytotoxic drug reactions, radiation pneumonitis, or lymphangitic spread of tumor.

The prevalence of pneumonia caused by *Pneumocystis jiroveci* has decreased because of widespread prophylaxis in immunocompromised patients with or without HIV infection, but it remains a major cause of morbidity and mortality. Once classified as a protozoan, the organism is now considered to be a fungus. The pneumonia it produces is acute and fulminating. The classic radiographic manifestation is initially a bilateral, perihilar or diffuse, symmetric interstitial pattern, which may have a finely granular, reticular, or ground-glass appearance. If left untreated, it may progress over 3 to 5 days to a homogeneous, diffuse alveolar consolidation (Fig. 4-6). Hilar adenopathy and pleural effusion are distinctly unusual. Computed tomography (CT), particularly high-resolution CT (HRCT), may show areas of disease due to *Pneumocystis* pneumonia when the appearance on a standard chest radiograph is normal. Involved areas of the lung show ground-glass opacification without obliteration of normal pulmonary vessels. Because it is not possible to culture these organisms, the diagnosis depends on morphologic identification of *Pneumocystis* in respiratory secretions obtained by bronchoalveolar lavage or from lung tissue.

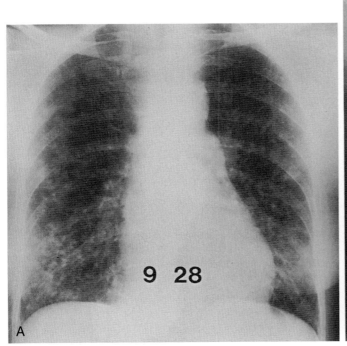
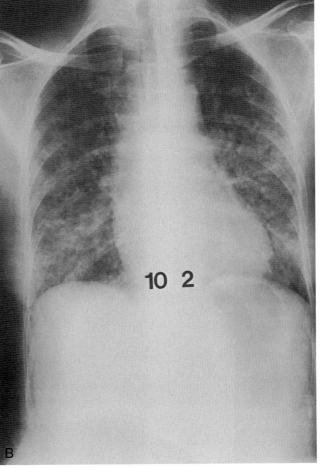

FIGURE 4-6. *Pneumocystis jiroveci* pneumonia in a renal transplant recipient. **A,** The original radiograph shows a diffuse reticulonodular pattern that is more pronounced at the bases. **B,** In 4 days, progression has occurred, producing a more confluent, consolidative pattern.

Viral pneumonias have not been common in immunocompromised patients. Most viral infections in this group are caused by herpes zoster or herpes simplex virus. However, organ transplant recipients are at high risk for viral pneumonia. By far, the most common agent of viral pneumonia in these patients is CMV. Radiographically, CMV pneumonia is characterized by a symmetric, diffuse, bilateral, linear or nodular pattern (Fig. 4-7). It may begin in the lower lobes peripherally and extend superiorly and centrally. Occasionally, unilateral consolidation or a solitary

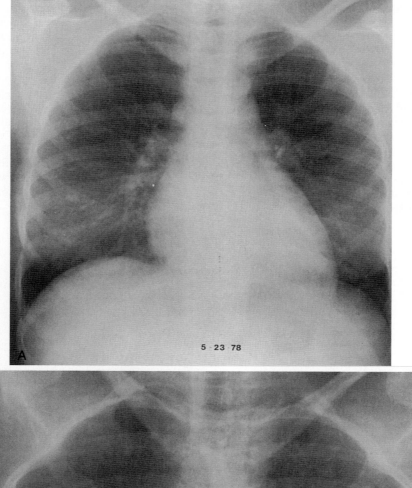

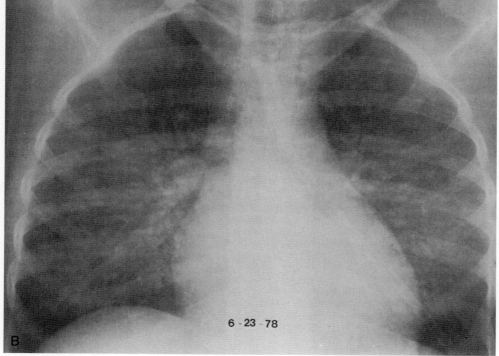

FIGURE 4-7. Cytomegalovirus pneumonia in a renal transplant recipient. **A,** The baseline radiograph is normal. **B,** The posteroanterior radiograph 1 month later demonstrates bilateral reticulonodular opacities in both lungs.

nodule may be identified. Confirmation of the diagnosis usually requires lung biopsy with identification of characteristic intranuclear inclusion bodies or isolation of virus directly from lung tissue.

Other viral organisms, especially RSV, are an important cause of respiratory infection among immunosuppressed patients, especially after hematopoietic stem cell transplantation. The most common CT patterns of RSV infection are extensive ground-glass opacities or a mixture of findings, including ground-glass attenuation, small nodules, and bronchial wall thickening. CT findings may be used to direct bronchoalveolar lavage procedures to enhance their diagnostic yields.

Differential Diagnosis

The noninfectious causes that produce fever and interstitial disease in immunocompromised hosts include lymphangitic spread of tumor, radiation pneumonitis, drug-induced lung toxicity, and the rather ill-defined entity called *nonspecific interstitial pneumonitis*.

Diagnostic and Therapeutic Approach

Two major factors help to narrow the differential diagnosis of fever and new lung disease in the compromised host: the underlying disease process, along with its risk factors and its therapy, and the radiographic patterns of the new lung disease. When these considerations are taken into account and a noninvasive workup is carried out, many patients may be successfully managed without an invasive procedure.

The time course for heightened susceptibility to specific infections is important among certain compromised hosts, especially patients who have received a solid organ or hematopoietic stem cell transplantation. As reviewed in Box 4-1, these subgroups exhibit characteristic periods of susceptibility to specific pathogens.

Standard chest radiography is the basic imaging technique used to detect and evaluate respiratory disease in the immunocompromised patient. In many instances, however, CT may provide additional useful information. CT is more sensitive than standard radiography in identifying early disease and the number of lesions in the lungs. In the immunocompromised host, focal abscesses may be identified on CT in areas that are difficult to evaluate with plain radiographs, including the apical, retrocardiac, and subdiaphragmatic lung. CT also provides a cross-sectional mapping of the extent of the disease; in the immunocompromised patient with diffuse lung disease, this may be useful, particularly as a guide to transbronchial or open lung biopsy.

When bacterial infection is clinically suspected, especially if a focal area of lobar or segmental consolidation is seen on the radiograph, empiric, broad-spectrum antibiotic coverage is recommended for the first 48 hours. If after that time there is no response and if the patient's clinical status permits an invasive procedure, a lung biopsy or lavage is frequently performed. The procedure should be carried out even sooner if there are nodules or cavitary lesions likely to be the result of fungal infection. Fungal and peripheral lesions are best approached by percutaneous needle biopsy; larger areas of consolidation are assessed by needle biopsy or transbronchial biopsy with the use of a fiberoptic bronchoscope. The radiologist therefore

Box 4-1. Time Course for Susceptibility to Specific Organisms after Solid Organ and Hematopoietic Stem Cell Transplantation

SOLID ORGAN TRANSPLANTATION

1 month
    Nosocomial bacterial infections (e.g., gram-negative bacilli, *Staphylococcus aureus*)
2 to 6 months
    Viruses (e.g., cytomegalovirus) and opportunistic fungi (e.g., *Aspergillus*, *Pneumocystis*)
>6 months
    Community-acquired bacterial pneumonia
    Opportunistic infections less common unless coexisting graft-versus-host disease present

HEMATOPOIETIC STEM CELL TRANSPLANTATION

1st month (early neutropenic phase after marrow ablative therapy)
    Opportunistic fungi (e.g., *Aspergillus*)
    Nosocomial bacterial infections (especially gram-negative bacilli)
2 to 4 months (marrow engraftment and neutrophil recovery phase)
    Viruses (e.g., cytomegalovirus) and opportunistic fungi (e.g., *Aspergillus*, *Pneumocystis*)
>4 months
    Community-acquired bacterial pneumonia
    Opportunistic fungi (e.g., *Aspergillus*) in setting of chronic graft-versus-host disease

performs an important function in the diagnostic approach to focal, solid or cavitary lesions in the lung. For percutaneous biopsy, thin-walled, 18- to 22-gauge needles are preferred. Needle aspiration biopsies can be performed under fluoroscopic or CT guidance. These procedures are contraindicated in immunocompromised patients with low platelet counts.

Pneumocystis pneumonia is one of the leading diagnostic possibilities when bilateral, diffuse disease is viewed on the chest radiograph. An empiric course of trimethoprim-sulfamethoxazole can be employed, but a specific diagnosis often is required. Bronchial lavage or, less frequently, transbronchial and video-assisted lung biopsy are the preferred approaches.

■■■ PULMONARY DISEASE IN PERSONS WITH ACQUIRED IMMUNODEFICIENCY SYNDROME

Epidemiology

There are more than 1 million cases of acquired immunodeficiency syndrome (AIDS) in the United States, and one half of all new infections occur in people 25 years old or younger. Worldwide, more than 40 million people are living with HIV infection or AIDS, and nearly 75% of infected individuals are located in sub-Saharan Africa. The Centers for Disease Control and Prevention (CDC) defines active cases of AIDS by HIV seropositivity plus a number of accompanying conditions, including opportunistic infections, HIV encephalopathy, and the wasting syndrome. The definition also includes HIV seropositivity plus pulmonary tuberculosis, recurrent bacterial pneumonias, invasive cervical carcinoma, and a CD4 cell count less than 200 cells/mm².

Since the emergence of the AIDS more than 25 years ago, the most impressive therapeutic advance has been the introduction of highly active antiretroviral therapy (HAART), a combination therapy composed of a three-drug regimen of HIV protease inhibitors and nucleoside analogue reverse transcriptase inhibitors. HAART has been associated with a dramatic reduction in HIV-associated morbidity and mortality among patients with access to this treatment. By suppressing viral replication, it decreases the viral load and increases the CD4 cell count. Patients receiving HAART have a reduced prevalence of opportunistic infections and certain neoplasms. Table 4-2 summarizes the radiographic patterns in AIDS pulmonary disease.

Pulmonary Diseases

Major categories of disease involving the lungs include infections; neoplastic entities, such as Kaposi's sarcoma, lymphoma, and lung cancer; and lymphoproliferative disorders

Infections
Infections in AIDS patients are outlined in Box 4-2.

Fungal Infections
The most common fungal infection is *Pneumocystis jiroveci* pneumonia . Despite a substantial decline in prevalence because of widespread prophylaxis, *Pneumocystis* pneumonia is still the most common life-threatening opportunistic respiratory infection in patients with HIV or AIDS. It occurs predominantly in patients with a CD4 count less than 200 cells/mm². The diagnosis can often be made on induced sputum samples or bronchoalveolar lavage. Several polymerase chain reaction (PCR)–based molecular assays have been developed to aid the diagnosis of this organism, which cannot be grown in culture.

Radiographic features include most commonly a diffuse reticular or consolidative process, which may be perihilar or diffuse (Fig. 4-8). The CT appearance usually consists of diffuse ground-glass opacities, which may be identified even when the radiograph is normal (Fig. 4-9). Atypical manifestations include nodules, focal lesions, adenopathy, and miliary disease. Cystic lung disease occurs in at least 10%, and pneumothorax may be a complicating factor (Figs. 4-10 and 4-11). These pneumothoraces are often refractory to chest tube drainage and are associated with an increased mortality rate.

Other fungal infections are rare and account for less than 5% of pneumonias in HIV-positive patients, although a higher prevalence may be observed in endemic areas. They include infections with *Cryptococcus*, *Candida*, *Histoplasma*, *Aspergillus*, and *Coccidioides*, and they often take the form of disseminated disease. Radiologic findings are nonspecific, and pleural effusions are common, as is adenopathy, which is rare with *Pneumocystis* pneumonia and bacterial pneumonias. Cryptococcal infection is the fourth most common opportunistic infection and the most common fungal infection, occurring in 6% to 13% of AIDS patients. Meningoencephalitis is the most common form, and the lungs are the most common sites of involvement outside the central nervous system. Radiologic features include discrete nodules with or without cavitation. Pleural effusions are common, and adenopathy may occur. Histoplasmosis is important in the HIV-positive patient in endemic areas. *Histoplasma* lung disease usually represents a disseminated infection, and the typical radiographic pattern is micronodular (miliary).

Bacterial Infections
Bacterial respiratory infections, including infectious airways disease and pneumonia, are the most common cause of respiratory infections in HIV-infected individuals in developed countries. Bacterial pneumonia is often one of the earliest manifestations of HIV infection. However, it may affect patients at any stage of HIV infection, and the risk for bacterial infection increases with declining immune function.

TABLE 4-2 Radiographic Patterns of Pulmonary Disease in AIDS Patients

Diffuse Infiltrative Disease		Nodules	Effusion			Adenopathy			Focal or Lobar Consolidation	
Common	Less Common		Common	Less Common	Uncommon	Common	Less Common	Uncommon	Common	Uncommon
PCP	Disseminated MTb, MAC	KS	KS	Bacterial pneumonia	PCP	MTb	Fungal	PCP	Bacterial pneumonia	PCP
LIP	Viral	Septic infarcts	MTb	MAC	Viral	KS	MAC	Viral	MTb	MAC
KS	Disseminated fungal	MTb	Lymphoma		Fungal		Lymphoma	LIP ± cavitation		
	Strongyloides	Fungal						Fungal ± cavitation		
		Lymphoma								

KS, Kaposi's syndrome; LIP, lymphocytic interstitial pneumonitis; MAC, *Mycobacterium avium* complex; MTb, *Mycobacterium tuberculosis*; PCP, *Pneumocystis jiroveci* pneumonia.

Box 4-2. Infections in Persons with Acquired Immunodeficiency Syndrome

PNEUMOCYSTIS JIROVECI PNEUMONIA

Characteristics
Fungus
CD4 count < 200 cells/mm²
Incidence decreasing because of prophylaxis

Radiologic Features
Diffuse reticular or consolidative process
Ground-glass appearance early on CT
Atypical features
Nodules
Adenopathy
Miliary disease
Cysts

FUNGAL INFECTIONS

Characteristics
Less than 5% of pneumonias
Cryptococcus most common organism
Central nervous system involvement

Radiographic Features
Nodules with or without cavitation
Pleural effusions
Adenopathy
Disseminated disease: miliary pattern,
  histoplasmosis

BACTERIAL PNEUMONIAS

Characteristics
Most common respiratory infection in AIDS
patients
Streptococcus pneumoniae (pneumococcal disease),
  Haemophilus influenzae, *Staphylococcus*, gram-negative
  organisms

Radiographic Features
Focal consolidation
Cavitary nodules

MYCOBACTERIAL INFECTIONS

Tuberculosis

Characteristics
10% have CD4 count < 200 cells/mm²
Occasionally multidrug resistant
Dissemination common

Radiographic Features
CD4 count < 200 cells/mm²
  Adenopathy (CT-enhancing rim)
  Basilar consolidation
CD4 > 200 cells/mm²
  Pattern of reactivation
  Disseminated (miliary pattern)

Mycobacterium avium Complex (MAC)

Characteristics
Disseminated disease
Severe immunodeficiency
5% pulmonary involvement

Radiographic Features
Adenopathy
Nodules
Focal consolidation (cavitation)

VIRAL PNEUMONIAS

Cytomegalovirus

Characteristics
Usually not sole pulmonary pathogen
Radiographic Findings
Diffuse reticulonodular opacities
CT findings
  Ground-glass appearance
  Linear opacities
  Nodules
  Consolidation

Pathogens are of the common types seen in the general population. Community-acquired organisms, such as pneumococcus, *Haemophilus influenzae*, *Staphylococcus*, and gram-negative bacteria, are identified. *Pseudomonas* also has been recognized as an important cause of pulmonary infection among patients with a recent history of hospitalization, antibiotic use, or steroid therapy. Atypical pneumonias, such as those caused by *Legionella* and *Mycoplasma*, are only rarely seen in patients with HIV or AIDS. Two episodes of bacterial pneumonia within a 12-month period in an HIV-positive patient define the presence of AIDS. Similar to its presentation in the general population, bacterial pneumonia typically is seen radiographically as focal consolidation in a segmental or lobar distribution. However, in HIV-positive patients, there is a higher propensity for multilobar and bilateral disease. Bacterial infection may also manifest as cavitary nodules. This pattern usually results from infection with *Pseudomonas aeruginosa* or *Staphylococcus aureus*. The latter organism is usually responsible for septic emboli, which typically occur in patients with a history of intravenous drug use.

HIV-infected patients are also at increased risk for developing infectious airways disease, such as bacterial tracheobronchitis and bronchiolitis. Chest radiographs are usually normal, but they may demonstrate bronchial wall thickening or a subtle reticulonodular pattern. Chest CT, particularly HRCT, is more sensitive than radiographs for detecting inflammatory changes of the bronchi and bronchioles, and it may demonstrate bronchial wall thickening and a tree-in-bud pattern even when the chest radiograph appears normal.

Mycobacterial infections can be seen with tuberculosis or atypical mycobacteria, including *Mycobacterium avium-intracellulare* (MAC) and *Mycobacterium kansasii* organisms. Seventy percent of HIV-positive patients with tuberculosis have CD4 counts less than 200 cells/mm². Drug prophylaxis (i.e., isoniazid [INH]) is effective in preventing tuberculosis in HIV-positive patients. The radiologic pattern depends on early or late onset relative to waning immunity. In the late stages of full-blown AIDS, features are similar to primary tuberculosis with adenopathy and lower lobe disease. Hematogenous dissemination

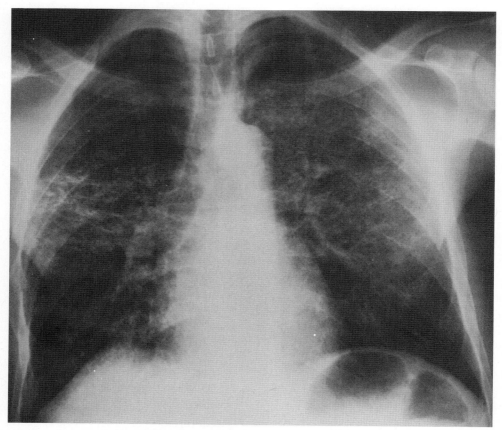

FIGURE 4-8. *Pneumocystis jiroveci* pneumonia in an AIDS patient. The posteroanterior view shows bilateral reticular opacities fanning out from the hila to the periphery.

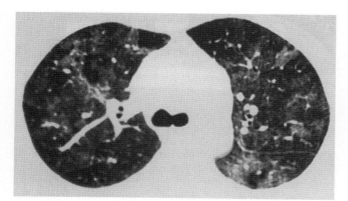

FIGURE 4-9. *Pneumocystis jiroveci* pneumonia in an AIDS patient. There are diffuse, patchy, ground-glass opacities. Notice that the pulmonary vessels can still be identified in the areas of opacification.

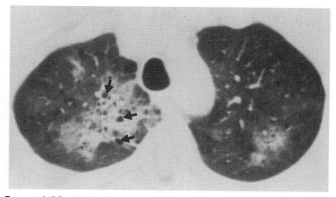

FIGURE 4-10. PCP pneumonia. CT of a patient with *Pneumocystis* pneumonia. There are small cysts in the more severely affected right upper lobe *(arrows)*. (Courtesy of Georgann McGuiness, M.D., New York University Medical Center, New York, NY.)

is common. On CT, the adenopathy often is characterized by an enhancing rim with a necrotic center (Fig. 4-12). In contrast, in patients with CD4 counts higher than 200 cells/mm², an upper lobe distribution similar to classic reactivation tuberculosis is frequently identified (Fig. 4-13). Compared with normal hosts, AIDS patients with tuberculosis are more likely to present with diffuse lung disease, bronchogenic spread, miliary disease, and

extrapulmonary disease. The chest radiograph may be normal for up to 20% of patients with tuberculosis who are in the advanced stages of AIDS.

MAC is a disseminated disease in persons with AIDS, with the gastrointestinal tract serving as the main entry site in most cases. Only 5% have pulmonary involvement. Radiologic manifestations include adenopathy, nodules, and focal consolidation with cavitation.

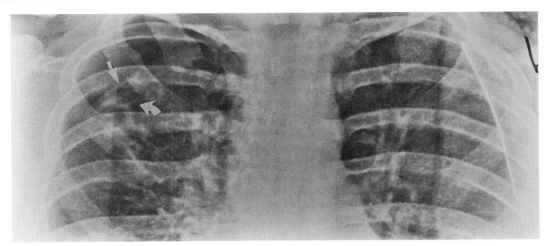

FIGURE 4-11. Pneumothorax complicating *Pneumocystis jiroveci* pneumonia. There is a right apical pneumothorax *(arrow)*. Multiple cysts can be identified in the underlying lung *(curved arrow)*.

Patients receiving HAART may exhibit a paradoxical symptomatic deterioration of preexisting untreated or partially treated opportunistic infections after HAART-induced recovery of the immune response. This phenomenon is referred to as immune reconstitution (or restoration) disease. Mycobacteria are the most commonly implicated infectious organisms in this syndrome. Immune reconstitution disease should be considered when a patient recently started on HAART develops fever accompanied by new thoracic abnormalities, such as lymphadenopathy, parenchymal consolidation, or pleural effusion. Treatment is aimed at the underlying infection, but severely symptomatic patients may also benefit from steroid therapy.

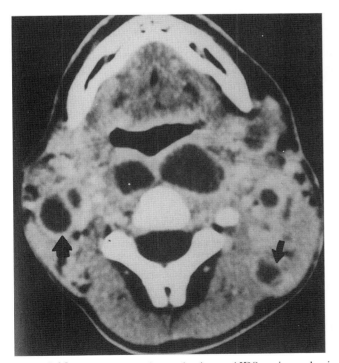

FIGURE 4-12. Tuberculous adenopathy in an AIDS patient who is severely immunocompromised (CD4 count = 100 cells/mm³). Contrast-enhanced CT of the neck shows many enlarged nodes with enhancing rims and necrotic centers *(arrows)*.

Viral Infection

Viral infections are a rare cause of significant clinical disease in HIV-positive patients. Most cases of viral disease are caused by CMV and are usually reactivations of latent infection. Although frequently recovered from the lungs, CMV is not considered a significant pathogen in most cases. Clinically significant cases of CMV pneumonitis may rarely occur, typically in the setting of advanced immune suppression and extrathoracic CMV infection. CT findings include ground-glass attenuation, dense consolidation, nodules, bronchial wall thickening or bronchiectasis, and diffuse linear opacities.

Neoplasms

Neoplasms occurring in AIDS patients are summarized in Box 4-3.

Kaposi's Sarcoma

Kaposi's sarcoma remains the most common malignancy in AIDS patients worldwide, but its prevalence has markedly declined in the Western world with the use of HAART. It is mostly seen in the homosexual population and is associated with the human herpesvirus 8 (HHV8), also referred to as Kaposi's sarcoma herpesvirus. One third of AIDS patients with Kaposi's sarcoma have pulmonary involvement, and in 10% to 15% of cases, it is clinically apparent. Pulmonary involvement is associated with mucocutaneous involvement in 85% of cases. Most patients with pulmonary involvement have CD4 counts less than 100 cells/mm².

Radiographic features include two major patterns: perihilar interstitial disease and multiple nodules (Figs. 4-14 and 4-15). Pleural effusions are common, and enhancing lymphadenopathy is a common feature. On HRCT, the pattern consists of an axial distribution of nodular or more confluent opacities, with thickening of the bronchovascular bundles. Thickened interlobular septa are frequently observed (see Fig. 4-15C).

Lymphoma

Lymphoma typically is seen in the late stages of AIDS and is usually disseminated at the time of diagnosis, involving

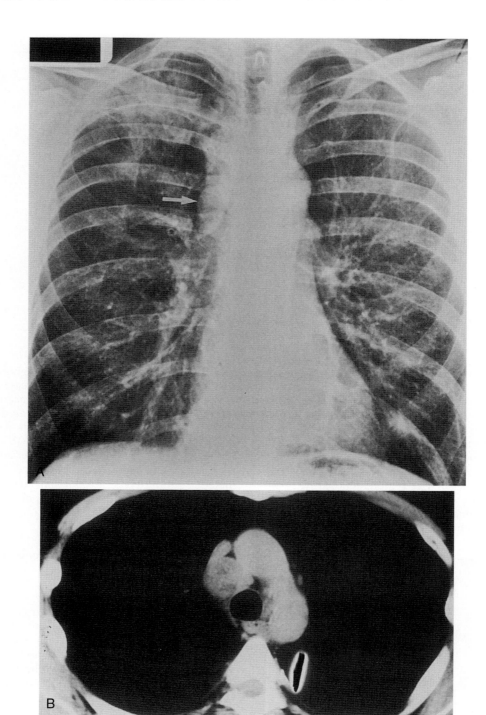

FIGURE 4-13. Tuberculosis in an AIDS patient. **A,** The standard radiograph demonstrates right apical opacity. There is also right paratracheal adenopathy *(arrow).* **B,** The adenopathy is confirmed on a CT scan. The CD4 count was 350 cells/mm³.

Box 4-3. **Neoplasms in AIDS Patients**

KAPOSI'S SARCOMA	LYMPHOMA
Characteristics	**Characteristics**
Most common malignancy	Disseminated disease
Homosexual population	Extranodal
Mucocutaneous involvement	B-cell malignancies
Radiographic Features	**Radiographic Features**
Perihilar interstitial disease (CT shows axial nodular thickening)	Bilateral diffuse opacities
Multiple nodules	Discrete nodules
Lymphadenopathy (enhancing)	Pleural effusion
Pleural effusion	Adenopathy less common

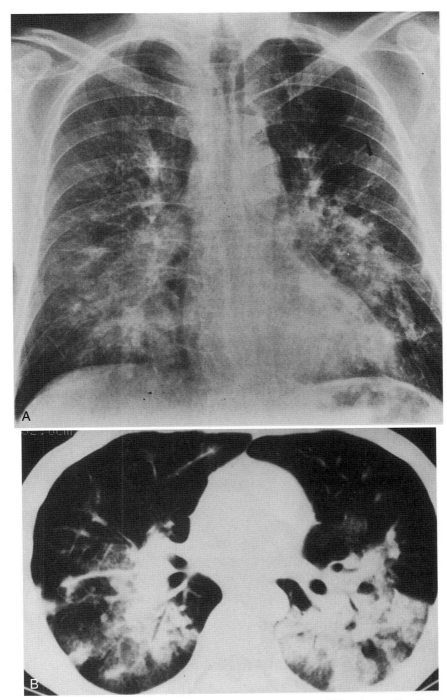

FIGURE 4-14. Kaposi's sarcoma. **A,** The standard posteroanterior radiograph demonstrates a diffuse abnormality characterized by central confluent opacities and ill-defined nodules. **B,** CT shows the central distribution of tumor, which is spreading from the hila along the bronchovascular bundles.

the central nervous system, liver, or gastrointestinal tract. It is usually extranodal in distribution, and 25% of patients have thoracic involvement. The prognosis is extremely poor. It is typically a B-cell lymphoma, associated with Epstein-Barr virus. Radiologically, lymphoma may manifest as nonspecific, bilateral, diffuse opacities; discrete nodules or masses; or pleural effusions. Mediastinal adenopathy may occur, but it is less common than in non-AIDS patients.

Lung Cancer
Although not considered an AIDS-related neoplasm, the overall rate of lung cancer is increased among patients infected with HIV with a history of cigarette smoking compared with the general population of smokers. Unlike Kaposi's sarcoma and lymphoma, there is no association with progressive immunosuppression. Lung cancer may occur at any stage of HIV infection. Patients with lung cancer and HIV infection are often younger and present at

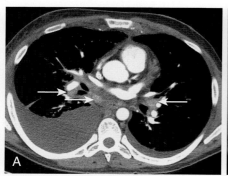
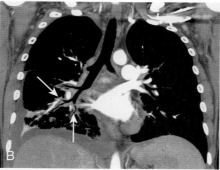
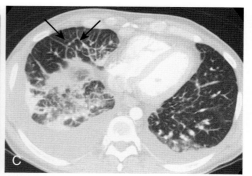

Figure 4-15. Kaposi's sarcoma. **A,** Axial CT shows enhancing hilar and subcarinal lymph nodes *(arrows)*. Notice the bilateral pleural effusions. **B,** Coronal reformation CT image shows characteristic thickening of bronchovascular bundles *(arrows)*. **C,** Axial CT (lung window setting) demonstrates marked interlobular septal thickening *(arrows)*.

a more advanced stage of disease compared with the general population. However, the thoracic radiologic manifestations of lung cancer in HIV are similar to those in the general population and include a lung nodule or mass, often accompanied by intrathoracic lymphadenopathy.

Lymphoproliferative Disorders

Lymphoproliferative disorders include lymphocytic interstitial pneumonitis (LIP) atypical lymphoproliferative disorder, and mucosa-associated lymphoid tissue (MALT).

LIP is a diffuse pulmonary disorder characterized by infiltration of the interstitium by lymphocytes, plasma cells, and histiocytes. It is thought to represent a lymphoid hyperplasia in response to chronic antigenic stimulus by the HIV. It is much more common in children. Radiologic findings include a diffuse pattern with nodules less than 3 mm in diameter or a reticulonodular pattern (Fig. 4-16). CT can reveal a variety of findings, including micronodules, thickening of the bronchovascular bundles and interlobular septa, and small cysts. Less common is patchy airspace disease. LIP is steroid responsive and not premalignant.

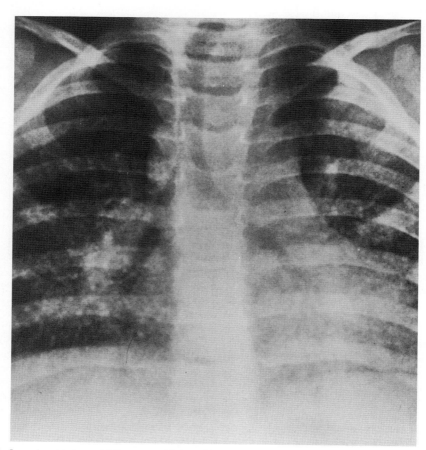

Figure 4-16. Lymphocytic interstitial pneumonitis in a child with AIDS. Diffuse, small nodules can be seen bilaterally.

Atypical lymphoproliferative disorder is characterized by infiltration of the interstitium by a polymorphous population of atypical cells. MALT is characterized by infiltration of the bronchial epithelium by atypical lymphoid tissue.

Other Pulmonary Disorders

Other pulmonary disorders that may be observed in patients with HIV infection or AIDS include nonspecific interstitial pneumonitis, bronchiolitis obliterans, cryptogenic organizing pneumonia, emphysema, and bronchiectasis. These entities have similar manifestations in HIV-infected patients and the general population, and they are discussed separately in other chapters.

▬ SUGGESTED READINGS

Albelda, S.M., Talbot, G.H., Gerson, S.L., et al., 1985. Pulmonary cavitation and massive hemoptysis in invasive pulmonary aspergillosis. Influence of bone marrow recovery in patients with acute leukemia. Am. Rev. Respir. Dis. 131, 115–118.

Aviram, G., Fishman, J.E., Boiselle, P.M., 2007. Thoracic infections in human immunodeficiency virus/acquired immune deficiency syndrome. Semin. Roentgenol. 42, 23–36.

Bergin, C.J., Wirth, R.L., Berry, G.J, et al., 1990. *Pneumocystis carinii* pneumonia: CT and HRCT observations. J. Comput. Assist. Tomogr. 14, 756–759.

Boiselle, P.M., Aviram, G., Fishman, J.E., 2002. Update on lung disease in AIDS. Semin. Roentgenol. 37, 54–71.

Castellino, R.A., Blank, R.N., 1979. Etiologic diagnosis of focal pulmonary infection in immunocompromised patients by fluoroscopically guided percutaneous needle aspiration. Radiology 132, 563–567.

Centers for Disease Control (CDC), 2006. HIV/AIDS Surveillance Report, 2005, US Department of Health and Human Services, CDC, Atlanta, pp. 1–46.

Cheung, M.C., Pantanowitz, L., Dezube, B.J., 2005. AIDS-related malignancies: emerging challenges in the era of highly active antiretroviral therapy. Oncologist 10, 412–426.

Curtis, A.M., Smith, G.J.W., Ravin, C.E., 1979. Air crescent sign of invasive aspergillosis. Radiology 133, 17–21.

Fanta, C.H., Pennington, J.E., 1981. Fever and new lung infiltrates in the immunocompromised host. Clin. Chest. Med. 2, 19–25.

Franquet, T., Rodriguez, S., Martino, R., et al., 2006. Thin-section CT findings in hematopoietic stem cell transplantation recipients with respiratory viral pneumonia. AJR. Am. J. Roentgenol. 187, 1085–1090.

Goodman, P.C., Broaduss, V.C., Hopewell, P.C., 1984. Chest radiographic patterns in the acquired immunodeficiency syndrome. Am. Rev. Respir. Dis. 129, 365.

Hirschtick, R.E., Glassroth, J., Jordan, M.C., et al., 1995. Bacterial pneumonia in persons infected with the human immunodeficiency virus. N. Engl. J. Med. 333, 845–851.

Huang, L., Morris, A., Limper, A.H., Beck, J.M., 2006. An official ATS workshop summary: recent advances and future directions in *Pneumocystis* pneumonia (PCP). Proc. Am. Thorac. Soc. 3, 655–664.

Kotloff, R.M., Ahya, V.N., Crawford, S.W., 2004. Pulmonary complications of solid organ and hematopoietic stem cell transplantation. Am. J. Respir. Crit. Care. Med. 170, 22–48.

Kuhlman, J.E., Kavuru, M., Fishman, EK, et al., 1990. *Pneumocystis carinii* pneumonia: spectrum of parenchymal CT findings. Radiology 175, 711–714.

Lerner, P.I., 1994. Pneumonia due to *Actinomyces*, *Propionibacterium* and *Nocardia*. In: Pennington, J.E. (Ed.), Respiratory Infections—Diagnosis and Management. third ed. Raven Press, New York, pp. 615–631.

McGuinness, G., Scholes, J.V., Garay, S.M., et al., 1994. Cytomegalovirus pneumonitis: spectrum of parenchymal CT findings with pathologic correlation in 21 AIDS patients. Radiology 192, 451–459.

McLoud, T.C., 1989. Pulmonary infections in the immunocompromised host. Radiol. Clin. North. Am. 27, 1059–1066.

McLoud, T.C., Naidich, D.P., 1992. Thoracic disease in the immunocompromised patient. Radiol. Clin. North. Am. 30, 525–554.

Ognibene, F.P., Pass, H.I., Roth, J.A., et al., 1988. Role of imaging and interventional techniques in the diagnosis of respiratory disease in the immunocompromised host. J. Thorac. Imaging. 3, 1–20.

Partnik, B.L., Leung, A.N., Herold, C.J., 2004. Pulmonary infections: imaging with MDCT. In: Schoepf, U.J. (Ed.), Multidetector-Row CT of the Thorax. Springer-Verlag, Berlin, pp. 107–120.

Patz, E.F., Goodman, P.C., 1992. Pulmonary cryptococcosis. J. Thorac. Imaging. 7, 51–55.

Sider, L., Gabriel, H., Curry, D.R., et al., 1993. Pattern recognition of the pulmonary manifestations of AIDS on CT scans. Radiographics 13, 771–784.

Singer, C., Armstrong, D., Rosen, R.P., et al., 1979. Diffuse pulmonary infiltrates in immunosuppressed patients: prospective study of 80 cases. Am. J. Med. 66, 110–114.

Thomas, C.F., Limper, A.H., 2004. *Pneumocystis* pneumonia. N. Engl. J. Med. 350, 2487–2498.

CHAPTER 5

Radiography for the Critical Care Patient

Beatrice Trotman-Dickenson

Introduction of the picture archiving and communication system (PACS) and advances in imaging technology have revolutionized intensive care radiology. PACS has significantly improved the quality of images, accessibility, delivery, and reporting time. The development of multidetector-row computed tomography (CT) scanners with very rapid acquisition times enables even dyspneic patients to be successfully imaged. CT imaging provides more accurate assessment of disease than the supine radiograph and frequently reveals unsuspected pathology. With the introduction of image-guided interventional procedures, the radiologist has become an increasingly active member of the intensive care patient's clinical team for diagnostic and therapeutic purposes.

The interpretation of the chest radiograph of the intensive care patient is a challenging exercise. A wide spectrum of pulmonary and pleural abnormalities may occur, and their radiographic appearances are complicated by several coexisting pathologies. Unraveling the various components is hindered by the supine projection of most radiographs, the variability of serial radiographs due to technique, and the multitude of tubes, lines, and other devices partially obscuring the underlying lungs.

For a safe and logical approach, the radiologist should first determine the nature and location of all the support devices, such as tubes and lines (Table 5-1). Incorrect positioning is an important cause of morbidity. A systematic review of the lungs, pleura, and mediastinum ensures that all important observations are made. Interpretation may be difficult, because the radiographic features are often nonspecific, and it is therefore important to have as much clinical information as possible and the aid of prior radiographs. Additional radiographic studies, such as decubitus views, ultrasound, or CT, often help to clarify a difficult interpretation or a suspected clinical problem.

■ SUPPORT DEVICES

Endotracheal Tube

Malposition occurs in about 15% of placements, with emergency intubation having the highest complication rates. Physical examination is an unreliable guide to correct tube location, and a chest radiograph is required for confirmation. Correct placement of the endotracheal tube can be determined by the location of the tube tip relative to the carina. Ideally, the tip should be within 5 to 7 cm of the carina, with the head in the neutral position (i.e., inferior border of the mandible projected over the C5 and C6 vertebra). During flexion and extension of the cervical spine, the tip of the endotracheal tube may vary by a distance of 2 cm. The endotracheal tube should be at least 3 cm distal to the cords. A location that is too high may result in inadvertent extubation or may damage to the vocal cords. A position that is too low results in endobronchial intubation, occurring on the right more frequently than the left (Fig. 5-1). This may result in overinflation and possibly pneumothorax on the intubated side and atelectasis of the opposite lung.

Esophageal intubation may be recognized by the margins of the endotracheal tube lying lateral to the tracheal air column and gaseous gastric distention. A right posterior oblique chest radiograph displaces the trachea to the right of the esophagus and allows recognition of the esophageal intubation (Fig. 5-2). The optimal width of the tube should be one half to two thirds of the width of the tracheal lumen, and the inflated cuff should not distend the tracheal wall. After a tracheostomy, the tube tip is ideally situated between one half and two thirds of the distance from the stoma to the carina. The width of the tube should be approximately two thirds of the width of the trachea, and the tip should not be wedged against the tracheal wall.

Tracheal laceration due to the endotracheal tube may result in pneumomediastinum, pneumothorax, or subcutaneous emphysema, singly or in combination. The tip of the endotracheal tube may be deviated to the right of the tracheal lumen.

TABLE 5-1 Correct Positioning for Tubes and Lines

Tube or Line	Location
Endotracheal tube	5 to 7 cm above the carina
Nasogastric tube	Side holes or tip below the left hemidiaphragm in the stomach
Central venous pressure catheter	Superior vena cava
Pulmonary artery line	Pulmonary artery within 2 cm of the hilum
Intra-aortic counterpulsation balloon catheter	Just below the superior aortic knob contour
Cardiac pacemaker (right ventricular lead)	Posteroanterior view: projected over the cardiac apex; lateral view: lies anterior and inferior (behind sternum)
Automatic implantable cardioverter-defibrillator	Proximal lead: superior vena cava; distal lead: right ventricle; patch: left chest wall or on pericardial surface
Pleural drainage tubes	Midaxillary, sixth to eighth interspace directed anterosuperiorly (pneumonectomy) or directed posteroinferiorly (effusion)

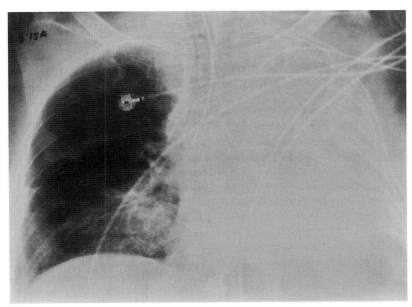

FIGURE 5-1. Right main bronchus intubation. The endotracheal tube lies within the right main bronchus, resulting in complete collapse of the left lung. The patient has right lower lobe pneumonia.

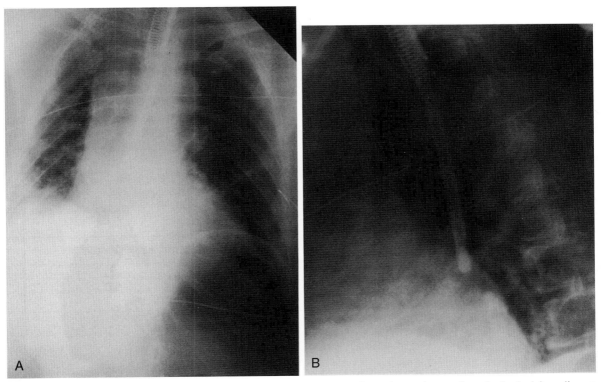

FIGURE 5-2. Endotracheal tube intubation of the esophagus. **A,** The anteroposterior radiograph reveals an endotracheal tube lying adjacent and parallel with an esophageal stethoscope and shows gross gastric gaseous distention. **B,** An oblique lateral radiograph confirms esophageal intubation with the endotracheal tube.

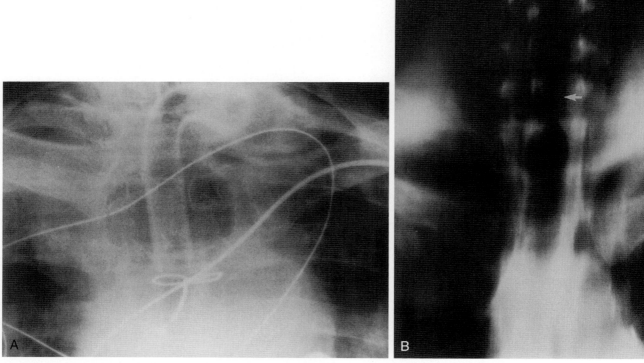

Figure 5-3. Tracheal stricture. **A,** The cuff of the tracheostomy tube is overinflated. **B,** Coronal tomogram shows that overinflation results in a tracheal stricture *(arrow).*

Inflation of the cuff by more than 2.8 cm (normal diameter is 2 to 2.5 cm) can cause tracheal laceration, as can positioning of the lower margin of the cuff at less than 1.3 cm from the tube tip (normal distance is 2.5 cm). Tracheal stenosis may occur at the tracheostomy stoma or at the endotracheal tube tip (Fig. 5-3). At the stoma, stenosis is caused by the formation of granulation tissue or by fibrosis with destruction of the tracheal cartilage. At the cuff site, stenosis results from a circumferential scar that is 1 to 4 cm long and that is typically 1.5 cm below the stoma.

Nasogastric Tube and Feeding Tube

Incorrect positioning of a nasogastric tube is the most common tube complication (Fig. 5-4). Radiographic confirmation of correct positioning is mandatory before suction or feedings begin. The tube may be seen lodged within the tracheobronchial tree or coiled with the larynx or pharynx. More commonly, the tube lies too high in the esophagus above the gastroesophageal junction (Fig. 5-5). On many tubes, the side holes extend for a distance of 10 cm from the tip, and at least 10 cm of tubing should be seen within the stomach. Side holes above the gastroesophageal junction place the patient at risk for aspiration of gastric contents. Feeding tubes should be positioned in the duodenum to reduce the risk of gastroesophageal reflux of feedings and aspiration. The enteroflex

tube is inserted over a wire, and perforation of the esophagus or stomach is a potential hazard. The stiff stylet may inadvertently enter the lung and cause a pneumothorax (Fig. 5-6). Complications associated with the nasogastric and feeding tubes are listed in Box 5-1.

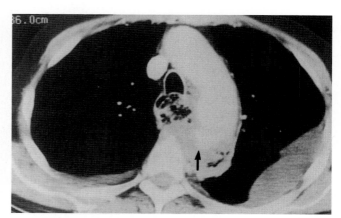

Figure 5-4. Esophageal perforation due to a nasogastric tube. Contrast-enhanced CT demonstrates a complex paraesophageal mass containing air and representing a mediastinal abscess. The abscess invades the posterior wall of the aortic arch, resulting in a mycotic aneurysm *(arrow).* Bilateral pleural effusions can be seen.

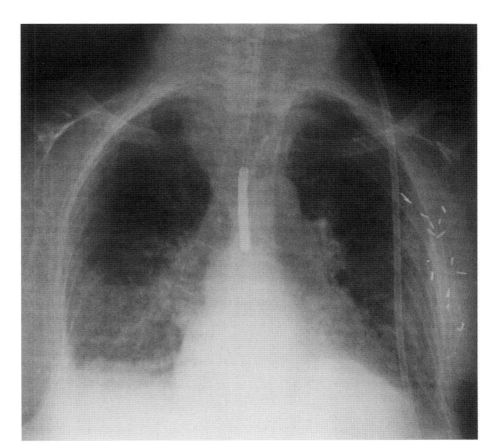

FIGURE 5-5. Intrathoracic nasogastric tube. The nasogastric tube lies too proximal, with the tip lying within the middle esophagus. Bilateral lower lobe consolidation is caused by aspiration pneumonia. Left axillary surgery has been performed.

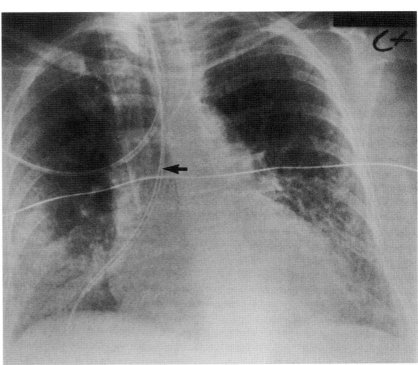

FIGURE 5-6. Endobronchial enteroflex feeding tube. The guidewire and feeding tube have passed through the right main bronchus *(arrow)* into the lower lobe bronchus and out through the diaphragmatic pleura. A follow-up radiograph showed a right pneumothorax. A right internal jugular catheter sheath lies with the tip within the superior vena cava.

Box 5-1. **Nasogastric and Feeding Tube Complications**

Aspiration pneumonia
Pulmonary abscess
Pneumothorax
Esophageal or gastric perforation

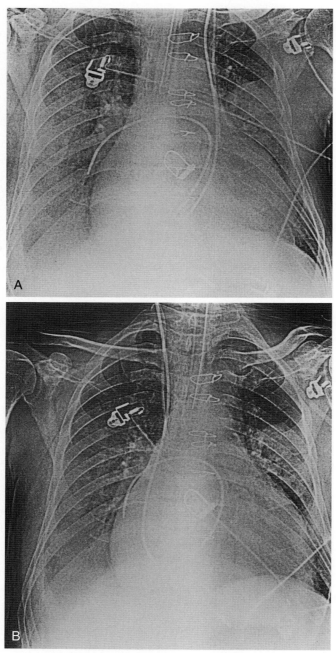

FIGURE 5-7. Digital photographs show a left-sided superior vena cava (SVC) with a right SVC. **A,** The pulmonary artery catheter has entered a left SVC and passed through the coronary sinus into the right atrium and out into the right pulmonary artery. **B,** In the same patient, a right internal jugular approach demonstrated a right SVC.

Central Venous Catheter

Central venous catheters are used routinely in the management of critically ill patients for venous access and measurement of intravascular blood volume (i.e., central venous pressure). Up to 40% of catheters are malpositioned. The catheters are usually placed through the subclavian or internal jugular vein. The optimal site for the catheter tip is within the superior vena cava, identified on the frontal view as at the level of the first anterior intercostal space. A catheter within the brachiocephalic veins produces inaccurate central venous pressure measurements due to interference by the proximal venous valves, and positioning within the right atrium is associated with a risk of cardiac perforation and arrhythmias. A catheter that follows a left anterior paramediastinal course is most likely in a left-sided superior vena cava (Fig. 5-7). This venous anomaly occurs in 0.3% of the population, and is usually associated with a right-sided superior vena cava. The left superior vena cava drains into the right atrium by way of the coronary sinus (Fig. 5-8). Catheter placement in an arterial vessel is usually clinically suspected because of the pulsatile flow through the catheter. This may be confirmed on the chest radiograph by the course of the catheter following the major arterial vessels.

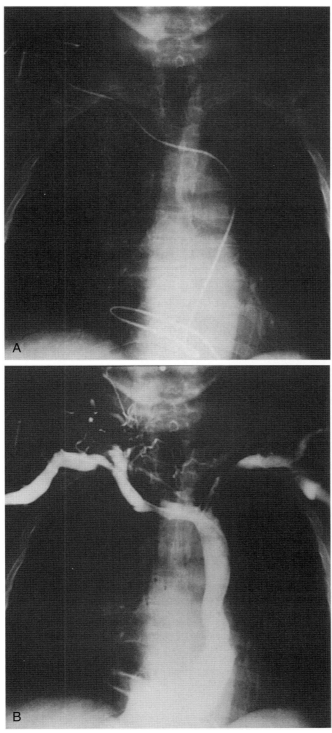

FIGURE 5-8. Left-sided superior vena cava (SVC) with an absent right SVC. **A,** The posteroanterior radiograph reveals a right pacing lead introduced with a right subclavian approach that crosses the midline and descends along the left mediastinal border before crossing over to the right at the base of the heart. **B,** Venogram confirms an absent right SVC, with the subclavian veins draining into a left SVC and then into the coronary sinus.

Pneumothorax is a common complication of line insertion, occurring in up to 5% of patients, particularly after using a subclavian approach. The pneumothorax is often difficult to detect clinically, and a chest radiograph with the patient preferably erect should be obtained after every line insertion. The pneumothorax may be evident immediately, hours, or rarely, days after insertion. Examination of the lung and pleura opposite to the line insertion is important because bilateral punctures may have been attempted.

Inadvertent puncture of the subclavian or carotid artery may result in an extrapleural hematoma, recognized as a small apical opacity or as mediastinal widening due to more extensive bleeding. Rarely, a pseudoaneurysm of these vessels may develop (Fig. 5-9).

Ectopic infusion of fluid into the mediastinal or pleural space through inadvertent placement of a line outside of a vein produces a radiographic appearance of mediastinal widening, suggesting significant intrathoracic bleeding. The diagnosis is suggested by the temporal relationship with the catheter insertion and is confirmed by thoracocentesis.

Central venous catheter placement is frequently associated with nonobstructing thrombus around the tip, and in

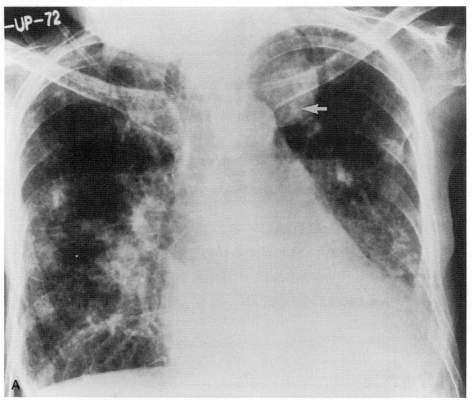

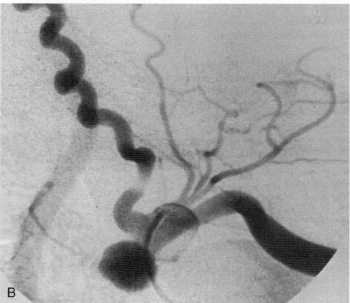

Figure 5-9. Left subclavian aneurysm. **A,** The posteroanterior radiograph shows a large, homogenous opacity in the left upper thorax *(arrow)* after attempted central line placement. The patient has a staphylococcal pneumonia and cardiomegaly. **B,** An angiogram with a selective injection into the origin of the left subclavian artery demonstrates an aneurysm, which was subsequently embolized.

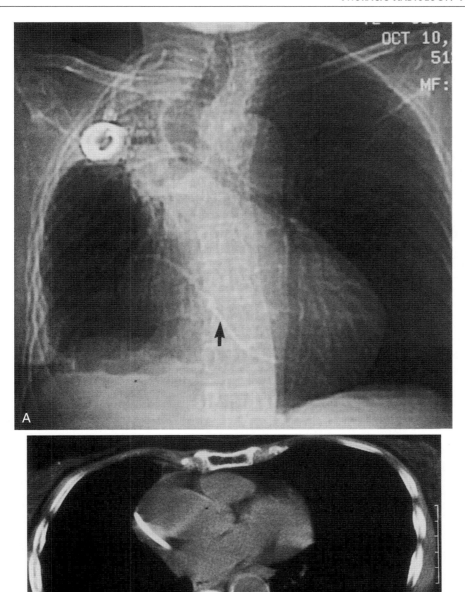

Figure 5-10. Intracardiac catheter fragment. **A,** An intravenous port catheter is positioned through the right subclavian vein. The catheter has fractured, and the distal fragment has migrated into the right atrium *(arrow).* **B,** It was confirmed on CT. The fragment was removed percutaneously through the right femoral vein with an angiographic snare.

15% of cases, a high-probability ventilation-perfusion scan for pulmonary emboli has been demonstrated.

Catheter fragmentation with subsequent central venous embolization is estimated to occur in 1% of catheter placements (Fig. 5-10). Many cases are unrecognized clinically and may be detected by the astute radiologist. The fragments typically migrate through the central veins and right heart chambers and into the pulmonary artery and its branches. Death, arrhythmias, cardiac or vessel perforation, sepsis, mycotic aneurysm, and pulmonary emboli may

result. In many cases, percutaneous retrieval devices can successfully remove the fragment.

Complications of line insertion in part reflect the expertise of the operator. For this reason, the femoral vein approach has gained popularity. There is no risk of a pneumothorax and access is direct and technically easier, and the puncture site is readily compressible. Bleeding from an inadvertent puncture of the femoral artery is easily controlled. Concern over the potentially increased risk of infection and thrombosis using this approach has proved

Box 5-2. **Central Venous Catheter Complications**

TECHNIQUE COMPLICATIONS
Inaccurate readings
Catheter fragmentation
CARDIAC COMPLICATIONS
Arrhythmias
Peripheral venous thrombosis
Vascular or cardiac perforation
PLEURAL COMPLICATIONS
Extrapleural hematoma
Pneumothorax
Hemothorax
SEPSIS COMPLICATIONS
Septic emboli
Mycotic aneurysm

to 5 F in diameter) and are routinely placed by way of the antecubital veins. Because of their fine caliber, they may be difficult to visualize radiographically, particularly in the mediastinum. There is obviously no risk of a pneumothorax, and the risk of infection and thrombosis is low. Because these lines are very flexible and may become displaced, they should be monitored by routine radiographs (Fig. 5-11).

Hickman lines are increasingly used in patients after organ transplantation or for prolonged chemotherapy because of the low incidence of line infections. These catheters are inserted surgically through the subclavian vein and are positioned in the distal superior vena cava or proximal right atrium. The catheter may become pinched at the junction of the clavicle and the first rib, resulting in difficult infusions (when the arms are down), thrombosis, or catheter fragmentation. Totally implantable venous access systems or infusaports consist of a disk placed just below the skin port and a catheter that should terminate in the superior vena cava. Infections are rare, but venous thrombosis may occur.

unwarranted. Complications associated with the central venous catheter are reviewed in Box 5-2.

Percutaneous intravascular central catheters (PICCs) are particularly useful for long-term access. They are small (2

Pulmonary Artery Catheter

Pulmonary artery catheters are frequently used to monitor the hemodynamic status of critically ill patients to aid

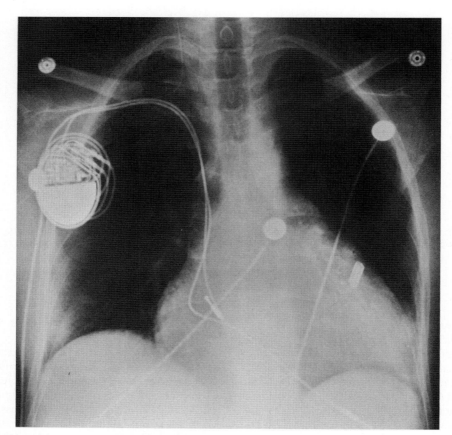

FIGURE 5-11. Incorrect position of the percutaneous intravascular central catheter. The catheter tip lies within the right internal jugular vein. The right-sided permanent pacemaker has atrial and ventricular leads.

differentiation of cardiogenic from noncardiogenic pulmonary edema. The complication rate associated with these catheters is low, but the complications may be fatal. The catheter is typically inserted through the subclavian or internal jugular vein and "floated" distal to the pulmonic valve to lie within the right or left main pulmonary artery. An inflatable balloon at the catheter tip is used to obtain a pulmonary capillary wedge pressure that reflects left atrial pressure and left end-diastolic volume. Balloon inflation is required only at the time of obtaining measurements and may be radiographically visible as a 1-cm, round lucency at the catheter tip. On inflation, the catheter floats distally into a smaller arterial vessel; when the balloon is deflated, the tip should lie in the right or left pulmonary artery within 2 cm of the hilum. Coiling or looping of the catheter within the atrium or ventricle may cause arrhythmias, right bundle branch block, complete heart block, or tricuspid valve rupture.

Pulmonary infarction is the most common serious complication; it results from a location of the catheter that is too peripheral or from excessively prolonged inflation of the balloon in a major peripheral pulmonary artery. Obstruction to distal flow results from the catheter itself or clot formation on or around the catheter tip. The extent of the infarct is determined by the size and distribution of the occluded vessel. Typically, infarction is recognized as patchy consolidation involving the region of the lung peripheral to the catheter. Management requires removal of the catheter, which is frequently a sufficient treatment.

Pulmonary hemorrhage, another complication, has a similar radiographic appearance and is more common in patients with pulmonary arterial hypertension and in those receiving anticoagulation (Fig. 5-12). It may be caused by pseudoaneurysm formation, a rare but potentially fatal complication resulting from rupture of the pulmonary artery (Fig. 5-13). A pseudoaneurysm of the pulmonary artery should be suspected in any patient with a Swan-Ganz catheter who develops hemoptysis or unexplained cardiorespiratory distress. A contrast-enhanced CT scan can demonstrate the aneurysm, which is often surrounded by airspace opacification due to alveolar hemorrhage (i.e., halo sign). Selected patients may require angiography and embolization or a thoracotomy. Other complications include bronchial-arterial fistula and uncontained pulmonary artery rupture.

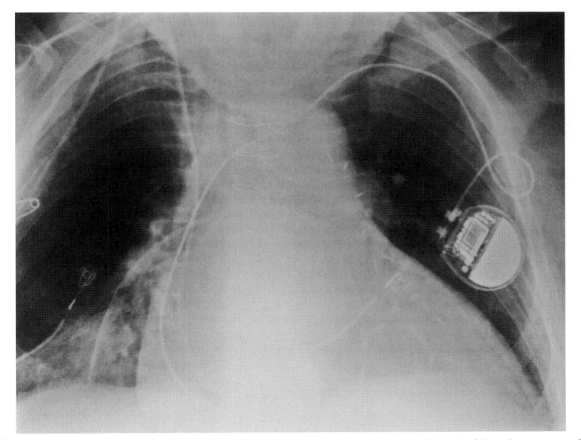

FIGURE 5-12. Pulmonary artery catheter-induced hemorrhage. The catheter tip, lying in a segmental basal branch of the pulmonary artery, is too distal. The surrounding airspace opacification represents hemorrhage. The in situ permanent left single pacemaker has a single right ventricular pacing lead.

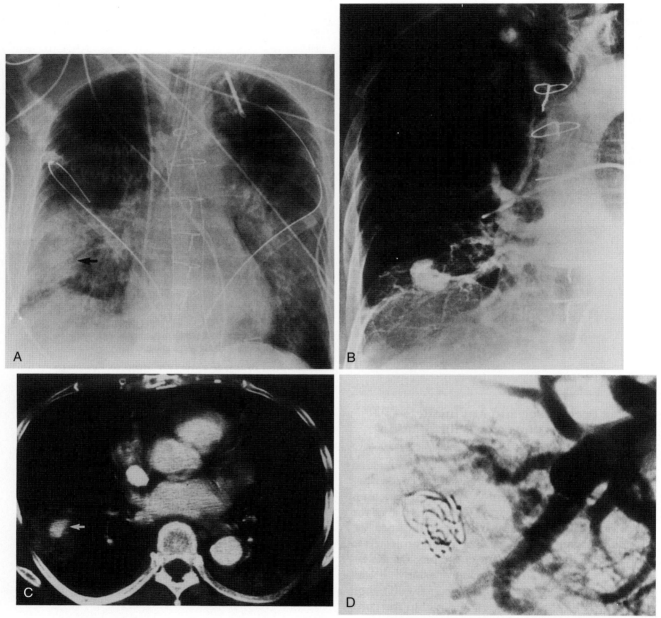

Figure 5-13. Pulmonary artery aneurysm. **A,** The supine anteroposterior radiograph reveals a densely opacified area in the periphery of the right lower lobe *(arrow)* with an absence of air bronchograms. A Swan-Ganz catheter lies in the proximal right pulmonary artery. **B,** Contrast-enhanced CT image at the level of the left atrium demonstrates an aneurysm of a basal segmental branch of the right pulmonary artery *(arrow)* with surrounding hemorrhage. **C,** An angiogram confirmed this finding, and the aneurysm was successfully occluded by embolization with coils. **D,** The aneurysm was attributed to pulmonary artery catheter-induced rupture from intraoperative placement that was too distal.

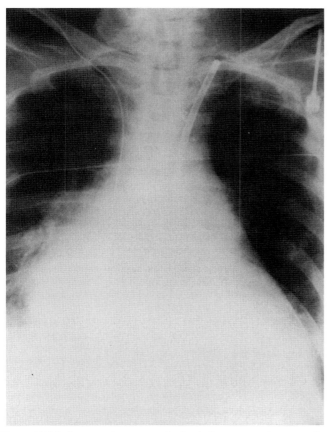

FIGURE 5-14. Intra-aortic counterpulsation balloon pump placement that is too high. The catheter tip lies in origin of left carotid artery.

Intra-aortic Counterpulsation Balloon Catheter

The intra-aortic counterpulsation balloon pump (IABP) is used to improve cardiac function after cardiac surgery or in the treatment of cardiogenic shock. The catheter has a 26- or 28-mm inflatable balloon at its tip. The balloon is inflated during diastole and deflated in systole in time with an electrocardiographic tracing to coincide with every cardiac cycle or every third to fourth cycle. The overall effect is increased oxygen delivery to the myocardium and decreased left ventricular work.

The catheter is inserted percutaneously through the femoral artery or surgically directly into the thoracic aorta. The tip is usually identified by a small, radiopaque, rectangular or circular marker, and it should lie distal to the left subclavian artery just below the superior contour of the aortic knob. A correctly positioned catheter may cross the ostia of the mesenteric and renal arteries. If the catheter is advanced too cephalad, it may obstruct the left subclavian or carotid artery, increasing the risk of cerebral embolism (Fig. 5-14). If the balloon lies too low, counterpulsation is less effective. Aortic dissection is a complication of insertion (Fig. 5-15). Patients with a tortuous aorta or extensive atherosclerotic disease are most at risk. The diagnosis may be indicated by the loss of contour of the descending thoracic aorta on the plain radiograph, and it can be confirmed by aortography or contrast-enhanced CT.

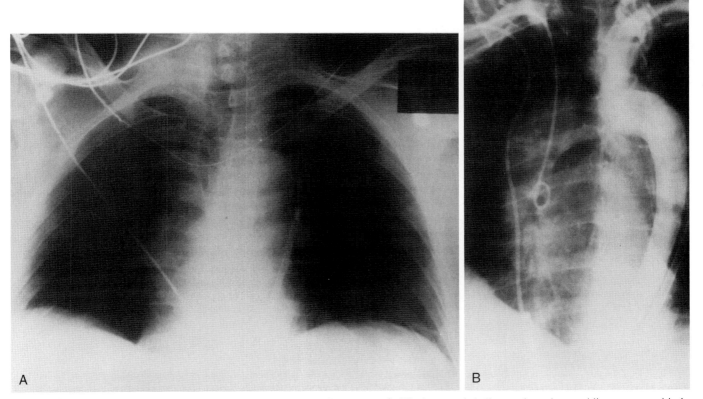

FIGURE 5-15. Aortic dissection by an intra-aortic counterpulsation balloon pump. **A,** The intra-aortic balloon catheter has an oblique course, with the tip overlying the region of the left pulmonary artery lateral to the aortic contour. **B,** An arch angiogram reveals aortic dissection, with the catheter lying outside the opacified true lumen and lying within the nonopacified false lumen of the dissection.

Cardiac Pacemakers and Automatic Implantable Cardioverter-Defibrillation Devices

Pacemakers are used for a variety of conduction abnormalities. The most commonly used pacemaker has a right ventricular lead, although sequential right atrial and right ventricular pacers are also in use. Insertion is achieved by a transvenous approach, with the electrode lying along the base of the right ventricle and the tip directed toward the apex. On the frontal radiograph, the pacemaker lead is projected to the left of the midline at the right ventricular apex. On the lateral view, the lead lies anteriorly and inferiorly. A lead directed upward and laterally on the frontal radiograph and posteriorly on the lateral view lies within the coronary sinus. Ideally, there should be a slight bend in the lead just proximal to the tip as a result of entrapment within the right ventricular trabeculae.

Fractures of the lead commonly occur at three locations: near the tip, near the pacemaker box, and at the venous access site. Sharp angulation, fixation, or flexion of the lead increases the risk of fracture. Myocardial perforation is uncommon and is recognized by the projection of the electrode tip beyond the cardiac border. Most perforations are clinically insignificant, but a pericardial effusion or tamponade may result.

The automatic implantable cardioverter-defibrillator (AICD) is used to prevent sudden death caused by ventricular fibrillation. The system is composed of a pulse generator and electrodes for arrhythmia sensing and for the delivery of pacing and defibrillator pulses to the myocardium. The AICD may be inserted through a thoracotomy

Box 5-3. Complications of Cardiac Pacemakers and Automatic Implantable Cardioverter-Defibrillators

CARDIAC PACEMAKERS
Fracture of pacing lead
Pneumothorax
Pericardial effusion
Cardiac rupture

AUTOMATIC IMPLANTABLE CARDIOVERTER-DEFIBRILLATORS
Lead fracture
Lead retraction

or with transvenous electrodes inserted through the subclavian or cephalic vein. Two electrodes are required: the proximal lead, positioned in the brachiocephalic vein or the superior vena cava, and the distal lead, positioned within the right ventricle. The electrodes may be on a single lead or on two separate leads (Fig. 5-16). If transvenous leads alone are insufficient to generate defibrillation, a subcutaneous patch can be inserted surgically along the left lateral chest wall or on the pericardium. Malfunction of the system is tested by routine device interrogation and chest radiography with frontal and lateral views. Fractures or retraction of the leads are uncommon, but the consequences may be fatal. Early detection of dislodgment allows repositioning before the electrode becomes adherent to the venous endothelium or endocardium. Complications associated with the cardiac pacemaker and the AICD are listed in Box 5-3.

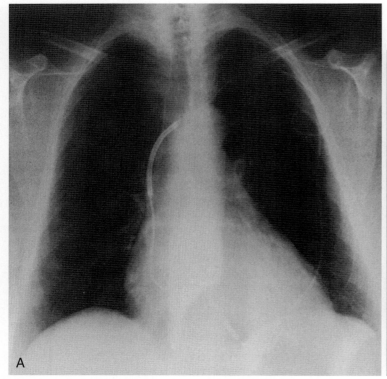
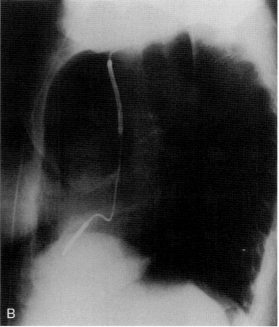

FIGURE 5-16. Automatic implantable cardioverter-defibrillator (AICD) electrode. The posteroanterior (**A**) and lateral (**B**) radiographs show a single transvenous lead with an electrode at the level of the superior vena cava and another in the right ventricle. In this patient, a patch over the left ventricle was not clinically necessary.

Pleural Drainage Tubes

Pleural drainage tubes (i.e., chest tubes) are used to evacuate air or fluid. To relieve a simple pneumothorax, the tube should be positioned near the lung apex and directed anterosuperiorly. To drain pleural fluid, the tube should be positioned posteroinferiorly through the sixth to eighth intercostal spaces in the midaxillary line. Loculated pleural air and fluid collections may require multiple drains positioned under radiologic guidance. Complications of tube drainage include bleeding due to the laceration of an intercostal artery and laceration of the liver, spleen, or stomach due to perforation through the diaphragm. Intraparenchymal placement may lead to hematoma, parenchymal laceration, and bronchopleural fistula. Reexpansion of the underlying lung that is too rapid may result in unilateral pulmonary edema.

Malfunction of the tube may occur from incorrect positioning within the extrapleural soft tissues or within the fissures. Failure to drain may be caused by blockage of the tube from blood or debris or by adhesions and multiloculations of the collection. An important adjunct to drainage is the use of intrapleural fibrinolytic therapy to break down adhesions and reduce the formation of a fibrin pleural peel.

▬ PULMONARY DISEASE

Atelectasis

Atelectasis, a common finding in the critically ill patient, represents areas of nonaerated lung that usually are caused

TABLE 5-2 Atelectasis: Distribution and Radiographic Appearance

Distribution	Radiographic Appearance
Subsegmental	Linear, bandlike
Segmental	Focal segmental opacification
Partial	Patchy opacification resembling pneumonia
Lobar	Dense, homogenous opacity conforming to the lobe with signs of volume loss (see Chapter 1)

by retained secretions. The extent may vary from linear bands of subsegmental atelectasis to more extensive patchy opacification to lobar collapse (Table 5-2). Air bronchograms may be seen, and the appearance is often indistinguishable from that of pneumonia. The presence of fever is not helpful, because it may be present in both conditions. However, atelectasis is usually basal, with a predominance in the left lower lobe, particularly after cardiac surgery (Fig. 5-17). Typically, atelectasis appears and resolves more rapidly than pneumonia and is associated with signs of volume loss.

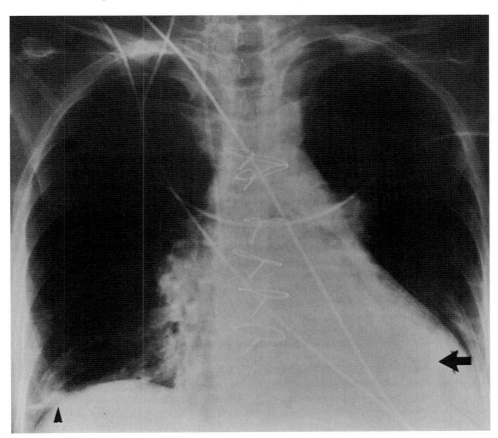

FIGURE 5-17. Atelectasis. The posteroanterior radiograph of a patient with postoperative coronary artery bypass grafts shows left lower lobe partial atelectasis *(arrow)* and right basal subsegmental atelectasis *(arrowhead)*. Mild cardiomegaly can be observed.

Aspiration

Aspiration is a common complication, and it is often unrecognized clinically. The radiographic appearance is determined by the volume and nature of the aspirate and by the position of the patient. Aspiration occurs into the dependent regions of the lung, and with the patient in the supine position, it involves the posterior segments of the upper lobes and the superior and occasionally basal segments of the lower lobes (Fig. 5-18). Three types of aspirate have been described with different radiologic outcomes (Table 5-3). The aspiration of acidic gastric contents produces a chemical pneumonitis, resembling pul-

TABLE 5-3 Aspiration Type and Radiologic Outcomes

Aspiration Type	Radiologic Outcome
Acidic gastric contents	Pulmonary edema
Bland fluids, small volume	Usually normal
Food, oral pathogens	Pneumonia

monary edema. The onset of symptoms occurs within minutes, and there is associated severe bronchospasm and hypotension. Fever and a leucocytosis are common. The chest radiograph shows bilateral perihilar opacification.

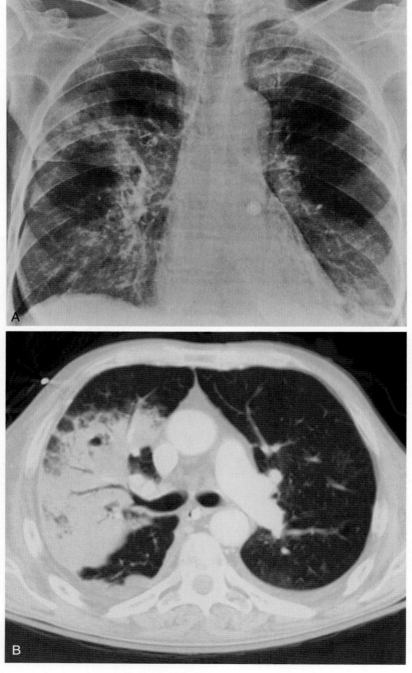

FIGURE 5-18. Aspiration pneumonia. **A,** The posteroanterior radiograph shows right upper lobe and bilateral lower lobe consolidation representing aspiration into the dependent regions of the lungs. **B,** CT performed because of persistent fever despite antibiotic therapy reveals a small air-fluid level representing early abscess formation in the densely consolidated right upper lobe and bibasal pleural effusions.

Clinical and radiographic resolution usually occurs within a couple of days. The aspiration of innocuous fluids such as blood or water is rarely clinically significant unless the fluid volume is large. The radiograph is typically normal, whereas the aspiration of food or oral pathogens results in pneumonia with the typical appearance of persistent airspace opacification in the dependent regions of the lung.

Pneumonia

Nosocomial pneumonia is the leading cause of death from hospital-acquired infection for critically ill patients, and it complicates the clinical course of up to 40% of ventilated patients, with a mortality rate as high as 80%. Nosocomial pneumonia is more likely to be complicated by emphysema or pulmonary abscess formation than is a community-acquired infection.

The diagnosis of pneumonia can be difficult (Table 5-4), but it is defined by the presence of a new or progressive airspace opacity on the chest radiograph that is associated with purulent sputum, fever, or leukocytosis developing in a patient 48 hours after admission to the hospital. However, fever and a leucocytosis may be absent, or the white cell count may be elevated from a number of other causes. The radiographic appearance may be similar to that of atelectasis, pulmonary edema, pulmonary hemorrhage, and pulmonary infarction. Atypical pulmonary edema due to underlying emphysema or asymmetric clearing of edema is particularly confusing. In the presence of acute respiratory distress syndrome (ARDS), the diffuse airspace opacification of the noncardiogenic edema may mask the appearance of pneumonia. The presence of positive sputum cultures may be misleading, merely representing colonization rather than infection. Colonization of the oropharyngeal and endotracheal tube by pathogenic bacteria occurs early, usually within 24 hours of intubation. The reliability of cultures from aspirated or expectorated tracheal sections is low, and protected brush catheter specimens obtained through a bronchoscope are essential for an accurate diagnosis of a lower respiratory tract infection.

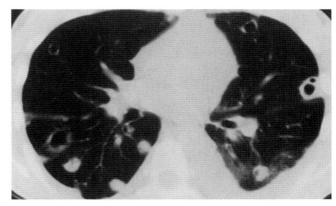

FIGURE 5-19. Septic emboli. CT scan through the middle chest shows multiple, peripheral, rounded pulmonary opacities, some of which are cavitating. They represent pulmonary infarcts in different stages of evolution.

Box 5-4. Common Intensive Care Unit Indications for Thoracic Computed Tomography

Sepsis of unknown origin
Evaluation of complications of thoracic surgery
Evaluation of drainage of pleural collections
Failure to wean from ventilator

Septic pulmonary emboli may arise from an infected catheter, an abscess, endocarditis, or pulmonary or urinary tract infection. The classic appearance of septic infarctions is of peripheral, often subpleural, wedge-shaped opacities and nodules with or without cavitation. They may be seen on the plain radiograph but are best demonstrated on CT (Fig. 5-19). Other radiographic features include the presence of bilateral patchy parenchymal opacification, which progresses slowly or more rarely occurs rapidly, mimicking pulmonary edema. CT evaluation is increasingly used in the evaluation of sepsis of unknown origin (Box 5-4). Unsuspected abscess formation or empyema may be detected. A negative CT result usually excludes the lungs as the sources of sepsis.

Pulmonary Thromboembolism

Critically ill patients are likely to have risk factors for venous thromboembolism. In a study of medical intensive care patients, 33% developed deep venous thrombosis despite prophylaxis, and most cases occurred within the first week. Approximately 10% of patients with deep venous thrombosis will develop pulmonary emboli, and 10% of these are fatal. Many thromboembolic episodes, however, are unrecognized. Autopsy studies report a prevalence ranging from 5% to more than 50%.

The introduction of pulmonary CT angiography has proved invaluable in the assessment of the dyspneic intensive care patient. CT angiography provides an accurate, noninvasive assessment of the pulmonary arteries by

TABLE 5-4 Airspace Opacification: Radiographic Distribution and Causes

Radiographic Distribution	Cause of Opacification
Diffuse, symmetric, perihilar; may be dependent	Cardiogenic pulmonary; edema
Patchy, asymmetric, peripheral; dependent, air bronchograms	Noncardiogenic pulmonary; edema (acute respiratory distress syndrome)
Patchy, asymmetric, peripheral; nondependent	Bronchopneumonia
Patchy, asymmetric; dependent	Aspiration pneumonia
Peripheral, wedge-shaped, cavitation	Septic infarcts

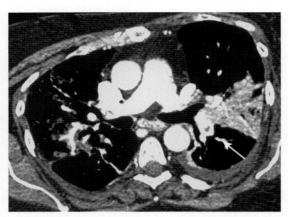

Figure 5-20. Pulmonary emboli and pneumonia. CT angiogram of the lungs in a breast cancer patient with known pneumonia was performed for evaluation of increasing dyspnea revealed a left lower lobe pulmonary embolus and confirmed the lingular consolidation associated with a small pleural effusion. Patchy consolidation is demonstrated in the right lung.

demonstrating even small peripheral emboli, and it allows identification of nonvascular causes of respiratory distress (Fig. 5-20). Studies have shown that up to two thirds of patients with an initial suspicion of pulmonary embolism have another diagnosis. The plain radiographic, scintigraphic, CT, and conventional pulmonary angiographic features are discussed elsewhere.

Pulmonary Edema

The chest radiograph provides an assessment of the systemic blood volume, pulmonary blood volume, pulmonary vascular flow patterns, and extravascular water. It is important to differentiate cardiogenic from noncardiogenic pulmonary edema due to fluid overload (renal) or increased permeability (ARDS) (Table 5-5). In the critical care setting, this is often difficult. Cardiomegaly, septal thickening, and pleural effusions are frequently seen in patients in cardiac failure.

The width of the vascular pedicle is the width of the superior mediastinum extending from the right lateral border of the superior vena cava at the point at which it crosses

TABLE 5-5 Radiographic Features of Cardiac versus Noncardiac Edema

Signs	Cardiac Features	Renal Features	Acute Respiratory Distress Syndro me
Cardiomegaly	Present	Present	Absent
Vascular redistribution	Present	Absent	Absent
Widened vascular pedicle	Present	Present	Absent
Pleural effusions	Present	Present	Absent
Kerley lines	Present	Present	Absent
Peribronchial cuffing	Present	Present	Absent
Airspace opacification	Diffuse perihilar	Central perihilar	Patchy peripheral

the right main bronchus to the left lateral margin, demarcated by the outer border of the left subclavian artery as it arises from the aortic arch. A serial change in the width of the vascular pedicle reflects circulating blood volume and provides a useful assessment of the patient's fluid status. In 95% of normal individuals, the vascular pedicle is between 38 and 58 mm wide. Because of the wide normal range, comparison of serial radiographs for an individual patient is more useful than an absolute measurement. However, similar radiographic positioning is required, and portable supine radiographs are rarely directly comparable. With fluid overload, the vascular pedicle typically increases in size, whereas in cases of cardiogenic edema, only one half of the patients have an abnormally wide vascular pedicle. Patients with permeability pulmonary edema (ARDS) have a normal or small pedicle.

Central venous pressure can be assessed by observing the relative width of the azygous vein seen end-on at the right tracheobronchial angle. The azygous vein responds directly to right atrial pressure rather than to changes in circulating blood volume. This vein normally is less than 1 cm wide on radiographs taken with the patient erect. Enlargement may be physiologic, as with a patient in the supine position and in a pregnant patient because of increased venous return, or it may be pathologic, as in patients with congestive cardiac failure.

Pulmonary blood flow can be estimated by assessing the caliber of the pulmonary vessels. In congestive cardiac failure, the arteries and veins dilate, and the nondependent vessels enlarge disproportionally. On the erect radiograph, this is seen as an increased diameter of the upper zone vessels relative to that of the lower lobe vessels (i.e., cephalization or redistribution of flow). In the supine patient, this gradient is anteroposterior and cannot be appreciated unless CT is performed. Arterial enlargement alone can be assessed on the supine radiograph. Normally, the size ratio between a pulmonary artery and its accompanying bronchus is 1:1, and an increase in this ratio indicates increased pulmonary flow. This increase is seen in fluid overload and left ventricular failure.

The Swan-Ganz catheter provides a reliable physiologic measurement of cardiac function. As the pulmonary capillary wedge pressure increases, transudation of fluid into the interstitium occurs with accumulation of fluid around the pulmonary vessels and bronchi. Radiographically, the vessels appear indistinct as a result of the perivascular cuffing, and the bronchial walls are thickened from peribronchial cuffing. Fluid accumulates within the interlobular septa and is seen as fine linear horizontal opacities extending to the pleural surface (Kerley B lines) or as perihilar linear opacities that are longer and central (Kerley A lines). Further increases in wedge pressure result in alveolar pulmonary edema and a perihilar bat wing distribution of the airspace opacification (Fig. 5-21).

The distribution of the airspace opacification of pulmonary edema is usually symmetric. Atypical patterns are seen in chronic underlying lung disease, such as in chronic obstructive pulmonary disease, in which the edema may be patchy or linear and asymmetric. Asymmetric pulmonary edema is usually caused by gravity and therefore patient position, but it may occur after aspiration or

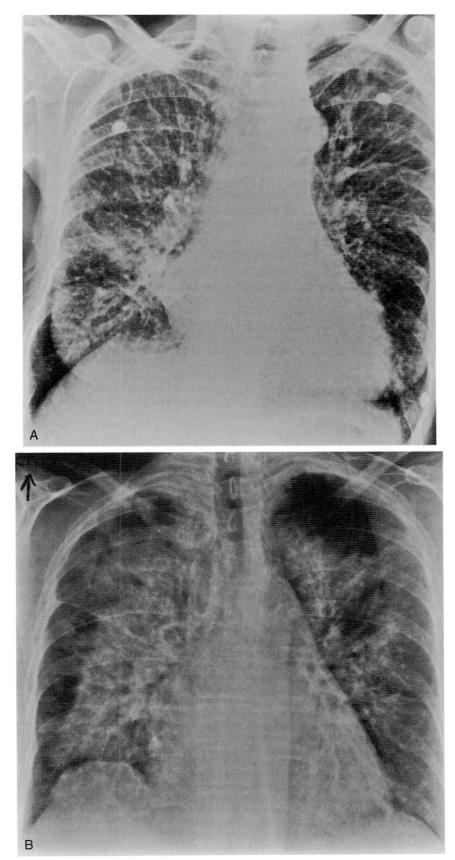

FIGURE 5-21. Cardiogenic pulmonary edema. **A,** In a case of interstitial pulmonary edema, the posteroanterior radiograph reveals multiple linear opacities throughout both lungs. These lines are composed of long, septal, perihilar opacities (Kerley A) and short, peripheral lines (Kerley B). **B,** In a case of alveolar pulmonary edema, the posteroanterior radiograph demonstrates a bat wing pattern of perihilar consolidation surrounded by a radiolucent peripheral zone of normal lung. Cardiomegaly is seen in both cases.

thoracocentesis. The latter is caused by reinflation of a collapsed lung that is too rapid. Pulmonary edema in the remaining lung is a well-recognized complication after pneumonectomy.

The posttherapeutic lag phase describes the discrepancy between the improving pulmonary capillary wedge pressure and the lack of radiographic resolution of edema. Although the wedge measurements may have returned to normal, it may still take hours or days for the reabsorption of large amounts of extracellular fluid and therefore clearing of the radiographic abnormality. This phenomenon is frequently seen in patients with left-sided heart failure.

Permeability edema (e.g., ARDS) results from the accumulation of a proteinaceous fluid in the extravascular space. Accumulation results from increased microvascular permeability.

Acute Respiratory Distress Syndrome

ARDS is a clinical diagnosis of acute respiratory failure characterized by profound hypoxia associated with a chest radiograph demonstrating widespread pulmonary opacification with air bronchograms. The risk factors for developing ARDS include multiple trauma, fat emboli, sepsis, severe pneumonia, aspiration of gastric contents, and multiple transfusions. Patients usually have more than one risk factor. The initiating event might have occurred hours or days before, as with sepsis or fat emboli, or ARDS might have developed acutely, as after gastric aspiration. The resultant diffuse alveolar damage causes a generalized permeability defect that produces noncardiogenic pulmonary edema.

The plain radiographic appearance is frequently distinguishable from other causes of pulmonary edema. Typically, the supine radiograph demonstrates extensive airspace opacification, which appears to uniformly involve both lungs (Fig. 5-22A). However, CT reveals the lung involvement as heterogeneous, with areas of normal lung in combination with areas of ground-glass opacification and areas of dense consolidation (see Fig. 5-22B). The normal lung is typically anterior, with the dense consolidation posterior and the ground-glass opacification between the two. In addition to the ventral dorsal gradient, the abnormal density of the lung increases in a cephalocaudal direction. The parenchymal pattern represents the generalized capillary leak (i.e., ground-glass opacification), the local lung injury (i.e., consolidation), and the dependent atelectasis from a prolonged supine position. Dense consolidation

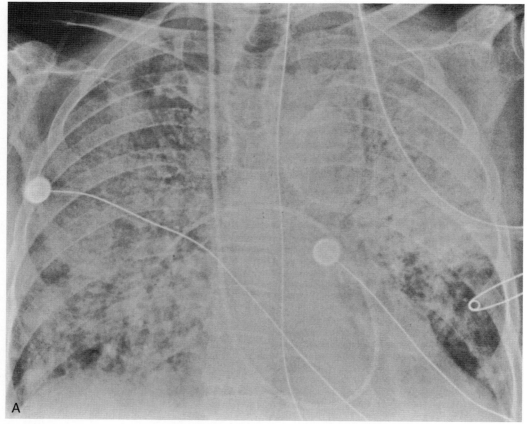

FIGURE 5-22. Acute respiratory distress syndrome (ARDS). **A,** The anteroposterior radiograph of an elderly woman demonstrates widespread consolidation with air bronchograms. The heart size is normal, and there are no pleural effusions.

(Figure continued on opposite page)

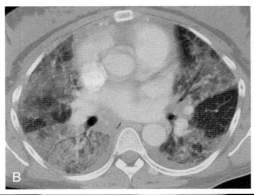

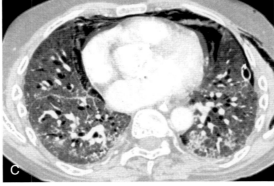

FIGURE 5-22. (cont'd) B, CT reveals the typical patchy distribution to the airspace abnormality with the ground-glass opacification interposed between normal lung tissues. Tiny pleural effusions can be seen. C, CT performed 1 month later reveals evidence of barotraumas with subcutaneous emphysema, pneumomediastinum, and a small, left pneumothorax. Reticular opacities and minor bronchiectasis superimposed on the ground-glass opacification suggest the development of pulmonary fibrosis.

predominates in patients with direct injury to the lung, such as pneumonia or aspiration, and ground-glass opacification (i.e., permeability edema) is the predominant finding in patients with alveolar damage from an extrapulmonary insult such as sepsis or hypotension. In contrast to cardiogenic, uremic, and hypervolemic edema, the vascular pedicle is not widened, and cardiomegaly and upper lobe vascular redistribution is absent. When visualized, the upper lobe vessesls are constricted rather than dilated. Septal lines are usually absent, as are pleural effusions. The lung volumes are reduced, although because of mechanical ventilation, this may not be apparent.

Bacterial pneumonia is a common and frequently missed complication of ARDS. The diffuse airspace opacification of ARDS often obscures the radiographic abnormality due to pneumonia. However, the CT finding of dense, nondependent consolidation should raise the suspicion of infection.

Most ARDS patients require mechanical ventilation for survival, often for prolonged periods and with high peak end-expiratory pressure (PEEP). Barotrauma is a well-recognized complication associated with a high mortality rate. The most common manifestation is the development of extra-alveolar air collections, particularly pneumothorax and pneumatocele formation (see Fig. 5-22C). Recovery from ARDS may be complicated by the development of fibrosis and cystic lung destruction.

ABNORMAL AIR COLLECTIONS

Subcutaneous Emphysema

Barotrauma from prolonged or high-pressure ventilation may result in subcutaneous emphysema, pulmonary interstitial emphysema (PIE), pneumomediastinum, and recurrent pneumothoraces (Fig. 5-23). Subcutaneous emphysema confined to the cervical region suggests possible injury to the upper airway or esophagus during intubation. Subcutaneous emphysema along the chest wall should alert the observer to the presence of a pneumothorax, with the lateralization indicated by the distribution of the emphysema. A continuous increase in the volume of subcutaneous air adjacent to a chest tube indicates a malfunctioning tube or improper wound dressing.

Pneumothorax

On a radiograph obtained with the patient erect, the pneumothorax edge is readily identified as a well-defined white line (i.e., visceral pleural edge) with an absence of vessels superiorly and laterally. On a radiograph obtained with the patient supine, pleural air preferentially collects anteriorly and surrounds the anterior mediastinal structures (Box 5-5). A suprahilar pneumothorax outlines the superior vena cava and azygos veins on the right and subclavian artery and superior pulmonary veins on the left. An infrahilar

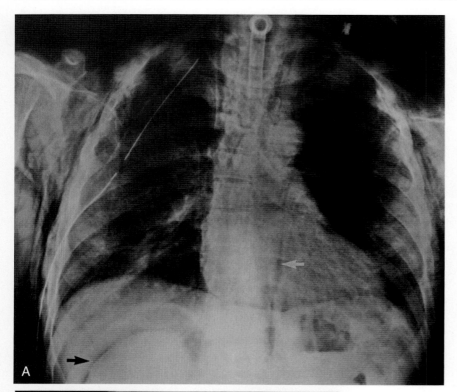

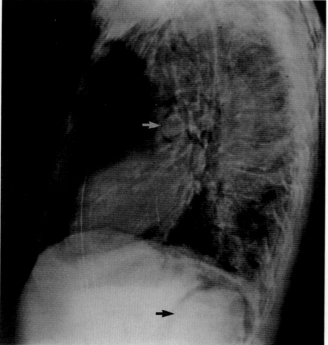

FIGURE 5-23. Abnormal air collections. Subcutaneous emphysema with pneumomediastinum and pneumoperitoneum. The anteroposterior radiograph of a trauma patient (**A**) reveals extensive subcutaneous emphysema. Pneumomediastinum outlines the contours of the aorta and pulmonary arteries *(white arrows)*. Pneumoperitoneum with retroperitoneal air (**B**) outlines the renal contours *(black arrows)*.

Box 5-5. **Radiographic Signs of Supine Anteromedial Pneumothorax**

SUPRAHILAR PNEUMOTHORAX
Right pneumothorax outlines
Superior vena cava
Azygous vein
Left pneumothorax outlines
Left subclavian artery
Superior pulmonary veins

INFRAHILAR PNEUMOTHORAX
Sharp delineation
Costophrenic deep sulcus sign
Diaphragmatic contour
Cardiac contour
Pericardial fat pad

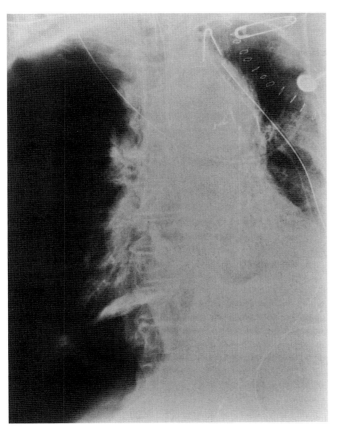

FIGURE 5-24. Tension pneumothorax with a subpulmonic component. A supine anteroposterior radiograph of a ventilated patient after aortic dissection repair reveals a large, right pneumothorax with contralateral mediastinal displacement. The subpulmonic distribution to the pneumothorax is shown by a deep sulcus sign.

finding known as the double diaphragm sign. The central infracardiac aspect of the diaphragm is normally not visible, but it can be seen in patients with pneumomediastinum or pneumoperitoneum. Loculated pneumothoraces can be difficult to identify in the supine patient, and in selected patients, a CT scan is indicated for diagnosis and drainage.

Pulmonary Interstitial Emphysema

PIE represents air dissecting around the pulmonary veins and lymphatics. Air may dissect along the axial interstitium medially, resulting in pneumomediastinum, which is rarely clinically significant, and pneumothorax. Radiographically, PIE (Box 5-7) is recognized as lucent streaks radiating from the hilum in a nonbranching, disorganized pattern that is most readily seen against a background of consolidation (e.g., ARDS). Larger radiolucencies seen in a perihilar or subpleural distribution represent air cysts (<5 mm) or pneumatoceles. Subpleural cysts increased the risk of pneumothorax.

Pneumomediastinum

Pneumomediastinum is usually a benign condition but may be the consequence of airway or esophageal rupture. Radiographically pneumomediastinum is seen as air outlining the contours of the mediastinal structures, specifically the medial border of the superior vena cava, the great vessels of the arch, around the pulmonary arteries, and along the thoracic aorta. Pneumothorax and pneumopericardium may be indistinguishable from pneumomediastinum. Decubitus views can differentiate these air collections, because air in the pleural space rises to the highest point, and air within the pericardium changes to a nondependent location around the heart, whereas the configuration of a pneumomediastinum remains unaltered.

pneumothorax produces the deep sulcus sign, with sharp delineation of the anterior costophrenic sulcus and adjacent diaphragmatic and cardiac contours (Fig. 5-24). A large, supine pneumothorax may result in hyperlucency of the affected hemithorax compared with the opposite lung. Decubitus views with the side of interest uppermost can confirm the diagnosis.

A subpulmonic pneumothorax (Box 5-6) appears as a hyperlucent upper quadrant of the abdomen and visualization of the superior contour of the diaphragm. A deep anterior costophrenic sulcus is also seen. The anterior and posterior diaphragmatic surfaces may be visualized, a

---

***Box 5-7.* Pulmonary Interstitial Emphysema**

Linear and mottled radiolucencies
Air cysts (<5 mm)
Pneumatoceles

***Box 5-6.* Radiographic Signs of Subpulmonic Pneumothorax**

Hyperlucent upper abdominal quadrant
Deep costophrenic sulcus (deep sulcus sign)
Sharp diaphragmatic contour
Double diaphragm sign

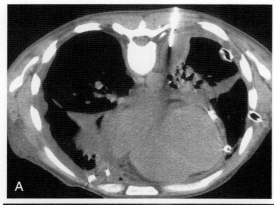

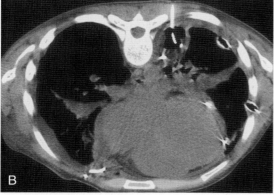

FIGURE 5-25. Loculated left posterior empyema. **A,** Under CT guidance with the patient prone, a diagnostic aspirate was performed of the loculated left paraspinal fluid collection. A loculated right empyema is drained by a separate pigtail catheter, and a large-bore left chest tube is seen lateral to the paraspinal collection. **B,** After pigtail catheter placement, an air-fluid level is seen because of a decrease in fluid.

■ PLEURAL FLUID COLLECTIONS

Most pleural effusions in intensive care patients are small and uncomplicated, and they occur postoperatively. Plain radiographs, sometimes supplemented by decubitus views, are usually sufficient to document a pleural effusion. Large, unilocular effusions; multilocular, parapneumonic effusions; empyemas; and hemothoraces require tube drainage.

Percutaneous image-guided catheter drainage has become the procedure of choice (Fig. 5-25). Sonography is typically reserved for diagnostic thoracentesis and for bedside catheter drainage of free-flowing pleural effusions. CT is particularly valuable in the evaluation of complex pleural-pulmonary disease. CT accurately depicts the size of a collection and the presence of loculation. CT also enables identification of associated complications, such as a lung abscess or bronchopleural fistula (see Chapter 18).

■ ABDOMINAL DISEASE

Evaluation of the upper abdomen is a bonus of thoracic CT examinations. Up to 27% of the studies reveal abdominal findings, and 5% have clinical significance (Fig. 5-26).

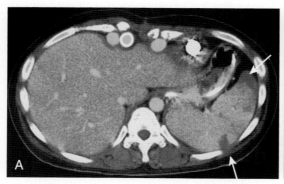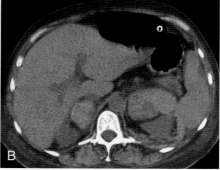

FIGURE 5-26. Unsuspected abdominal pathology. **A,** Septic splenic infarcts occurred in a patient with recurrent bacteremia and a biventricular cardiac assist device for cardiomyopathy. CT revealed multiple, wedge-shaped, peripheral opacities in the spleen. **B,** Bilateral adrenal hemorrhage occurred in an elderly woman with acute myelogenous leukemia who presented with fever, hypotension, and dyspnea. CT demonstrated bilateral, massive adrenal enlargements of high density that were consistent with recent hemorrhage.

■ SUGGESTED READINGS

Cascade, P.N., Kazerooni, E.A., 1994. Aspects of chest imaging in the intensive care unit. Crit. Care. Clin. 10 (2), 247–263.

Desai, S.R., Wells, A.U., Suntharalingam, G., et al., 2001. Acute respiratory distress syndrome caused by pulmonary and extra pulmonary injury: a comparative computed tomographic study. Radiology 218, 689–693.

Drucker, E.A., Brooks, R., Sweeney, M.O., et al., 1995. Malfunction of implantable cardioverter defibrillators placed by a nonthoracotomy approach: frequency of malfunction and value of chest radiography in determining the cause. AJR. Am. J. Roentgenol. 165, 275–279.

Fraser, R.G., Pare, J.A.P., Pare, P.D., 1991. Pulmonary hypertension and edema. In: Fraser, R.G., Pare, J.A.P., Pare, P.D. (Eds.), Diagnosis of Diseases of the Chest. third ed., vol. 3, WB Saunders, Philadelphia.

Goodman, L.R., Fumagalli, R., Tagliabue, P., et al., 1999. Adult respiratory distress syndrome due to pulmonary and extra pulmonary causes: CT, clinical, and functional correlations. Radiology 213, 545–552.

Goodman, L.R., Kuzo, R.S. (Eds.), 1996. Intensive care radiology [review]. Radiol. Clin. North Am. 34, 1–190.

Hirsch, D.R., Ingenito, E.P., Goldhaber, S.Z., 1995. Prevalence of deep venous thrombosis among patients in medical intensive care. JAMA. 274, 335–337.

Hull, R., Raskob, G.E., Ginsberg, J.S., 1994. A noninvasive strategy for the treatment of patients with suspected pulmonary embolism. Arch. Intern. Med. 154, 289–297.

Lefcoe, M.S., Fox, G.A., Lesa, D.J., et al., 1994. Accuracy of portable chest radiography in the critical care setting: diagnosis of pneumonia based on quantitative cultures obtained from protected brush catheter. Chest 105, 885–887.

Mattison, L.E., Coppage, L., Alderman, D.F., et al., 1997. Pleural effusions in the medical ICU: prevalence, causes, and clinical implications. Chest 111, 1018–1023.

McCarroll, K.A. (Ed.), 1994. Imaging in the intensive care unit. Crit. Care. Clin. 10 (2).

Miller Jr., W.T., Tino, G., Friedburg, J.S., 1998. Thoracic CT in the intensive care unit: assessment of clinical usefulness. Radiology 209, 491–498.

Milne, E.N., Pistolesi, M., Miniati, M., Giuntini, C., 1985. The radiologic distinction of cardiogenic and noncardiogenic edema. AJR. Am. J. Roentgenol. 144, 879–894.

Monreal, M., Ruiz, J., Fraile, M., et al., 2001. Prospective study on the usefulness of lung scan in patients with deep vein thrombosis of the lower limbs. Thromb. Haemost. 85, 771–774.

Moulton, J.S., 2000. Image-guided management of complicated pleural fluid collections. Radiol. Clin. North. Am. 38, 345–374.

Schoepf, U.J., Costello, P., 2004. CT angiography for diagnosis of pulmonary embolism: state of the art. Radiology 230, 329–337.

Snow, N., Bergin, K.T., Horrigan, T.P., 1990. Thoracic CT scanning in critically ill patients: information obtained frequently alters management. Chest 97, 1467–1470.

Talgiabue, M., Casella, T.C., Zincone, G.E., et al., 1994. CT and chest radiography in the evaluation of adult respiratory distress syndrome. Acta. Radiol. 35, 230–234.

Zarshenas, Z., Sparschu, R.A., 1994. Catheter placement and misplacement. Crit. Care. Clin. 10, 416–435.

Ziter Jr., F.M.H., Westcott, J.L., 1981. Supine subpulmonary pneumothorax. AJR. Am. J. Roentgenol. 137, 699–701.

CHAPTER 6

Thoracic Trauma

Beatrice Trotman-Dickenson and Stephen Ledbetter

Chest injuries are responsible for 25% of all trauma-related deaths. Injuries are classified as *blunt trauma* if the chest wall remains intact and *penetrating injury* if the chest wall is breached. Blunt traumatic injury comprises approximately 90% of cases and is most frequently caused by motor vehicle accidents and falls. These injuries are related to the deceleration force at impact. In penetrating injury, the major risk is to mediastinal vascular structures along the path of the projectile or other penetrating object. Although penetrating injury represents only about 10% of chest trauma, it may have a higher prevalence in urban trauma centers.

The plain chest radiograph, as part of the trauma series (i.e., anteroposterior chest radiograph, anteroposterior pelvis radiograph, and cross-table lateral view of the cervical spine) is typically the initial means of diagnostic imaging for all cases of trauma. The trauma series identifies injuries that have the potential for being immediately life threatening (e.g., tension pneumothorax) or iatrogenic insults that may occur from the injudicious placement of tubes and lines during resuscitation (e.g., right mainstem bronchus intubation) (Box 6-1). However, the importance of chest radiography for clearing major chest trauma victims has considerably diminished, and computed tomography (CT) has become the primary imaging modality for all hemodynamically stable trauma patients. This represents a rather significant change in practice compared with less than a decade ago.

CT realized significant gains in speed, accuracy, and utility with the advent of volumetric scanning (i.e., spiral, helical CT) in the early 1990s. Further major advances have occurred in the past decade with multidetector CT (MDCT) imaging. These gains have proved extraordinarily beneficial in the evaluation of trauma patients. Consequently, CT is often requested despite a relatively unremarkable chest radiograph, particularly for the multitrauma patient for whom CT of the head, cervical spine, abdomen and pelvis has become routine. CT images of the chest should be acquired after the administration of intravenous contrast material (IVCM) using an injection rate of at least 2 to 3 mL/sec and with collimation no greater than 1 to 3 mm, although images may be reconstructed at greater thickness (e.g., 5 mm). As further advances in CT speed develop, the trauma series, including the chest radiograph, may be replaced by primary evaluation with CT.

■ INJURIES TO THE CHEST WALL

Rib Fractures

Injuries to the chest wall, particularly rib fractures, are common (Box 6-2). The complications of rib fractures, such as pneumothorax and splenic injury, are often of greater consequence than the fractures themselves. Rib fractures are frequently not detected on the initial chest radiograph because an undisplaced or minimally displaced fracture, or a costovertebral separation are radiographically occult. Multiple rib views are not necessary because the treatment for clinically suspected rib fractures is the same whether they are shown by radiography or not. In children, rib fractures are uncommon because of the elasticity of the cartilage. The presence of multiple rib fractures, particularly if of various ages or if posteriorly located is strongly suggestive of child abuse. In adults, multiple, bilateral, healed or healing fractures are often associated with repeated falls and frequently indicate alcoholism or chronic drug use.

Rib fractures are an important indicator of the trauma mechanism, providing information about the vector and severity of the applied forces, as well as indicating the possible complications (Fig. 6-1). Fractures of the first three ribs raise concern for more severe traumatic injury since these can be associated with airway, spinal, or vascular injury (Table 6-1). Ninety percent of patients with tracheobronchial injury have rib fractures at this site. However, only 3% to 15% of patients with upper rib fractures have brachial plexus or vascular injury; CT's ability to effectively screen for these injuries permits the highly selective use of other modalities. For example, angiography is reserved for those patients for whom clinical or CT findings are inconclusive or warrant a more specific approach to investigation. Fractures of the lower three ribs should raise suspicion for splenic, hepatic, or renal trauma (Fig. 6-2) and should prompt an abdominal CT study to evaluate for these solid visceral injuries (Fig. 6-3).

Several plain chest radiographic findings may indicate splenic trauma. Displacement of the gas-filled fundus of the stomach medially and anteriorly by hematoma and/or signs of left diaphragmatic rupture indicate a greater likelihood of splenic injury. Segmental rib fractures involving more than three contiguous ribs or single fractures involving five consecutive ribs constitute a flail chest (Fig. 6-4). Severe respiratory compromise may develop as a result of the paradoxical movement of the flail segment during respiration. For this reason some institutions have begun to perform open reduction internal fixation (ORIF) of flail segments using hardware plates.

Extrapleural hematomas frequently accompany rib fractures. On the chest radiograph, the hematoma may appear as a focal, lobulated opacity that has a convex margin with the lung. Unlike pleural fluid, these hematomas do not alter configuration with changes in patient position. Extrapleural hematoma at the apices may be caused by subclavian vessel hemorrhage as a result of the initial trauma or after central line placement (Fig. 6-5). Aortic injury can also result in a left apical extrapleural hematoma, manifest as increased opacity above the left lung apex. More inferiorly, extrapleural hematoma is usually the result of injury to intercostal vessels. Hemorrhage from intercostal vessels may result in a rapidly developing hemothorax, or even exsanguination. Angiography with embolization can be life saving (Fig. 6-6).

Box 6-1. **Life-Threatening Injuries**

Tracheal rupture
Tension pneumothorax
Hemothorax
Cardiac tamponade
Aortic transection

Box 6-2. **Frequency of Thoracic Injuries Identified by Computed Tomography**

MOST COMMON
Pneumothorax
Lung contusion
Rib fractures
Hemothorax
Spinal fractures

LESS COMMON
Sternal fracture
Diaphragmatic injury
Vascular injury
Bronchus fracture

TABLE 6-1 Rib Fractures

Location	Associations or Complications
First three pairs	Spinal or vascular injury, tracheobronchial rupture
Last three pairs	Hepatic, splenic, renal injury
Multiple sites	Flail chest
Multiple healed, adult	Alcoholism
Multiple healed, child	Child abuse

Sternal Fractures

Sternal fractures occur in less than 10% of patients with major thoracic trauma and may be associated with injury to the mediastinal vascular structures or myocardial contusion, the diagnosis was most easily made on the lateral chest radiograph (Fig. 6-7A). Today, coronal or sagittal reformations or three-dimensional renderings of the chest CT readily show sternal fracture as well as the degree of fracture displacement (see Fig. 6-7B). Sternoclavicular dislocations can be difficult to identify on the chest radiograph, but CT can readily show them. Most dislocations

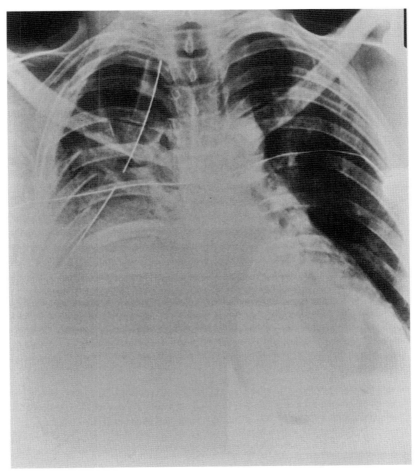

FIGURE 6-1. Upper rib fractures. A posteroanterior, erect chest radiograph reveals multiple right upper rib fractures and a right basal pleural effusion. A right pneumothorax has resolved after tube placement.

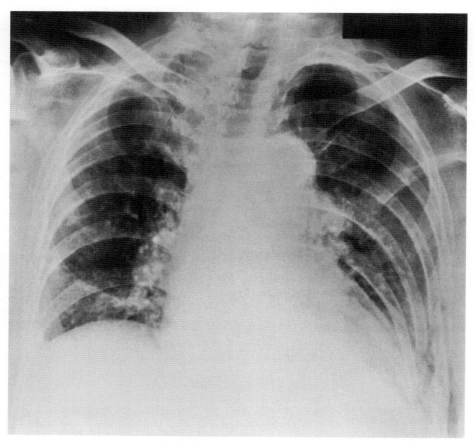

FIGURE 6-2. Lower rib fractures. A supine, anteroposterior radiograph reveals multiple left lower rib fractures and subcutaneous emphysema along the lower lateral left chest wall. The left hemidiaphragm is not seen because of a pleural effusion and left lower lobe atelectasis. Evaluation for splenic trauma is mandatory.

are anterior and are of little clinical significance. Posterior dislocations are more concerning given their greater association with injuries to adjacent mediastinal vessels, trachea, and esophagus.

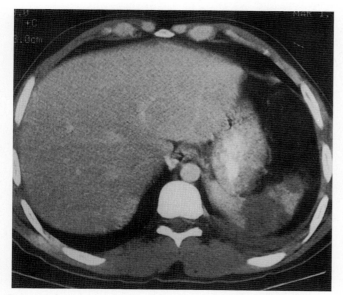

FIGURE 6-3. Splenic laceration. Contrast-enhanced CT scan through the upper abdomen shows multiple, low-density lesions within the spleen due to lacerations. A small, left hemothorax can be seen posteriorly.

Spinal Injury

Spinal injury is common in cases of high-velocity trauma where up 30% of patients with significant thoracic trauma have spinal injuries. More than 60% of fracture dislocations in the thoracic spine are associated with neurologic defects. This compares with a prevalence of 32% in the cervical spine and 2% in the lumbar spine (Box 6-3). Early identification of spinal fractures may prevent irreversible and potentially devastating cord injury. Thoracic spine radiographs are not necessary for trauma patients who have undergone volumetric chest CT. Studies have shown that coronal and sagittal reformatted images are more sensitive, specific, and accurate for detecting and characterizing spinal injuries. Most fracture dislocations occur at the thoracolumbar junction (Fig. 6-8). Multiple fractures are found in 10% of patients and eighty percent of these injuries are noncontiguous. The radiologic features to be considered include abnormal vertebral shape, location, size, and density. The "rule of 2 s" applies (Box 6-4).

INJURY TO THE TRACHEA AND MAJOR AIRWAYS

Tracheobronchial Rupture

Tracheobronchial injury is frequently associated with fractures or dislocations to the upper thoracic cage. The tear may be partial or complete. The diagnosis is frequently delayed, resulting in tracheal or bronchial stenosis from partial healing.

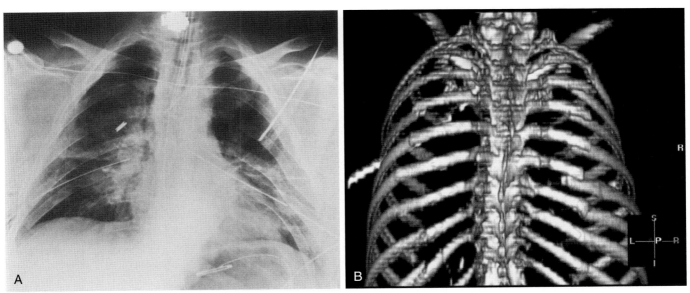

FIGURE 6-4. Flail chest. **A,** Supine, anteroposterior radiograph reveals segmental fractures involving multiple, contiguous left ribs. The patient has a small, right pneumothorax and widespread pulmonary contusion. **B,** 3D CT reconstruction, posterior view in a different patient, reveals multiple bilateral posterior rib fractures confirming bilateral flail chest.

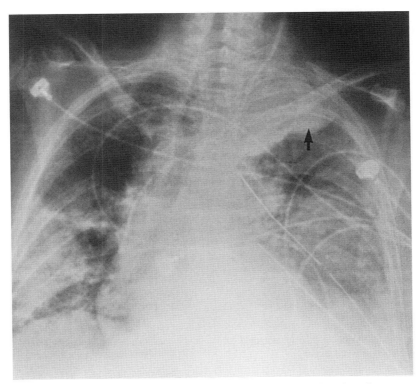

FIGURE 6-5. Left extrapleural hematoma *(arrow).* After placement of an internal jugular central line, there is a new convex opacity in the left apex. Notice the extensive bilateral pulmonary contusion.

The early diagnostic features include persistent severe pneumomediastinum, subcutaneous emphysema, and pneumothorax (Box 6-5). Uncommon signs of rupture include the fallen lung sign, bayonet deformity of the trachea, and ectopic position of the endotracheal tube or balloon cuff.

Bronchial Rupture

Bronchial rupture occurs within 2.5 cm of the carina in 80% of patients. Right-sided rupture is more common than left, and most patients develop a pneumothorax.

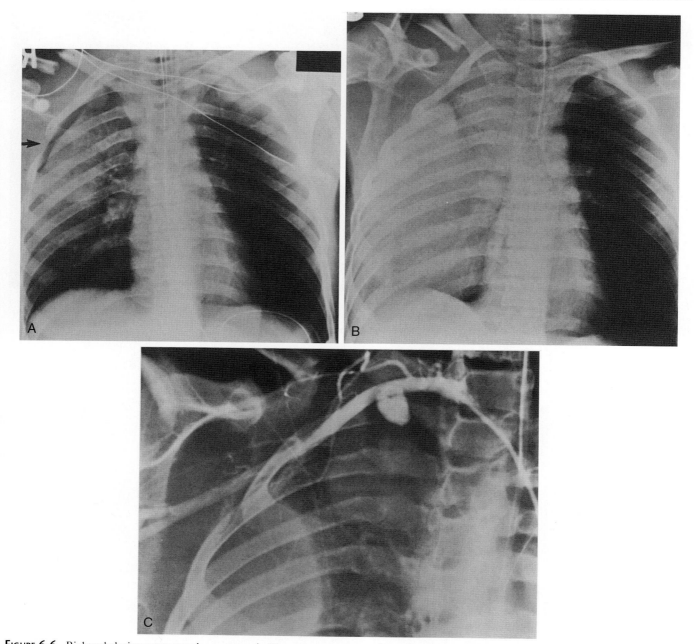

FIGURE 6-6. Right subclavian artery pseudoaneurysm. **A,** The anteroposterior, supine radiograph reveals a pneumothorax *(arrow)*, right upper lobe pulmonary contusion, and a fracture dislocation of the right clavicle. **B,** Within hours, a hemothorax rapidly developed, opacifying the entire right hemithorax. **C,** The arteriogram reveals a pseudoaneurysm of the right subclavian artery at the site of bony injury. Bleeding was successfully controlled with embolization.

Pneumomediastinum, however, may be the only finding, particularly with injury to the left main bronchus, which has a longer extrapleural course in the mediastinum. Bronchial rupture that occurs within the pleural space leads to pneumothorax that is usually large and fails to resolve despite tube drainage because of the persistent air leak (Fig. 6-14). The fallen lung sign occurs with complete disruption of the main stem bronchus (Fig. 6-9). The detached lung segment falls inferiorly and laterally to the base of the hemithorax. This contrasts with a pneumothorax from a partial bronchial tear, for which the lung typically collapses medially and centrally toward its attachment. In both instances the lung fails to reexpand on chest tube drainage. A missed partial bron-

chial tear should be suspected if there is persistent lobar atelectasis or air trapping in the affected lung.

ESOPHAGEAL RUPTURE

Esophageal disruption is very uncommon after blunt trauma. Iatrogenic causes such as endoscopic dilation of a stricture are more likely etiologies, but still uncommon. Severe pneumomediastinum is a manifestation of rupture. Other nonspecific findings include pneumothorax, left pleural effusion, and mediastinal widening due to hemorrhage or mediastinitis. Leakage of oral contrast detected by a contrast swallow or by thoracic CT confirms the diagnosis.

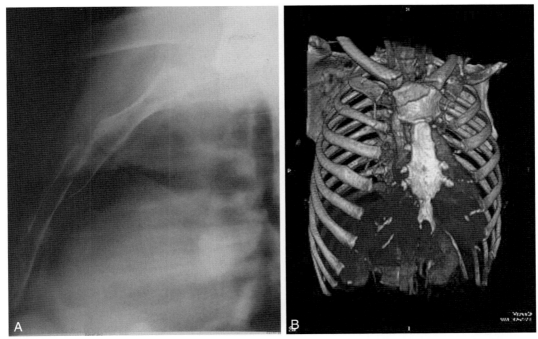

FIGURE 6-7. Sternomanubrial fracture. **A,** The lateral chest radiograph reveals a displaced sternal fracture with overlapping fragments just distal to the sternomanubrial junction. **B,** Three-dimensional image rendered from chest CT data in a different patient reveals a fracture across the manubrium. Courtesy of Peter Clarke, MD, Brigham and Women's Hospital, Boston, MA.

Box 6-3. Thoracic Spinal Injury

Occurs frequently with high-velocity injury
10% of patients have multiple fractures
80% of multiple fractures are noncontiguous
60% of fracture dislocations are associated with
complete neurologic defect
10% of spinal cord injuries occur after admission

▬ PLEURAL ABNORMALITIES

Pneumothorax

A pneumothorax occurs twice as often in patients with blunt trauma as in those with a penetrating injury. The identification of even a small pneumothorax is important, because a rapid increase in size of the pneumothorax may occur in mechanically ventilated patients. Because most chest radiographs are performed with the patient in the supine position, it may be difficult to recognize even a large pneumothorax. Air collects in the most nondependent regions; in the supine position air collects in an anterior and often inferior location and results most commonly in the deep sulcus sign (Box 6-6 and Fig. 6-10). On an erect radiograph, identification of the visceral pleural edge with absence of lung vessels peripherally is diagnostic (Fig. 6-11). A tension pneumothorax is a medical emergency (Box 6-7 and Fig. 6-12). Pneumothoraces are frequently associated with severe extrathoracic trauma. One study found that a pneumothorax occurred in 52% of patients with closed

head injury. The lung bases should always be reviewed on abdominal CT scans, which enable easy identification of an unsuspected pneumothorax. Pneumothoraces are rather conspicuous on chest CT.

Pneumomediastinum

Pneumomediastinum is a frequent finding after blunt trauma. The most common cause is disruption of the lung parenchyma and interstitial dissection of air due to sudden chest compression followed by reexpansion. Pneumomediastinum also can be seen during a prolonged or sudden increase in intrathoracic pressure (e.g., asthmatic attacks, barotrauma). It is often associated with a pneumothorax. Tracheobronchial rupture accounts for less than 1.5% of cases. The radiograph may show thin, streaky radiolucencies within the mediastinum that represent air and sharpening of mediastinal contours at the air interface (Fig. 6-13). The parietal pleura can be seen as a sharp line adjacent to the air lucency. Pneumomediastinum is most clearly identified on the left; it creates a sharply defined aortic contour that often can be followed inferiorly into the abdomen, and it produces a continuous diaphragm sign seen underlying the cardiac contour. The air may dissect superiorly into the neck through the fascial planes, inferiorly into the retroperitoneum or peritoneum, or subcutaneously (Fig. 6-14).

Pneumomediastinum alone is rarely clinically significant, although it may be exacerbated by positive pressure ventilation. Like any abnormal air collection, pneumomediastinum and its cause usually are easily identified and characterized by chest CT.

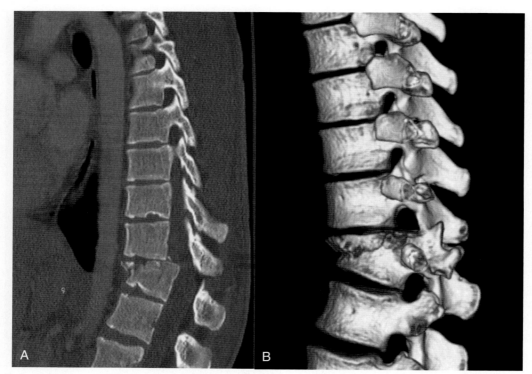

Figure 6-8. **A,** Sagittal CT image with **B,** 3D reconstruction demonstrates a T12 compression fracture with subluxation of T12 resulting in 50% compromise in the spinal canal. Case courtesy of Dr. Peter Clarke, Brigham and Women's Hospital, Boston, MA.

Box 6-4. **Rule of 2s for Normal Spinal Dimensions**

Posterior vertebral height is less than 2 mm greater than the anterior height (except T11 and T12).
Facet joint width is less than 2 mm.
Transverse interpedicular distance of contiguous vertebrae has a less than 2 mm difference.
Vertical interpedicular distance of contiguous vertebrae has a less than 2 mm difference.
Interspinous distance of adjacent vertebrae has a less than 2 mm difference.

Box 6-5. **Diagnostic Features of Rupture of the Trachea and Major Bronchus**

Pneumomediastinum
Persistent pneumothorax despite drainage
Fallen lung

Pleural Effusions

Most pleural collections after trauma result from hemorrhage. Surgery is required in less than 10% of cases of hemothorax. The principal indication is bleeding at a rate greater than 200 mL/hour or an effusion of more than 1 L at presentation. A rapidly expanding pleural effusion is most likely arterial in origin and may be life threatening. The usual cause is laceration of intercostal or internal mammary arteries or large mediastinal vessels. The admission radiograph may show complete opacification of the hemithorax, with contralateral mediastinal displacement due to the large volume of hemorrhage (see Fig. 6-6). Venous hemorrhage is usually self-limited because the expanding hemothorax compresses the underlying lung, causing pulmonary tamponade and hemostasis. The effusion may vary in size and may have a well-defined meniscus (Box 6-8). A hemothorax may result from laceration of the pleura by fractured ribs (occurring with or without a pneumothorax) or from closed chest trauma without evidence of rib fractures. Hemothorax is common when aortic rupture is present, and it is invariably left sided; it should not be erroneously attributed to left-sided rib fractures.

A left-sided pleural effusion or a hydrothorax or pyopneumothorax frequently develops after rupture of the esophagus. Identification of ingested material within the pleural fluid is diagnostic.

On the erect radiograph, an uncomplicated pleural effusion demonstrates a well-defined superior border; convex downward with widening of the lateral pleural stripe; and blunting of the costophrenic sulcus. On the supine radiograph, the pleural effusion layers in the dependent part of the pleural space, resulting in uniform, hazy opacification of the hemithorax. This is most easily recognized with unilateral collections.

Subpulmonic effusions may collect in the erect patient, with elevation and flattening of the apparent hemidiaphragm and a shift of the midpoint peak laterally. Fluid may collect in the mediastinal pleura space, resulting in a paraspinal opacity, or it may track into the fissure. Air and

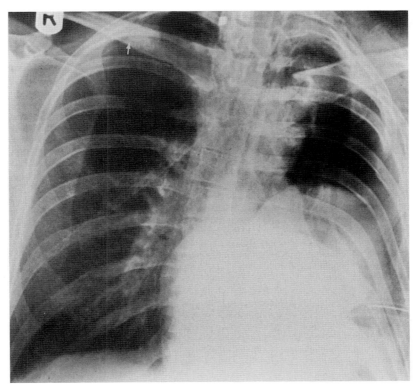

FIGURE 6-9. Fallen lung. Erect, anteroposterior radiograph of a patient ultimately found to have rupture of the left main bronchus reveals a large, left pneumothorax that persists despite tube drainage. A small, right apical pneumothorax *(arrow)* and subcutaneous emphysema can be seen in the left chest wall. Notice the multiple left rib fractures and left sternoclavicular dislocation.

Box 6-6. *Supine Radiographic Features for Identifying Pneumothorax*

Deep sulcus sign
Hyperlucency of hemithorax
Double diaphragmatic contour
Sharp mediastinal and cardiac contours (e.g., right cardiophrenic region, cardiac apex)

---

blood in the pleural effusion may result from a traumatic pneumothorax or a bronchopleural fistula.

Loculated Pleural Effusions

Loculated pleural collections may be subtle, and when bilateral, they are difficult to identify in the supine patient. CT or ultrasound, which can be performed at the bedside, can confirm the clinical suspicion and permit accurate tube placement.

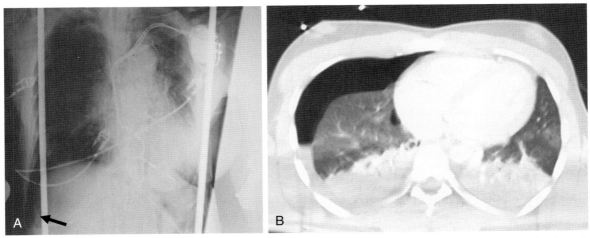

FIGURE 6-10. Pneumothorax. **A,** Portable, anteroposterior radiograph of a patient on a trauma board illustrates the deep sulcus sign *(arrow)* that can be observed when patients are imaged in a supine position. **B,** The CT image shows the right-sided pneumothorax.

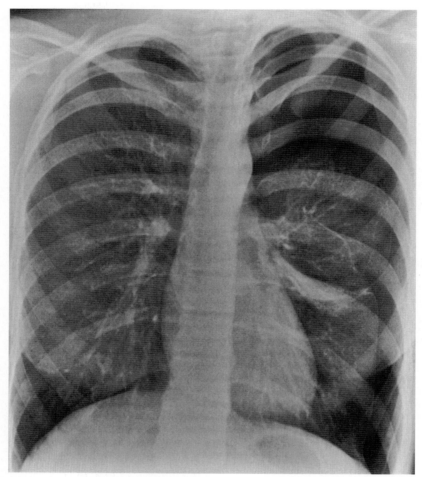

FIGURE 6-11. Pneumothorax. The erect, posteroanterior radiograph demonstrates a large, left pneumothorax.

Box 6-7. **Signs of Tension Pneumothorax**

Flattening of ipsilateral hemidiaphragm
Spreading of the ipsilateral ribs
Contralateral mediastinal displacement

Rupture of the Thoracic Duct

Rupture of the thoracic duct is rare and is usually the result of a penetrating injury or inadvertent injury to the duct during surgery. Treatment is surgical ligation of the duct. A chylous effusion typically develops over several days and may become very large. Most chylous effusions have a negative attenuation value. However, the chylous nature of the fluid may not be readily appreciated in the fasting patient or when the fluid is mixed with blood; in these instances, a high degree of suspicion is required to make the diagnosis.

■ PULMONARY PARENCHYMAL INJURY

Pulmonary parenchymal injury may be widespread and bilateral. It is usually most severe at the sites of skeletal injury because of the transmission of the injurious forces through the chest wall to the lung parenchyma. In most patients, the pulmonary injury resolves without complication. CT should be performed for any trauma patient with abnormal parenchymal opacification seen on chest radiography.

Contusion

Contusion (i.e., pulmonary hemorrhage) is the most frequent parenchymal injury, and it is usually radiographically evident within 6 hours of trauma. Initial clearing is relatively rapid, and it may be complete within 24 to 48 hours, but it more typically resolves over 72 hours. Contusions appear as nonsegmental homogenous opacities, which are frequently peripheral in location and often associated with a few millimeters of subpleural sparing (Fig. 6-15). Pulmonary contusion may or may not be associated with fractures. Contusions may be multifocal, solitary, unilateral, or bilateral. Occasionally, very severe contusion may result in acute respiratory distress syndrome (ARDS). Air bronchograms are an atypical finding because the bronchi are usually filled with blood. Airspace opacification that is slow to resolve or increases in extent suggests an additional complication such as infection, pulmonary edema, or ARDS.

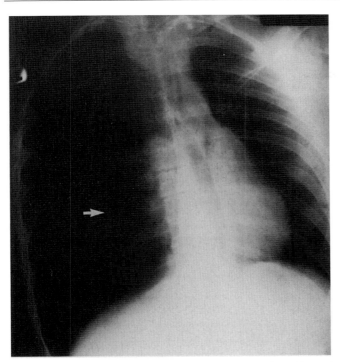

FIGURE 6-12. Tension pneumothorax. The posteroanterior radiograph reveals a large, right pneumothorax (*arrow* marks the pleural edge), with flattening of the right hemidiaphragm and contralateral mediastinal displacement indicating a mass effect.

Laceration

More severe trauma causes disruption of the parenchymal architecture, resulting in laceration. Pulmonary lacerations commonly accompany contusion and may initially be masked by the surrounding hemorrhage. An ovoid radiolucency with a surrounding pseudomembrane forming a pneumatocele is characteristic (Fig. 6-16A). Hemorrhage into the cavity can produce a gas-fluid level

or an air-crescent sign if the blood has clotted (see Fig. 6-16B). This appearance is most easily recognized on CT (Fig. 6-17). Pneumatoceles that result after resorption of the intracavitary hemorrhage are usually small (<5 mm), but lesions greater than 10 mm may occur. Typically, lacerations resolve slowly over weeks, but the hematoma may produce a solitary nodule or mass that persists for months. In the absence of an appropriate history, the latter may be mistaken for a carcinoma. Other complications of laceration include bronchopleural fistula and infection, which may require surgical intervention.

▬ DIAPHRAGMATIC RUPTURE

Diaphragmatic rupture is often associated with other severe injuries and is seen in 1% to 6% of major blunt chest trauma victims. The high mortality rate results from associated injuries (Box 6-9). The diaphragm is typically torn in the area of the central tendon or posteriorly at the musculotendinous insertion. Injury is more often left sided because of the protective effects of the liver subjacent the right hemidiaphragm. Right-sided rupture may be under recognized for this reason. Rupture into the pericardium is rare.

Diaphragmatic rupture is missed on the initial chest radiograph in up to two thirds of patients, but it is more readily recognized if the injury is recent and the tear is large and left sided (Fig. 6-18), permitting bowel or stomach to ascend into the left hemithorax. Delayed diagnosis is associated with increased morbidity and mortality from bowel strangulation and obstruction. The radiographic features are typically subtle and nonspecific and may include elevation of the hemidiaphragm with contour irregularity, contralateral mediastinal displacement, rib fractures, and left pleural effusion or hemothorax. The demonstration of a gas-containing abdominal viscus within the thorax by a contrast swallow provides the definitive diagnosis in most cases of left-sided rupture. However, this examination is often difficult to perform in the acute setting. Passage of a nasogastric tube during the initial resuscitation may provide

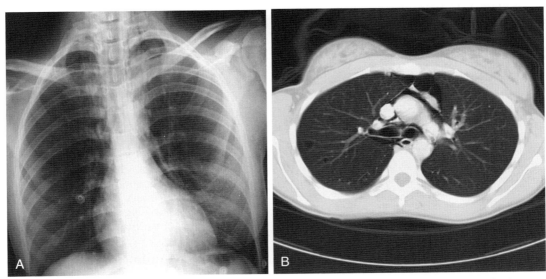

FIGURE 6-13. Pneumomediastinum. **A,** The posteroanterior radiograph reveals a streaky lucency within the superior mediastinum and sharpening of the left superior cardiac border *(arrow)* in a patient whose airbag deployed as a result of a low-speed collision. **B,** The corresponding CT image readily shows air outlining mediastinal structures.

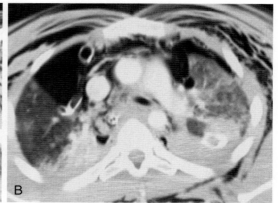

Figure 6-14. Pneumomediastinum and airway injury. **A,** Coronal CT image shows a large persistent right pneumothorax despite placement of two right chest tubes, smaller left pneumothorax, pneumomediastinum and subcutaneous emphysema. **B,** Axial image reveals avulsion of the right main stem bronchus, later confirmed by bronchoscopy; Case courtesy of Dr. Bharti Khurana, Brigham and Women's Hospital, Boston, MA.

Box 6-8. **Differentiation of Pleural Effusions**

Arterial injury: rapid onset, develops in minutes, life-threatening condition
Venous injury: slowly progressive, develops over hours, self-limited condition
Thoracic duct injury: chylous effusion, develops over several days, chronic condition

---

the necessary confirmation of the intrathoracic position of the stomach. Herniation of abdominal viscera such as the liver or spleen may be more difficult to recognize, particularly on chest radiography. Many of these features may be mimicked or masked by traumatic lung cysts, pulmonary contusion, atelectasis, or pleural fluid collections. Chronic conditions such as hiatal hernia, diaphragmatic eventration, and chronic hemidiaphragmatic elevation may also mimic diaphragmatic injury.

MDCT imaging with coronal and sagittal reformations has greatly increased the sensitivity and specificity for the diagnosis of diaphragmatic injury. MRI is most commonly reserved for problematic cases for which CT or serial radiography is nondiagnostic. CT-specific signs for diaphragmatic injury include the collar sign and the dependent viscera sign. The collar sign is identified when a hollow viscus, most commonly the stomach, appears to reside partially within the thorax and is kinked or collared as it passes through the expected plane of the diaphragm (Fig. 6-19). Herniation of the liver through the diaphragm with resulting constriction of the liver is also known as the collar sign or sometimes called the cottage loaf sign (Fig. 6-20 A, B, C). Recognition of this sign is greatly aided by coronal and sagittal reformations. The dependent viscera sign is identified on axial imaging when the upper third of the liver or spleen is in contact with the posterior thoracic wall. These structures are normally suspended away from the posterior wall in their superior extent by the presence of an intact diaphragm (Fig. 6-20 D)

Intrathoracic splenosis is a curious complication of diaphragmatic rupture. Fragments of the ruptured spleen may implant within the pleural cavity, enlarge, and produce an intrathoracic mass or masses. A radionucleotide splenic scan can confirm the cause of the mass or masses.

▬ LUNG HERNIATION OR TORSION

Herniation of lung through the chest wall due to separation of the ribs and injury to the intercostal muscles is an infrequent complication and is of little clinical significance. Lung torsion, however, is usually a surgical emergency. Torsion of either a lobe or the complete lung may occur and result in pulmonary infarction. Fortunately, this injury is rare; it is, however, more likely to occur in children.

Recognition of torsion may be very difficult. It is suspected when a collapsed or consolidated lung lies in an unusual position and there is malposition of the hilar structures, fissures, or the pulmonary vessels. Serial radiographs may be diagnostic because they demonstrate the changing position of a readily identifiable opacity (Fig. 6-21).

▬ TRAUMA TO THE AORTA

Causes and Survival

Motor vehicle accidents are the most common cause of deceleration injury to the thoracic aorta. After complete transection, most victims die at the site of the accident. The survivors have incomplete tears, with the surrounding adventitia maintaining some degree of integrity of the aorta (Box 6-10). The typical site of injury is at the aortic isthmus, the transition zone between the relatively mobile aortic arch and the tethered proximal descending thoracic aorta. Less common sites of injury include other points of aortic fixation, such as the aortic root, great vessel origins, and diaphragmatic hiatus. Without surgical repair, more than one half of patients with aortic injury succumb within the first 24 hours. Untreated, most survivors die in the following weeks. Only 2% survive long term with a chronic pseudoaneurysm.

Radiographic Findings

Plain film findings of aortic trauma (Box 6-11), although relatively sensitive, are not very specific (Fig. 6-22) and may be difficult to interpret. The anteroposterior, supine

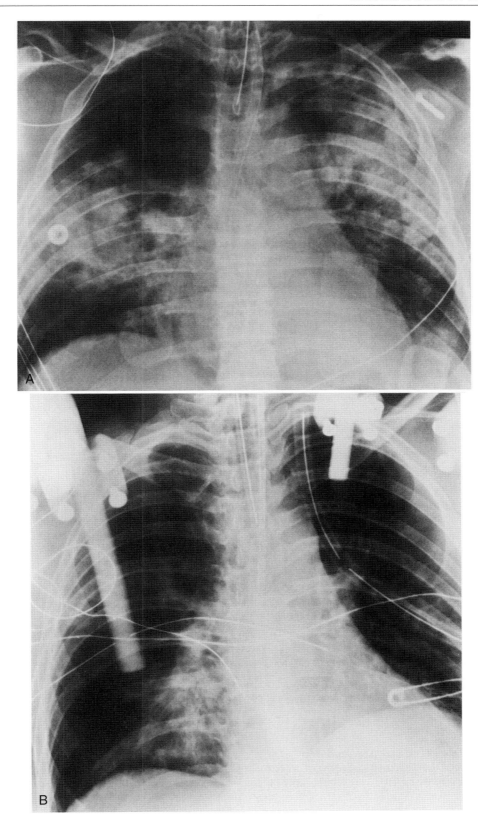

FIGURE 6-15. Pulmonary contusion. **A,** Admission radiograph reveals extensive, bilateral airspace opacification and a fracture dislocation of the right clavicle. **B,** Six days later, there has been significant clearing of the pulmonary contusion, with persistent right lower lobe opacification due to atelectasis. There has been interval placement of a left-sided chest tube.

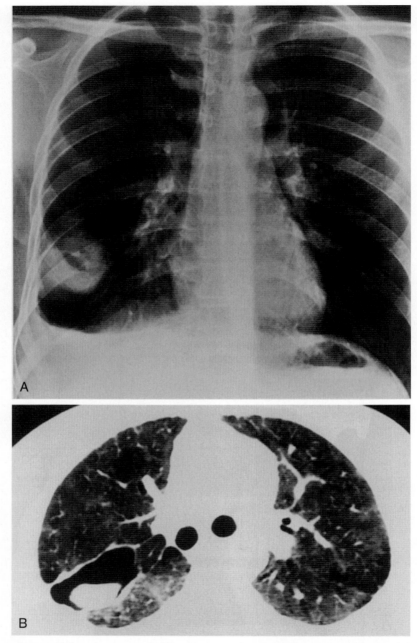

FIGURE 6-16. Pulmonary laceration containing a hematoma. **A,** The posteroanterior chest radiograph reveals a rounded, right lower lobe opacity with a central lucency and a small, right pleural effusion. The appearance mimics a pulmonary abscess or tumor. The history of recent right-sided trauma provides the diagnosis. **B,** CT scan at the level of the carina (lung windows) shows a large pneumatocele in the right upper lobe abutting the fissure. The cavity contains a hematoma, which may persist for months and may resemble a pulmonary tumor.

projection magnifies the mediastinum and may cause apparent rather than real mediastinal widening. Layering pleural effusions are more difficult to recognize and may obscure mediastinal contours. For this reason, CT is recommended for most trauma patients with any abnormalities detected by chest radiography, and it is often performed for patients with a significant trauma mechanism, even in the presence of a fairly unremarkable chest radiograph.

Aortography is rarely required. CT is able to diagnose the presence or absence of aortic tears with a high degree of accuracy (Table 6-2). CT scanning should always include the intrathoracic portion of the great vessels. Scanning should begin at the thoracic inlet rather than just above the aortic arch. In a few cases, CT findings are indeterminate for technical reasons (e.g., poorly timed bolus, intravenous contrast extravasation, motion artifact) or because of nonspecific findings, or anatomic reasons such as a periaortic hematoma, ductus diverticulum, or coarse atherosclerosis. In most cases, CT can definitively determine the absence or presence of aortic injury and obviate the need for aortography.

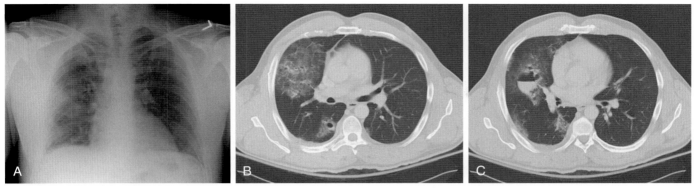

FIGURE 6-17. Pulmonary contusion and laceration. **A,** Chest radiography reveals a patchy parenchymal opacity in the right lung that is consistent with pulmonary contusion. **B,** CT image reveals a multifocal pulmonary contusion and laceration in the right lung that is subjacent to the site of trauma. **C,** More inferiorly, CT reveals a larger pulmonary laceration with a layering hemorrhage that was not seen prospectively by chest radiography.

Box 6-9. Diaphragmatic Rupture

70% involve the left hemidiaphragm
50% are missed clinically
50% have no initial radiologic findings
50% are identified at exploratory surgery

Aortic injury most commonly occurs as a transverse tear and can be segmental or circumferential. The severity of the aortic injury may range from a minimal intimal flap to frank rupture with active extravasation. An indirect finding of aortic injury is the presence of a mediastinal hematoma. The importance of the hematoma depends on the location. Blood within the mediastinum with a preserved fat plane with the aorta is not from aortic injury and is usually venous

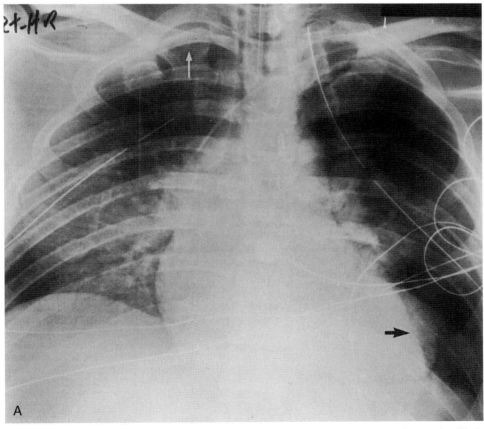

FIGURE 6-18. Left diaphragmatic rupture. **A,** The supine admission radiograph reveals a dense, left retrocardiac opacity *(black arrow)* with an oblique contour. The left diaphragmatic contour is absent medially. There are multiple, bilateral rib fractures and a small, right apical pneumothorax *(white arrow)*. The right lower lobe and left perihilar opacification represents contusion.

(Continued)

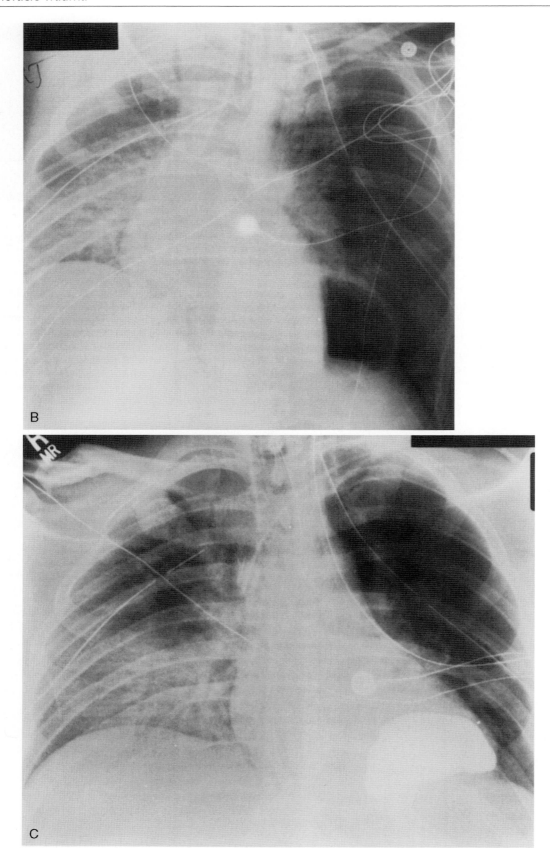

FIGURE 6-18, cont'd.   B, A right-side-down decubitus radiograph demonstrates an air-fluid level in the left retrocardiac region. C, Contrast material administered through the nasogastric tube confirms intrathoracic extension of the stomach through a partial left diaphragmatic tear.

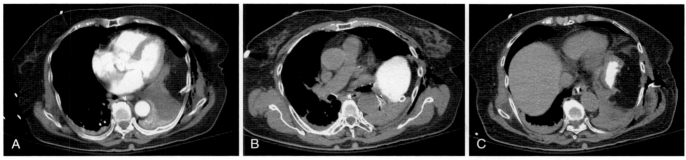

FIGURE 6-19. Left diaphragmatic rupture. **A,** CT reveals an unusual fluid collection anterior to lung parenchyma in a patient with multiple, left rib fractures and extensive subcutaneous emphysema. **B,** Repeat CT after administration of oral contrast material through a nasogastric tube shows the "collection" to be a fluid-filled stomach. **C,** CT image several slices lower shows the stomach being "collared" as it passes through the diaphragmatic tear.

in etiology due to bleeding from mediastinal veins and/or due to sternal or spinal injury. While periaortic hematoma may be venous in etiology, aortic injury needs to be considered, which may manifest as an occult intimal aortic tear.

Traumatic aortic injuries, when evaluated with multidetector CT (MDCT) can be graded (Fig. 6-23). The grading of aortic injury has implications for clinical management. MDCT grades 0 and 1 reliably exclude aortic injury and do not require aortography. MDCT grades 3 and 4 reliably confirm aortic injury. Only MDCT grade 2 injuries require aortography to confirm or exclude the

diagnosis of aortic injury (Fig. 6-24). Grade 3 injuries may, at the discretion of the surgeon, progress to aortography as a means of preoperative evaluation.

■ CARDIAC INJURY

Pneumopericardium

Pneumopericardium is usually the result of penetrating trauma. Pneumomediastinum may lead to pneumopericardium from air tracking along the adventitia of the pulmonary veins and into the pericardial space. Air outlines the cardiac contour and

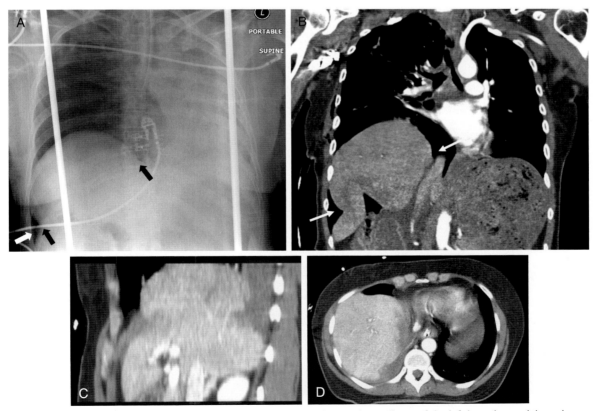

FIGURE 6-20. Right diaphragmatic rupture. **A,** Portable chest radiograph reveals complete collapse of the left lung due to right main stem bronchus intubation. The right-sided "deep sulcus" sign (black arrows) confirms a right pneumothorax, which improves visualization of the "collar" sign around a partially herniated liver (white arrow), indicating right diaphragmatic rupture. **B,** Coronal CT image confirms rupture of the right hemidiaphragm with herniation of the liver into the thorax. The resulting "collar" sign (white arrows) results from diaphragmatic constriction around the herniated liver. **C,** Sagittal MR image in a different patient reveals a similar injury with the liver demonstrating the "cottage loaf" sign. **D,** Axial image shows the dependent viscera sign.

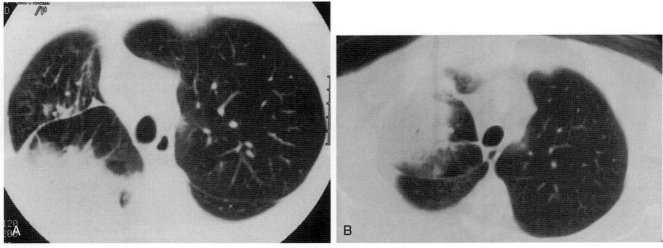

FIGURE 6-21. Lung torsion. Pneumonia in the right upper lobe, which is posterior on the supine CT scan (**A**), moves anteriorly on the prone scan (**B**). The rapid change in location confirms lung torsion.

Box 6-10. **Aortic Rupture Survival**
8% succumb immediately (i.e., complete transection)
50% of those surviving (i.e., incomplete tears), if untreated, will experience a rupture within 24 hours
2% of survivors succumb every hour
2% survive long term with a pseudoaneurysm

Box 6-11. **Radiographic Findings for Aortic Rupture**
Mediastinal width increased by more than 8 cm
Mediastinal widening of more than 25% of the thoracic diameter at the arch
Effacement of the aortic arch contour
Left apical cap or pleural effusion
Deviation of the trachea and nasogastric tube to the right
Depressed left main bronchus

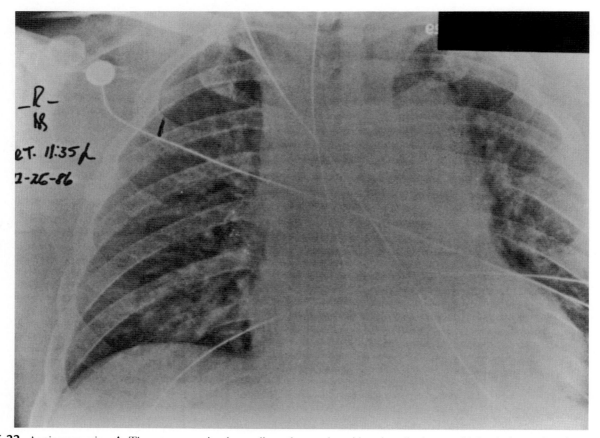

FIGURE 6-22. Aortic transection. **A,** The anteroposterior chest radiographs reveals a widened mediastinum and left apical extrapleural cap.

TABLE 6-2 Grading of Aortic Injury by Computed Tomography and Role of Aortography

Grade	Description and Role of Aortography
0	Normal aorta, normal mediastinum; no aortography
1	Normal aorta, mediastinal hematoma present but not contiguous with aorta; no aortography
2	Periaortic hematoma and/or indeterminate intrinsic abnormalities of the aorta; aortography
3	Confined aortic injury; aortography discretionary
4	Traumatic aortic disruption; aortography likely contraindicated

extends to the pericardial reflection at the level of the origin of the aortic great vessels (Fig. 6-25). Unlike pneumomediastinum, air in the pericardium shifts with the patient's position and assumes a nondependent location. Pneumopericardium is rarely clinically significant, although there are reports of tamponade following tension pneumopericardium.

Hemopericardium

Hemopericardium may occur as a result of blunt trauma, but it more typically follows a penetrating injury. Cardiac tamponade may develop and rapidly become life threatening. The chest radiograph may demonstrate a normal cardiac contour, and a high index of clinical suspicion is required to make the diagnosis. The diagnosis is more readily made if the cardiac size is large or increasing on serial radiographs. Echocardiography can rapidly confirm the presence of pericardial fluid. CT can demonstrate the high density of the fluid and may confirm the clinical findings of tamponade by showing periportal edema, transit delay of intravenous contrast material through the heart, and distention of the inferior vena cava, hepatic veins, and renal veins.

Pericardial rupture is rare and usually fatal. The diaphragmatic or mediastinal pleurae may also be involved. Left-sided pericardial-pleural rupture can result in herniation of an abdominal viscus into the pericardial cavity. Pneumothorax and pneumopericardium are associated findings.

Myocardial Contusion

Cardiac contusion is common and is frequently asymptomatic. Most cases are unrecognized. Cardiac monitoring can identify contusion-related arrhythmias. Radionuclide ventriculography can detect wall-motion abnormalities. Right ventricular dysfunction is most common because of the right ventricle's immediate retrosternal location. Ventricular dysfunction is usually reversible unless myocardial infarction has occurred.

■ INDIRECT PULMONARY COMPLICATIONS OF TRAUMA

Acute Respiratory Distress Syndrome

ARDS may complicate trauma. The initial chest radiograph often is normal. A characteristic delay of up to 12 hours from the clinical onset of respiratory failure to the appearance of radiographic abnormalities is well recognized. Progressive opacification from an interstitial appearance to widespread consolidation develops. Interstitial emphysema leading to tiny cysts and larger pneumatoceles and pneumothorax are frequent complications. The severity of ARDS varies from complete recovery within days to prolonged assisted ventilation with residual permanent lung damage or death from respiratory failure. Pulmonary edema from fluid overload, pneumonia, and atelectasis may complicate the syndrome (see Chapter 5).

Fat Embolism Syndrome

Fat embolism is common, but fortunately, fat embolism syndrome is rare (Box 6-12). It is most likely to occur after severe bony injury, usually involving a long bone such as the femur. The syndrome encompasses pulmonary and systemic manifestations involving the brain, kidneys, and skin. Fat emboli are thought to originate at the site of fractures and to enter the intramedullary veins. The circulating fat globules are then trapped within the pulmonary vasculature. This causes obstruction and chemical injury from the released fatty acids. The resultant endothelial damage leads to leakage of fluid, hemorrhage, and inflammation. There is a typical lag time of 12 to 72 hours before the syndrome develops, which allows differentiation from the other complications of trauma that usually present immediately. Fat embolism syndrome is a cause of ARDS, and identification of fat globules allows the differentiation of this cause of ARDS from the many others. Prevention of fat embolism syndrome includes early immobilization of fractures and the recognition that patients with closed fractures are most at risk.

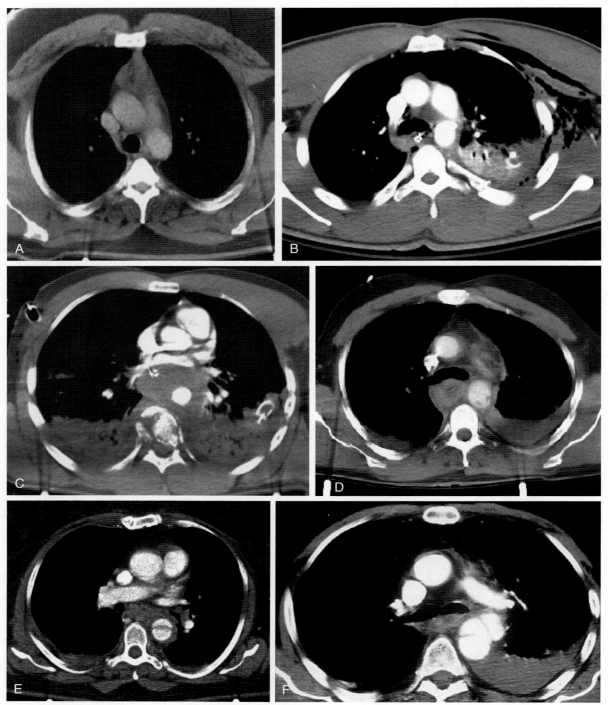

FIGURE 6-23. CT for aortic injury. **A,** CT image reveals abnormal anterior mediastinal soft tissue attenuation that is consistent with hematoma. However, the fat plane between the hematoma and the aorta is preserved (grade 1), and aortography is not needed. **B,** CT image of a different patient shows a subtle contour abnormality of the aortic arch at the isthmus, later confirmed by angiography to represent aortic injury. **C,** Extensive posterior mediastinal hematoma surrounding and contiguous with the aorta, but the aorta itself appeared normal on CT (grade 2). Notice the thoracic spine fracture. Aortography was indicated, but the result was negative for aortic injury. **D,** CT image of another patient reveals a slightly oval shape to the proximal descending thoracic aorta and intraluminal filling defects within the contrast material, confirming aortic injury (grade 3). Mediastinal hematoma is present, but there is no active contrast extravasation. Aortography is discretionary before definitive repair. **E,** Axial CT image shows a small pseudoaneurysm on the anterior wall of proximal descending thoracic aorta at the location of the ligamentum arteriosum. The abnormal aortic contour, periaortic mediastinal hematoma and classic location are diagnostic of aortic injury. Case courtesy of Dr. Peter Clarke, Brigham and Women's Hospital, Boston, MA. **F,** CT of yet another patient shows traumatic aortic disruption with contrast material extending beyond the normal confines of the aorta and a moderate-sized left hemothorax (grade 4). Delay for aortography before definite repair carries a significant risk of exsanguination and death and is likely contraindicated.

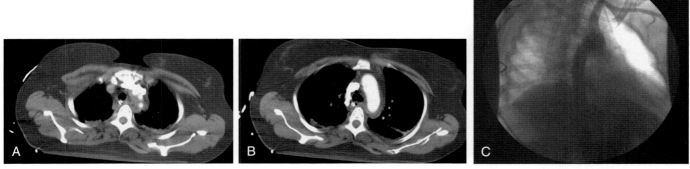

FIGURE 6-24. Aortic injury. **A** and **B,** Two CT images at the level of the aortic arch and great vessel origins reveal a small amount of periaortic hematoma that is contiguous with the posterior arch and surrounds the proximal great vessels, although the aorta appears normal (grade 2). **C,** Aortography confirmed the presence of aortic injury, and the patient underwent emergent surgical repair.

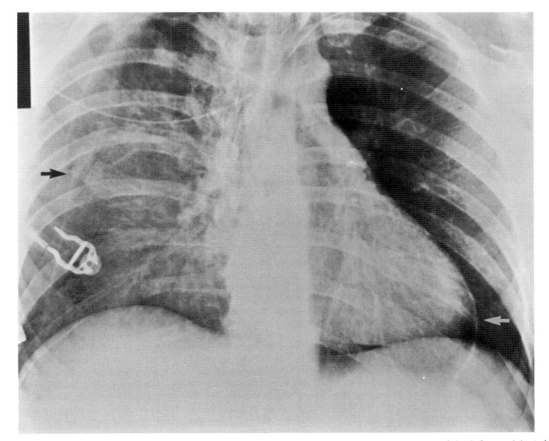

FIGURE 6-25. Pneumopericardium. The anteroposterior, supine radiograph demonstrates air around the apex of the left ventricle *(white arrow)* and a large, right pneumothorax *(black arrow)*. Air outlines the aortic knob confirming pneumomediastinum.

Box 6-12. **Diagnosis of Fat Embolism Syndrome**

Severe bony injury
Hypoxia or tachypnea
Widespread pulmonary opacification
Fat globules in sputum or urine
Petechia in skin and optic fundi
Delirium, convulsions, and coma

■ SUGGESTED READINGS

Daffner, R., 1988. Imaging of vertebral Trauma, Aspen, Rockville, IL.

Dee, P.M., 1992. The radiology of chest trauma [review]. Radiol. Clin. North. Am. 30, 291–306.

Fishman, J.E., 2000. Imaging of blunt aortic and great vessel trauma. J. Thorac. Imaging. 15, 97–103.

Fraser, R.G., Pare, J.A.P., Pare, P.D., 1991. Diagnosis of Diseases of the Chest, third ed., vol. 4, WB Saunders, Philadelphia, pp. 2481–2518.

Gavant, M., 1999. Helical CT grading of traumatic aortic injuries. Radiol. Clin. North. Am. 37, 553–574.

Gavant, M.L., Menke, P.G., Fabian, T., 1995. Blunt traumatic aortic rupture detection with helical CT of the chest. Radiology 197, 125–133.

Gavelli, G., Canini, R., Bertaccini, P., et al., 2002. Traumatic injuries: imaging of thoracic injuries. Emerg. Radiol. 12, 1273–1294.

Groskin, S.A., 1992. Selected topics in chest trauma [review]. Radiology 183, 605–617.

Hauser, C.J., Visvikis, G., Hinrichs, C., et al., 2003. Prospective validation of computed tomographic screening of the thoracolumbar spine in trauma. J. Trauma. 55, 228–234.

Jelly, L.M.E., Evans, D.R., Easty, M.J., et al., 2000. Radiography versus spiral CT in the evaluation of cervicothoracic junction injuries in polytrauma patients who have undergone intubation. Radiographics 20, S251–S259.

Kerns, S.R., Gay, S.B., 1990. Computed tomography of blunt trauma. AJR. Am. J. Roentgenol. 156, 273–279.

Kuhlman, J.E., Pozniak, M.A., Collins, J., et al., Radiographic and CT findings of blunt chest trauma: aortic injuries and looking beyond them. Radiographics 18, 1085–1108.

Mirvis, S.E., Templeton, P., 1992. Imaging in acute thoracic trauma [review]. Semin. Roentgenol. 27, 184–210.

Murphey, M., Batmitzky, S., Bramble, J., 1989. Diagnostic imaging of spinal trauma. Radiol. Clin. North. Am. 27, 855–872.

Patel, N.H., Stephens, K.E., Mirvis, S.E., et al., 1998. Imaging of acute thoracic aortic injury due to blunt trauma: a review. Radiology 209, 335–348.

Richardson, P., Mirvis, S.E., Scorpio, R., 1991. Value of CT in determining the need for angiography when the findings of mediastinal hematoma on chest radiographs are equivocal. AJR. Am. J. Roentgenol. 156, 273–279.

Sheridan, R., Peralta, R., Rhea, J., et al., 2003. Reformatted visceral protocol helical computed tomographic scanning allows conventional radiographs of the thoracic and lumbar spine to be eliminated in the evaluation of blunt trauma patients. J. Trauma. 55, 665–669.

Stark, P., Jacobson, F., 1992. Radiology of thoracic trauma [review]. Curr. Opin. Radiol. 4, 87–93.

Trerotola, S.C., 1995. Can helical CT replace aortography in thoracic trauma [editorial]?. Radiology 197, 13–15.

Van Hise, M.L., Primack, S.L., Israel, R.S., et al., 1998. CT in blunt chest trauma: indications and limitations. Radiographics 18, 1071–1084.

Wintermark, M., Mouhsine, E., Theumann, N., et al., 2003. Thoracolumbar spine fractures in patients who have sustained severe trauma: depiction with multidetector row CT. Radiology 227, 681–689.

Wintermark, M., Wicky, S., Schnyder, P., 2002. Imaging of acute traumatic injuries of the thoracic aorta. Eur. Radiol. 12, 431–442.

CHAPTER 7

Interstitial Lung Disease

Theresa C. McLoud and Subba R. Digumarthy

Many chronic diseases can produce diffuse opacities in the lung. Some are primarily lung disorders, and some others are manifestations of diseases arising elsewhere. Although these disorders have frequently been referred to as *interstitial lung diseases*, many also involve the alveolar spaces. More than 150 such disorders have been described, and a comprehensive list is provided in Box 7-1. Despite the large number, approximately 15 to 20 constitute 90% of such disease states, and these are the entities that are discussed in this chapter. Pneumoconioses and vascular disorders are discussed in Chapters 8 and 9.

■ CLINICAL PRESENTATION

Patients usually present (Box 7-2) with dyspnea as the predominant symptom. Physical examination frequently finds only dry rales or crackles. Physiologically, the abnormalities primarily affect gas exchange and result in hypoxemia. Reduced lung volumes may result in a restrictive pattern identified on pulmonary function tests.

The standard chest radiograph remains the basic and, in some cases, the only imaging technique that is useful. The chest radiograph, however, is often nonspecific. Development of high-resolution computed tomography (HRCT) has resulted in markedly improved accuracy in diagnosing interstitial lung disease. The following are the main technical components: 0.625- to 1.25-mm-thick sections, use of a high-resolution algorithm, targeted reconstruction to a single lung (optional), and prone scans to evaluate early or minimal basal disease. Prone scans are necessary to differentiate dependent atelectasis, a physiologic phenomenon that usually occurs posteriorly in the basal areas of the lungs, from true early interstitial lung disease. Gallium scanning and positron emission tomography

---

Box 7-1. Diffuse Interstitial (Parenchymal) Lung Diseases

INFECTIONS
Viral and mycoplasma pneumonia
Miliary tuberculosis
Fungal
Parasitic

IMMUNOLOGIC AND CONNECTIVE TISSUE DISORDERS
Progressive systemic sclerosis
Lupus erythematosus
Rheumatoid lung
Dermatomyositis
Ankylosing spondylitis
Drug reactions
Chronic eosinophilic pneumonia
Wegener's granulomatosis
Idiopathic pulmonary hemorrhage
Goodpasture's syndrome

ENVIRONMENTAL DISORDERS
Allergic alveolitis (hypersensitivity pneumonitis)
Silicosis
Coal worker's pneumoconiosis
Asbestosis
Berylliosis
Other pneumoconioses

IDIOPATHIC INTERSTITIAL PNEUMONIAS
Idiopathic pulmonary fibrosis
Nonspecific interstitial pneumonia
Desquamative interstitial pneumonia

Lymphocytic interstitial pneumonia
Respiratory bronchiolitis interstitial lung disease
Organizing pneumonia
Pneumonia resulting from irradiation
Pneumonia resulting from neurofibromatosis

SARCOIDOSIS

OTHER SPECIFIC DISORDERS
Histiocytosis X (Langerhans cell histiocytosis)
Lymphangioleiomyomatosis
Gaucher's disease
Pulmonary alveolar microlithiasis
Pulmonary alveolar proteinosis
Amyloidosis

NEOPLASTIC DISEASE
Metastatic carcinoma, lymphangitic carcinomatosis
Bronchioloalveolar carcinoma
Leukemia
Lymphoma

CARDIOVASCULAR DISEASE
Pulmonary edema
Hemosiderosis, chronic passive congestion

PULMONARY VASCULAR DISEASE
Veno-occlusive disease
Arteriolitis
Fat embolism
Embolism from oily contrast media
Multiple emboli and idiopathic pulmonary hypertension

Box 7-2. **Clinical Presentation**

SYMPTOMS
Dyspnea
Dry rales or crackles
Reduced lung volumes

EVALUATION
Chest radiography
Computed tomography (CT)
Gallium 67 scanning
Positron emission tomography (PET)

(PET) have also been used in the evaluation of interstitial lung disease and are discussed in more detail in *Nuclear Medicine: The Requisites.*

▬ PATTERN RECOGNITION

Classification

Pattern recognition in diffuse interstitial lung disease has been the subject of controversy for many years. Traditional interpretation of chest radiographs separates these processes into two groups: diseases that radiographically appear to involve the terminal airspaces or alveoli and those that appear to involve the interstitium. However, several problems limit this approach to differential diagnosis. Many pulmonary diseases produce pathologic changes in both compartments, and disease processes that are pathologically classified as interstitial may produce an alveolar pattern on the radiograph.

A graphic or morphometric classification is a better approach and is enumerated in Box 7-3. The patterns are described as nodular, irregular or linear, cystic, ground-glass, and parenchymal consolidation. Most patterns can be readily identified on standard radiographs, but ground-glass and cystic disease patterns are much more readily appreciated on HRCT. Many diseases demonstrate more than one pattern (see Box 7-3).

Pattern Characteristics

The nodular pattern (Fig. 7-1) is composed of multiple, small nodules that range from 1 mm to 1 cm in diameter. Irregular linear opacities (Fig. 7-2) frequently form a reticular pattern that may be fine or coarse. There are two types of cystic patterns: thin-walled cysts (Fig. 7-3) and honeycombing. Honeycomb spaces usually are 1 cm or less in diameter with relatively thick walls (>2 mm), and they are a pathologic correlate of end-stage lung disease with fibrosis (Fig. 7-4). Ground-glass attenuation is a term used almost exclusively with CT. It consists of an amorphous opacification or increase in attenuation, which is mildly severe and is not sufficient to obliterate the pulmonary vessels. Parenchymal consolidation, which has been referred to as alveolar or airspace disease, is characterized by dense opacification often with air bronchograms (Fig. 7-5). This opacification obliterates the pulmonary vasculature. Septal lines are a common feature of many interstitial lung disorders but are particularly predominant in lymphangitic spread of carcinoma and in congestive heart failure.

Other features should be considered in the differential diagnosis. They include distribution of disease, pleural

---

Box 7-3. **Patterns of Opacities in Interstitial Lung Disease**

NODULAR OR RETICULAR NODULAR PATTERN (SMALL, ROUNDED OPACITIES)
Silicosis
Coal worker's pneumoconiosis
Hypersensitivity pneumonitis
Histiocytosis X
Lymphangitic carcinomatosis
Sarcoidosis*
Pulmonary alveolar microlithiasis

LINEAR PATTERN (SMALL, IRREGULAR, RETICULAR OPACITIES)
Usual interstitial pneumonitis (idiopathic pulmonary fibrosis)*
Nonspecific interstitial pneumonitis
Lymphocytic interstitial pneumonitis
Sarcoidosis
Radiation fibrosis
Fibrosis associated with collagen vascular disease
Asbestosis
Drug reactions
Lymphangitic carcinomatosis

CYSTIC PATTERN
Idiopathic pulmonary fibrosis (honeycombing)
Lymphangioleiomyomatosis

Histiocytosis X
Lymphocytic interstitial pneumonitis

GROUND-GLASS ATTENUATION
Hypersensitivity pneumonitis
Acute interstitial pneumonitis
Desquamative interstitial pneumonitis
Nonspecific interstitial pneumonitis
Alveolar proteinosis*
Idiopathic pulmonary fibrosis

PARENCHYMAL CONSOLIDATION (AIRSPACE OR ALVEOLAR DISEASE)
Cryptogenic organizing pneumonia
Chronic eosinophilic pneumonia
Bronchioloalveolar carcinoma
Lymphoma
Alveolar proteinosis
Vasculitis
Pulmonary hemorrhage
Septal Lines
Lymphangitic carcinomatosis
Congestive heart failure (interstitial edema)

*Pattern that is predominant or usually associated with a specific disorder.

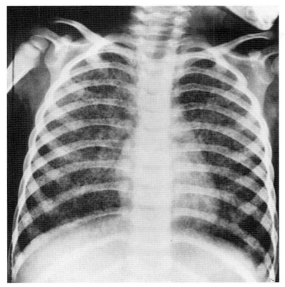

FIGURE 7-1. Nodular pattern of miliary tuberculosis. Multiple, small (1 to 3 mm) nodules are distributed diffusely throughout the lungs.

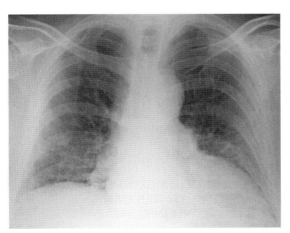

FIGURE 7-2. Linear opacities of nonspecific interstitial pneumonia. The posteroanterior view shows coarse linear opacities distributed more in the lower lungs than upper areas.

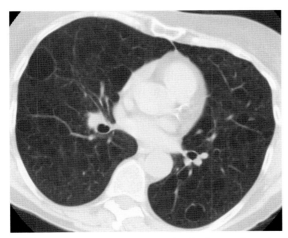

FIGURE 7-3. Thin-walled cysts are seen in the lungs of a patient with lymphangioleiomyomatosis.

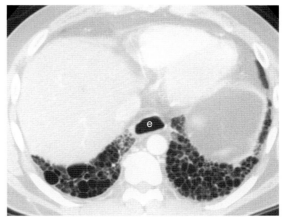

FIGURE 7-4. Honeycombing pattern in the usual interstitial pneumonitis of scleroderma. Thick-walled cysts are seen in the both lung bases. Notice the dilated esophagus (e).

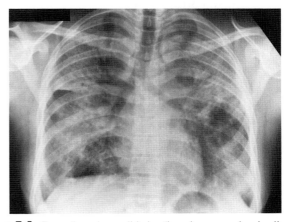

FIGURE 7-5. Parenchymal consolidation (i.e., airspace or alveolar disease). Confluent, diffuse consolidation and air bronchograms in both upper lobes can be seen in this example of an alveolar pattern in a patient with interstitial lung disease (i.e., sarcoidosis).

abnormalities, the size of the lungs, the presence of pulmonary arterial hypertension, and mediastinal and hilar adenopathy.

Zonal Distribution

Diseases have zonal preferences in the lungs (Box 7-4), although severe diseases often become diffuse. For example, histiocytosis, sarcoidosis, silicosis, and coal worker's pneumoconiosis typically favor the upper lobes, whereas idiopathic pulmonary fibrosis and fibrosis associated with collagen vascular disease tend to be a lower-zone phenomenon. Pleural disease may take one of several forms (Box 7-5). Pneumothorax may be seen as a complication of any cause of end-stage lung, but it may be identified early in the course of diseases such as histiocytosis X and lymphangioleiomyomatosis, in which there is a high prevalence of pneumothorax. Similarly, pleural effusions and diffuse thickening are often associated with collagen vascular disease and asbestos exposure. Pleural plaques, an uncommon feature, are produced almost exclusively by asbestos exposure. Adenopathy (Box 7-6), which is recognized on

Box 7-4. Zonal Preference

UPPER ZONES
Silicosis
Coal worker's pneumoconiosis
Sarcoidosis
Ankylosing spondylitis
Histiocytosis X

LOWER ZONES
Chronic interstitial pneumonias
Idiopathic pulmonary fibrosis
Asbestosis
Fibrosis due to collagen vascular disease

CENTRAL AREA
Pulmonary edema
Pulmonary alveolar proteinosis
Some lymphangitic tumors (Kaposi's sarcoma)
Lymphoma

PERIPHERAL AREA
Chronic interstitial pneumonias, idiopathic
    pulmonary fibrosis
Organizing pneumonia
Chronic eosinophilic pneumonia

Box 7-5. Pleural Disease

PNEUMOTHORAX
Lymphangioleiomyomatosis
Histiocytosis X
End-stage honeycombing

PLEURAL EFFUSION
Lymphangioleiomyomatosis
Collagen vascular disease
Lymphangitic carcinomatosis
Pulmonary edema

PLEURAL THICKENING
Asbestosis (plaques or diffuse)
Collagen vascular disease

Box 7-6. Adenopathy

STANDARD RADIOGRAPHY
Silicosis
Sarcoidosis
Lymphoma
Lymphangitic carcinomatosis

COMPUTED TOMOGRAPHY*
Idiopathic pulmonary fibrosis
Nonspecific interstitial pneumonitis
Hypersensitivity pneumonitis
Fibrosis associated with collagen vascular disease
Lymphangioleiomyomatosis

*More sensitive in detection of adenopathy than radiography.

Box 7-7. Lung Volumes

REDUCED
Idiopathic pulmonary fibrosis (usual interstitial
    pneumonitis)
Nonspecific interstitial pneumonitis
Asbestosis
Collagen vascular disease

NORMAL
Sarcoidosis
Histiocytosis

INCREASED
Lymphangioleiomyomatosis

standard radiographs, is associated with silicosis and sarcoidosis, lymphangitic carcinomatosis, and lymphoma. CT is more sensitive in the identification of adenopathy and may demonstrate mildly enlarged lymph nodes in idiopathic pulmonary fibrosis, hypersensitivity pneumonitis, fibrosis associated with the collagen vascular diseases, and lymphangioleiomyomatosis.

The size of the lung (i.e., lung volumes) may be a clue to the differential diagnosis (Box 7-7). The fibrotic disorders are characterized by marked restriction, and small lungs invariably are seen in idiopathic pulmonary fibrosis and related disorders. However, histiocytosis X and sarcoidosis in the early stages are usually associated with normal lung volumes, but lymphangioleiomyomatosis produces air trapping with large lung volumes. Pulmonary arterial hypertension usually indicates end-stage disease with pronounced obliteration of the pulmonary vasculature. Except for pulmonary vascular diseases, signs of pulmonary arterial hypertension are rarely identified.

▬ HIGH-RESOLUTION COMPUTED TOMOGRAPHY FEATURES OF INTERSTITIAL LUNG DISEASE

The five classifications of patterns of diffuse parenchymal lung disease on HRCT are linear or reticular opacities, nodular opacities, cystic lesions, ground-glass opacification, and parenchymal consolidation (i.e., alveolar or airspace disease). Webb and colleagues describe such HRCT findings in interstitial lung disease further in their work (see Suggested Readings).

Reticular or Linear Opacities

Reticular opacities usually are caused by interstitial thickening by cells, fluid, or fibrous tissue (Box 7-8).

Box 7-8. High-Resolution Computed Tomography Findings for Linear Opacities

Thickening of bronchovascular bundles (axial)
Interlobular septal thickening (septal lines)
Intralobular interstitial thickening
Honeycombing
Subpleural lines
Centrilobular abnormalities

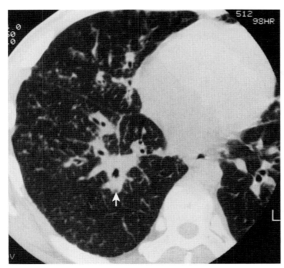

FIGURE 7-6. Axial interstitial thickening in a patient with sarcoidosis. Bronchial wall thickening *(white arrow)* and small nodules are seen subpleurally along the fissures and lateral chest wall.

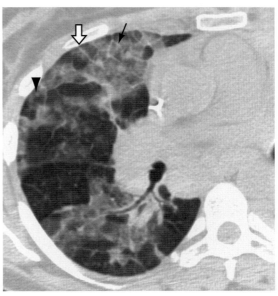

FIGURE 7-7. Septal thickening in lymphangitic carcinomatosis. Central septal lines outline the secondary pulmonary lobule, which appears as a polyhedral structure *(thin arrow)*. Peripheral septal lines lie perpendicular to the pleural surface *(open arrow)*. A central dot in the lobule is prominent, and the intralobular bronchiole is visible *(arrowhead)*.

Axial Interstitial Thickening

Thickening of the axial interstitium (i.e., interstitium in a peribronchovascular location) (Fig. 7-6) occurs in many diseases, such as lymphangitic spread of carcinoma, pulmonary fibrosis, and sarcoidosis. It is manifested by bronchial wall thickening and apparent enlargement of central pulmonary vessels. The thickening may be smooth or nodular. This appearance must be differentiated from a primary airway problem, bronchiectasis. In bronchiectasis, the bronchi show evidence of bronchial wall thickening, but they also are dilated and larger than adjacent pulmonary artery branches. This results in the appearance of large ring shadows. In patients with isolated bronchiectasis, there are no other signs of lung disease.

Interlobular Septal Thickening

Thickening of the interlobular septa (Fig. 7-7) is common in many interstitial lung diseases. In the peripheral lung, it appears as 1- to 2-cm lines that extend perpendicularly from the pleural surface into the substance of the lung. In the more central portion of the lung, the thickened septa can outline the secondary pulmonary lobules, producing polygonal structures that are 1 to 2.5 cm in diameter. These structures typically have a central dot that represents the pulmonary artery. Occasionally, lines that are 2.5 cm long and that outline more than one lobule can be identified, particularly in the periphery of the lung. They have been called *parenchymal bands* and *long lines*.

Centrilobular Abnormalities

Prominence of the central dot (Fig. 7-8) within the secondary pulmonary lobule (i.e., centrilobular vessel) may occur in a number of interstitial lung diseases. The intralobular bronchiole often becomes visible when there is centrilobular thickening. Centrilobular abnormalities can also be seen in patients with diseases of the peripheral airways (i.e., bronchioles).

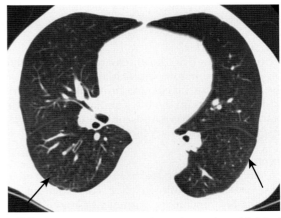

FIGURE 7-8. Centrilobular nodules in respiratory bronchiolitis. In the lower lobes, there are multiple, small, centrilobular ground-glass nodules. Notice the subpleural sparing at the fissures.

Intralobular Interstitial Thickening

Involvement of the interstitium within the lobule around the central artery and bronchiole or related to the interlobular septum may produce a fine reticular pattern within the lobule itself (Fig. 7-9). This usually extends from the centrilobular vessel peripherally to join a thickened septum.

Subpleural Lines

A subpleural line may be defined as a curvilinear opacity that is less than 1 cm from the pleural surface. It parallels the pleura and is a few millimeters thick (see Chapter 8). First described in asbestosis, a subpleural line occasionally is seen in normal lungs and results from dependent atelectasis.

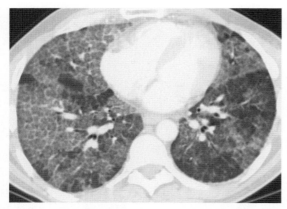

FIGURE 7-9. Intralobular interstitial thickening (i.e., reticular opacities) in pulmonary alveolar proteinosis. Thickened interlobular septa (hexagons) and a fine reticular pattern are visible within the lobules.

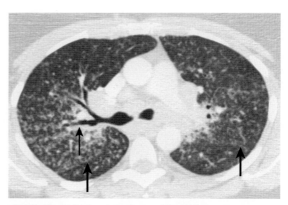

FIGURE 7-10. Interstitial nodules in sarcoidosis. Small nodules up to 4 mm in diameter are identified in both lungs. There is also thickening of the axial interstitium along the bronchi *(arrow)* and nodules along the fissures *(thick arrows)*.

Nodules and Nodular Opacities

Some investigators have attempted to differentiate interstitial from airspace or acinar nodules on HRCT. Because the anatomy of the secondary pulmonary lobule can be readily observed on HRCT, this distinction often may be possible, even though overlap in the appearance of interstitial and alveolar nodules occurs and many disease processes involve both compartments.

Interstitial Nodules

Interstitial nodules (Fig. 7-10) tend to be well defined and can be seen in numerous interstitial lung diseases. They may be located in the axial interstitium along the peribronchovascular bundles, in the interlobular septa in a subpleural location adjacent to fissures, and in the central portion of the secondary pulmonary lobule.

Airspace Nodules

Ill-defined nodules that are 6 mm to 1 cm in diameter may be associated with airspace consolidation around the peripheral bronchioles, particularly around the terminal bronchiole in the center of the secondary pulmonary lobule. They are not truly acinar but may be considered airspace nodules (Fig. 7-11). They may be associated with more confluent areas of airspace consolidation with air bronchograms. These nodules may be seen in patients with lobular pneumonia, endobronchial spread of tuberculosis, or bronchioloalveolar carcinoma.

Masses of Fibrosis or Conglomerate Masses

Large masses of fibrous tissue may occur, usually in the central or axial interstitium (Fig. 7-12). They are usually associated with architectural distortion and volume loss. They typically produce traction bronchiectasis centrally in the bronchi that they encompass. This appearance is typical for silicosis and for coal worker's pneumoconiosis, but it may also occur in end-stage sarcoidosis.

Cystic Pattern

Cystic abnormalities include honeycombing, traction bronchiectasis, lung cysts, and cavitary nodules. Findings

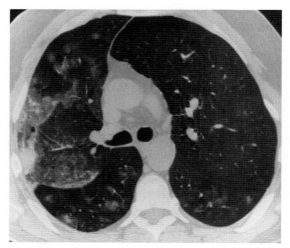

FIGURE 7-11. Airspace nodules in bronchioloalveolar carcinoma. Ill-defined nodules up to 1 cm in diameter are identified in both lungs. There is ground-glass opacification and more confluent consolidation in the right lung.

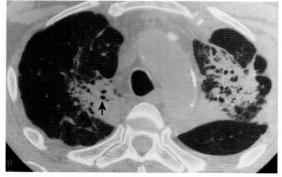

FIGURE 7-12. Masses of fibrosis in end-stage sarcoidosis. Large masses of fibrous tissue seen centrally in the upper lobes are associated with traction bronchiectasis *(arrow)*.

related to emphysema and small airways disease (e.g., bronchiolitis, which may cause decreased lung opacity) are discussed in Chapters 10 and 13.

Honeycombing

Honeycombing is produced pathologically by the dissolution of alveolar walls with the formation of randomly distributed airspaces that are lined by fibrous tissue. Honeycombing represents an end-stage lung that is destroyed by fibrosis. The typical appearance of honeycombing is that of thick-walled cystic spaces that are usually less than 1 cm in diameter (Fig. 7-13). Honeycombing typically is in the peripheral portions of the lungs subpleurally, particularly in idiopathic pulmonary fibrosis. It is often accompanied by other signs of interstitial lung disease, especially the patterns associated with reticular opacities and architectural distortion.

Traction Bronchiectasis

Traction bronchiectasis (Fig. 7-14) is a phenomenon that occurs in the presence of severe lung fibrosis and distortion of lung architecture, in which the fibrous tissue produces traction on the bronchial walls, resulting in irregular bronchial dilation. It usually involves the more central bronchi.

Lung Cysts

On HRCT, the term *lung cyst* refers to a thin-walled (usually < 2 mm), well-defined and circumscribed, air-containing lesion that is 1 cm or more in diameter (Fig. 7-15). These cysts can be differentiated from honeycombing because of their thinner walls and the lack of other signs of fibrosis. Emphysematous bullae are focal areas of emphysema that are 1 cm or more in diameter and that have a wall less than 1 mm thick. Although they may be difficult to distinguish from true lung cysts, they are most frequently associated with other signs of extensive emphysema.

Cavitary Nodules

Cavitary nodules have much thicker and more irregular walls than lung cysts. Among the interstitial lung diseases, they are typically seen in histiocytosis X (Fig 7-16).

Ground-Glass Opacity

Ground-glass opacity is an ill-defined area of increased attenuation in the lung that does not obscure the underlying vessels (see "Airspace Consolidation") (Fig. 7-17). Ground-glass opacity may occur as a predominant finding, or it may be associated with other patterns. Physiologically, it may result from disease in the interstitium with alveolar wall thickening or disease in the alveoli of minimal severity, or both.

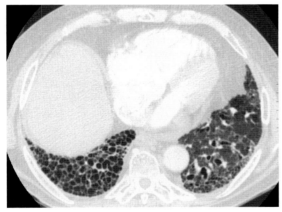

FIGURE 7-13. Honeycombing in idiopathic pulmonary fibrosis. Thick-walled cystic spaces can be seen subpleurally in the bases.

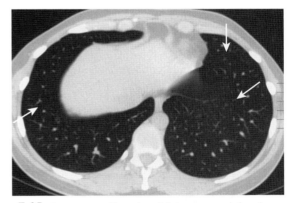

FIGURE 7-15. Lung cysts of lymphangioleiomyomatosis in tuberous sclerosis. Thin-walled, air-containing cysts are visualized in the lungs *(arrows)*. There is no evidence of architectural distortion or fibrosis.

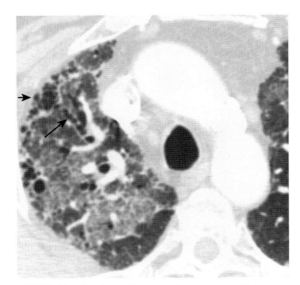

FIGURE 7-14. Traction bronchiectasis of usual interstitial pneumonitis in scleroderma. Notice the dilated bronchus in the right upper lobe *(thin arrow)* and the subpleural honeycomb cysts *(thick arrow)*.

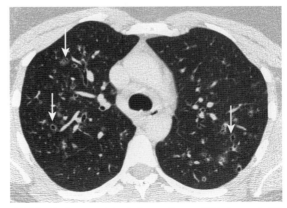

FIGURE 7-16. Cavitary nodules in Langerhans cell histiocytosis. The cavitary nodules *(arrows)* in the bilateral upper lungs have thick and irregular walls compared to cysts.

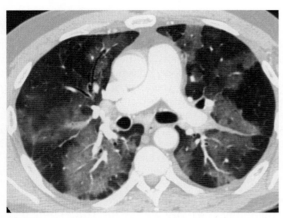

FIGURE 7-17. Ground-glass opacification in antiphospholipid antibody vasculitis. The increased attenuation in the lungs has a patchy distribution, but the pulmonary vessels are not obscured.

Ground-glass opacity may reflect an ongoing and potentially treatable process, such as active alveolitis in desquamative interstitial pneumonitis or an active infection such as *Pneumocystis jiroveci* pneumonia or fine fibrosis in usual interstitial pneumonitis. Pulmonary edema and hemorrhage may produce similar appearances. Areas showing ground-glass opacification are good sites for lung biopsy because they are more likely to yield active diagnostic material.

Airspace Consolidation

Airspace consolidation is increased opacification that results in the obscuration of vessels and is frequently characterized by the presence of air bronchograms (Fig. 7-18). Disease processes producing this appearance usually are

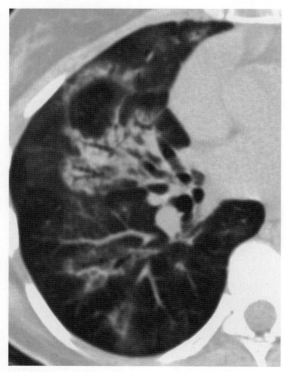

FIGURE 7-18. Airspace consolidation in cryptogenic organizing pneumonia. Patchy areas of consolidation containing air bronchograms are visualized in the right lung, and the blood vessels are obscured.

characterized by a replacement of alveolar air by fluid, cells, or other material.

▬ DISEASES CHARACTERIZED BY A NODULAR OR RETICULONODULAR PATTERN

Sarcoidosis

Sarcoidosis (Box 7-9) is difficult to define, but it is a systemic disorder of unknown cause that is characterized pathologically by widespread noncaseating granulomas. These granulomas are not unique to sarcoidosis and may appear in many other conditions. The diagnosis therefore must be based on consistent clinical and laboratory findings, tissue biopsy, and exclusion of other diseases, particularly granulomatous infections. The noncaseating granulomas may resolve spontaneously or may progress to fibrosis.

Most patients are young (20 to 40 years old), and at least one half of them are asymptomatic. The disease is more common among blacks. When symptoms occur, they are usually systemic rather than respiratory.

Radiographic Findings

The chest radiograph is abnormal in more than 90% of patients. Lymph node enlargement, parenchymal abnormalities, or a combination of the two constitute the major radiographic changes. Intrathoracic lymphadenopathy appears in 75% to 85% of patients with sarcoidosis at some time during the course of their disease. On the initial chest

---

Box 7-9. Sarcoidosis

CHARACTERISTICS
Cause unknown
Clinical features
  20 to 40 years old
  50% asymptomatic
Elevated angiotensin-converting enzyme (ACE) levels
Pathologic features
  Noncaseating granulomas

RADIOGRAPHIC FEATURES
Standard Radiography
Symmetric adenopathy
Nodular or reticular nodular opacities
Upper lung zones
Fibrosis
  Upper lobes, hilar retraction
  Bullae

High-Resolution Computed Tomography
Axial interstitial thickening
Nodular thickening along lymphatics
Interlobular septa, fissures, subpleural zones
Reticular opacities
Fibrosis
  Upper lobes: architectural distortion
  Fibrotic masses
  Traction bronchiectasis

DIFFERENTIAL DIAGNOSIS
Granulomatous infections
Silicosis: progressive massive fibrosis

radiograph, approximately one half of the patients have this finding exclusively; the others have lymphadenopathy plus parenchymal disease. Bilateral hilar adenopathy is the most frequent finding, and it occurs in up to 98% of cases with nodal enlargement (Fig. 7-19). Bilateral, symmetric mediastinal adenopathy is also common. The parenchymal lung disease in sarcoidosis typically consists of a nodular or a reticulonodular pattern, which is more predominant in the upper lung zones (Fig. 7-20). It is common for the adenopathy to decrease as the parenchymal disease becomes worse. For about 25% of patients, the radiographic findings may be atypical and can include diffuse airspace disease or large parenchymal nodules simulating cannonball metastases.

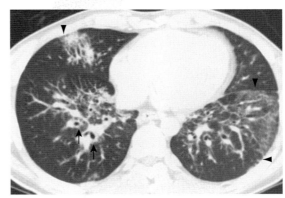

FIGURE 7-21. Granulomas in sarcoidosis. The granulomas have a perilymphatic distribution along the bronchovascular bundles *(thin arrows)* and along the subpleural interstitium *(arrowheads)*.

Sarcoid granulomas are distributed primarily along the lymphatics in the peribronchovascular bundles emanating from the hila in an axial distribution and, to a lesser extent, in the interlobular septa and subpleural lymphatics peripherally and along the fissures. This distribution is much more easily recognized on CT than on plain radiographs (Fig. 7-21). On HRCT, the classic pattern consists of small nodules identified along the axial interstitium (i.e., emanating from the hila along the bronchovascular bundles), within the interlobular septa, adjacent to the major fissures, and in the subpleural regions. The nodules vary from 2 mm to 1 cm in diameter. Confluence of granulomas may result in large opacities with ill-defined contours, some of which may appear nodular and others of which may contain air bronchograms.

Approximately 20% of patients with radiographic evidence of interstitial lung disease eventually develop fibrosis. The fibrosis in sarcoidosis is quite characteristic (Fig. 7-22). It is typically identified in the upper lobes, which show evidence of hilar retraction and bullae. The fibrosis is more

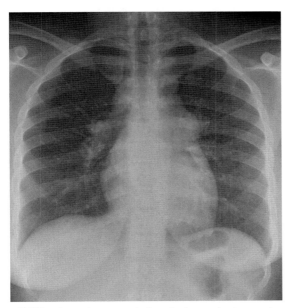

FIGURE 7-19. Bilateral, symmetric lymphadenopathy in a patient with sarcoidosis. There is typical distribution of adenopathy in the right paratracheal and bilateral hilar areas (i.e., 1, 2, 3 sign).

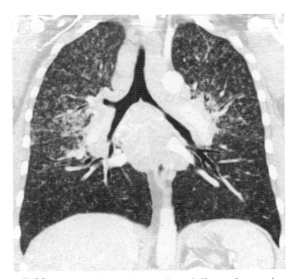

FIGURE 7-20. Adenopathy and parenchymal disease in a patient with sarcoidosis. There are diffuse nodular opacities that are more profuse in the upper lungs. Notice the symmetric lymphadenopathy.

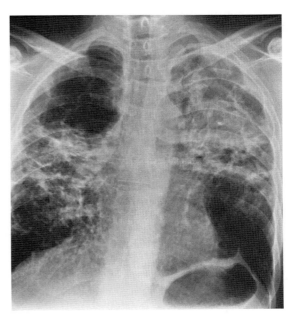

FIGURE 7-22. End-stage sarcoidosis. The posteroanterior chest radiograph shows right perihilar and left upper lobe fibrosis, with straightening of the left main bronchus due to hilar retraction. There are bullae in the right upper lobe.

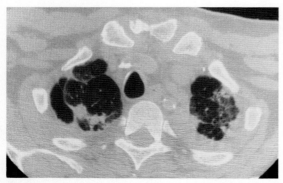

FIGURE 7-23. End-stage sarcoidosis. High-resolution CT shows coarse linear opacities in both upper lobes and multiple bullae.

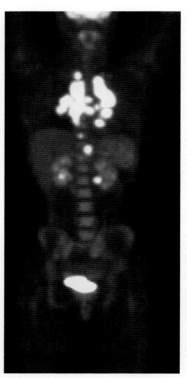

FIGURE 7-24. FDG-PET for diagnosing sarcoidosis. Increased ^{18}F-fluorodeoxyglucose uptake can be seen in the lymph nodes.

pronounced in the apical and posterior portions of the upper lobes and the superior segments of the lower lobes. HRCT (Fig. 7-23) can show the fibrosis as irregular, reticular opacities, which are usually more predominant along the bronchovascular bundles. Loss of volume in the upper lobes occurs with distortion of lung architecture. Large masses of fibrous tissue may develop centrally along the perihilar bronchi and vessels, particularly in the upper lobes; this is often associated with traction bronchiectasis (see Fig. 7-12). Because of this appearance, silicosis and tuberculosis must be considered in the differential diagnosis.

Other Imaging Modalities

Gallium (^{67}Ga) citrate has been used to assess activity in sarcoidosis, and ^{18}F-fluorodeoxyglucose positron emission tomography (FDG-PET) is also useful for assessing activity of disease. There is observable uptake in the lymph nodes and the lung parenchyma (Figs. 7-24 and 7-25) (see *Nuclear Medicine: The Requisites*). There are no specific laboratory tests for the diagnosis of sarcoidosis, although elevation of the serum level of angiotensin-converting enzyme (ACE) in patients with active sarcoidosis is common, but ACE levels may be elevated in other diseases. Diagnosis is usually made by bronchoscopy with transbronchial biopsy, which has an extremely high yield because of the close relationship of the noncaseating granulomas and peripheral bronchi.

The prognosis of sarcoidosis is related to the findings on chest radiograph at the time of the initial presentation. The lungs of most patients with adenopathy alone will clear completely, but approximately 15% to 25% of patients with parenchymal abnormalities on the initial chest radiograph will develop progressive pulmonary fibrosis.

Lymphangitic Carcinomatosis

Pulmonary lymphangitic carcinomatosis (Box 7-10) is characterized by metastatic tumor involving the lymphatic system of the lungs. It occurs most commonly in patients with carcinoma of the lung, breast, stomach, or

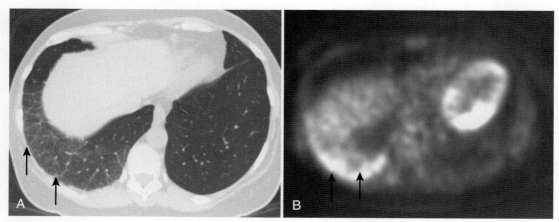

FIGURE 7-25. FDG-PET for diagnosing sarcoidosis. Interstitial opacities in the right lower lobe (**A**, *arrows*) show increased ^{18}F-fluorodeoxyglucose uptake (**B**, *arrows*).

Box 7-10 Lymphangitic Carcinomatosis

CHARACTERISTICS
Sites: colon, lung, breast, stomach

RADIOGRAPHIC FEATURES
Reticular-nodular pattern
Adenopathy
Effusions

HIGH-RESOLUTION CT FINDINGS
Nodular axial thickening
Septal thickening
Nodular thickening of fissures
Polygonal structures
Normal lung architecture

DIFFERENTIAL DIAGNOSIS
Lymphoma
Sarcoidosis
Kaposi's sarcoma

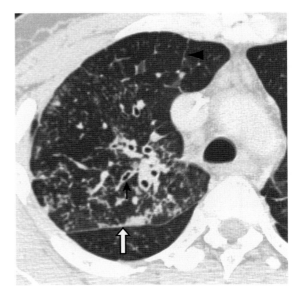

FIGURE 7-27. Lymphangitic carcinomatosis. Nodular thickening of the axial interstitium *(thin arrow)*, septal lines *(arrowhead)*, and fissural thickening *(open arrow)* are visualized.

colon and in those with metastatic adenocarcinoma from unknown primary sites. Patients usually have dyspnea and dry cough.

Radiographic Findings
Standard chest radiographs may show a constellation of findings (Fig. 7-26), including diffuse reticular nodular or linear opacities, septal lines, hilar and mediastinal adenopathy, and pleural effusions. Frequently, only one or two of these features are identified, and the signs are often nonspecific. HRCT provides more specific findings (Fig. 7-27). The pattern is related to the distribution of lymphatics in the lung. Features include smooth or nodular axial interstitial thickening along the bronchovascular bundles, septal thickening, smooth or nodular thickening of the fissures, normal lung architecture, and identification of polygonal structures (i.e., secondary pulmonary

lobules). Given the correct clinical history in a symptomatic patient, these findings are virtually pathognomonic.

One of the most characteristic findings is polygonal arcades or polygons, seen in about 50% of patients with lymphangitic spread of carcinoma (Fig. 7-28). These structures usually contain a central dot that is visible on HRCT. The cross-sectional appearance is caused by thickened interlobular septa surrounding secondary lobules. The central dot represents the intralobular central artery branch surrounded by axial interstitium that is thickened by tumor.

Differential Diagnosis
The differential diagnosis must include other diseases that may be characterized by nodules, septal thickening, and an axial distribution (i.e., those that have a perilymphatic distribution of abnormalities). These diseases

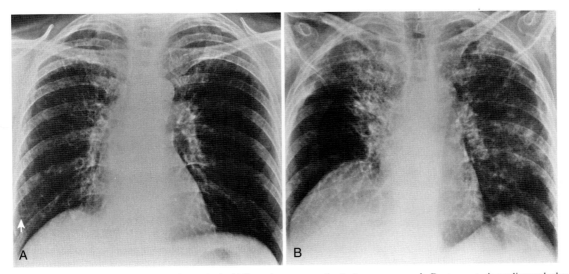

FIGURE 7-26. Lymphangitic carcinomatosis in a patient who had bilateral mastectomies for breast cancer. **A,** Posteroanterior radiograph shows fine linear opacities in both lungs and Kerley B lines *(arrow).* **B,** Chest radiograph 3 months later shows more confluent opacities and bilateral pleural thickening.

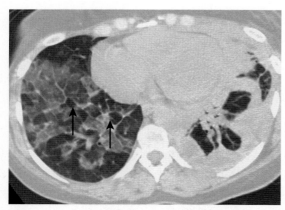

Figure 7-28. Lymphangitic carcinomatosis. There are prominent polygons with central dots *(arrows)* in the right lower lobe. Notice the left pleural metastases.

include sarcoidosis, lymphoma when it involves the lung, and Kaposi's sarcoma.

The most effective means of making the diagnosis is transbronchial biopsy with use of the fiberoptic bronchoscope. As in sarcoidosis, the proximity of the lesions to the bronchi results in high diagnostic accuracy rates.

■ DISEASES CHARACTERIZED BY AN IRREGULAR LINEAR PATTERN

A linear or a reticular pattern of opacities is found in a large number of interstitial lung diseases. The most important of these are the idiopathic pulmonary fibrosis and other idiopathic interstitial pneumonias (Box 7-11).

Idiopathic Interstitial Pneumonias

Terminology
In the past few decades, the lack of an international standard resulted in variable and confusing diagnostic criteria

---

Box 7-11. Classification of Diffuse Parenchymal Lung Disease

1. Diffuse parenchymal lung disease (DPLD) of known cause, such as drug-induced and connective tissue diseases
2. Idiopathic interstitial pneumonia (IIP)
   Idiopathic pulmonary fibrosis (IPF)
   Idiopathic interstitial pneumonias other than IPF
      Desquamative interstitial pneumonia (DIP)
      Acute interstitial pneumonia (AIP)
      Nonspecific interstitial pneumonia (NSIP)
      Respiratory bronchiolitis interstitial lung disease (RBILD)
      Cryptogenic organizing pneumonia (COP)
      Lymphocytic interstitial pneumonia (LIP)
3. Granulomatous DPLD, such as sarcoidosis
4. Other forms of DPLD, such as Langerhans cell histiocytosis and lymphangioleiomyomatosis

Modified from American Thoracic Society and European Respiratory Society: American Thoracic Society/European Respiratory Society international multidisciplinary consensus classification of the idiopathic interstitial pneumonias. Am J Respir Crit Care Med 165:277–304, 2002.

Box 7-12. Histologic and Clinical Classification of Idiopathic Interstitial Pneumonias

Histologic Pattern	Clinical-Radiologic-Pathologic Diagnosis
Usual interstitial pneumonia	Idiopathic pulmonary fibrosis
Nonspecific interstitial pneumonia	Nonspecific interstitial pneumonia
Organizing pneumonia	Cryptogenic organizing pneumonia
Diffuse alveolar damage	Acute interstitial pneumonia
Respiratory bronchiolitis with interstitial inflammation	Respiratory bronchiolitis interstitial lung disease
Desquamative interstitial pneumonia	Desquamative interstitial pneumonia
Lymphocytic interstitial pneumonia	Lymphocytic interstitial pneumonia

Modified from American Thoracic Society and European Respiratory Society: American Thoracic Society/European Respiratory Society international multidisciplinary consensus classification of the idiopathic interstitial pneumonias Am J Respir Crit Care Med 165:277–304, 2002.

and terminology for the classification of diffuse idiopathic interstitial pneumonias. An International Consensus Statement defining the clinical manifestations, pathology, and radiologic features of patients with idiopathic interstitial pneumonia was issued and adopted by The American Thoracic Society and European Respiratory Society (ATS/ERS) in 2001. The idiopathic interstitial pneumonias are classified broadly as idiopathic pulmonary fibrosis and idiopathic interstitial pneumonias other than idiopathic pulmonary fibrosis. Diffuse parenchymal disease due to known causes and associations such as drugs and connective tissue diseases are not considered idiopathic (Box 7-12).

Types
Idiopathic Interstitial Fibrosis
Idiopathic interstitial fibrosis (i.e., idiopathic pulmonary fibrosis) is a distinct type of chronic fibrosing interstitial lung disease confined to lungs. The histologic pattern is that of usual interstitial pneumonia. The histologic features consist of subpleural architectural distortion, often with honeycombing and the presence of fibroblastic foci. Heterogeneity alternates with areas of fibrosis and honeycombing, interstitial inflammation, and normal lung. Even within the fibrosis, there is temporal heterogeneity with areas of dense acellular collagen and scattered fibroblastic foci. Areas of relatively normal lung should be included in surgical biopsy specimens to exclude other interstitial diseases.

Idiopathic pulmonary fibrosis is slightly more common in men than women and is seen in people older than 50 years. The dominant clinical symptoms are progressive dyspnea and nonproductive cough. In late stages, this leads to right heart failure. The median survival time after diagnosis is

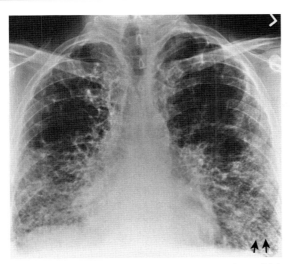

FIGURE 7-29. Idiopathic pulmonary fibrosis or usual interstitial pneumonia. The posteroanterior radiograph shows coarse reticular opacities predominating at the bases. There is also evidence of honeycombing *(arrows)*.

Box 7-13. Idiopathic Pulmonary Fibrosis

CHARACTERISTICS
Clinical features
    40 to 60 years old
    Dyspnea, dry cough
Histologic features
    Temporal heterogeneity

RADIOGRAPHIC FINDINGS
Linear opacities
Lower zones
Honeycombing
Small lungs

HIGH-RESOLUTION CT FINDINGS
Septal thickening
Intralobular thickening
Honeycombing
Bronchiolectasis
Traction bronchiectasis
Peripheral and subpleural

between 2.5 and 3.5 years. Occasionally, periods of rapid decline occur because of intercurrent infections or accelerated disease.

The plain radiographic features are low lung volumes with coarse reticular opacities and honeycombing in the lung bases (Fig. 7-29). If emphysema is present, the lung volumes may be normal. The CT features consist of bilateral, patchy, subpleural, and basilar reticular opacities that often are associated with architectural distortion, traction bronchiectasis, and honeycombing (Fig 7-30). The presence of honeycombing is the single best characteristic of idiopathic pulmonary fibrosis. There may be ground-glass opacities that are less prominent than reticular opacities. The ground-glass opacity on CT represents histologic fibrosis below the limits of CT resolution (Box 7-13). The

radiologic pattern of usual interstitial pneumonia seen in idiopathic pulmonary fibrosis may be indistinguishable from that of other causes, such as asbestosis, connective tissue diseases, drug toxicity, familial idiopathic pulmonary fibrosis, Hermansky-Pudlak syndrome, and chronic hypersensitivity pneumonitis.

The presence of pleural plaques suggests asbestosis, whereas occasional nodules and sparing of lung bases suggest hypersensitivity pneumonitis. Hermansky-Pudlak syndrome is a rare autosomal recessive disease produced by lysosomal accumulation of ceroid lipofuscin. This syndrome is characterized by oculocutaneous albinism, platelet abnormalities, and pulmonary fibrosis.

There is no effective treatment for idiopathic pulmonary fibrosis. Lung transplantation is offered for advanced disease.

Nonspecific Interstitial Pneumonia
Idiopathic nonspecific interstitial pneumonia (NSIP) is a distinct clinical entity that has very good prognosis and responds to steroid treatment. NSIP is associated with connective tissue diseases, drug-induced pneumonitis, hypersensitivity pneumonitis, infection, and immunodeficiency, including that caused by human immunodeficiency virus (HIV) infection.

The histologic features consist of various amounts of interstitial inflammation and fibrosis with a uniform appearance. There are two distinct types: cellular NSIP, with mild to moderate inflammation and little fibrosis, and fibrosing NSIP, with interstitial thickening by uniform fibrosis and preservation of alveolar architecture. The fibrosis is of the same age, unlike the temporal heterogeneity seen in usual interstitial pneumonia. Honeycombing is not a feature. Organizing pneumonia may be seen, but it affects less than 10% to 20% of specimens. Inflammation may be seen around the airways.

NSIP is more common in women, and is diagnosed at an average age of 50 years. The disease is seen in smokers and

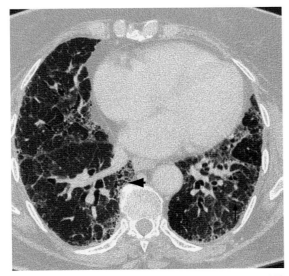

FIGURE 7-30. Idiopathic pulmonary fibrosis. High-resolution CT shows diffuse, predominantly subpleural, reticular opacities with associated architectural distortion, traction bronchiectasis *(thin arrow)*, and honeycombing *(arrowhead)*.

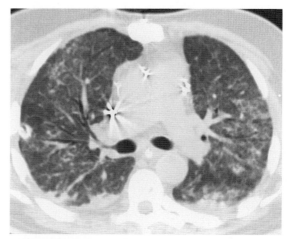

FIGURE **7-32.** Acute interstitial pneumonia. CT shows diffuse ground-glass opacities and dependent consolidation. Notice the chest tube in the right major fissure.

Box 7-14. Nonspecific Interstitial Pneumonitis

CHARACTERISTICS
Clinical features
    Average age of 50 years
    More women than men affected
    Dyspnea, dry cough
Histologic features
    Temporal homogeneity

RADIOGRAPHIC FINDINGS
Linear opacities
Lower zones
Absent or rare honeycombing
Small lungs

HIGH-RESOLUTION CT FINDINGS
Reticular opacities
Traction bronchiectasis
Ground glass opacity
Peripheral with or without subpleural sparing

---

nonsmokers. The common symptoms are dyspnea, cough, and weight loss.

The plain radiographic features consist of reticular opacities in the lower lungs without honeycombing (Box 7-14 and see Fig 7-2). The HRCT features consist of bilateral, predominantly lower lung, reticular opacities with traction bronchiectasis and volume loss. A subpleural distribution may or may not be visualized (Fig 7-31). Ground-glass opacification may be seen in up to 50% of patients, but consolidation is rare. Honeycombing is rare and is seen in less than 5% of patients.

The prognosis for this disease is very good, with an estimated mortality rate of less than 18% at 5 years. The cellular NSIP has better prognosis than fibrosing NSIP.

Acute Interstitial Pneumonia

Acute interstitial pneumonia is a rapidly progressive interstitial pneumonia with a poor prognosis. Histologically, the disease is characterized by diffuse alveolar damage and hyaline membrane formation and is indistinguishable from acute respiratory syndrome (ARDS).

The mean age at disease diagnosis is 50 years, and both sexes are affected equally. Patients usually have a preceding flulike illness and develop rapidly progressive dyspnea in a few weeks.

Radiography in the acute phase shows bilateral, diffuse consolidation with a normal heart size and absence of pleural effusions. On HRCT in the acute phase, there is predominantly diffuse ground-glass opacification with foci of lobular sparing. If there is consolidation in the dependent lungs, findings may also be diffuse (Fig 7-32). Subpleural reticular opacities and honeycombing may occur in some patients. In the organizing phase, there is architectural distortion, traction bronchiectasis, and replacement of consolidation by ground-glass opacities. In patients who survive, ground-glass opacities and consolidation resolve, but residual reticular opacities, cysts, and areas of hypoattenuation may be observed in the nondependent lungs (Box 7-15). Radiologically and clinically, acute interstitial pneumonia should be differentiated from ARDS from other causes, diffuse alveolar damage superimposed on usual interstitial pneumonia, infection, and acute eosinophilic pneumonia.

There is no effective treatment for acute interstitial pneumonia. It has a mortality rate exceeding 50%.

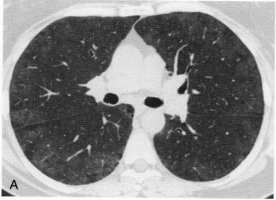
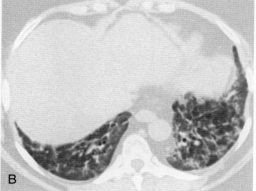

FIGURE **7-31.** Nonspecific interstitial pneumonia. **A,** High-resolution CT shows diffuse, predominantly subpleural ground-glass opacities **B,** Prone, high-resolution CT of another patient shows subpleural reticular and ground-glass opacities and traction bronchiectasis.

Box 7-15. Acute Interstitial Pneumonia

CHARACTERISTICS
Clinical features
    Average age of 50 years
    More women than men affected
    Rapidly progressive dyspnea, flulike illness
    High mortality rate
Histologic features
    Diffuse alveolar damage
    Hyaline membranes

RADIOGRAPHIC FINDINGS
Bilateral, diffuse consolidation

HIGH-RESOLUTION CT FINDINGS
Acute phase: diffuse ground-glass opacity or
    consolidation
Organizing phase: traction bronchiectasis,
    architectural distortion

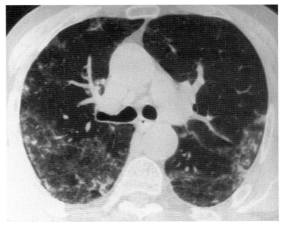

FIGURE 7-33. Desquamative interstitial pneumonitis. High-resolution CT shows ground-glass opacities in the peripheral lung zones. There is no architectural distortion or honeycombing.

Desquamative Interstitial Pneumonia

Desquamative interstitial pneumonia is primarily a disease seen in smokers. It affects women twice as often as men, and it is typically diagnosed in the fourth or fifth decade of life. The common symptoms are progressive dyspnea and dry cough.

The histology consists of intra-alveolar accumulation of macrophages and inflammatory infiltrate in the alveolar septa. The macrophages contain a dusty brown pigment.

The standard radiograph is insensitive for detecting desquamative interstitial pneumonia, and results appear to be normal in up to 40% of cases. Ground-glass opacities may be seen in the lower lungs. On HRCT, the predominant finding is ground-glass opacities in the lower lobes that may be diffuse, peripheral, or patchy in distribution. Reticular opacities are less common. Limited peripheral honeycombing may be seen in some cases (Box 7-16 and Fig. 7-33).

Lymphocytic interstitial pneumonia and respiratory bronchiolitis are discussed in Chapters 9 and 13.

Collagen Vascular Disease, Asbestosis, and Drug Reactions

The collagen vascular diseases have features that are almost identical to those of idiopathic pulmonary fibrosis and NSIP on standard radiography and HRCT. The parenchymal fibrosis due to asbestos exposure (i.e., asbestosis) radiologically and pathologically resembles idiopathic pulmonary fibrosis. More details about these entities are provided in Chapters 8 and 9. Similarly, reactions in the lung to drugs may be allergic in origin and occasionally may induce pulmonary fibrosis (see Chapter 9).

▬ CYSTIC PATTERN

Lymphangioleiomyomatosis

Lymphangioleiomyomatosis (Box 7-17) is a rare cystic disease of the lungs that occurs in women between menarche and menopause. It can occur as a rare sporadic disease, with a prevalence of 1 in 1,000,000, or as a manifestation of tuberous sclerosis, with a prevalence of 40% in females with this genetic disease. Sporadic disease is seen exclusively in women, whereas the genetic form also affects men.

The pathologic feature is accumulation and proliferation of abnormal smooth muscle cells. These lymphangioleiomyomatosis cells contain receptors for estrogen and progesterone. The cells form nodules and progressively accumulate in the airways and lymphatics. Cystic change likely results from tissue destruction from lymphangioleiomyomatosis cell–derived matrix metalloproteinases (MMPs). In the lymphatics, lymphangioleiomyomatosis cells form haphazard clumps of cells, leading to thickening of lymphatic walls, obliteration of the vessel lumen, and cystic dilatation. Nodules may compress venules and capillaries. The lymphangioleiomyomatosis lesions are lined with type II pneumocytes, and in patients with tuberous sclerosis, focal proliferations of type II pneumocytes (i.e., multifocal micronodular pneumocyte hyperplasia [MMPH]) may occur.

Box 7-16. Desquamative Interstitial Pneumonia

CHARACTERISTICS
Clinical features
    Primarily in smokers and rarely in nonsmokers
    Age between 40 and 50 years
    Women affected twice as often as men
    Progressive dyspnea and dry cough
    Better prognosis (responds to smoking cessation
        and steroids)
Histologic features
    Intra-alveolar macrophages and inflammatory
        infiltrate of interlobular septa

RADIOGRAPHIC FEATURES
Lower zones
Ground-glass opacities

HIGH-RESOLUTION CT FINDINGS
Lower zones
Ground-glass opacification and reticular opacities

Box 7-17. Lymphangioleiomyomatosis

CHARACTERISTICS

Clinical features

Young women, reproductive age, tuberous sclerosis

Chylothorax

Pneumothorax

Hemoptysis

Pathologic features

Proliferation of immature smooth muscle

RADIOGRAPHIC FINDINGS

Linear pattern

Thin-walled cysts

Normal or increased lung volumes

HIGH-RESOLUTION CT FINDINGS

Thin-walled cysts

Diffuse

Otherwise normal parenchyma

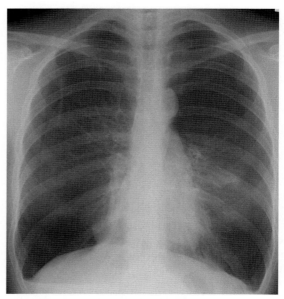

FIGURE 7-34. Lymphangioleiomyomatosis. The posteroanterior chest radiograph of a young woman shows bilateral spontaneous pneumothoraces. Cysts and linear opacities are difficult to appreciate on this standard film.

Most patients present with progressive dyspnea or pneumothorax. Less common presentations are cough, hemoptysis, or chylous pleural effusions due to compression of airways, lymphatics, and venules. The clinical course of lymphangioleiomyomatosis is highly variable; the 10-year survival rate is between 55% and 71%. The pulmonary complications increase during pregnancy.

Standard radiographic features include a diffuse linear pattern that may be associated with thin-walled cysts. The lung volumes are normal or increased. The increase in lung volumes correlates with evidence of airway obstruction on pulmonary function testing. Pneumothorax occurs in 40% of patients, and 60% may develop chylous pleural effusions (Fig. 7-34). The HRCT findings are striking (Fig. 7-35) and show thin-walled cysts that may be difficult to recognize on standard radiography. On HRCT, they are distributed diffusely throughout the lungs, in contrast to honeycombing, in which the cysts are thicker walled and are predominant in the subpleural zones. The lung parenchyma between the cysts usually is normal, and there is no evidence of lung distortion, although there may be occasional septal thickening and increased linear opacities or ground-glass opacities. Nodules are extremely unusual, but adenopathy occurs occasionally. However, nodules due to MMPH are seen in patients with tuberous sclerosis (Fig. 7-36).

The prognosis for lymphangioleiomyomatosis has improved as a result of treatment with progesterone and oophorectomy. Severe disease is treated with lung transplantation.

Adult Pulmonary Langerhans Cell Histiocytosis

Langerhans cell histiocytosis (LCH) represents diverse group diseases of unknown origin that affect several organs with different clinical outcomes. These diseases can affect single or multiple organs. Multiorgan involvement is seen in children and adolescents. The acute disseminated form (i.e., Letterer-Siwe disease) is seen in young children

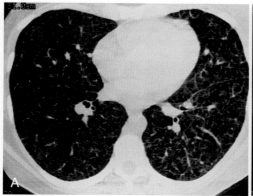 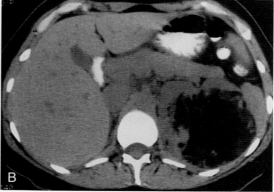

FIGURE 7-35. Lymphangioleiomyomatosis in tuberous sclerosis in a young woman with recurrent pneumothoraces. **A,** High-resolution CT demonstrates multiple, thin-walled cysts distributed uniformly throughout the lungs without architectural distortion or small opacities. **B,** CT of the upper abdomen demonstrates a large angiomyolipoma (a tumor common in tuberous sclerosis) in the left kidney. There is abundant lipid in the lesion, as demonstrated by the low-attenuation area.

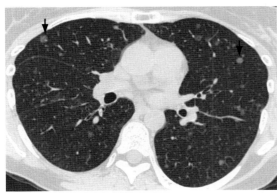

FIGURE 7-36. Multifocal micronodular pneumocyte hyperplasia in tuberous sclerosis. High-resolution CT demonstrates multiple nodules *(arrows)* throughout the lungs but no cysts.

and carries a poor prognosis. Multifocal LCH (i.e., Hans-Schüller-Christian disease) affects older children and adolescents and has a more favorable prognosis. Single-system LCH can affect bone, lung, or skin, has a more benign course, and can regress spontaneously. Isolated pulmonary involvement in adults is characterized by distinct clinical, epidemiologic, and radiologic features (Box 7-18).

Langerhans cells in the lungs are confined to tracheobronchial epithelium. In patients with pulmonary Langerhans cell histiocytosis (PCLH), these cells infiltrate the interstitium around the terminal and respiratory bronchioles and form granulomas, eventually destroying the bronchioles. The granulomas are focal and patchy, with normal intervening lung parenchyma. The alveoli contain macrophages and resemble respiratory bronchiolitis interstitial lung disease and desquamative interstitial pneumonia changes. The adjacent arterioles may be involved. Later in the disease, cavitary nodules develop, representing the destroyed bronchiolar lumens. In the advanced stage, the nodules are replaced by fibrotic scars, and there is confluence of adjacent cavities forming large cysts. There is a strong epidemiologic association with smoking, but the exact mechanism is unknown.

Box 7-18. Histiocytosis

CHARACTERISTICS
Clinical features
  Young adults
  Smokers
Pathologic features
  Benign proliferation of histiocytes
  Granulomas

RADIOGRAPHIC FEATURES
Reticulonodular pattern
Predominance in upper zone
Pneumothorax
Cysts

HIGH-RESOLUTION CT FINDINGS
Thin-walled cysts
Nodules with or without cavitation
Predominance in upper zone

PCLH is an uncommon disease that occurs in young and middle-aged adults, and more than 90% of the patients are smokers. The presenting symptoms usually consist of dyspnea and nonproductive cough. The natural history of disease is variable and unpredictable. One half of patients have a favorable outcome, with regression of symptoms spontaneously or with cessation of smoking. Between 30% and 40% have persistence or progression of symptoms and progression of radiologic findings. In 10% to 20%, respiratory failure and recurrent pneumothoraces may occur.

Features seen on standard radiographs (Fig. 7-37) include a reticulonodular pattern. These findings are bilateral and symmetric. The apical areas are affected, with relative sparing of the bases and particular sparing of the costophrenic sulci. The lung volumes are normal or increased. Occasionally, thin-walled cysts can be recognized. Pneumothorax is a common complication, occurring in 20% to 30% of cases, and it may be recurrent.

HRCT findings (Fig. 7-38) include centrilobular peribronchial nodules that measure 1 to 10 mm in diameter early in the disease. The disease is focal, with normal intervening lung parenchyma. With disease progression, thin-walled lung cysts are seen, usually measuring less than

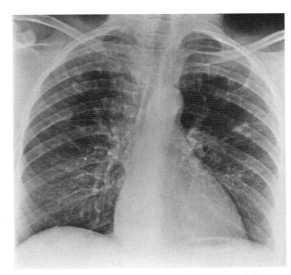

FIGURE 7-37. Histiocytosis X. There is a reticular nodular pattern in the upper lobes. The lung volumes are preserved.

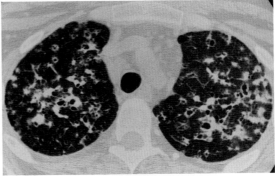

FIGURE 7-38. Histiocytosis X. High-resolution CT shows multiple, irregular nodules, some of which are cavitating. There are also some thin-walled cysts.

1 cm in diameter. Longitudinal studies have shown evolution of nodules to cavitated nodules and then to thick- and thin-walled cysts. The cysts may have bizarre shapes. The nodules and cavitated nodules can resolve, whereas cysts persist or progress. There is upper lobe predominance of the disease and sparing of costophrenic angles.

The differential diagnosis includes primarily lymphangioleiomyomatosis, but the presence of nodules is a highly useful distinguishing feature. As in lymphangioleiomyomatosis, the cysts must be differentiated from the emphysema and honeycombing seen in pulmonary fibrosis. The differential diagnosis includes other diseases characterized by nodules, and if cysts are not present, differentiation may be difficult.

The treatment consists primarily of smoking cessation. In some cases, glucocorticoid therapy is successful.

GROUND-GLASS ATTENUATION

Ground-glass opacity is a nonspecific finding that may occur in several disease processes. In most instances, it represents an active and potentially reversible or treatable process, although in a few cases, it may signify fibrosis. Many interstitial lung diseases demonstrate areas of ground-glass opacity interspersed with other patterns of disease that tend to be more predominant. These areas likely represent active alveolitis or active parenchymal disease. Hypersensitivity pneumonitis characteristically shows areas of ground-glass opacification on HRCT (see Chapter 9).

Alveolar Proteinosis

Pulmonary alveolar proteinosis (Box 7-19) is a disease characterized pathologically by accumulation of large amounts of a proteinaceous material in the alveoli with little or no tissue reaction. The cause of the disease is unknown, although it has been suggested that excessive production or impaired removal of surfactant may be the mechanism underlying the alveolar filling process. The material in the alveoli stains positively with the periodic acid–Schiff

(PAS) reaction. Most cases are idiopathic, although some cases may result from overwhelming exposure to silica or immunologic disturbances due to hematologic and lymphatic malignancies such as lymphoma or chemotherapy. The disease predominantly affects men between 30 and 50 years old. Symptoms include nonproductive cough and dyspnea.

The chest radiographic findings are often dramatic (Fig. 7-39). The pattern is bilateral and symmetric, and it is identical in distribution and character to that of pulmonary edema. It consists of alveolar consolidation and ground-glass opacification in a typical butterfly or bat wing pattern. Occasionally, there is a localized lobar consolidation or nodular pattern. This process can be differentiated from congestive heart failure by the absence of cardiomegaly and Kerley B lines. Features on HRCT (Fig. 7-40) include primarily ground-glass opac-

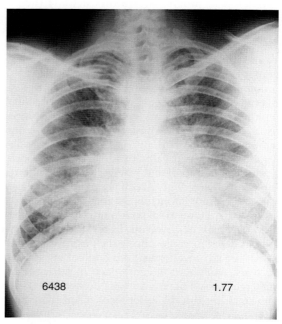

FIGURE 7-39. Pulmonary alveolar proteinosis. Ground-glass opacification and airspace consolidation can be seen centrally in a pattern similar to that of pulmonary edema.

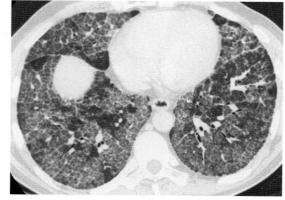

FIGURE 7-40. Pulmonary alveolar proteinosis. High-resolution CT demonstrates septal thickening and intralobular linear opacities with a crazy-pavement appearance. Notice the diffuse ground-glass opacification.

Box 7-19. Alveolar Proteinosis

CHARACTERISTICS
Clinical features
  Cause unknown
  Affects men more than women
  Patients 30 to 50 years old
Pathologic features
  Lipo proteinaceous material in alveoli

RADIOGRAPHIC FEATURES
Consolidation or ground-glass opacities
Bilateral, symmetric pattern
Central location

HIGH-RESOLUTION CT FINDINGS
Ground-glass opacity
Septal lines
Patchy distribution
Crazy-paving pattern

ity, although dense consolidation can be seen. The distribution often is geographic, with sharp demarcation of normal from abnormal areas. Thickening of the interlobular septa by edema may produce prominent septal lines. If smooth septal thickening is superimposed on the ground-glass opacification, it produces a pattern commonly referred to as crazy paving.

The prognosis for this disease has been improved by the use of bronchoalveolar lavage. However, relapse may occur after lavage, and repeated lavages may be necessary. The course of alveolar proteinosis may be complicated by certain types of pulmonary infections, particularly *Nocardiosis* and infection with *Aspergillus* or *Mucormycetes*.

■ PARENCHYMAL CONSOLIDATION

Several diffuse interstitial lung diseases may cause parenchymal consolidation or what has been referred to as *alveolar or airspace disease*. They may be chronic interstitial disorders or acute diseases that often have an infectious cause (see Chapters 3 and 11).

Organizing Pneumonia and Cryptogenic Organizing Pneumonia

Organizing pneumonia is mainly intra-alveolar but is considered a form of interstitial pneumonia due to the presence of interstitial inflammation in involved areas. Organizing pneumonia can be associated with several other entities or may be truly idiopathic (Box 7-20). The diagnosis of cryptogenic organizing pneumonia (COP) requires the exclusion of any underlying cause. COP is recognized as a distinct interstitial pneumonia by the ATS/ERS consensus classification of idiopathic interstitial pneumonias. The term bronchiolitis obliterans organizing pneumonia (BOOP) has been abandoned because bronchiolitis obliterans is only a minor finding and occasionally may be absent.

The hallmark of organizing pneumonia is the presence of intra-alveolar plugs consisting of fibroblasts and myofibroblasts. These extend between the alveoli through the interalveolar pores of Kohn. The buds may also extend into bronchioles and obstruct their lumens. Some interstitial inflammation can be seen in the involved areas.

Men and women are affected equally, with mean age of onset between 50 and 60 years. The typical history is weeks to months of nonproductive cough, progressive dyspnea, malaise, and a history of a flulike illness, but wheezing is rare.

Box 7-20. Causes of Organizing Pneumonia

Idiopathic (cryptogenic organizing pneumonia)
Infections
Drugs
Radiation therapy
Aspiration
Middle lobe syndrome
Connective tissue diseases
Hematologic malignancies and lymphoma
Inflammatory bowel disease
Immunoglobulin deficiency syndromes

The imaging features fall into three categories: multiple alveolar opacities (i.e., typical COP), solitary opacity (i.e., focal COP), and interstitial opacities (i.e., infiltrative COP). Typical COP is the most frequent type and consists of multiple alveolar opacities with air bronchograms. They vary in size from a few centimeters to a whole lobe. These opacities are often subpleural and occasionally migratory (Fig. 7-41). The periphery may appear denser than the center, which is called the reverse halo or atoll sign (Fig. 7-42). Focal COP manifests as a persistent solitary nodule or mass, which occasionally may cavitate. The diagnosis is often made after excision. Infiltrative COP is seen as interstitial opacities with superimposed alveolar opacities. The features may overlap with other interstitial pneumonias, such as usual interstitial pneumonia and NSIP.

The other imaging features of COP include multiple nodules of various sizes and consolidation along the central bronchovascular bundles. Pleural effusions and adenopathy are rare findings. The larger opacities can be seen on standard radiographs, but HRCT is required to see subtle findings and to assess the distribution of disease (Box 7-21).

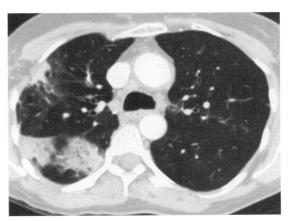

FIGURE 7-41. Cryptogenic organizing pneumonia. CT shows areas of subpleural consolidation in the right upper and lower lobes.

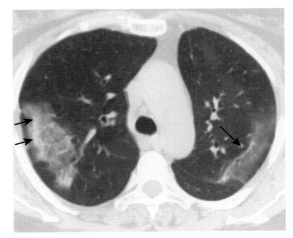

FIGURE 7-42. Cryptogenic organizing pneumonia. CT shows areas of subpleural ground-glass opacification and consolidation in the bilateral upper lobes. Notice the peripheral increased opacity *(arrows)* in the right and left upper lobes (i.e., atoll sign).

Box 7-21. Cryptogenic Organizing Pneumonia

CHARACTERISTICS

Clinical features
  Cough, dyspnea and flulike illness
  Middle-aged patients
  Responds to steroids

RADIOGRAPHIC FINDINGS

Bilateral consolidation and airspace opacities
Focal opacity or mass
Multiple nodules

HIGH-RESOLUTION CT FINDINGS

May be peripheral or bronchocentric
Bilateral patchy consolidation; reverse halo
Focal opacity
Nodules
Combined interstitial and airspace opacities

Corticosteroid treatment results in rapid clearing of opacities. However, relapses are common after cessation of therapy, and prolonged treatment may be required.

◼ SUGGESTED READINGS

American Thoracic Society, 2008. Idio pathic nonspecific interstitial pneumonia: report of an American Thoracic Society project. Am. J. Respir. Crit. Care. Med. 177, 1338–1347.

American Thoracic Society and European Respiratory Society, 2002. American Thoracic Society/European Respiratory Society international multidisciplinary consensus classification of the idiopathic interstitial pneumonias. Am. J. Respir. Crit. Care. Med. 165, 277–304.

Carrington, C.B., Gaensler, E.A., Coutu, R.E., et al., 1978. Natural history and treated course of usual and desquamative interstitial pneumonia. N. Engl. J. Med. 298, 801–809.

Cordier, J.F., 2006. Cryptogenic organizing pneumonia. Eur. Respir. J. 28, 422–446.

Epler, G.R., Colby, T.V., McLoud, T.C., et al., 1985. Idiopathic bronchiolitis obliterans with organizing pneumonia. N. Engl. J. Med. 312, 152–159.

Epler, G.R., McLoud, T.C., Gaensler, E.A., et al., 1978. Normal chest roentgenograms in chronic diffuse infiltrative lung disease. N. Engl. J. Med. 298, 934–939.

Friedman, P.J., Liebow, A.A., Sokoloff, S., 1981. Eosinophilic granuloma of lung: clinical aspects of primary pulmonary histiocytosis in the adult. Medicine (Baltimore) 60, 385–396.

Godwin, J.D., Müller, N.L., Takasugi, J.E., 1988. Pulmonary alveolar proteinosis: CT findings. Radiology 169, 609–613.

Heitzman, E.R., 1984. Sarcoidosis. Mosby–Year Book, St. Louis.

Janower, M.L., Blennerhasset, J.B., 1971. Lymphangitic spread of metastatic tumor to lung. Radiology 101, 267–273.

Johnson, S.R., 2006. Lymphangioleiomyomatosis. Eur. Respir. J. 27, 1056–1065.

Lynch, D.A., Webb, W.R., Gamsu, G., 1989. Computed tomography in pulmonary sarcoidosis. J. Comput. Assist. Tomogr. 13, 405–410.

Mathisen, J.R., Mayo, J.R., Staples, C.A., et al., 1989. Chronic diffuse infiltrative lung disease: comparison of diagnostic accuracy of CT and chest radiography. Radiology 171, 111–116.

McLoud, T.C., 1991. Diffuse infiltrative lung disease. In: Putman, C.E. (Ed.), Pulmonary diagnosis: imaging and other techniques. Appleton Communications, New York, pp. 125–153.

McLoud, T.C., Carrington, C.B., Gaensler, E.A., 1983. Diffuse infiltrative lung disease: a new scheme for description. Radiology 149, 353–363.

Moore, A.D., Godwin, J.D., Müller, N.L., et al., 1989. Pulmonary histiocytosis X: comparison of radiographic and CT findings. Radiology 172, 249–254.

Müller, N.L., Chiles, C., Kullnig, P., 1990. Pulmonary lymphangioleiomyomatosis: correlation of CT with radiographic and functional findings. Radiology 175, 335–339.

Müller, N.L., Miller, R.R., 1990. Computed tomography of chronic diffuse infiltrative lung disease. Part I. Am. Rev. Respir. Dis. 142, 1206–1215.

Müller, N.L., Miller, R.R., 1990. Computed tomography of chronic diffuse infiltrative lung disease. Part II. Am. Rev. Respir. Dis. 142, 1440–1448.

Müller, N.L., Miller, R.R., Webb, W.R., et al., 1986. Fibrosing alveolitis: CT-pathologic correlation. Radiology 160, 585–588.

Stein, M.G., May, J., Müller, N., et al., 1987. Pulmonary lymphangitic spread of carcinoma. Appearances on CT scans. Radiology 162, 371–375.

Tazi, A., 2006. Adult pulmonary Langerhans' cell histiocytosis. Eur. Respir. J. 27, 1272–1285.

Webb, W.R., 1989. High resolution CT of the lung parenchyma. Radiol. Clin. North. Am. 27, 1085–1097.

Webb, W.R., Müller, N.L., Naidich, D.P., 1992. High resolution CT of the lung. Raven Press, New York.

Ziessman, H.A., O'Malley, J.P., Thrall, J.H., 2008. Nuclear Medicine: The Requisites, 3rd edition, Mosby, Philadelphia.

CHAPTER 8

The Pneumoconioses

Theresa C. McLoud and Subba R. Digumarthy

Many respiratory disorders can be occupationally induced. The most important of these are the pneumoconioses. A pneumoconiosis is a diagnosable disease produced by the inhalation of dust (i.e., particulate matter in the solid phase, excluding living organisms). Mineral dust can be classified as fibrogenic, such as asbestos and silica, or inert, such as iron, tin, or barium. The metal dusts include beryllium and cobalt, which are associated with granulomatous pneumonitis and giant cell pneumonitis, respectively (Table 8-1). Most pneumoconioses produce diffuse opacities on the chest radiograph that are similar to those seen in other interstitial lung disorders.

▬ INTERNATIONAL LABOUR ORGANIZATION CLASSIFICATION OF PNEUMOCONIOSES

The International Labour Organization (ILO) classification of the radiographic appearances of the pneumoconioses is a standardized, internationally accepted system used to codify the radiographic changes in the pneumoconioses in a reproducible manner (Box 8-1). The advantage of the system is that it provides graphic and morphometric terms to describe diffuse lung patterns. The classification includes conventions of small, rounded (nodules) and small, irregular (linear and reticular) opacities (Fig. 8-1). The small, rounded opacities are classified according to the approximate diameter of the predominant opacity: p (up to 1.5 mm in diameter), q (1.5 to 3 mm in diameter), and r (3 to 10 mm in diameter). Small, irregular opacities are classified on the basis of thickness and appearance: s (fine, up to 1.5 mm thick), t (medium, 1.5 to 3 mm thick), and u (coarse or blotchy, 3 to 10 mm thick).

The ILO scheme also quantifies the radiographic severity, or *profusion*, on a 12-point scale. There are four basic categories: 0, normal; 1, slight; 2, moderate; and 3, advanced. The distribution and extent of opacities are recorded in six zones. The convention for large opacities describes the conglomerate masses identified in some of the pneumoconioses. The 1980 ILO classification also includes detailed categorization of pleural thickening that is quantified and classified as diffuse or circumscribed (i.e., plaque).

▬ SILICOSIS

General Description

Silicosis (Box 8-2) is a fibrotic disease of the lungs caused by inhalation of dust containing free crystalline silica or silicon dioxide. It is the predominant constituent of the earth's crust. Silica dust may be encountered in almost any mining, quarrying, or tunneling operation. Occupations at risk therefore include the mining of heavy metals, such as gold, tin, copper, silver, nickel, and uranium, and to a lesser extent, coal mining; the pottery industry; sandblasting;

foundry work; and stone masonry. Silicosis is usually a chronic, slowly progressive disease that occurs with a latency period of at least 20 years.

Simple Silicosis

Simple silicosis (Box 8-3) has no symptoms and is not associated with any significant changes in pulmonary function.

Pathologic Findings

The pathologic findings of simple silicosis consist of fibrotic nodules with a typical whorled appearance that have the greatest profusion in the apical and posterior regions of the upper and apical region of the lower lobes.

Radiographic Findings

Classic radiographic findings of simple silicosis consist of multiple nodules or small, rounded opacities 1 to 10 mm in diameter (Fig. 8-2A). Larger nodules often predominate, and they typically are distributed more in the upper lung zones. Occasionally, the nodules calcify. Enlargement of lymph nodes is common and may precede the appearance of diffuse nodularity. Calcification of the periphery of hilar and mediastinal nodes may occur. This is called *eggshell calcification*, and it has a characteristic appearance (Fig. 8-3).

Computed Tomography Findings

Because silicosis and coal worker's pneumoconiosis exhibit a nodular pattern, conventional computed tomography (CT) and high-resolution CT (HRCT) should be used. CT clearly depicts the characteristic nodules in patients with simple silicosis, and it is more sensitive in the detection of these nodules than conventional radiographs (see Fig. 8-2B). Conventional 10-mm CT is preferred because the thin sections in HRCT may lead to underestimation of the

TABLE 8-1 Dust Diseases

Agent	Examples	Disorders
Mineral dusts	Asbestos Silica Coal	Pneumoconioses
Metal dusts	Iron Tin Barium	"Inert dust" pneumoconioses
Metal dusts	Beryllium Cobalt	Granulomatous pneumonitis Giant cell pneumonitis
Biologic dusts	Spores Mycelia Bird droppings	Hypersensitivity pneumonitis (allergic alveolitis)

Box 8-1. International Labour Organization (ILO) Classification of Pneumoconioses

OPACITIES
Small
    Rounded (p, q, r)*
    Irregular (s, t, u)
Large
    A (1-5 cm)
    B (cm² = RU)
    C (cm² > RU)

ZONES

RU	LU
RM	LM
RL	LL

PROFUSION (SEVERITY)
0 (normal: 0/–, 0/0, 0/1)
1 (slight: 1/0, 1/1, 1/2)
2 (moderate: 2/1, 2/2, 2/3)
3 (severe: 3/2, 3/3, 3/+)
* The size of small, round opacities is characterized by a diameter of p (≤1.5 mm), q (1.5-3 mm), or r (3-10 mm). Irregular, small opacities are classified by width and appearance as s (≤1.5 mm, fine), t (1.5-3 mm, medium), or u (3-10 mm, coarse or blotchy).
  LL, left lower; LM, left middle; LU, left upper; RL, right lower; RM, right middle; RU, right upper.

Box 8-2. Silicosis

CHARACTERISTICS
Occupations
    Mining heavy metals
    Foundry work
    Pottery industry
    Sandblasting
Latency period of 20 years
TYPES
Simple
Complicated
Acute or accelerated
Caplan's syndrome

Box 8-3. Simple Silicosis

CHARACTERISTICS
Pathology: fibrotic nodules
No changes in pulmonary function
RADIOLOGIC FEATURES
Small nodules
Upper zones
Occasional calcification
Adenopathy, eggshell calcification

R		mm	I	
p	. • .	–1, 5	ʹ ∫ ⌐	s
q	• ● ●	1, 5 –3	✦ ✦ ◆	t
r	● ● ●	3 –10	▬ ▬ ▬	u

FIGURE 8-1. Diagrammatic representation of small opacities in the International Labour Organization (ILO) classification. The small, rounded nodules (R) are divided in to p, q, and r subsets based on size. The small, irregular (linear and reticular) lesions (I) are divided in to s, t, and u subsets based on thickness in millimeters (mm).

prevalence of nodules, and it is often difficult to differentiate small nodules from normal pulmonary vessels. However, conventional scans should be supplemented with thin-section HRCT to depict fine parenchymal detail. These scans can be limited and performed at preselected levels. The study should include at least three slices through the upper lung zones, where nodules of silicosis predominate.

Complicated Silicosis

Characteristics
Complicated silicosis (Box 8-4) is characterized by the appearance of one or more areas in which the silicotic nodules have become confluent (>1 cm in diameter). These areas may contain obliterated blood vessels and bronchi.

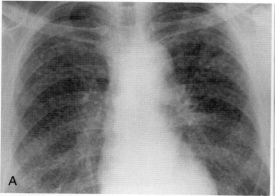
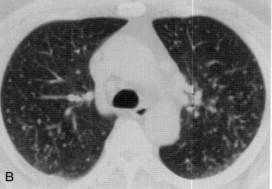

FIGURE 8-2. Simple silicosis. **A,** Multiple, small (2- to 4-mm) nodules are distributed throughout the lungs, with an upper lobe predominance. **B,** CT in a different patient shows multiple, randomly distributed nodules in the upper lungs.

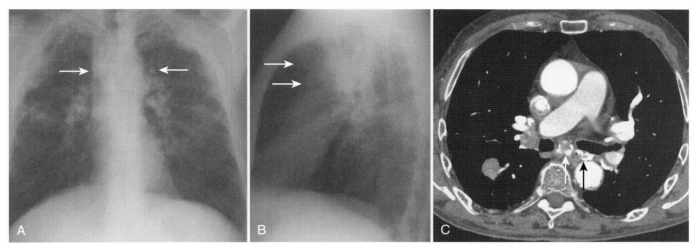

FIGURE 8-3. Eggshell calcification. The posteroanterior (**A**) and lateral (**B**) chest radiographs shows multiple, calcified nodes, some with peripheral calcification *(arrows)*, **C,** CT of another patient with silicosis demonstrates eggshell calcification in the subcarinal nodes.

<table>
<tr><td>

Box 8-4. **Complicated Silicosis**

CHARACTERISTICS
Confluent fibrosis
Lesions diameter > 1 cm
Associated with symptoms, dyspnea, cough
Complication: tuberculosis

RADIOLOGIC FEATURES
Upper or middle zones
Periphery migrating to hilum
Surrounding emphysema
Vertical orientation
Cavitation (ischemia or tuberculosis)

COMPUTED TOMOGRAPHY FEATURES
Earlier detection of coalescence
Better detection of emphysema

</td></tr>
</table>

Complicated silicosis is associated with symptoms and often with disability.

Radiographic Findings

On the chest radiograph, the opacities of complicated silicosis appear in the middle zone or in the periphery of the lung in the upper lobes (Fig. 8-4A). They tend to migrate to the hilum, leaving overinflated emphysematous lung tissue in the surrounding lung, particularly at the bases. The more extensive the progressive massive fibrosis, the less the apparent the nodularity in the remaining lungs.

As conglomeration develops, the lungs gradually lose volume, and cavitation of the masses may result from ischemic necrosis. In this setting, tuberculosis or infection with atypical mycobacteria may supervene. Superimposed tuberculosis may be difficult to detect radiographically; findings such as cavitation of conglomerate masses, pleural reaction at the apices, or other rapid radiographic changes are suggestive (Fig. 8-5). The diag-

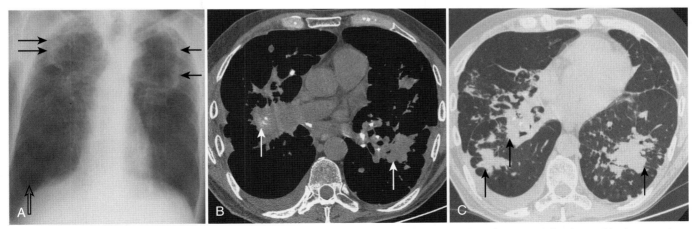

FIGURE 8-4. A, In a case of complicated silicosis with progressive massive fibrosis, large, vertically oriented masses can be observed in the upper lung zones midway between the hila and lateral pleura *(arrows)*. Notice the emphysema in the lung bases *(open arrow)*. CT using mediastinal (**B**) and lung (**C**) windows of a different patient shows masslike, confluent fibrosis *(arrows)* in the posterior upper and lower lobes that contain calcification *(arrow)*. Notice the calcified mediastinal and hilar nodes.

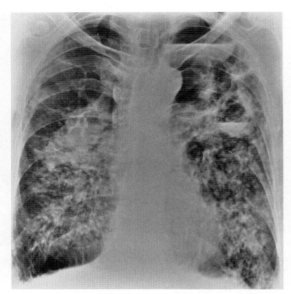

Figure 8-5. Silicotuberculosis. Areas of massive fibrosis are present in the right perihilar area and left upper lobe, and there are cavities with air-fluid levels in the left upper lobe. The sputum culture was positive for *Mycobacterium tuberculosis.*

nosis of supervening tuberculosis, however, is bacteriologic rather than radiologic.

Computed Tomography Findings

CT features are similar to those seen on standard radiographs, but coalescence of nodules and the development of conglomerate masses can often be detected at an earlier stage (see Fig. 8-4B and C). Conglomerate masses of complicated silicosis can be associated with disruption of normal vessels and bulla formation (Fig 8-6). CT is better at revealing gross disruption of the pulmonary parenchyma in the upper lung zones in complicated disease.

Accelerated Silicosis and Acute Silicosis

Accelerated Silicosis

Accelerated silicosis (Box 8-5) often occurs after exposure to high concentrations of silica over a relatively short

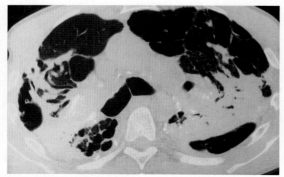

Figure 8-6. Complicated silicosis. Large masses identified in the upper lobes are associated with architectural distortion, bullae, and paracicatricial emphysema.

Box 8-5. Accelerated and Acute Silicosis

ACCELERATED TYPE
High concentration of silica
Exposure over short period of time
Simple silicosis

ACUTE TYPE
Characteristics
    Few weeks' exposure
    Lipoproteinaceous fluid in alveoli (proteinosis)
    Rapidly progressive, high mortality
Radiologic features
    Airspace consolidation, perihilar
    Identical to pulmonary alveolar proteinosis

---

period, usually a few years. The radiographic and CT features are similar to those in simple silicosis.

Acute Silicosis

Acute silicosis or silicoproteinosis (see Box 8-5) usually occurs as a consequence of exposure to large quantities of fine particulate silica in enclosed spaces over a period of a few weeks. Pathologically, the alveoli are filled with an eosinophilic and lipid-rich exudate, which is periodic acid–Schiff (PAS) stain positive. The disease rapidly progresses, and death is caused by respiratory failure.

The radiographic appearance of acute silicosis is quite different from that of classic simple silicosis. Acute silicosis has a pattern of diffuse consolidation or airspace disease with a perihilar distribution and air bronchograms. Radiographic and pathologic findings are similar to those in alveolar proteinosis. Mycobacterial infection is quite prevalent (25%), and one half of the cases are caused by atypical organisms.

Caplan's Syndrome

Silicosis is associated with increased prevalence of several connective tissue diseases, including progressive systemic sclerosis, rheumatoid arthritis, Caplan's syndrome, and systemic lupus erythematosus. Caplan's syndrome (Box 8-6) consists of large, necrobiotic nodules (i.e., rheumatoid nodules) superimposed on a background of simple silicosis or coal worker's pneumoconiosis (Fig. 8-7).

Box 8-6. Caplan's Syndrome

CHARACTERISTICS
Simple silicosis or coal worker's pneumoconiosis
Rheumatoid nodules

RADIOLOGIC FEATURES
Multiple nodules, 0.5 to 5 cm in diameter
Cavitation
Calcification

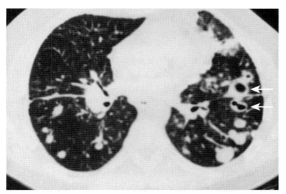

FIGURE 8-7. Caplan's syndrome. CT shows multiple nodules larger than 1 cm in diameter, some of which are cavitated *(arrows)*. The background of smaller nodules results from simple coal worker's pneumoconiosis.

It is a manifestation of rheumatoid lung disease, and it is seen more commonly in coal worker's pneumoconiosis than in silicosis. The nodules are 0.5 to 5 cm in diameter, and they may cavitate and calcify. Although they most often develop concomitantly with the joint disease, their formation may precede the onset of arthritis by months or years.

■ COAL WORKER'S PNEUMOCONIOSIS

Coal worker's pneumoconiosis is a compensable occupational disease in the United States. This disease is particularly common in underground miners. In studies of coal worker's pneumoconiosis in this population, prevalences between 9% and 27% have been reported.

Simple Coal Worker's Pneumoconiosis

Causes and Pathology
Simple coal worker's pneumoconiosis (Box 8-7) results from the retention of coal dust alone. Pathologically, the hallmark of coal worker's pneumoconiosis is the coal macule. It consists of aggregations of dust around dilated respiratory bronchioles. Fibrosis is minimal. Simple coal worker's pneumoconiosis is not associated with any significant functional impairment, and workers are usually asymptomatic.

Box 8-7. **Simple Coal Worker's Pneumoconiosis**

CHARACTERISTICS
Causative agent: coal dust alone
Pathology: coal macule
Minimal fibrosis

RADIOLOGIC FEATURES
Small nodules
Upper zones
Lymphadenopathy
Eggshell calcification

COMPUTED TOMOGRAPHY FEATURES
Parenchymal and subpleural micronodules
Pseudoplaques
Centrilobular emphysema

Radiographic Findings
The findings on the chest radiograph consist of small nodules, which are predominant in the upper lobes. In contrast to silicosis, after the exposure to coal dust subsides or ceases, the nodules become stable without further evidence of progression.

Computed Tomography Findings
The CT findings for simple coal worker's pneumoconiosis include parenchymal and subpleural micronodules (<7 mm in diameter) (Fig. 8-8). The nodules show an upper-zone and right-sided predominance. When they occur in the subpleural zones, they may become confluent, forming pseudoplaques, which consist of subpleural focal linear areas of increased attenuation that are less than 7 mm wide. Larger nodules that are between 7 and 20 mm in diameter can be seen scattered on a background of micronodules.

Hilar and Mediastinal Lymph Nodes
Eggshell calcification of hilar and mediastinal lymph nodes is a feature of coal worker's pneumoconiosis. Adenopathy may occur in any of the mediastinal lymph node groups, but it seldom exceeds more than 2 cm in diameter.

Complicated Coal Worker's Pneumoconiosis

General Description
Complicated coal worker's pneumoconiosis (Box 8-8) is also called *progressive massive fibrosis*. It occurs on a background of

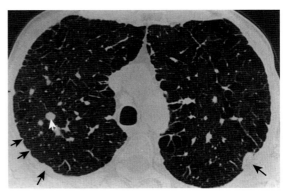

FIGURE 8-8. Coal worker's pneumoconiosis. High-resolution CT shows micronodules less than 7 mm in diameter subpleurally *(small black arrows)*. In some areas, they have become confluent, forming pseudoplaques *(large black arrows)*. Larger nodules can be seen deep in the lung parenchyma *(white arrow)*. (Courtesy of Martine Remy-Jardin, MD, Lille, France.)

Box 8-8. **Complicated Coal Worker's Pneumoconiosis**

CHARACTERISTICS
Progressive massive fibrosis
Lesion diameter > 1 cm
Upper lobes and superior segments of lower lobes
Respiratory impairment

RADIOLOGIC FEATURES
Similar to complicated silicosis
Scar emphysema
Cavitation (tuberculosis)

---

simple coal worker's pneumoconiosis. Progressive massive fibrosis may result from additional exposure to silica, it may develop many years after exposure has ceased, and it may progress in the absence of further exposure. It is associated with respiratory impairment, disability, and premature death.

Radiographic Findings

The radiologic features consist of large opacities that are identical to those described for silicosis. The ILO classification recognizes complicated coal worker's pneumoconiosis when a single opacity on the chest radiograph is more than 1 cm in diameter. Massive lesions tend to occur in the upper lobes or apical parts of the lower lobes, and they may cavitate.

Computed Tomography Findings

CT can identify two categories of lesions of progressive massive fibrosis. The first category is masses with irregular borders that are usually associated with gross disruption of the pulmonary parenchyma and scar emphysema, occasionally with bulla formation (Fig. 8-9). The second category is masses with regular borders and without emphysema. Aggregation and fusion of groups of smaller fibrotic nodules probably produce the first group. There is a typical predilection for the upper and posterior portions of the lung. Cavitation may occur and may be complicated by infections such as tuberculosis or intracavitary aspergilloma.

Emphysema

Coal miners have all types of emphysema, including panacinar, paraseptal, centrilobular, and scar. Centrilobular is the most common type, and it is considered an integral part of the lesion of coal worker's pneumoconiosis. It is defined by a zone of enlarged airspaces within and around the coal dust macule. The two major forms of emphysema in coal workers are particularly visible on CT. The first type is scar emphysema, which consists of bullae and paracicatricial lesions around progressive, massive fibrotic lesions (see Fig. 8-9). The second type is nonbullous emphysema, which is centrilobular emphysema characterized by areas of low attenuation without definable walls. Centrilobular emphysema may occur in coal workers with nodular opacities independent of smoking history.

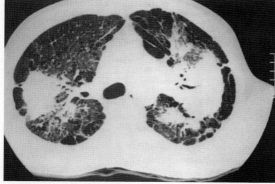

FIGURE 8-9. Complicated coal worker's pneumoconiosis. High-resolution CT demonstrates large masses in the upper zones with irregular borders and associated paracicatricial emphysema.

ASBESTOS-RELATED DISEASE

Public Health Interest

Exposure to asbestos is an important public health hazard in all industrial societies. The problem is of widespread public interest, in part because of the ubiquity of the material in daily life and because of the association of pulmonary fibrosis and malignant disease with the inhalation of fibers. *Asbestos* is the generic term for several fibrous silicate minerals that share the property of heat resistance. There are two large groups: the serpentines and the amphiboles. Chrysotile is the only asbestos mineral in the serpentine group, and it accounts for more than 90% of asbestos used in the United States. The amphiboles include crocidolite (i.e., blue asbestos), amosite (i.e., brown asbestos), anthophyllite, and tremolite.

Although the use of asbestos has declined precipitously since the late 1970s, its use was widespread earlier in the 20th century. Major sources of exposure to asbestos have included primary occupations, such as asbestos mining and its processing in a mill, and secondary occupations, such as insulation manufacturing, textile manufacturing, construction, shipbuilding, and the manufacture and repair of gaskets and brake linings. High levels of exposure in the United States ceased after the late 1970s because of federal regulations and strict industrial hygiene.

General Description

There is a 20-year latency period between initial exposure and the development of many asbestos-related diseases. Pleural changes are the most common finding, but there also may be interstitial fibrosis (i.e., asbestosis) and benign masses in the lung that are usually associated with pleural thickening. A variety of related malignancies can occur.

Pleural Manifestations

Pleural Plaques

Pleural plaques (Box 8-9) are the most common manifestation of asbestos exposure and are seldom seen before 20 years after first exposure. They do not produce any symptoms, and they are incidentally discovered. They appear as focal, irregular areas of pleural thickening that involve the parietal pleura and occasionally involve the fissures. They are composed of dense bands of avascular collagen and are

---

Box 8-9. **Plaques**

CHARACTERISTICS
Most common finding
Latency period of 20 years
No symptoms or respiratory impairment
Parietal pleura, fissures

RADIOGRAPHIC FEATURES
Localized, smooth or nodular, interrupted
Seen en face or in profile
Bilateral, lower chest

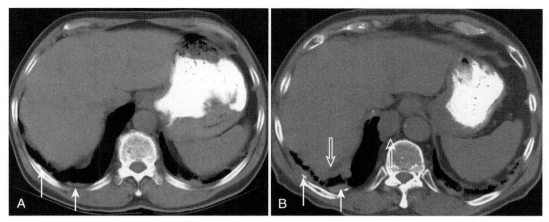

FIGURE 8-10. Progression of pleural plaques. **A,** Axial CT shows bilateral pleural plaques and calcification *(arrows).* B, Axial CT 5 years later shows progression of pleural plaques *(arrows)* and development of new plaques *(open arrows).*

not considered premalignant. The number and thickness of plaques increases with time (Fig. 8-10).

On the chest radiograph, plaques are identifiable as localized, limited, plateau-like, smooth, and nodular areas of pleural thickening (Fig. 8-11). They may be seen in profile or en face. A plaque seen in profile appears as a well-marginated, dense band of soft tissue that is 1 to 10 mm thick and that parallels the inner margin of the lateral thoracic wall. Plaques are usually bilateral, often symmetric, and more prominent in the lower half of the thorax between the sixth and ninth ribs. The apices and costophrenic angles are usually spared. When seen en face, a pleural plaque appears as a faint, ill-defined, veil-like opacity with irregular edges.

CT is more sensitive than standard radiographs in the detection of plaques and typically shows more pleural plaques and calcification (Fig. 8-12). It is also associated with fewer false-positive readings of plaques than on standard films.

Diffuse Pleural Thickening

Diffuse pleural thickening (Box 8-10) is uncommon. It is characterized by a uniformly homogeneous density, by smooth contours (i.e., no nodularity), and frequently by obliteration of the costophrenic angle (Fig. 8-13). It is often a residual of a previous benign asbestos effusion or pleurisy. It may be associated with clinical symptoms and physiologic abnormalities that are comparable in severity to that resulting from fibrothorax from other causes.

Subcostal fat may mimic pleural thickening in obese individuals. Typically, it appears as a symmetric, smooth, soft tissue density that parallels the chest wall and that is thickest over the lung apices. CT may help to differentiate fat from diffuse thickening, to identify localized fat, and to assess patients with a combination of fat and plaques. CT easily shows subcostal fat because of its low attenuation (Fig. 8-14).

Diffuse pleural thickening can be identified on CT when it extends more than 8 cm craniocaudally, is more

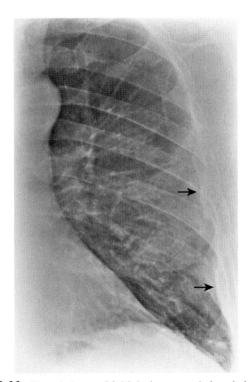

FIGURE 8-11. Pleural plaques. Multiple, interrupted pleural plaques can be identified adjacent to the lateral chest wall *(arrows).* The apices and costophrenic angle are spared.

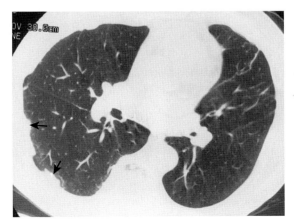

FIGURE 8-12. Pleural plaques. CT demonstrates multiple plaques on the right side *(arrows).*

Box 8-10. Diffuse Pleural Thickening

CHARACTERISTICS
Less common than plaques
Symptoms and respiratory impairment

RADIOLOGIC FEATURES
Smooth, extensive
Involves costophrenic angle

COMPUTED TOMOGRAPHY FEATURES
Lesions > 8 × 5 × 3 cm
Parenchymal bands

DIFFERENTIAL DIAGNOSIS
Subcostal fat
Malignant mesothelioma
Other causes of fibrothorax

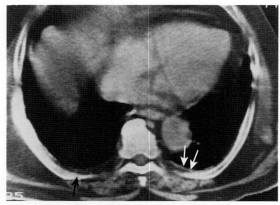

FIGURE 8-14. Extrapleural fat. CT demonstrates extrapleural fat *(black arrow)* deep to the posterior ribs bilaterally and a pleural plaque on the left *(white arrows)*. Notice the prominent pericardial fat pad, which can often be seen in these patients, and there may be associated mediastinal lipomatosis.

than 5 cm wide, and is more than 3 cm thick. Diffuse pleural thickening invariably involves the visceral pleura and the underlying lung parenchyma, producing fibrous bands. It can include calcification, and it may be associated with focal pleural disease.

Benign Asbestos Pleural Effusion
A diffuse exudative pleural reaction after asbestos exposure (Box 8-11) may occur before other manifestations of asbestos-related disease (often within 10 years). The effusion may be unilateral, bilateral, or recurrent, and the diagnosis is made by exclusion of other diseases, particularly malignant mesothelioma. Occasionally, the effusion may be bloody.

Most benign asbestos effusions are easily detected on standard posteroanterior and lateral chest radiographs. Decubitus films may be help to demonstrate free-flowing fluid. Residual diffuse pleural thickening, usually with a blunted angle, occurs in roughly one half of the patients with a benign asbestos pleurisy as the effusion resolves (Fig. 8-15).

Pleural Calcification
Pleural calcification (Box 8-12) is a later manifestation of asbestos exposure, often seen 30 to 40 years after the onset

Box 8-11. Benign Asbestos Effusion

CHARACTERISTICS
Exposure less than 10 years
Exudate, may be bloody
Unilateral, bilateral, recurrent
Diagnosis of exclusion

RADIOLOGIC FEATURES
Effusion
Often leaves residual thickening

of exposure. It occurs within pleural plaques and occasionally within diffuse pleural thickening. Calcifications can be identified along the chest wall, diaphragm, or cardiac border. Viewed en face, they have an irregular, unevenly dense pattern likened to the fringe of a holly leaf. The posteroanterior and lateral chest radiographs best show pleural calcifications (Fig. 8-16). Oblique views and CT may help to differentiate calcified pleural plaques seen en face from underlying pulmonary parenchymal nodules.

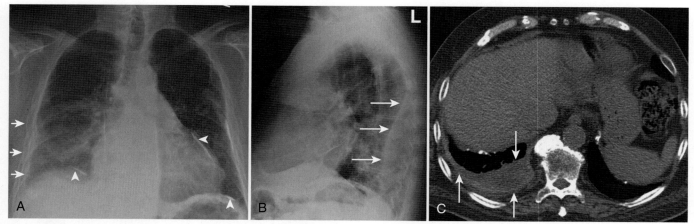

FIGURE 8-13. Diffuse pleural thickening. The posteroanterior (**A**) and lateral (**B**) chest radiographs demonstrate haziness of the right lower lung and blunting of the costophrenic angle due to diffuse pleural thickening *(arrows)*. Notice the pleural calcification *(arrowheads)*. **C,** CT shows diffuse thickening of the parietal and visceral layers of right pleura *(arrows)*, and there are pleural calcifications.

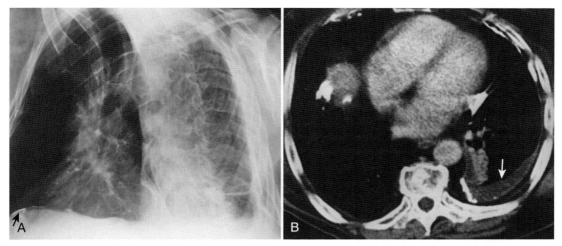

FIGURE 8-15. Benign asbestos pleurisy. Former shipyard worker with biopsy-proven, recurrent, benign asbestos effusion. **A,** Right anterior oblique chest radiograph demonstrates diffuse pleural thickening on the left and calcified plaques along the right hemidiaphragm *(arrow).* **B,** CT shows calcified pleural thickening on the left and a new left effusion *(arrow).*

Box 8-12. **Pleural Calcification**

CHARACTERISTICS
Plaques or thickening
Diagnosed 30 to 40 years after exposure

RADIOGRAPHIC FEATURES
Bilateral
Chest wall, diaphragm, cardiac border

Box 8-13. **Asbestosis**

CHARACTERISTICS
Pulmonary fibrosis
Latency period of 20 years
Respiratory impairment

RADIOGRAPHIC FEATURES
Fine to coarse linear opacities
Opacities predominate in bases
Shaggy heart sign
Plaques or diffuse thickening

COMPUTED TOMOGRAPHY FEATURES
Early detection
Features
    Curvilinear subpleural lines
    Thickened interstitial short lines
    Subpleural dependent density
    Parenchymal bands
    Honeycombing

Lung Manifestations

Diffuse interstitial fibrosis (i.e., asbestosis) is the most significant change that occurs in the lung after asbestos exposure. Several other benign radiographic changes may be seen in the lungs of these individuals.

Asbestosis

The term *asbestosis* (Box 8-13) refers only to the pulmonary fibrosis that occurs in asbestos workers. Most workers in

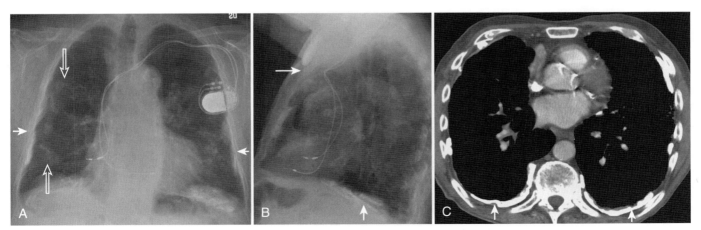

FIGURE 8-16. Pleural calcifications. **A** and **B,** Standard radiographs show extensive calcifications *(arrows),* many of which appear en face *(open arrows),* reflecting calcified plaques along the anterior and posterior chest walls. **C,** CT scan confirms the presence of calcified plaques.

whom pulmonary fibrosis develops have been exposed to high dust concentrations for a prolonged period, and there is a definite dose-effect relationship. Symptoms include dyspnea and dry cough. Functional abnormalities consist of progressive reduction of vital capacity and diffusing capacity.

On pathologic examination, pulmonary fibrosis is usually evident when there are 10 million asbestos fibers per gram of pulmonary tissue. The parenchymal fibrosis begins in and around the respiratory bronchioles in the lower lobes adjacent to the visceral pleura, where asbestos fibers tend to accumulate. Progression of fibrosis may lead to honeycombing and complete destruction of the alveolar architecture.

Standard radiographic findings include small, linear or reticular opacities that predominate in the lung bases (Fig. 8-17). They may progress from a fine reticulation to a coarse linear pattern with honeycombing. A combination of parenchymal and pleural changes leads to partial obscuration of the heart border, the so-called shaggy heart sign. Radiographic findings are similar to those

seen in idiopathic pulmonary fibrosis. The presence of pleural thickening or plaques lends support to the diagnosis of asbestosis, although plaques are not invariably present. Because lung biopsy is usually not warranted in individuals with asbestos exposure, the diagnosis of asbestosis rests on a combination of the history of exposure; restrictive pulmonary impairment, including basilar crackles on physical examination; and radiographic evidence of small, linear opacities. However, the standard radiographic appearance may be normal in the presence of disease, and it may be further compromised by associated pleural disease, emphysema, and other parenchymal abnormalities.

CT is superior to radiography in characterizing and quantifying parenchymal abnormalities and in the detection of early asbestosis. It is the best noninvasive method to assess gross pathologic morphology. HRCT with 1- to 2-mm collimation is preferred, and it is performed through the bases of the lungs with the patient in prone and supine positions (Fig. 8-18). All of the findings described on HRCT

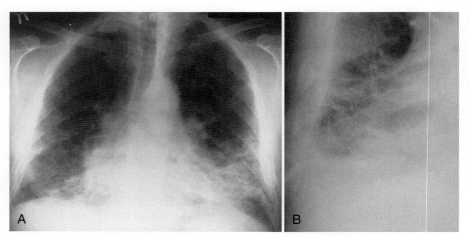

FIGURE 8-17. Asbestosis A, The posteroanterior radiograph shows coarse, linear opacities at both lung bases that obscure the cardiac borders. **B,** Cone-down view at the right base demonstrates associated pleural thickening.

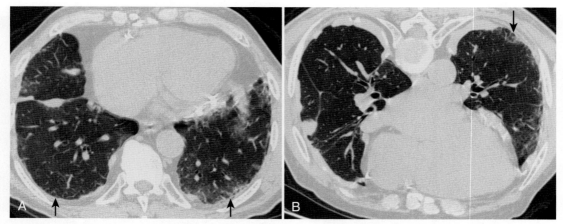

FIGURE 8-18. Asbestosis. **A,** Axial HRCT of the patient in the supine position shows bilateral, subpleural, reticular opacities *(arrows)* and pleural thickening. **B,** Axial CT with the patient in the prone position shows no reticular opacities on the right, suggesting dependent atelectasis and persistent reticular opacities on the left *(arrow)*. Notice the diffuse pleural thickening.

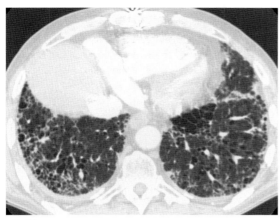

FIGURE 8-19. High-resolution CT shows asbestosis. There is evidence of subpleural dependent density, interstitial lines, and honeycombing.

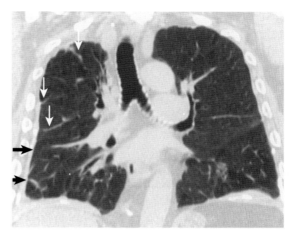

FIGURE 8-21. Parenchymal bands. Coronal CT image demonstrates long, linear bands bilaterally that extend into the lung parenchyma *(white arrows)*. There is underlying pleural thickening on both sides *(black arrows)*.

are nonspecific and may be seen in other interstitial lung disorders. Five major parenchymal abnormalities are identifiable on HRCT (Fig. 8-19): curvilinear subpleural lines; thickened, interstitial short lines; subpleural dependent density; parenchymal bands; and honeycombing.

A subpleural curvilinear line is defined as a linear density of variable length within 1 cm and parallel to the chest wall. However, these lines may be observed in individuals without asbestos exposure; as a single finding, they are not diagnostic of asbestosis (Fig. 8-20). CT may show thickened interlobular septa that consist of lines 1 to 2 cm

long in the peripheral lung that extend to the pleura (see Chapter 1 and 7). These are the most common abnormalities in asbestosis, and they may be in combination with thickened core structures around the centrilobular bronchovascular bundles. A subpleural dependent density consists of a band of increased density that is 2 to 20 mm thick and that borders the dependent pleura. Parenchymal bands (Fig. 8-21) or linear densities that are 2 to 5 cm long and that course through the lung are usually in contact with the pleura. These parenchymal bands likely results from pleural thickening and may represent atelectasis or fibrosis related to pleural disease rather than progressive interstitial fibrosis. Typical honeycombing occurs with advanced asbestosis.

In an asbestos-exposed individual with a normal chest radiographic appearance, the presence of the previously described findings suggests the diagnosis of asbestosis but is not confirmatory. A combination of findings rather than isolated features is more likely to be conclusive.

Benign Parenchymal Lesions
In addition to asbestosis, other parenchymal abnormalities may occur in the lung parenchyma in individuals exposed to asbestos. These abnormalities include rounded atelectasis, benign fibrotic masses, and transpulmonary bands.

Rounded Atelectasis
The most common of the benign parenchymal lesions is rounded atelectasis (Box 8-14), a form of peripheral lobar collapse that develops in patients with pleural disease. On a standard chest radiograph, rounded atelectasis appears as a rounded, sharply marginated mass abutting the pleura. The mass, which has an intrapulmonary location as manifested by an acute angle between it and the pleura, usually occurs at the base of the lung. There is always pleural thickening, and it often has greatest dimensions near the mass. The mass often has a curvilinear tail, frequently referred to as comet tail sign. This is produced by the crowding together of bronchi and blood vessels that extend from the lower border of the mass to the hilum, creating a whorled appearance of the bronchovascular bundle. Occasionally, findings

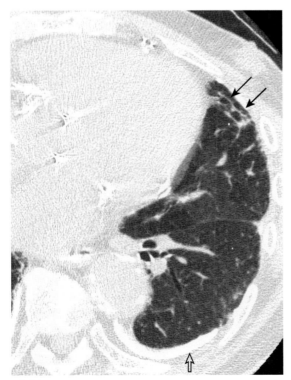

FIGURE 8-20. Subpleural, curvilinear opacity. High-resolution CT of the patient in the prone position shows a single, short line paralleling the chest wall *(arrows)*. As an isolated finding it is not diagnostic of asbestosis. Note also calcified pleural plaque *(open arrow)*.

Box 8-14. Rounded Atelectasis

CHARACTERISTICS
Peripheral location
Pleural disease

**RADIOGRAPHIC AND COMPUTED
TOMOGRAPHY FEATURES**
Well-marginated mass
Occurs at base of lung
Pleural thickening
Comet tail sign

of volume loss may be associated with rounded atelectasis, although they are usually minimal. This mass should be differentiated from bronchogenic carcinoma, which occurs commonly in individuals exposed to asbestos. The features can be appreciated on standard posteroanterior and lateral radiographs, but oblique views may help to demonstrate the relationship of the peripheral mass to a thickened pleura. CT, however, is often required to make a definitive diagnosis (Fig. 8-22).

Other Benign Fibrotic Masses

Other focal benign fibrotic masses may occur in asbestos-exposed individuals. The masses are usually in a subpleural or occasionally in a more central intraparenchymal location (see Fig. 8-22). They may be wedge shaped, lentiform, or rounded, and they may be associated with parenchymal bands that radiate into the surrounding lung. Bronchogenic carcinoma must be excluded in patients with a parenchymal mass or nodules and with known exposure to asbestos. A needle biopsy should be done instead of radiographic follow-up because of the very high degree of correlation between bronchogenic carcinoma and asbestos exposure.

Transpulmonary Bands

Transpulmonary or parenchymal bands consist of linear opacities crossing the lungs that are usually found in the lower lobes (Fig. 8-23 and see Fig. 8-21). They may be identified on standard radiographs, although they were originally described on CT. Frequently associated with visceral or parietal pleural thickening, they are thought

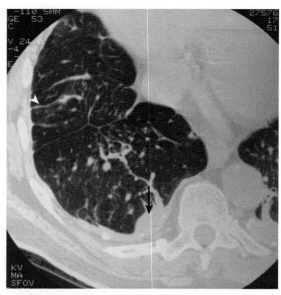

FIGURE 8-23. Benign fibrotic mass. CT shows a lentiform mass *(thin arrow)* in the right lower lobe. There is associated pleural thickening, calcification, and parenchymal bands. Note also parenchymal bands *(arrowhead).*

to represent fibrotic projections that have merged with the pleura. The bands may be involved with the development of rounded atelectasis because they serve as tethers to the atelectatic lung and the pleura-based mass. When the bands are multiple and radiate from a single point on the pleura, they may produce a crow's feet appearance.

Malignant Neoplasms

Bronchogenic Carcinoma

Bronchogenic carcinoma is estimated to develop in 20% to 25% of heavily exposed asbestos workers, and it is a major cause of death in that group. Asbestos workers who smoke are at greater risk, perhaps as much as 80 to 100 times that of the nonsmoking, nonexposed population. The clinical presentation and radiographic features of asbestos workers with lung cancer are not different from those of other patients with this tumor (see Chapter 11).

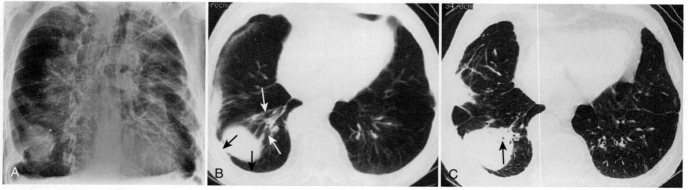

FIGURE 8-22. Rounded atelectasis. **A,** Oblique view of the chest demonstrates a right lower lobe mass abutting pleural thickening. **B,** Standard CT demonstrates rounded atelectasis as a peripheral mass associated with pleural thickening *(black arrows).* Vessels and bronchi medial to the mass are crowded together, forming a comet tail pattern *(white arrows).* **C,** High-resolution CT demonstrates loculations of air in the mass (i.e., pseudocavitation) *(arrow).*

Malignant Mesothelioma

Malignant mesothelioma is an uncommon and fatal neoplasm of the pleural cavity or peritoneum, or both. It is highly associated with asbestos exposure, and the risk of mesothelioma developing in an asbestos worker is approximately 10% over his or her lifetime.

■ TALCOSIS

General Description

Talc is magnesium silicate hydroxide, and it is usually contaminated with other substances such as silica and asbestos. Talc exposure is seen in two groups: in those working in the talc industry, who inhale it, and in intravenous drug abusers, who inject crushed oral tablets containing talc. The pathologic findings consist of foreign body granulomatous reaction and interstitial fibrosis. Talc can be identified in specimens as birefringent particles (Box 8-15).

Clinical and radiologic findings vary in the two groups. In intravenous drug abusers, talc may cause acute respiratory symptoms and respiratory failure. In the occupational inhalational group, symptoms are insidious and consist of worsening dyspnea, weight loss, and eventually respiratory and right heart failure caused by interstitial fibrosis.

Radiographic Findings

In intravenous drug abusers, initial findings consist of diffusely distributed, small nodules and consolidation. Later, the nodules coalesce and form conglomerate parahilar masses. There may be high-density material within the masses. The findings in the inhalational group resemble those of the contaminant silica (i.e., talcosilicosis) or asbestos (i.e., talcoasbestosis). Pure talc is much less fibrogenic than the contaminated form.

Computed Tomography Findings

In intravenous drug abusers, diffusely distributed, small nodules may appear in a centrilobular distribution (Fig. 8-24). The late findings consist of parahilar masses containing high-density talc with architectural distortion. The CT findings in inhalational talcosis are similar to those of silicosis or asbestosis, depending on the contaminant.

Box 8-15. Talcosis

CHARACTERISTICS
Exposure
    Talc industry workers, who inhale it
    Intravenous drug abusers, who inject crushed talc-
        containing tablets
Pathology: respiratory failure, foreign body
    granuloma, and fibrosis

RADIOLOGIC FEATURES
Intravenous form: diffuse, small nodules; parahilar
    conglomerate masses
Inhalational form: talcosilicosis and talcoasbestosis

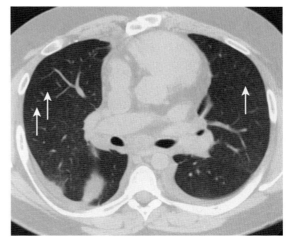

FIGURE 8-24. Talcosis in intravenous drug abuser. Axial CT shows diffuse, small nodules in a centrilobular distribution.

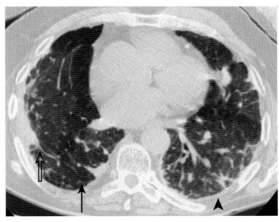

FIGURE 8-25. Inhalational talcosis. Coronal CT shows parenchymal bands *(open arrow)* and subpleural reticular opacities *(thin arrow)* similar to those of asbestosis. Pleural thickening *(arrowhead)* can be seen.

In talcoasbestosis, the findings are pleural thickening and calcification, parenchymal bands, and interstitial fibrosis (Fig. 8-25). In talcosilicosis, diffuse, small nodules; parahilar conglomerate masses; and lymph node calcification predominate.

■ CHRONIC BERYLLIUM DISEASE

General Description

Beryllium-related disease was first described in workers in fluorescent lamp industries. It is caused by exposure to dust, fumes, or aerosols of beryllium metal or its salts (Box 8-16). Currently, beryllium exposure is seen in workers in nuclear facilities and in aeronautic, telecommunication, x-ray tube, computer, and electronics manufacturing. Beryllium-related disease can be classified as beryllium sensitization, chronic berylliosis, or acute toxic chemical pneumonitis.

Beryllium sensitization occurs in 2% to 10% of individuals exposed to beryllium, and it may be seen within few weeks after exposure. The diagnosis is established by abnormal proliferation of lymphocytes in response to

> *Box 8-16.* **Chronic Beryllium Disease**
>
> **CHARACTERISTICS**
> Multisystem disorder
> Chronic granulomatous pulmonary disease
> Latency period of 10 to 20 years
> Pathology: noncaseating granulomas
>
> **RADIOGRAPHIC FEATURES**
> Small nodules
> All lung zones affected
> Hilar adenopathy
> Linear opacities
> Conglomerate masses
> Upper lobe fibrosis

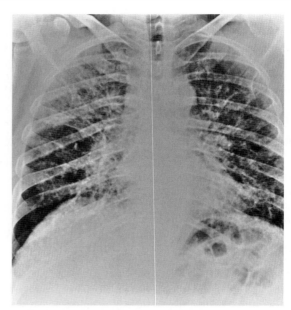

FIGURE 8-26. Chronic berylliosis. Diffuse, reticular-nodular opacities are associated with right hilar and right paratracheal adenopathy.

beryllium (i.e., beryllium lymphocyte proliferation test [BeLPT]). Individuals are asymptomatic and have no radiologic or clinical abnormalities. However, continued exposure leads chronic berylliosis. Regular screening of high-risk workers with BeLPT is done to identify sensitized individuals and prevent further exposure.

Chronic berylliosis is seen after continued exposure to beryllium for months to years after sensitization. The characteristic histologic finding is the noncaseating granuloma, which is similar to the pattern in sarcoidosis. The granulomas are found in the bronchial mucosa and interstitium along the bronchovascular bundles and in the lymph nodes. Other organs, such as liver, spleen, and bone marrow, are affected. Clinically, patients have progressive dyspnea, fatigue, weight loss, and arthralgias. Acute severe exposure to beryllium results in pulmonary edema due to acute chemical pneumonitis.

The treatment of chronic berylliosis consists of long-term corticosteroids and close monitoring. There is no treatment for beryllium sensitivity apart from removal of workers from further exposure.

Radiographic Findings

The radiographic findings in chronic beryllium disease closely resemble those of sarcoidosis (Fig. 8-26). The most common finding is a nodular pattern or small, rounded opacities; occasionally, reticulonodular opacities involving all lung zones are seen. Very small nodules up to 2 mm in diameter occur most commonly, and they can produce a granular or sandpaper appearance. The small opacities may gradually decrease over time, and after treatment with steroids, the chest radiograph may show dramatic clearing.

In addition to small opacities, conglomerate masses occasionally develop. Radiographically, they are similar in appearance to the conglomerate masses in patients with silicosis. Hilar lymphadenopathy is also common with chronic beryllium disease. In long-standing disease, pulmonary fibrosis and contraction of the upper lobes may be associated with emphysematous bullae. The opacities in the lung are usually linear at this stage. Pleural thickening may develop, usually in the upper and middle zones of the thorax.

Computed Tomography Findings

The few reports of CT findings in berylliosis describe them as resembling those of sarcoidosis. Prominent thickening of the bronchovascular bundles may be found, and in the end stage, thin- and thick-walled cysts with traction bronchiectasis and lung distortion may be seen, particularly in the upper lobes (Fig. 8-27).

◾ HARD METAL DISEASE

Hard metal disease is seen in workers manufacturing hard metal tools or using these tools for grinding, machining, and sharpening processes, which create small metal particles. Individuals may be exposed to compounds containing cobalt, tungsten, and small quantities of other metals. The prevalence of disease is extremely low.

The characteristic pathologic finding is giant cell pneumonitis with pathognomonic giant cells. The other histologic findings resemble desquamative interstitial pneumonitis, cryptogenic organizing pneumonia, and usual interstitial pneumonitis. The workers may present with acute respiratory symptoms, which often improve after removal from the workplace, or chronic symptoms with progressive shortness of breath and findings of right heart failure. Radiographic findings include small nodules that occur predominantly in the lower lungs, ground-glass opacities, consolidation, and pulmonary fibrosis with honeycombing.

◾ ALUMINUM EXPOSURE

The incidence of lung toxicity is extremely low. The pathologic mechanism is not clearly understood but likely requires high levels of exposure to cause fibrosis. Aluminum exposure is one of the causes of granulomatous pneumonitis. The pathologic and radiologic findings resemble those of desquamative interstitial pneumonitis and usual interstitial pneumonitis.

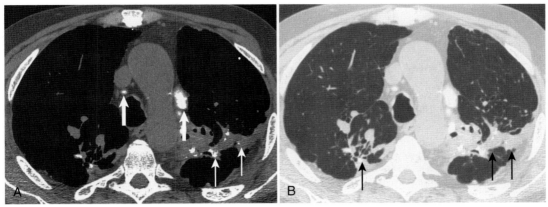

FIGURE 8-27. Chronic berylliosis. **A,** Axial CT in mediastinal windows shows calcified nodes *(thick arrows)* and parenchymal calcifications *(thin arrows)*. **B,** Axial CT in lung windows shows architectural distortion and confluent fibrosis in the posterior upper lobes *(arrows)*.

▬ NONFIBROGENIC DUSTS AND THEIR EFFECTS

Iron

Workers who inhale dust containing a high content of iron, usually in the form of iron oxide, may develop *siderosis*, a condition that is not associated with fibrosis or functional impairment. Workers at risk include those involved in the mining and processing of iron ore, manufacture of metallic pigments, and welding.

The radiographic pattern is a combination of lines and nodules creating a reticulonodular appearance involving all lung zones. The opacities may disappear partly or completely when patients are removed from dust exposure.

Tin

Pneumoconiosis caused by inhalation of tin is called *stannosis*. Workers at risk include those who are employed in the handling of tin after it has been mined, especially in industries in which tin oxide fumes are created. The condition is not of any functional significance.

The radiographic findings are striking because of the high density of tin. Typically, small nodules of high density, about 1 mm in diameter, are distributed evenly throughout the lungs.

Barium

Pulmonary disease caused by exposure to barium and its salts, particularly barium sulfate, is known as *baryto-*

sis. Because of the high density of barium (atomic number 56), the discrete opacities are extremely opaque. The apices and bases are usually spared, and large opacities do not occur. The lesions are usually nodular and characteristically regress after the patient is removed from the dust-filled environment.

▬ SUGGESTED READINGS

Akira, M., Kozuka, T., Yamamoto, S., et al., 2007. Inhalational talc pneumoconiosis: radiographic and CT findings in 14 patients. AJR. Am. J. Roentgenol. 188, 326–333.

Aronchick, J.M., Rossman, M.D., Miller, W.T., 1987. Chronic beryllium disease: diagnosis, radiographic findings, and correlation with pulmonary function tests. Radiology 163, 677–682.

International Labour Office, 1980. Guidelines for the Use of the ILO International Classification of Radiographs of Pneumoconioses. International Labour Office, Geneva.

Kim, J.S., Lynch, D.A., 2002. Imaging of non-malignant occupational lung disease. J. Thorac. Imaging 17, 238–260.

Maier, L.A., 2002. Clinical approach to chronic beryllium disease and other non-pneumoconiotic interstitial lung disease. J. Thorac. Imaging 17, 273–284.

McLoud, T.C., 1992. Conventional radiography in the diagnosis of asbestos-related disease. Radiol. Clin. North. Am. 30, 1177–1189.

Morgan, W.R.C., Seaton, A., 1984. Occupational Lung Disease. WB Saunders, Philadelphia.

Remy-Jardin, M., Degreef, J.M., Beuscart, R., et al., 1990. Coal worker's pneumoconiosis: CT assessment in exposed workers and correlation with radiographic findings. Radiology 177, 363–371.

Shipley, R.T., 1992. The 1980 ILO classification of radiographs of the pneumoconioses. Radiol. Clin. North. Am. 30, 1135–1145.

Staples, C.A., 1992. Computed tomography in the evaluation of benign asbestos-related disorders. Radiol. Clin. North. Am. 30, 1191–1207.

Staples, C.A., Gamsu, G., Ray, C.S., et al., 1989. High resolution computed tomography and lung function in asbestos-exposed workers with normal chest radiographs. Am. Rev. Respir. Dis. 139, 1502–1508.

Stark, P., Jacobsen, F., Shaffer, K., 1992. Standard imaging in silicosis and coal worker's pneumoconiosis. Radiol. Clin. North. Am. 30, 1147–1154.

CHAPTER 9

Diseases of Altered Immunologic Activity

Theresa C. McLoud, Phillip M. Boiselle and Beatrice Trotman-Dickenson

Several pulmonary disorders are associated with systemic or local bronchopulmonary immunologic alterations. Some of these disorders primarily involve the lung, and in others, the pulmonary manifestations result from disease arising elsewhere. The choice of diseases included in this chapter is somewhat arbitrary. For example, asthma is addressed elsewhere with chronic obstructive pulmonary disease. Some of the infiltrative lung diseases such as sarcoidosis and occupational lung diseases such as silicosis and asbestosis are associated with multiple immunologic aberrations, but they are also discussed elsewhere.

▪ IMMUNE REACTIONS

There are four basic types of immunologic reaction, all of which may be responsible for diseases in the lung. These reactions are not mutually exclusive, and the development of one type may be accompanied by the simultaneous or subsequent development of another (Box 9-1).

Type I:
- Involves immediate hypersensitivity mediated by nonprecipitating antibody IgE or reagin.
- Takes place on the surface of the mast cells.
- Leads to the release of histamine and other mediators.
- May manifest as allergic asthma, the classic prototype in the lung.
- Is immediate and cause local infiltration with eosinophils.

Type II:
- Depends on cytotoxic tissue-specific antibodies.
- Usually has complement that reacts with cells or other tissue elements.
- Causes pathologic changes or the death of cells.
- Includes Goodpasture's syndrome involving the lung, the hemolytic anemias, and thrombocytopenic purpura.

Type III:
- Involves the formation of circulating immune complexes composed of antigen and antibody of the IgG or IgM type.
- Activates complement.
- Results in tissue damage of various types, such as vasculitis, pneumonitis, and granulomatosis.
- Results in a vasculitis if the complexes are precipitated within the endothelium of small vessels.
- Is identifiable in collagen vascular disorders, such as systemic lupus erythematosus (SLE), rheumatoid arthritis, and polyarteritis nodosa.
- Usually has a reaction time of 2 to 4 hours.

- Is referred to as Arthus reactions.
- Includes allergic bronchopulmonary aspergillosis (sometimes associated with type I reaction), hypersensitivity pneumonitis, and possibly interstitial fibrosis.

Type IV:
- Is referred to as delayed (or tuberculin) hypersensitivity.
- Typically develops 24 to 48 hours after contact with the antigen.
- Is mediated by sensitized T lymphocytes.
- Involves neither circulating antibodies nor complement.
- Usually features granulation formation.
- Includes infectious and noninfectious granulomatous disease (i.e., tuberculosis and hypersensitivity pneumonitis).

▪ GOODPASTURE'S SYNDROME

Characteristics

Goodpasture's syndrome (Box 9-2) is a disorder of unknown origin that is characterized by repeated episodes of pulmonary hemorrhage, iron deficiency anemia, and glomerulonephritis. It is often rapidly progressive. The immunopathologic nature of the disease is apparent because of the linear deposits of immunoglobulins, which can be demonstrated in the glomerular basement membrane and alveolar septa.

Pathology

Goodpasture's syndrome is an autoimmune disease in which the renal and pulmonary lesions are mediated by an anti-glomerular basement membrane (anti-GBM) antibody that cross-reacts with lung basement membrane. Most patients with Goodpasture's syndrome have circulating anti-GBM antibodies.

Clinical Features

The syndrome is classically a disease of young men. The initial and most common symptom is hemoptysis. Iron deficiency anemia is invariably present. Pulmonary hemorrhage commonly antedates the clinical manifestations of renal disease. Anti-GBM antibodies can be identified in the sera of patients with the disease.

Radiographic Features

The classic radiographic appearance of Goodpasture's syndrome consists of diffuse, homogeneous consolidation or

Box 9-1. **Types of Immune Reactions**

Type I immediate hypersensitivity
Type II cytotoxic
Type III immune complexes
Type IV delayed or tuberculin

Box 9-2. **Goodpasture's Syndrome**

CHARACTERISTICS
Pulmonary hemorrhage
Iron-deficiency anemia
Glomerulonephritis

PATHOLOGY
Autoimmune
Anti-glomerular basement membrane (anti-GBM)
  antibody

CLINICAL FEATURES
Young men
Hemoptysis
Anemia
Anti-GBM in serum

RADIOGRAPHIC FEATURES
Diffuse, homogeneous consolidation
All lung zones affected
Irregular, linear opacities during resolution

alveolar opacities distributed fairly uniformly throughout all lung zones (Fig. 9-1). These changes are characteristic of the early stages of the disease and the development of acute pulmonary hemorrhage. Although the radiographic pattern is similar to that of cardiogenic pulmonary edema,

conspicuously absent features are cardiomegaly, Kerley B lines, and pleural effusions. In the later stages, the changes depend on the time sequence and the number of hemorrhages that have occurred in the past. The alveolar consolidation seen during the acute episode may resolve in 2 to 3 days. Irregular or linear opacities often persist for an extended period. If bleeding is continuous or repetitive, these linear and occasionally nodular opacities become permanent as increasing amounts of hemosiderin are deposited within the interstitial tissue. Goodpasture's syndrome must be differentiated from pulmonary hemorrhage due to other causes, such as idiopathic pulmonary hemorrhage (i.e., hemosiderosis) and numerous causes of vasculitis. Hemorrhage may occur rarely in patients receiving systemic anticoagulants.

Therapy

Treatment consists of a combination of immunosuppressive therapy with cyclophosphamide, prednisone, and plasmapheresis, which reduces the level of circulating anti-GBM antibodies. Prognosis, however, remains guarded.

■ CONNECTIVE TISSUE DISEASES

The connective tissue or collagen vascular diseases are a group of immunologically mediated disorders characterized by inflammation of joints, serosal membranes, connective tissue, and blood vessels in various organs. Pathologically, alterations occur in the connective tissue ground substance, which contains elastin, collagen, and reticulin. Edema, fibrinoid degeneration, and vascular lesions are characteristic.

Rheumatoid Disease

Characteristics
Rheumatoid arthritis is a subacute or chronic disease that primarily affects the joints with a symmetric inflammatory arthritis. Constitutional symptoms are common, and

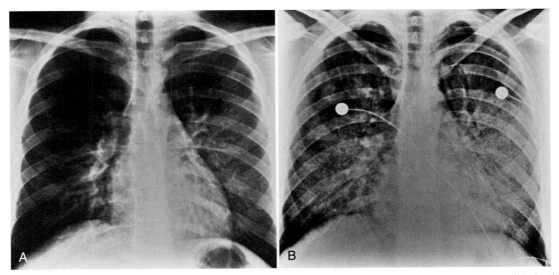

FIGURE 9-1. Goodpasture's syndrome. The posteroanterior chest radiographs obtained several days apart demonstrate consolidation in the left lung (**A**), which progressed to diffuse alveolar disease (i.e., consolidation) (**B**).

laboratory abnormalities include an elevated erythrocyte sedimentation rate and a high level of rheumatoid factor. Occasionally, rheumatoid arthritis may involve other organs and tissues, including the lungs and pleura.

Six pleuropulmonary abnormalities are associated with rheumatoid disease: pleurisy with or without effusion; diffuse interstitial pneumonitis or fibrosis; pulmonary (necrobiotic) nodules; Caplan's syndrome (i.e., pneumoconiotic nodules); pulmonary hypertension resulting from rheumatoid vasculitis, and airways disease (i.e., bronchiectasis, obliterative bronchiolitis, and follicular bronchiolitis).

Rheumatoid Pleurisy

Pleural involvement is the most common thoracic manifestation of rheumatoid disease (Box 9-3). Clinical evidence of rheumatoid pleurisy appears in about 20% of patients, but only 5% have radiologic evidence of effusions. In contrast, pleural involvement may be found in 50% of autopsy series. Pleural disease occurs much more frequently in men than in women with rheumatoid disease. Rheumatoid pleurisy usually occurs in the sixth decade of life and is associated with moderate to severe arthritis. Rheumatoid factor is present in the serum and the pleural fluid in high titers. The pleural fluid is exudative and characterized by a low glucose concentration and low pH.

The chest radiograph usually shows a small- to medium-sized pleural effusion. It is typically unilateral, with a slight predominance on the right. Rheumatoid effusions tend to remain unchanged for many months or even years. Other manifestations of rheumatoid lung disease, such as interstitial fibrosis, are usually absent. The effusions may be recurrent and occasionally result in a diffusely thickened pleura or fibrothorax (Fig. 9-2).

Interstitial Fibrosis and Pneumonitis

Interstitial lung disease (Box 9-4) may be seen in a variety of collagen vascular diseases. Histopathologically, the abnormalities may take the form of any of the various idiopathic interstitial pneumonias, including usual interstitial pneumonitis (UIP), nonspecific interstitial pneumonitis (NSIP), cryptogenic organizing pneumonia (COP), and lymphocytic interstitial pneumonia (LIP). Whereas NSIP is the most common histopathologic pattern in most collagen vascular disorders, UIP predominates in patients with rheumatoid arthritis. The prevalence may be as high as 30%. Immunologically mediated injury most likely plays a central role in this interstitial pneumonitis, and immune

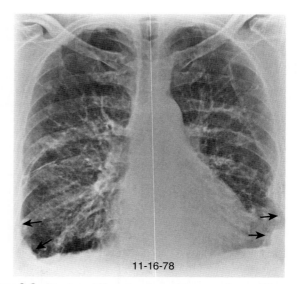

11-16-78

FIGURE 9-2. Rheumatoid lung is a pleuropulmonary disease. The posteroanterior chest radiograph shows linear opacities diffusely distributed in both lungs, indicating interstitial fibrosis. There is bilateral pleural thickening (*arrows*) with blunting of both costophrenic angles. The patient had recurrent bilateral rheumatoid pleurisy with effusions.

Box 9-4. Rheumatoid Interstitial Fibrosis and Pneumonitis

CHARACTERISTICS
Type III reaction
Dyspnea and restrictive impairment

RADIOGRAPHIC FEATURES
Linear opacities
Affects lung bases
Honeycombing

COMPUTED TOMOGRAPHY FEATURES
Reticular opacities
Subpleural zones
Thickened interlobular septa
Ground-glass attenuation
Honeycombing

---

complexes (i.e., type III reaction) containing rheumatoid factor have been identified in alveolar walls and pulmonary capillaries by immunofluorescence.

The interstitial lung disease may occur before, after, or with the onset of arthritis. The classic symptom is progressive dyspnea, and pulmonary function tests show evidence of restrictive ventilatory impairment.

The radiologic features of rheumatoid interstitial disease are usually identical to those seen in UIP (Fig. 9-3) and NSIP. In the early stages, a pattern of fine linear or irregular opacities can be identified predominantly in the bases, which may progress to coarse reticulation with end-stage cystic changes and honeycombing. CT findings include reticular opacities located predominantly in the subpleural regions in the lung bases; ground-glass attenuation (especially in NSIP) (Fig. 9-4); irregular pleural and mediastinal interfaces; thickened interlobular septa; and honeycomb cysts (especially in UIP). Progressive loss of

---

Box 9-3. Rheumatoid Pleurisy

CHARACTERISTICS
Pleural effusion in 5% of cases
Men affected more than women
Pleural fluid: low pH, low glucose level, positive for rheumatoid factor

RADIOGRAPHIC FEATURES
Small to moderate effusion
Unilateral
Often chronic

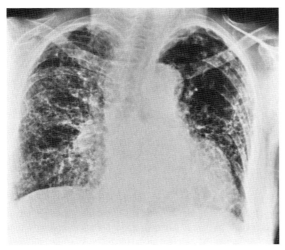

FIGURE 9-3. Rheumatoid interstitial fibrosis. Advanced disease is characterized by a diffuse, coarse linear pattern and evidence of honeycombing.

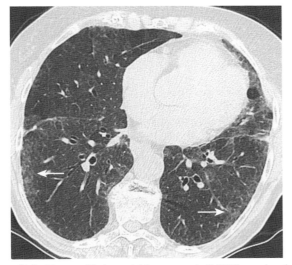

FIGURE 9-4. Nonspecific interstitial pneumonia (NSIP) associated with rheumatoid arthritis. Axial HRCT of the lung bases demonstrates a subpleural distribution of ground-glass attenuation *(arrows)* and reticulation. Honeycombing is notably absent.

volume ("shrinking lungs") may be observed on serial studies. Pleural effusion or thickening may be present. Occasionally, other features of rheumatoid disease may be observed in the bony thorax, including typical arthritic changes in the shoulder, joints, and tapering of the distal clavicles.

Necrobiotic Nodules

The intrapulmonary rheumatoid or necrobiotic nodule is pathologically identical to the subcutaneous nodule in rheumatoid arthritis. It may occur in the pleura and pericardium in addition to the lung parenchyma. It is an uncommon manifestation of pulmonary rheumatoid disease, and it is usually associated with the presence of advanced arthritis and subcutaneous nodules.

Radiographically, these lesions appear as multiple, well-circumscribed pulmonary nodules that are usually located in the periphery of the lungs (Fig. 9-5). Cavitation is common, and the walls are usually thick and smooth. Changes in the size of nodules may be observed; these correlate with the activity and treatment status of the disease. Although nodules usually cause no symptoms, they may rarely lead to complications, including pleural effusion, pneumothorax, bronchopleural fistula, hemoptysis, and infection.

On pathologic examination, these lesions are identical to the subcutaneous rheumatoid nodule, and they contain a central zone of fibrinoid necrosis surrounded by a zone of palisading fibroblasts oriented at right angles to the zone of necrosis. External to the palisade is a zone of cellular granulation tissue.

Caplan's Syndrome

Caplan's syndrome is described in Chapter 8.

Pulmonary Vasculitis and Hypertension

In rare cases, pulmonary vasculitis may cause pulmonary hypertension in rheumatoid arthritis; more commonly, pulmonary hypertension is caused by end-stage fibrosis. The radiographic features consist of enlargement of the right side of the heart and dilation of central pulmonary arteries, with rapid tapering of peripheral branches.

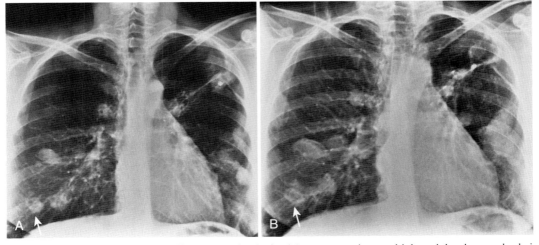

FIGURE 9-5. Rheumatoid necrobiotic nodules. **A** and **B**, Radiographs obtained 4 years apart show multiple nodules that are slowly increasing in size. Some of the nodules are cavitated *(arrows)*. An open lung biopsy was performed for a nodule in the left upper lobe.

Airways Disease

Bronchiectasis has been reported in up to 30% of patients with rheumatoid arthritis. In most cases, it is not clinically significant. Obliterative bronchiolitis may be caused by rheumatoid arthritis or several drugs used to treat this condition, including D-penicillamine, gold, and sulfasalazine. This disorder is discussed separately in Chapter 13. Patients with rheumatoid arthritis may also develop follicular bronchiolitis, a benign condition characterized by lymphoid hyperplasia of bronchus-associated lymphoid tissue (BALT). This entity is discussed separately at the end of this chapter.

Progressive Systemic Sclerosis: Scleroderma

Characteristics

Progressive systemic sclerosis or scleroderma (Box 9-5) is a connective tissue disease characterized by fibrosis and atrophy of the skin, lungs, gastrointestinal tract, heart, and kidneys. Patients are usually affected in the fourth to sixth decade of life, and the disease is three times more common in women than in men.

After the esophagus, the lung is the second most frequently involved visceral organ. Chest radiographic abnormalities have been reported in up to 25% of cases. The pulmonary manifestations of scleroderma may take one of three forms; interstitial fibrosis is the most common, but pulmonary vascular disease and pleural changes may also occur. Although the pathogenesis of interstitial lung disease is unknown, an immunologic mechanism is likely. Vascular disease involving the arterioles and capillary bed frequently occurs in the lungs of scleroderma patients. These changes appear to be unrelated to the interstitial fibrosis and may occur independently. Pulmonary hypertension may develop as a consequence of these lesions.

Clinical Features

Clinical symptoms include dyspnea and nonproductive cough. Pulmonary function abnormalities consist of restrictive pattern with a diminished diffusing capacity. Signs of cor pulmonale may occur at a later stage. Pulmonary hypertension is a frequent complication of scleroderma, and it appears to be independent of the duration of the disease or the severity of the interstitial fibrosis. It results from primary lesions in the small- and medium-sized pulmonary arteries that are characterized by intimal proliferation with myxomatous changes. In contrast to interstitial lung disease, pulmonary hypertension usually is a late complication of systemic sclerosis. Severe pulmonary hypertension is also found in patients with the CREST syndrome (i.e., calcinosis cutis, Raynaud's phenomenon, esophageal dysfunction, sclerodactyly, and telangiectasia). It is a benign variant of scleroderma. Pulmonary symptoms may also occur as a result of recurrent aspiration pneumonia because of disturbances of esophageal motility and distal esophageal strictures.

Radiographic Features

The radiographic pattern is usually identical to that seen in NSIP or UIP and may be indistinguishable from rheumatoid lung. NSIP is the most common histopathologic pattern in patients with systemic sclerosis. A fine linear pattern of small, irregular opacities can be identified, with predominant involvement at the bases and often accompanied by ground-glass attenuation. As the disease progresses, the opacities become coarser, and eventually, traction bronchiectasis and honeycomb cysts develop. The latter pattern is a typical feature of UIP. Progressive loss of volume occurs over several years. Pleural involvement, however, is uncommon. On high-resolution CT (Fig. 9-6), findings are similar to those described in rheumatoid lung disease. In patients with systemic sclerosis, interstitial lung disease is frequently accompanied by thoracic lymphadenopathy, which tends to increase as the profusion of lung disease worsens.

Other nonpulmonary manifestations of scleroderma may be identified on the chest radiograph. Calcinosis may be present in the skin and subcutaneous tissue of the thorax, particularly about the shoulders. Atrophy and atony of the esophagus that results in absent peristalsis may also lead to dilation of the esophagus. On chest radiography and CT, this is manifested by the presence of gas without an air-fluid level in a distended esophagus, the so-called air esophagram (see Fig. 9-6). Dilation of the central pulmonary arteries with rapid tapering of peripheral vessels is characteristic of pulmonary arterial hypertension (Fig. 9-7).

Systemic Lupus Erythematosus

SLE is a chronic disease of unknown origin that affects the components of connective tissue of many organs, including the lungs. The vascular system, the epidermis, and serous and synovial membranes are the most commonly involved

---

Box 9-5. Scleroderma or Progressive Systemic Sclerosis

CHARACTERISTICS
Fibrosis and atrophy
  Skin
  Lung (second most common site)
  Gastrointestinal tract (esophagus most common)

CLINICAL FEATURES
Women affected more than men
Age: 40 to 70 years
Dyspnea, cough, restrictive disease
Pulmonary hypertension
Recurrent aspiration

RADIOGRAPHIC FEATURES
Fibrosis
Ground-glass attenuation
Linear opacities
Lung bases
Calcinosis (soft tissues)
Air esophagram
Pulmonary arterial hypertension
  Dilated central arteries
  Rapid tapering
Chronic aspiration
  Basilar opacities
  Bronchiectasis

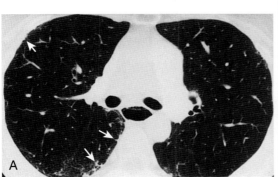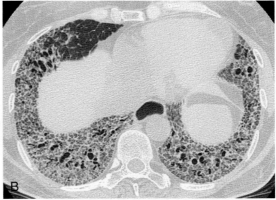

Figure 9-6. Progressive systemic sclerosis. **A,** High-resolution CT shows extensive, basilar ground-glass attenuation, intralobular and interlobular thickening, and traction bronchiectasis, as well as a dilated esophagus. **B,** Coronal reformation image demonstrates subpleural and basilar distribution.

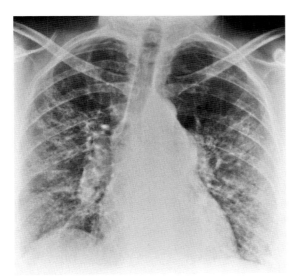

Figure 9-7. Scleroderma with pulmonary arterial hypertension. Enlargement of the central pulmonary arteries and diffuse, linear opacities in both lungs are indicative of interstitial fibrosis.

sites. The diagnosis of SLE is established by clinical and laboratory phenomena, including a positive antinuclear antibody test result and the lupus cell (i.e., LE cell phenomenon). SLE is the prototype of disease caused by a type III immunologic reaction.

Young women are affected four times as often as men. Renal and central nervous system involvement and various infections are common determinants of survival. The lungs and pleura are involved more frequently in SLE than in any other collagen vascular disease, with the prevalence ranging from 30% to 70% in several series.

The clinical manifestations of pleural pulmonary lupus vary. Symptoms include pleuritis and cough with or without dyspnea. Pleuritis occurs in 35% to 40% of patients and is often painful and accompanied by fever. Patients occasionally have hemoptysis associated with pulmonary hemorrhage. The radiographic manifestations may be classified in six categories (Box 9-6), and patient may have more than one of these entities.

Pleuritis and/or Effusion

Separately or combined, pleuritis and effusion are the most common pleuropulmonary abnormalities in SLE. Pleuritis is often an early manifestation of disease and may

---

Box 9-6. **Systemic Lupus Erythematosus**

CHARACTERISTICS
Type III reaction
Positive antinuclear antibodies
Vascular system, epidermis, serous and synovial
  membranes
Young women more than men
Lungs and pleura
  Affected in 30% to 70% cases
  Pleuritis

RADIOGRAPHIC FEATURES
Pleuritis or effusion, or both
  Most common
  Early
  Bilateral, small
  Pericardial effusion
Atelectasis
  Subsegmental
  Bases
Uremic pulmonary edema
  Central alveolar opacities
  Cardiac enlargement
Acute lupus pneumonitis
  Uncommon
  Vasculitis, hemorrhage
  Widespread consolidation
  Focal opacities at bases
Diffuse interstitial disease
  Uncommon
  Appearance identical to idiopathic pulmonary
    fibrosis
Diaphragmatic dysfunction
  Low lung volumes
  Elevated hemidiaphragms

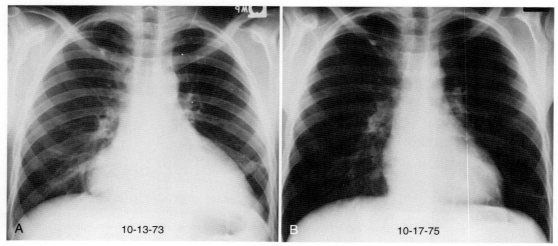

FIGURE 9-8. Lupus pleurisy and pericarditis. **A,** The posteroanterior radiograph shows enlargement of the cardiac silhouette, suggesting a pericardial effusion, and a small, left pleural effusion. **B,** Four days later after steroid therapy, the pericardial and pleural effusion have resolved.

have exacerbations. The effusions are commonly bilateral and small, although they may be massive. Pericardial effusions may also be present (Fig. 9-8). The fluid is an exudate with a high protein content and normal glucose concentration.

Atelectasis
Atelectasis, usually of the subsegmental variety, can be identified on chest radiographs in patients with SLE. These areas appear as horizontal-line opacities usually occurring at the bases. They may be migratory and fleeting. These areas are often associated with pleural effusion or diaphragmatic dysfunction.

Uremic Pulmonary Edema
Uremic pulmonary edema is seen in the presence of severe renal failure in patients with SLE. The chest radiograph reveals evidence of cardiac enlargement and central alveolar opacities in a classic butterfly or bat's wing distribution.

Acute Lupus Pneumonitis
Acute lupus pneumonitis is an uncommon but well-recognized manifestation of SLE. It is characterized by severe dyspnea, nonproductive cough, fever, and hypoxia. The radiographic features (Fig. 9-9) consist of poorly defined focal areas of increased opacity at the bases or widespread, extensive, unilateral or bilateral consolidation. These pulmonary opacities usually respond to steroids or cytotoxic drugs. The pathogenesis of this disorder is unclear, but histologic alterations include vasculitis and hemorrhage.

Diffuse Interstitial Lung Disease
Unlike other collagen vascular diseases, chronic interstitial lung disease in SLE is distinctly uncommon. Estimates of prevalence vary from 1% to 6%. Clinical symptoms and pulmonary function tests are identical to those found in other collagen vascular diseases with interstitial fibrosis. The radiographic changes are identical to other causes of UIP or NSIP.

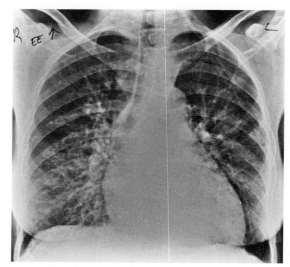

FIGURE 9-9. Acute lupus pneumonitis. Patchy consolidation is evident in the right lung. Biopsy showed vasculitis and hemorrhage.

Diaphragmatic Dysfunction
Diaphragmatic dysfunction with loss of lung volume is related to a diffuse myopathy affecting the diaphragmatic muscles. The chest radiograph shows evidence of elevated hemidiaphragms and loss of lung volume. On fluoroscopic examination, diaphragmatic movement is sluggish.

Pleural effusions and pulmonary disease may be seen in cases of drug-induced lupus-like syndromes. Unlike cases of idiopathic SLE, the prognosis is excellent after the offending agent is discontinued.

Polymyositis or Dermatomyositis

Characteristics
Polymyositis and dermatomyositis (Box 9-7) include a group of autoimmune disorders characterized by diffuse inflammatory and degenerative changes in striated muscle. Fewer cases are associated with underlying malignancy. Symptoms include dyspnea on exertion and nonproductive

Box 9-7. Polymyositis or Dermatomyositis

CHARACTERISTICS
Autoimmune
Weakness, pain, atrophy of proximal muscle
Violaceous rash in about 50% of cases
Affects women twice as often as men
Occurs in the first, fifth, and sixth decades
Types of lung disease
  Chronic interstitial pneumonia (<5%)
  Aspiration pneumonia
  Hypostatic pneumonia

RADIOGRAPHIC FEATURES
Basilar linear opacities
Small lung volumes
Patchy, subpleural foci of consolidation
Unilateral or bilateral aspiration pneumonia
Soft tissue calcification

cough. There is evidence of restriction on pulmonary function testing, and there may be a profound weakness of the muscles of respiration. The cause is unknown, and unlike other collagen vascular diseases, there are no circulating immune complexes.

Three types of pulmonary disease can be identified in this disorder: chronic interstitial pneumonitis, aspiration pneumonia due to a hypotonic esophagus, and hypostatic pneumonia due to chest wall involvement with resultant hypoventilation. The prevalence of interstitial pneumonitis is low, estimated to be about 5%.

Dermatomyositis or polymyositis is twice as common in women as in men. A peak incidence occurs in the first decade and in the fifth and sixth decades.

Radiologic Features

The radiologic features consist of diffuse linear opacities of varied coarseness that predominate at the bases, similar to other collagen vascular diseases, and correlate histopathologically to UIP or NSIP. However, many patients may have normal chest radiographs. CT findings may include multifocal areas of patchy, subpleural consolidation accompanied by parenchymal bands and bronchovascular thickening. Areas of peripheral consolidation correlate histopathologically with COP. These findings are potentially reversible after treatment with corticosteroids or other immunosuppressant therapy, or both.

When polymyositis involves the muscles of respiration, diaphragmatic elevation with small lung volumes and areas of subsegmental atelectasis are apparent. Unilateral or bilateral aspiration pneumonia may result when pharyngeal muscle paralysis is a feature. Diffuse soft tissue calcification may be identified on the chest radiograph, a finding more often seen in children than in adults.

Mixed Connective Tissue Disease

Mixed connective tissue disease is a rheumatic disease syndrome that overlaps features of SLE, polymyositis, and scleroderma. It is distinguished from other collagen vascular diseases by the presence of a specific antibody to an extractable nuclear antigen (ENA) in the serum. Many patients with this disorder have had interstitial lung disease. The pulmonary involvement may be mild and responsive to steroids, but rapidly progressive fibrosis and pulmonary hypertension occasionally develop.

Ankylosing Spondylitis

Involvement of the thoracic spine is common in ankylosing spondylitis. Between 1% and 2% of patients also may develop pleuropulmonary manifestations, most commonly in the form of upper lobe fibrotic and bullous disease (Fig. 9-10).

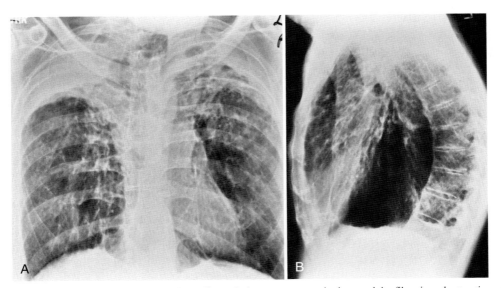

FIGURE 9-10. Ankylosing spondylitis. **A,** The posteroanterior radiograph demonstrates marked upper lobe fibrosis and retraction with bullae and pleural thickening. **B,** The lateral chest radiograph shows the typical features of ankylosing spondylitis of the thoracic spine. Notice the calcification of the anterior longitudinal ligament.

Although it is rare, ankylosing spondylitis should be considered in the differential diagnosis of chronic infiltrative lung disorders that cause upper lobe scarring and fibrosis.

▬ VASCULITIDES AND GRANULOMATOSES

Characteristics

Any disease characterized pathologically by an inflammatory response within blood vessels may be considered a vasculitis. If the inflammation produces destruction of vessel walls, the process is called a *necrotizing vasculitis*. Most vascular diseases are systemic, although there often is a target organ. The lungs commonly are involved by several types of vasculitis. Box 9-8 provides a classification that divides these disorders into four groups. This section deals with diseases in category 1, those that histopathologically have a granulomatous appearance and have been characterized by Liebow as pulmonary angiitis and granulomatosis. In all these diseases, the lung is the major site of involvement. These granulomatous vasculitides include classic and limited Wegener's granulomatosis, lymphomatoid granulomatosis, allergic granulomatosis (i.e., Churg-Strauss syndrome), necrotizing sarcoid angiitis and granulomatosis, and bronchocentric granulomatosis.

Box 9-8. Classification of the Pulmonary Vasculitides

GRANULOMATOUS VASCULITIS
Classic Wegener's granulomatosis
Lymphomatoid granulomatosis
Allergic granulomatosis and angiitis
Necrotizing sarcoidal angiitis and granulomatosis
Bronchocentric granulomatosis

HYPERSENSITIVITY VASCULITIS
Anaphylactoid purpura
Essential mixed cryoglobulinemia with
    leukocytoclastic vasculitis
Vasculitis associated with malignancy, infection, or
    drugs
Hypersensitivity pneumonitis

PULMONARY VASCULITIS ASSOCIATED WITH CONNECTIVE TISSUE DISEASES
Rheumatoid disease
Systemic lupus erythematosus
Progressive systemic sclerosis
Dermatomyositis/polymyositis
Mixed connective tissue disease

VASCULITIS ASSOCIATED WITH PULMONARY ARTERY ANEURYSM
Behçet's disease
Hughes-Stovin syndrome

From Dreisin RB: Pulmonary vasculitis. Clin Chest Med 3:607–618, 1982.

Box 9-9. Wegener's Granulomatosis

CHARACTERISTICS
Upper respiratory tract, lungs, kidneys
Women are affected more than men
Occurs in middle age
Cough, hemoptysis
Positive for antineutrophil cytoplasmic antibody

RADIOLOGIC FEATURES
Multiple nodules or masses
    Cavitation
    Peripheral location
Focal or diffuse consolidation

Wegener's Granulomatosis

Characteristics

Wegener's granulomatosis (Box 9-9) usually consists of a disease triad of necrotizing vasculitis that involves the upper respiratory tract, lungs, and glomeruli of the kidneys. However, the limited form of Wegener's is confined to the lungs.

In Wegener's granulomatosis, the mean age of onset is 40 years, and there is a female-to-male ratio of 2:1. Symptoms are usually related to the upper respiratory tract, such as sinus pain and rhinorrhea. Pulmonary symptoms include cough with mild sputum production and occasionally hemoptysis. Renal involvement in classic Wegener's granulomatosis is usually asymptomatic and revealed only on subsequent evaluation. There is no single laboratory test that is diagnostic of Wegener's granulomatosis. However, elevated levels of antineutrophil cytoplasmic antibody (ANCA) in the serum are suggestive. There is also striking elevation of the erythrocyte sedimentation rate. Wegener's granulomatosis can often be successfully treated with a combination of steroids and cyclophosphamide.

Radiologic Findings

The radiologic features of Wegener's granulomatosis are varied. The most common and characteristic pattern is that of multiple, rounded nodules or masses that usually are well defined and that range in size from a few millimeters to 9 cm in diameter. They may cavitate (Fig. 9-11), and they are commonly bilateral and multiple. The cavities have thick and irregular walls. The nodules may be peripheral in location and may simulate pulmonary infarcts. CT may demonstrate a peripheral distribution of pulmonary opacities that are wedge shaped and associated with a feeding vessel, suggesting an angiocentric process. It is not uncommon to see focal or diffuse areas of consolidation that are transient and fleeting in nature; these areas most likely result from associated pulmonary hemorrhage (Fig. 9-12). This type of involvement is usually more fulminating and more severe. Hilar and mediastinal adenopathy and pleural effusions are rare. However, CT may demonstrate slightly enlarged nodes in a minority of patients. CT may show bronchial wall thickening in the segmental and subsegmental airways and, less commonly, bronchiectasis.

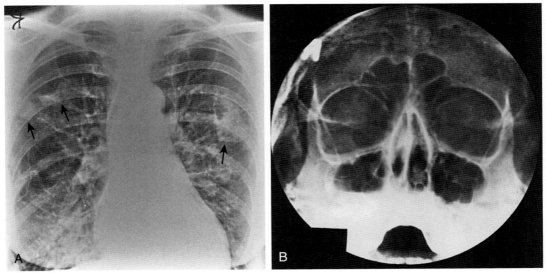

FIGURE 9-11. Wegener's granulomatosis. **A,** The posteroanterior chest radiograph shows multiple pulmonary nodules *(arrows)*. The one on the left is cavitated, and there is consolidation in the right base. **B,** Sinus radiograph shows disease in both maxillary antra and an air-fluid level on the right.

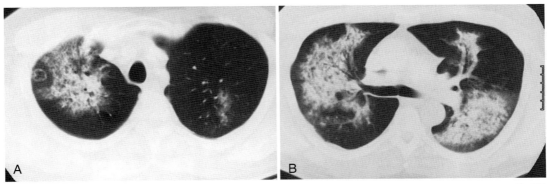

FIGURE 9-12. Wegener's granulomatosis. **A,** CT shows a peripheral cavitary nodule abutting the pleura in the right upper lobe. **B,** CT shows bilateral airspace consolidation with air bronchograms due to pulmonary hemorrhage.

Lymphomatoid Granulomatosis

Characteristics

Lymphomatoid granulomatosis (Box 9-10) is a systemic disease characterized by an angiocentric, angiodestructive, lymphoreticular, granulomatous vasculitis that primarily involves the lungs but frequently involves the kidneys, skin, and central nervous system. For many years, lymphomatoid granulomatosis was considered to represent a continuum from a more benign lymphocytic angiitis to frank lymphoma. There is currently general agreement that this disease entity is a frank lymphoma of the B-cell variety with rich T-cell components.

Presentation and Diagnosis

Lymphomatoid granulomatosis usually occurs in patients in early middle age. There is a male-to-female predominance of 2:1. Symptoms such as cough and dyspnea may be present and may be accompanied by neurologic or systemic symptoms or cutaneous lesions. The radiographic features are similar to those of Wegener's. The most common radiographic presentation consists of multiple

---

Box 9-10. Lymphomatoid Granulomatosis

CHARACTERISTICS
Granulomatous vasculitis
Considered to be a B-cell lymphoma
Occurs in middle age
Men affected more than women

RADIOGRAPHIC FEATURES
Multiple nodules or masses
   Numerous
   Cavitation

---

pulmonary nodules that range in size from 1 to 10 cm (Fig. 9-13). The nodules are often much more numerous than in Wegener's granulomatosis and may simulate advanced metastatic disease. On CT, the nodules have a perilymphatic distribution, clustering along bronchovascular bundles and interlobular septa. The lower lung

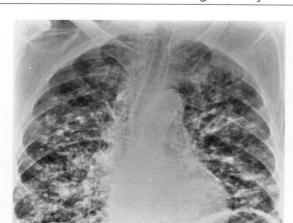

FIGURE 9-13. Lymphomatoid granulomatosis. The posteroanterior chest radiograph shows multiple, ill-defined nodules, some of which are cavitated. The nodules are smaller and much more numerous than in Wegener's granulomatosis.

zones are more frequently involved, and the nodules may be ill defined initially. The occasionally coalesce, producing a more pneumonic appearance. Cavitation is common, and hilar adenopathy is rare. Thin-walled cystic lesions may also be observed.

The diagnosis is usually made by open lung biopsy. Treatment decisions are based on a combination of the patient's symptoms, extent of extrapulmonary involvement, and histopathologic grade of the lesion. Therapy usually consists of a combination of steroids and cyclophosphamide, with approximately one half of patients achieving complete remission after therapy. Combination chemotherapy may also be employed. In the absence of treatment, the disease is usually progressive, and the prognosis is poor. However, about 20% of patients may achieve spontaneous remission without therapy.

Allergic Angiitis and Granulomatosis (Churg-Strauss Syndrome)

Characteristics

Allergic angiitis and granulomatosis (i.e., Churg-Strauss syndrome) is a disease characterized by inflammation and vascular necrosis of many organs, including the heart, lungs, skin, nervous system, and kidneys (Box 9-11). It occurs almost exclusively in patients with a history of asthma, and it is accompanied by pronounced peripheral eosinophilia. Many patients have signs of a systemic necrotizing vasculitis that may be indistinguishable from periarteritis nodosa. The disease is very similar to periarteritis nodosa, but its distinguishing characteristics include pulmonary disease and eosinophilia.

Patients may develop symptoms at any age, with extreme manifestations of atopy. They always have asthma or a history of asthma. Systemic symptoms are common and include fever, anemia, and weight loss accompanied by pronounced peripheral eosinophilia. The patient's asthma may clear as the vasculitis develops.

The American College of Rheumatology has developed six diagnostic criteria: asthma; peripheral eosinophilia greater than 10%; mononeuropathy or polyneuropathy;

Box 9-11. Allergic Angiitis and Granulomatosis*

CHARACTERISTICS
Affects heart, lungs, skin, nervous system, kidneys
Asthma history
Pronounced eosinophilia
Occurs at any age

RADIOGRAPHIC FEATURES
Patchy areas of consolidation
Multiple nodules
Fleeting opacities

---

* Also called Churg-Strauss syndrome.

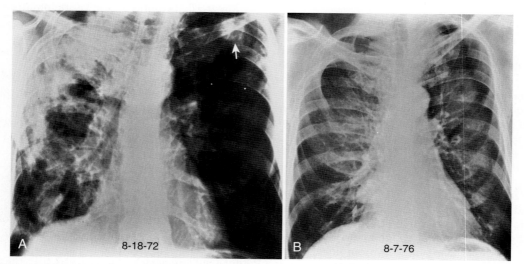

FIGURE 9-14. Allergic angiitis and granulomatosis. **A,** The initial posteroanterior chest radiograph demonstrates peripheral airspace consolidation in the right lung and a nodule *(arrow)* in the left upper lobe in this asthmatic patient. **B,** Four years later, the radiograph documents a recurrent episode by showing a nodule is in the right middle lobe *(arrow)*.

pulmonary opacities; paranasal sinus abnormalities; and extravascular eosinophilic infiltration on biopsy findings. The presence of four of six criteria is 85% sensitive and 99.7% specific for Churg-Strauss syndrome. The syndrome remains a clinical diagnosis, which should be considered in patients with asthma, peripheral eosinophilia, and pulmonary opacities. Although pathologic confirmation of tissue eosinophilia or vasculitis is helpful, an invasive biopsy is not always feasible in acutely ill patients requiring prompt initiation of therapy. When feasible, biopsy is usually performed of skin lesions; however, lung biopsy may be required in some cases. Histologic examination shows fibrinoid, necrotizing, and eosinophilic granulomatous lesions with frequent involvement of the pulmonary arteries.

Treatment consists of systemic corticosteroid therapy for a minimum of 1 year. Adjuvant cyclophosphamide is indicated for patients with severe end-organ vasculitis and for those who relapse or fail to respond to corticosteroids.

Cyclophosphamide increases the rate and rapidity of remission, but it has not been shown to improve 10-year survival.

Radiologic Findings

The radiographic features vary (Fig. 9-14). The most common presentation consists of nonsegmental areas of consolidation with no zonal predominance. The areas of consolidation typically demonstrate a characteristic peripheral distribution. The opacities may be fleeting, and new lesions may appear while older lesions are resolving. Complete regression of pulmonary lesions with corticosteroid therapy may occur. Less common findings include pulmonary nodules, diffuse reticulonodular opacities, and bronchial wall thickening. Diffuse alveolar opacities, if present, may represent alveolar hemorrhage. Pleural effusions are present in 30% of cases.

Necrotizing Sarcoid Granulomatosis

Necrotizing sarcoid granulomatosis probably represents a vascular manifestation of disseminated or localized sarcoidosis. Patients are often asymptomatic, and the disease is discovered on an incidental chest radiograph. The radiographic findings consist of multiple, bilateral, and often confluent nodules. Hilar and mediastinal adenopathy is usually absent, although nodes are often involved pathologically. The diagnosis is made by lung biopsy, and the prognosis is excellent, with a marked response to corticosteroid therapy.

Bronchocentric Granulomatosis

Although bronchocentric granulomatosis is classified as a vasculitis, the predominant pathologic feature is a necrotizing granulomatous reaction of the bronchial wall that only secondarily invades accompanying vessels. It is thought to represent a nonspecific response to airway injury and is seen characteristically in atopic and asthmatic patients who have bronchopulmonary aspergillosis and mucoid impaction. In other cases, it is usually idiopathic, but it may also be associated with a variety of infectious and inflammatory conditions. Alone, it causes few symptoms and is usually diagnosed by biopsy of a lung mass discovered radiographically. The radiologic features, similar to

those of bronchopulmonary aspergillosis, consist of lobar and segmental consolidation, atelectasis, and branching central "gloved finger" opacities due to mucoid impaction in abnormal bronchi. Single or multiple lung nodules may also be observed.

■ EOSINOPHILIC LUNG DISEASE

Characteristics

The term *pulmonary eosinophilia* was originally used to describe a group of diseases in which radiographic abnormalities were seen in association with blood eosinophilia. The descriptive term of pulmonary infiltration with eosinophilia, or *PIE syndrome*, is sometimes used to identify these disorders. However, eosinophilic infiltration of the lung can exist in the absence of blood eosinophilia. The classification of these disorders is discussed in the sections which follow.

Loeffler's Syndrome

General Description

Loeffler's syndrome (i.e., simple pulmonary eosinophilia) consists of fleeting radiographic opacities associated with blood eosinophilia (Box 9-12). Most patients have a background of atopy. Loeffler's syndrome may occur without an exciting extrinsic agent or allergen, but it may occur in response to infestations with parasites or drug therapy. In the original cases, *Ascaris lumbricoides* was a common finding. Drug-related eosinophilia is described later in this chapter.

Patients may be asymptomatic, and the syndrome is discovered incidentally on a chest radiograph. When present, symptoms are usually mild and consist of cough, slight fever, and chest pain. A low-level eosinophilia can be identified in the peripheral blood.

Radiologic Findings

Radiographic features are highly characteristic in Loeffler's syndrome (Fig. 9-15). These consist of single or multiple areas of opacity that are usually ill defined but homogeneous, typically occurring in the peripheral or axillary portions of the lungs. The areas of consolidation

---

Box 9-12.* Loeffler's Syndrome

CHARACTERISTICS
Atopy
Causes
  Idiopathic
  Parasites
  Drug-induced
Mild symptoms and eosinophilia

RADIOGRAPHIC FEATURES
Peripheral consolidation
Fleeting opacities
Photographic negative of pulmonary edema

---

* Also called simple pulmonary eosinophilia.

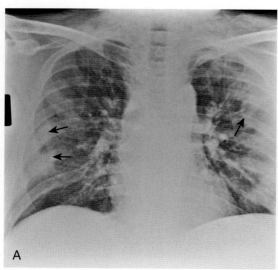
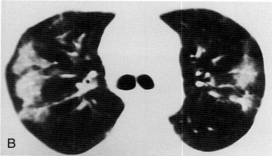

FIGURE 9-15. Loeffler's syndrome. **A,** The posteroanterior chest radiograph shows multiple, ill-defined radiographic opacities *(arrows).* **B,** CT confirms the peripheral location of the patchy consolidation.

are transient and frequently shift from one area to another, although stability may occur over several days. Cavitation, pleural effusion, and lymphadenopathy do not occur.

CT typically shows ground-glass attenuation and consolidation in the upper and middle lung regions, with a subpleural distribution. Single or multiple, small nodules with a ground-glass halo (similar in appearance to nodules associated with angioinvasive *Aspergillus* infection) may be seen in some cases.

The prognosis is excellent, and the opacities and blood eosinophilia usually resolve spontaneously. Careful search for a parasitic or drug reaction should be undertaken and the underlying disease treated.

Chronic Eosinophilic Pneumonia

Characteristics

Chronic eosinophilic pneumonia (Box 9-13) is a serious disease that requires treatment. Most patients are middle-aged women. Prominent symptoms include dyspnea, fever, chills, night sweats, and weight loss. Asthma is present in only 50% of cases. The disease is often insidious. Peripheral blood eosinophilia (>6% of total white cell count) occurs in most patients, but it is often mild or moderate.

Radiographic Patterns

The typical radiographic pattern is said to be virtually diagnostic of this disorder (Fig. 9-16). There are typically dense opacities with ill-defined margins and without lobar or segmental distribution peripherally apposed to the pleura. The opacities are usually in an apical or axillary location, but they occasionally may be basal. When the opacities surround the lung, the appearance is that of a photographic negative or reversal of opacities usually seen in pulmonary edema. The opacities sometimes disappear and recur in exactly the same location. Oblique or vertical lines with no anatomic reference occasionally appear during resolution. CT shows peripheral consolidation even when the chest radiograph fails to show the peripheral location of the opacities (Fig. 9-17). Less common CT findings, which are typically seen in the later stages of this condition, include ground-glass opacities, nodules, and reticular opacities. One half of patients have mediastinal adenopathy on CT that is also not apparent on standard radiographs. Tuberculosis should be considered in the differential diagnosis because of the apical or upper lobe location. Histologic examination demonstrates eosinophil and leukocyte accumulation in the alveoli and in the interstitium with thickened alveolar walls.

Outcomes

The prognosis for patients with this disease is excellent, although if untreated, it is likely to be protracted and may be fatal. One of the characteristic features of chronic eosinophilic pneumonia is a dramatic response to corticosteroid treatment, with clinical improvement occurring in hours and radiographic resolution occurring within a few days. A trial of corticosteroids may be used as a diagnostic tool.

Box 9-13. Chronic Eosinophilic Pneumonia

CHARACTERISTICS
Middle-aged women
Mild or moderate eosinophilia
More severe disease than Loeffler's, insidious onset
Rapid response to steroids

RADIOGRAPHIC FEATURES
Peripheral consolidation
Upper zones
Photographic negative of pulmonary edema
Differential diagnosis: tuberculosis

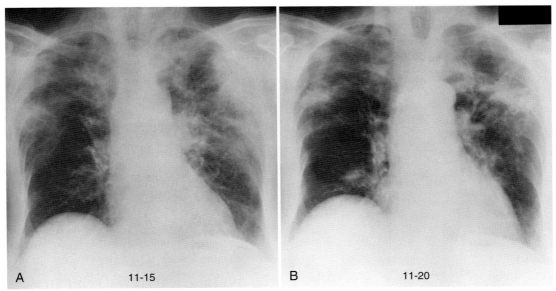

FIGURE 9-16. Chronic eosinophilic pneumonia. **A,** The posteroanterior chest radiograph demonstrates peripheral consolidation in the upper axillary zones of both lungs (i.e., photographic negative of pulmonary edema). **B,** Five days later after steroid therapy, there is significant improvement.

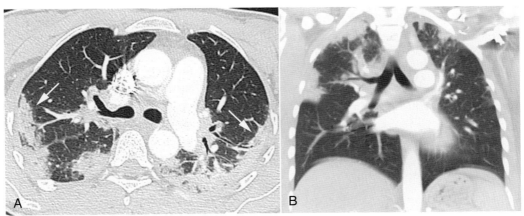

FIGURE 9-17. Chronic eosinophilic pneumonia. **A,** Axial CT demonstrates extensive peripheral foci of consolidation *(arrows)*. **B.** Coronal reformation image demonstrates upper lobe foci.

Acute Eosinophilic Pneumonia

Characteristics

Idiopathic acute eosinophilic pneumonia (Box 9-14) was first described in 1989 and represents a clinical entity distinct from other idiopathic eosinophilic lung disease, such as chronic eosinophilic pneumonia. Diagnostic criteria include an acute febrile illness of less than 5 days' duration; respiratory failure; eosinophils greater than 25% on bronchoalveolar lavage; absence of parasitic, fungal, or other infection; prompt and complete response to corticosteroids; and failure to relapse after discontinuation of corticosteroids. Patients do not usually have a history of atopy or asthma.

Radiologic Findings

Radiographic findings usually include subtle linear opacities, which progress to a consolidative pattern that is usually bilateral and extensive and involves all lobes. Unlike chronic eosinophilic pneumonia and many of the

> **Box 9-14.** Acute Eosinophilic Pneumonia
>
> **CHARACTERISTICS**
> Acute febrile illness
> Respiratory failure
> Complete response to steroids
> Absence of atopic history
>
> **RADIOGRAPHIC FEATURES**
> Diffuse consolidation
> Not peripheral
>
> **COMPUTED TOMOGRAPHY FEATURES**
> Diffuse parenchymal consolidation
> Septal thickening
> Effusion
> No lymphadenopathy

other eosinophilic syndromes, the opacities are usually not located peripherally. CT shows diffuse parenchymal consolidation, ground-glass attenuation, pleural effusions, pronounced thickening of the interlobular septa, and normal-size lymph nodes. Less commonly, focal areas of consolidation or poorly defined nodules may be seen.

Diagnosis and Treatment

The cause of this disease is unknown, but it may represent an acute hypersensitivity phenomenon to an unidentified inhaled antigen. In the differential diagnosis, infectious disease must be excluded. Patients respond rapidly to high doses of corticosteroids, usually within 24 to 48 hours. If untreated, they may progress rapidly to acute respiratory failure.

Idiopathic Hypereosinophilic Syndrome

Characteristics

Idiopathic hypereosinophilic syndrome (Box 9-15) is a rare and fatal disorder characterized by blood eosinophilia of greater than 1500 cells/mL for more than 6 months and an absence of parasitic or other causes of secondary eosinophilia. Initially, this disease was called *eosinophilic leukemia.*

The disease usually occurs in the third or fourth decades of life, and there is marked 7:1 male-to-female predominance. Symptoms include night sweats, anorexia, weight loss, cough, and fever. There is a profound peripheral eosinophilia of 30% to 70%, with a total white cell count greater than 10,000 cells/mL. Cardiac involvement may occur, and it is a major cause of morbidity and mortality. Pulmonary involvement occurs in up to 40% of patients and typically manifests with cough. It is usually caused by pulmonary edema related to cardiac failure.

Radiologic Findings

The chest radiograph shows interstitial linear or nodular opacities that are nonlobar in distribution, and approximately one half of patients have pleural effusions. CT findings include septal thickening, ground-glass attenuation, and alveolar opacities related to pulmonary edema. CT may show poorly defined nodules, with or without surrounding ground-glass attenuation. Thromboembolic disease occurs in two thirds of patients. About one half of the patients have a good clinical response to steroids alone, but others may require cytotoxic therapy.

Asthma, Allergic Bronchopulmonary Aspergillosis, Bronchocentric Granulomatosis, Allergic Angiitis, and Granulomatosis

Asthma is discussed in Chapter 10, and allergic bronchopulmonary aspergillosis is discussed in Chapter 13. Bronchocentric granulomatosis, allergic angiitis, and granulomatosis are discussed earlier in this chapter.

Parasitic Infections

Many parasites can cause pulmonary consolidation with blood or alveolar eosinophilia, or both. Those causing infection in the United States include *Strongyloides, Ascaris, Toxocara,* and *Ancylostoma.* Radiographic features for most of parasitic infections are typically those of fleeting and migratory peripheral areas of consolidation. Tropical pulmonary eosinophilia is caused by filarial worms.

■ HYPERSENSITIVITY PNEUMONITIS

Characteristics

Hypersensitivity pneumonitis (Box 9-16), also known as extrinsic allergic alveolitis, describes a spectrum of granulomatous and interstitial pulmonary disorders associated with intense and often prolonged exposure to a wide range

---

Box 9-16. Hypersensitivity Pneumonitis

CHARACTERISTICS
Causes
  Inhaled organic dust
  Occupational antigens
  Animal proteins
  Saprophytic fungi
  Dairy and grain products
  Water vaporizers
Stages
  Acute (4 to 6 hours)
  Subacute: after resolution of acute stage, between episodes
  Chronic: fibrosis, occurring months or years after exposure
Diagnosis
  History related to exposure
  Precipitating antibodies
  Positive inhalational challenge

RADIOGRAPHIC FEATURES
Acute
  Airspace consolidation (diffuse)
  Rapid clearing
Subacute
  Nodular or reticular nodular opacities
  Upper zones
  Centrilobular nodules on CT
  Ground-glass opacity on CT
Chronic
  Medium to coarse linear opacities
  Honeycombing
  Upper zones

Box 9-15. Idiopathic Hypereosinophilic Syndrome

CHARACTERISTICS
High rate of chronic eosinophilia (30%–70%), previously called eosinophilic leukemia
Occurs in third and fourth decades
Marked male predominance

RADIOGRAPHIC FEATURES
Reticular nodular opacities

COMPUTED TOMOGRAPHY FEATURES
Ground-glass appearance
Consolidation
Septal thickening

of inhaled organic dust and related occupational antigens. The site of inflammatory host response in these disorders is located primarily in the alveolar air exchange portion of the lung and not in the large conducting airways that are involved in asthmatic diseases.

A variety of organic antigens may cause hypersensitivity pneumonitis. These antigens, usually disseminated as aerosol dust, can be derived from animal dander and proteins; saprophytic fungi (i.e., spores) in contaminated vegetables, wood, bark or water reservoir vaporizers; and dairy and grain products. The diseases and the major inciting antigens are listed in Table 9-1.

The exposure is often occupational. The organic antigen may be a microbial organism, and the most commonly incriminated is thermophilic *Actinomyces*, a ubiquitous bacterium that has the morphologic features of a fungus. This is the offending antigen in one of the most common types of hypersensitivity pneumonitis, farmer's lung.

Stages of Disease

Three stages of the disease can be identified: acute, subacute, and chronic. Acute disease usually results from heavy exposure to the inciting antigen and occurs 4 to 6 hours after exposure. The subacute stage is seen after resolution of acute abnormalities or between episodes of acute exposure, and the chronic stage is characterized by the presence of fibrosis, which may develop months or years after initial exposure.

TABLE 9-1 Agents Causing in Hypersensitivity Pneumonitis

Major Antigens	Exposure or Source	Disease
Thermophilic Bacteria		
Saccharopolyspora rectivirgula (formerly *Micropolyspora faeni*)	Moldy hay	Farmer's lung
Thermoactinomyces vulgaris	Moldy grain	Grain handler's lung
S. rectivirgula, T. vulgaris	Mushroom compost	Mushroom worker's lung
Thermoactinomyces sacchari	Moldy sugar cane (bagasse)	Bagassosis
T. vulgaris, Streptomyces candidus, S. rectivirgula	Heated water reservoirs	Humidifier or air conditioner lung
Other Bacteria		
Bacillus subtilis	Water	Detergent worker's lung
Bacillus cereus	Water reservoir	Humidifier lung
Nontuberculous Mycobacteria		
Mycobacterium avium complex	Contaminated water	Hot tub lung
True fungi		
Cryptostroma corticale	Moldy bark	Maple bark stripper's lung
Aspergillus clavatus	Moldy malt, barley	Malt worker's lung
Aureobasidium pullulans and *Graphium* sp.	Moldy redwood dust	Sequoiosis
Mucor stolonifer	Moldy paprika pods	Paprika splitter's lung
Sitophilus granarius	Infested wheat flour	Wheat weevil's disease
Penicillium casei	Cheese mold	Cheese worker's lung
Penicillium frequentans	Moldy cork dust	Suberosis
Aspergillus spores	Water reservoir	Aspergillosis
Animal Proteins		
Avian proteins (serum and excreta)	Pigeons, parakeets	Bird breeder's lung
Chicken feathers, serum	Chickens	Chicken handler's lung
Turkey feathers, serum	Turkeys	Turkey handler's lung
Duck feathers	Ducks	Duck fever
Rat urine, serum	Rats	Rodent handler's disease
Porcine and bovine pituitary protein	Pituitary snuff	Pituitary snuff–taker's lung
Amebae		
Acanthamoeba	Water	Humidifier lung
Bacterial Products		
Endotoxin (?)	Cotton bract	Byssinosis
Streptomyces verticillus glycopeptides	Bleomycin	Bleomycin hypersensitivity lung (in contrast to fibrosis)

From Reynold HY: Hypersensitivity pneumonitis. Clin Chest Med 3:503, 1982.

Presentation and Diagnosis

The first clue to the diagnosis of hypersensitivity pneumonitis is a good clinical history that suggests the temporal relationship between the patient's symptoms and certain activities, including hobbies and occupations. The acute form of the disease is characterized by cough, dyspnea, and fever, which usually begin 4 to 6 hours after exposure to large quantities of the causative agent. There is often a leukocytosis, and pulmonary function studies reveal restrictive dysfunction. Usually characterized by dyspnea and chronic cough, subacute and chronic disease associated with low-grade exposure to the offending antigen may be confused with other forms of interstitial lung disease. Laboratory studies consistent with the diagnosis include precipitating antibodies reactive to the offending dust antigen and a positive inhalational challenge that can reproduce the symptoms.

Radiologic Findings

The radiographic features vary with the stage of the disease. In the acute form, the chest radiograph may be normal, but after heavy exposure to the appropriate antigen, alveolar consolidation may be observed, especially in the lower lung zones. This reflects pathologic findings of alveolar filling by polymorphonuclear leukocytes, eosinophils, lymphocytes, and large mononuclear cells. This airspace consolidation may be quite extensive, simulating pulmonary edema, but it is transitory and usually clears within hours or days. The subacute form is characterized by a fine nodular or reticulonodular pattern that tends to predominate in the upper lung zones (Fig. 9-18). This nodular appearance corresponds pathologically with alveolitis, interstitial infiltration, small granulomas, and some degree of bronchiolitis. Histologic abnormalities are usually most severe in a peribronchiolar distribution. CT may be helpful in the diagnosis of the subacute form (Fig. 9-19). The findings usually consist of small nodular opacities often distributed in a centrilobular location and areas of ground-glass opacity. Air trapping is seen on expiratory CT images.

In the chronic stage of hypersensitivity pneumonitis, when there is continued exposure to the antigen, the diffuse reticulonodular pattern is replaced by changes characteristic of diffuse interstitial fibrosis: medium to coarse linear opacities, with loss of lung volume and honeycombing. The fibrosis tends to be more pronounced in the upper zones. Similar reticular opacities can be identified on CT scans, which may also demonstrate expiratory air trapping (Fig. 9-20).

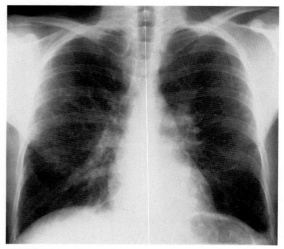

Figure 9-18. Subacute stage of hypersensitivity pneumonitis: humidifier lung. Small nodular opacities are more predominant in the upper lung zones.

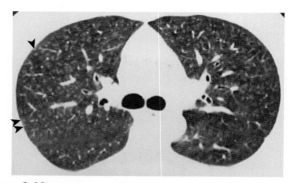

Figure 9-19. Hypersensitivity pneumonitis in a fish-plant worker. High-resolution CT shows multiple, ill-defined, low-attenuation nodules. In the subpleural zones, the nodules occupy a centrilobular location 2 to 3 mm deep to the pleural surface *(arrowheads)*. (Courtesy of Victoria General Hospital, Halifax, Nova Scotia.)

Treatment

If the environmental source of the inhaled antigen is identified, simple avoidance is sufficient treatment; the acute form of the disease abates without specific therapy. With chronic forms of disease, a trial of corticosteroids can be given.

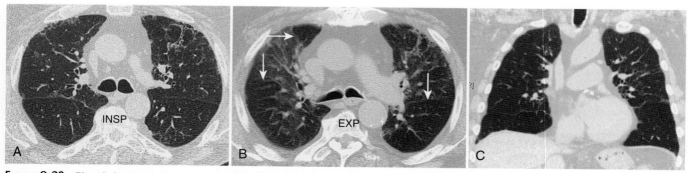

Figure 9-20. Chronic hypersensitivity pneumonitis: "baker's lung" due to exposure to moldy flour. **A,** Axial, end-inspiratory (INSP) HRCT shows interstitial fibrosis with subpleural and peribronchovascular distribution. **B,** Axial, end-expiratory (EXP) HRCT at similar level shows extensive air trapping *(arrows)*, with regions of lung that fail to demonstrate the expected expiratory increase in lung attenuation. **C,** Coronal reformation image demonstrates upper and middle lung distribution, with relative sparing of lower lungs.

Specific Diseases

Farmer's Lung

Farmer's lung was the first occupationally related form of hypersensitivity pneumonitis to be clearly described and understood. *Thermoactinomyces vulgaris* is the most important antigen in farmer's lung. It is found in moldy hay that has been improperly dried for storage.

Farmer's lung typically affects men between 40 and 50 years old. The disease occurs in late winter or early spring, when the lower levels of hay, which have had the longest time to compost, are reached. A classic acute onset occurs in one third of cases, but a more common clinical presentation is insidious and is characterized by gradual progression of cough and dyspnea, weight loss, and fever. Prevalence of the syndrome among farmers is estimated to be between 1% and 10%.

Humidifier Lung

Equipment used to heat, humidify, or cool air may harbor microorganisms responsible for hypersensitivity pneumonitis. Humidifier lung can develop in unsuspecting people who do not have obvious known exposure, and it may affect large numbers of people in an epidemic form. The diagnosis may be obvious when exposure occurs at home. However, contamination of heating and air conditioning or humidifying equipment with microorganisms in an office or commercial establishment is difficult to prove. The causative agents are usually thermophilic *Actinomyces* species. An accurate diagnosis requires a thorough history and detailed environmental probing, including a visit to suspicious areas and cultures from contaminated appliances.

Pigeon Breeder's Lung

Pigeon breeder's lung (i.e., bird fancier's disease) differs from farmer's lung or humidifier lung in that it is caused by inhaled proteins rather than microbial antigens and spores. Exposure to excreta and proteinaceous material from pigeons and other fowl and birds provokes the disease. It may produce an acute or chronic reaction.

Hot Tub Lung

Water within hot tubs may be contaminated by nontuberculous mycobacterial organisms that may become aerosolized and inhaled, resulting in a hypersensitivity pneumonitis. *Mycobacterium avium* complex is by far the most common type of nontuberculous mycobacteria found on culture in affected patients, with other species only rarely detected. This condition is reportedly more common after exposure to enclosed indoor hot tubs, which are at greater risk for contamination than those located outdoors.

■ DRUG-INDUCED LUNG DISEASE

Drug-induced lung toxicity is common and may result from complex chemotherapeutic regimens or the abuse of elicit drugs. Many drugs may produce a similar clinical syndrome, and individual drugs may cause a variety of reactions. Many drug reactions are immunologically mediated, although some may occur as a result of direct toxicity. Direct toxicity is usually dose related. The pathologic reaction consists of permeability pulmonary edema, which may progress to diffuse alveolar damage and pulmonary fibrosis. The injury may be mediated by the generation of reactive oxygen species. Hypersensitivity reactions are not dose related and require prior sensitization to the drug. This reaction is the result of the interaction between the drug and humeral antibodies or sensitized lymphocytes. Idiosyncratic toxicity is not dose related and does not require prior sensitization. These reactions are usually acute, manifesting with noncardiogenic pulmonary edema.

Patterns of Injury

Noncardiogenic Pulmonary Edema

Noncardiogenic pulmonary edema is a common complication of a variety of drugs, particularly cytotoxic agents, such as interleukin, methotrexate, cytosine, and arabinoside. The pulmonary edema typically occurs within hours of administration. It is a well-recognized complication of opiate (heroin) and salicylate overdose.

Pulmonary Hemorrhage

Pulmonary hemorrhage is most commonly a complication of anticoagulant therapy or drug-induced thrombocytopenia. Penicillamine may rarely cause a pulmonary renal syndrome similar to Goodpasture's syndrome. Acute and even fatal pulmonary hemorrhage has been reported with nitrofurantoin therapy, but more commonly, this drug is associated with hypersensitivity pneumonitis or pulmonary fibrosis. Cocaine abuse is increasingly recognized as a cause of intra-alveolar hemorrhage.

Pulmonary Fibrosis

Pulmonary fibrosis usually develops as a chronic insidious process and is typically seen with a wide variety of cytotoxic and noncytotoxic drugs, such as busulfan and bleomycin. Several new chemotherapy agents, including gemcitabine, have been associated with pulmonary fibrosis.

Eosinophilic Pneumonia

Drug reactions are one of the most commonly reported causes of pulmonary opacities associated with blood or alveolar eosinophilia (Box 9-17). One of the most common is sulfasalazine, which is used for inflammatory bowel disease. Eosinophilia-myalgia syndrome is an interesting multiorgan disorder caused by contaminants found in batches of L-tryptophan that were manufactured in the late 1980s. The disease involved approximately one half of the persons ingesting the contaminated drug, who developed acute peripheral blood eosinophilia accompanied by severe myalgias. Approximately one half of the patients had respiratory symptoms. Typical peripheral pulmonary consolidation was identified on chest radiographs.

Drug-induced eosinophilia may be mild or manifest as a fulminant, acute eosinophilic pneumonia–like syndrome. Most patients respond to withdrawal of the drug, although steroid therapy may be necessary.

Exogenous Lipoid Pneumonia

Exogenous lipoid pneumonia has been described as a complication of accidental aspiration of mineral oil. Endogenous phospholipoidosis induced by amiodarone is an important cause of pulmonary toxicity.

Drug-Induced Lupus Syndrome

Drug-induced lupus syndrome is more common than the idiopathic form of SLE. It has, however, a more benign course and is usually reversible. Common manifestations

---

Box 9-17. **Drugs and Biologic Chemicals that Cause Eosinophilic Lung Disease**

Ampicillin	Naproxen
Beclomethasone dipropionate (inhaled)	Nickel
Bleomycin	Nitrofurantoin
Carbamazepine	Para-aminosalicylic acid
Chlorpromazine	Penicillin
Clofibrate	Pentamidine (inhaled)
Cocaine (inhaled)	Phenytoin
Cromolyn (inhaled)	Pyrimethamine
Desipramine	Rapeseed oil
Diclofenac	Sulfadimethoxine
Fenbufen	Sulfadoxine
Glafenine	Sulfasalazine
Ibuprofen	Sulindac
Interleukin 2	Tamoxifen
Interleukin 3	Tetracycline
Iodinated contrast dye	Tolazamide
Mephenesin carbamate	Tolfenamic acid
Methotrexate	L-tryptophan
Methylphenidate	Vaginal sulfonamide cream
Minocycline	

---

include pleural and pericardial effusions. Subsegmental atelectasis and basilar consolidation are typical radiographic findings. Drugs implicated include hydralazine, procainamide, and phenytoin. Most patients have a positive antinuclear antibody (ANA) result.

Bronchiolitis Obliterans

Bronchiolitis obliterans is characterized pathologically by the proliferation of granulation tissue in the small airways and obliteration of their lumens. It is an uncommon drug-induced complication, most frequently associated with penicillamine therapy prescribed for rheumatoid arthritis.

Illicit Drug Use

The pulmonary manifestations of drug abuse include a wide variety of infectious and inflammatory complications. The adverse effects are related to the route of administration and to the type of drug. Talcosis results from intravenous injection of aqueous solutions of oral preparations contaminated by talc. Talc is a filler used in the manufacture of tablets to prevent them from sticking to the mouth. When injected, the talc particles become lodged in peripheral pulmonary arterioles and capillaries, producing pulmonary hypertension and vasculitis.

Radiologic Features

Clinical and radiologic features of drug-induced lung disease are summarized in Box 9-18.

Hydrochlorothiazide

Hydrochlorothiazide produces noncardiogenic pulmonary edema due to a hypersensitivity reaction. Reported cases have occurred in women, and the radiographic features consist of bilateral, diffuse airspace opacities.

Interleukin 2

Interleukin 2 is used to treat advanced malignant disease. Pulmonary edema has been reported in up to 70% of patients and usually occurs within a week of commencing therapy. The radiographic findings consist of mild, interstitial or frank alveolar pulmonary edema that is often associated with pleural effusions and ascites.

Amiodarone

Amiodarone is a tri-iodinated compound used in the treatment of cardiac arrhythmias. Pulmonary toxicity is a common complication, occurring in up to 18% of patients. Toxicity appears to be dose related. The onset is usually subacute. Several forms of pulmonary toxicity have been reported among patients treated with amiodarone. The most common presentation is a chronic interstitial pneumonitis with imaging features of reticular opacities that may be difficult to distinguish from congestive heart failure. If the diagnosis is delayed, the interstitial process may progress to end-stage pulmonary fibrosis. In some cases, patchy alveolar and interstitial opacities may be present diffusely. Upper lobe predominance has been described in some cases, which can be helpful for differentiating this condition from congestive heart failure. A less common presentation is solitary or multiple peripheral areas of consolidation or nodules, or both, that may mimic cryptogenic organizing pneumonia, chronic eosinophilic pneumonia, and pulmonary infarction. A rare but potentially fatal form of pulmonary toxicity is acute respiratory distress syndrome (ARDS). A pleural reaction may occur, but effusions are uncommon. CT may demonstrate the characteristic high density of the pleuropulmonary lesions as a result of the iodine content of amiodarone (Fig. 9-21). When areas of consolidation or nodules, or both, with high attenuation are seen on unenhanced CT scans, amiodarone pulmonary toxicity should be considered. Because amiodarone therapy is frequently associated with high attenuation of the liver, evaluation of the hepatic parenchyma may provide an important clue that a patient is receiving amiodarone.

Box 9-18. Clinical and Radiologic Features of Drug- and Chemical-Induced Lung Disease

HYDROCHLOROTHIAZIDE
Noncardiogenic pulmonary edema

INTERLEUKIN 2
Noncardiogenic edema
Pleural effusions and ascites

AMIODARONE
Treatment of cardiac arrhythmias
Patchy alveolar and diffuse linear opacities
Upper lobe and peripheral distribution
Solitary or multiple nodules and consolidation
High attenuation (iodine) on CT

NITROFURANTOIN
Urinary tract infections
Eosinophilia
Patchy and peripheral airspace consolidation
Fibrosis (with chronic use)

METHOTREXATE
Treatment of inflammatory diseases and malignancy
Allergic response
Diffuse, reticulonodular opacities or widespread
    consolidation

Adenopathy
Distribution in lung bases and middle zones

BUSULFAN
Treatment chronic granulocytic leukemia
Diffuse, reticulonodular opacities

BLEOMYCIN
Treatment of lymphoma, solid tumors
Dose-related effects
Pulmonary fibrosis
Linear subpleural basilar opacities

CYCLOSPORINE
Prevention of transplant rejection
Lymphoproliferative disorder (3% to 5%)
Lungs, nodes, gastrointestinal tract distribution
Solitary mass, multiple nodules, with or without
    adenopathy

ASPIRATED OILY SUBSTANCES
Lipoid pneumonia
Chronic multifocal basal areas of consolidation
Air bronchograms
Attenuation of fat on CT

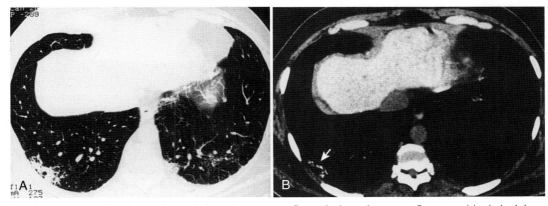

FIGURE 9-21. Amiodarone toxicity. **A,** CT using lung windows demonstrates fine reticular and some confluent opacities in both lower lobes subpleurally. **B,** Mediastinal windows reveal high attenuation of the pulmonary opacities *(arrow)* and a high-attenuation liver.

Nitrofurantoin
Nitrofurantoin is a drug widely used in the treatment of urinary tract infections. It is an important cause of pulmonary eosinophilia, which occurs in the majority of patients. It may cause acute onset of pneumonitis and chronic interstitial pneumonia. The chest radiograph demonstrates bilateral, patchy, and occasionally peripheral airspace consolidation (Fig. 9-22). Pleural effusions may occur. Pulmonary fibrosis develops with prolonged use of nitrofurantoin, and the fibrosis probably results from chronic drug toxicity rather than a hypersensitivity reaction.

Methotrexate
This drug is used to treat a variety of inflammatory diseases, such as rheumatoid arthritis and psoriasis, and

malignant disorders. Methotrexate toxicity is unique is several respects. Discontinuation of the drug is not always required for recovery, and reintroduction of the drug is not necessarily associated with recurrent symptoms. Toxicity may occur with low-dose therapy, and it appears to be related to the frequency of administration. The features are usually that of an allergic response with a subacute illness associated with pulmonary eosinophilia. A typical radiographic appearance is that of diffuse reticulonodular opacities, but there may be widespread consolidation with hilar and mediastinal lymphadenopathy (Fig. 9-23). A predilection for the lung bases and middle zones has been described. Most patients recover completely, even if the drug is continued, and residual pulmonary fibrosis is uncommon.

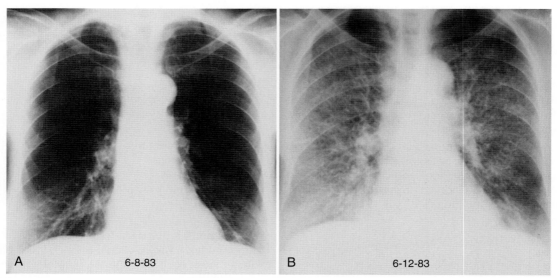

FIGURE 9-22. Nitrofurantoin reaction. **A,** Baseline radiograph is normal. **B,** Several days after administration of the drug for a urinary tract infection, diffuse, bilateral reticular opacities and areas of consolidation are visualized on the radiograph. There is no evidence of a peripheral distribution.

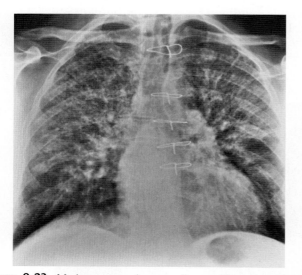

FIGURE 9-23. Methotrexate pulmonary disease. The posteroanterior radiograph shows diffuse reticulonodular and patchy opacities.

Busulfan

Busulfan is used almost exclusively in the treatment of chronic granulocytic leukemia. Pulmonary toxicity is usually related to the duration of therapy and is increased with combination chemotherapy. The chest radiograph usually shows a diffuse reticulonodular appearance. The prognosis is poor, with a mortality rate of about 50%.

Bleomycin

Bleomycin is used in the treatment of lymphomas, squamous cell cancer, and testicular tumors. Pulmonary toxicity occurs in about 4% of patients and is an important factor limiting dosage. The incidence of toxicity is related to the cumulative dose. Pulmonary fibrosis is the most serious complication, although acute hypersensitivity reaction has been described. The chest radiograph may be normal or may show typical basal subpleural reticular opacities similar to those seen in idiopathic pulmonary fibrosis (Fig. 9-24). CT may demonstrate abnormalities even when

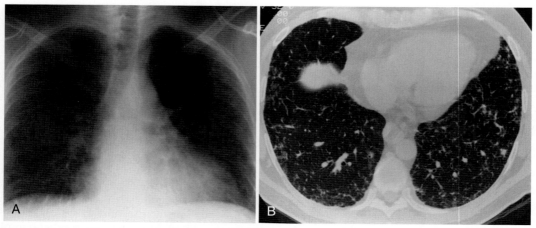

FIGURE 9-24. Bleomycin lung. **A,** The posteroanterior radiograph shows fine reticular opacities at the lung bases. **B,** High-resolution CT shows linear opacities with intralobular lines and septal thickening that are most pronounced in the subpleural basal lung.

the chest radiograph is normal. In the early stages of the disease, regression may occur after stopping therapy, but fibrosis may progress, resulting in death.

Cyclosporine

Cyclosporine inhibits cytotoxic T cells and is used to control rejection in transplant recipients. Approximately 3% to 5% of patients treated with cyclosporine develop a drug-induced lymphoproliferative disorder, typically within 4 to 6 months of commencing therapy. The lungs, lymph nodes, and gastrointestinal tract may be involved. All reported patients have evidence of Epstein-Barr virus infection. This virus selectively affects B cells, causing B-cell proliferation that is normally controlled by cytotoxic T cells. Pulmonary radiologic manifestations include a solitary mass, multiple pulmonary nodules, and hilar adenopathy (Fig. 9-25).

Lipoid Pneumonia

Lipoid pneumonia usually occurs as the result of inadvertent aspiration of oily substances, such as mineral oil. It usually results in multifocal areas of consolidation, typically at the bases of the lungs. The areas of consolidation tend to be chronic, with prominent air bronchograms (Fig. 9-26). The diagnosis can be made on CT. The CT density numbers for the areas of consolidation are in the range of fatty tissue and are therefore pathognomonic for lipoid pneumonia (Fig. 9-27).

▬ PULMONARY LYMPHOPROLIFERATIVE DISORDERS

Characteristics

Several nonlymphomatous lymphoproliferative disorders may occur in the lung. There is considerable overlap between these disorders and lymphoma. The normal lung contains abundant lymphoid tissue. Lymph nodes are present within the hila and along the tracheobronchial branches, and there is submucosal lymphoid tissue along the respiratory tract at the level of the pulmonary acinus. Lymphoid clusters can be found at the level of the distal respiratory bronchiole. There is also a chain of subpleural lymphatics abutting the visceral pleura. The benign lymphoid disorders of the lung are thought to represent hyperplasia of the pulmonary lymphoid system in response to chronic antigenic stimulation. They are associated with an abnormality of immune response. These pulmonary extranodal and lymphoid disorders include plasma cell granuloma, pseudolymphoma, lymphocytic interstitial pneumonitis, lymphomatoid granulomatosis, follicular bronchiolitis, mucosa-associated lymphoid tissue (MALT) lymphoma, and lymphoproliferative disorders associated

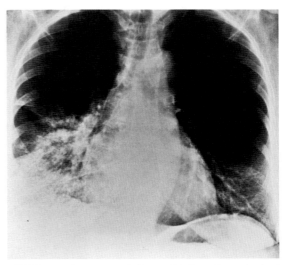

FIGURE 9-26. Lipoid pneumonia in an elderly patient who had taken mineral oil regularly for chronic constipation. There is consolidation with air bronchograms at the base of the right lung.

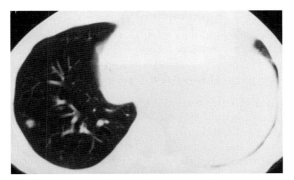

FIGURE 9-25. Lymphoproliferative disorder after cardiac transplantation and cyclosporine therapy. CT shows a solitary nodule in the right lower lobe.

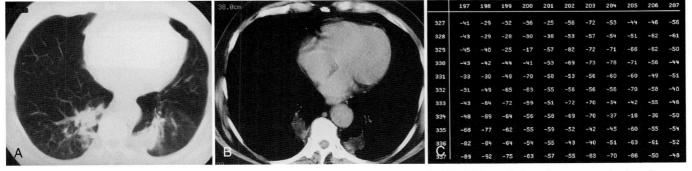

FIGURE 9-27. Lipoid pneumonia in a patient who had been a regular user of oily nose drops. **A,** CT with lung windows demonstrates focal patchy areas of consolidation in the basal segments of both lower lobes. **B,** Mediastinal windows show areas of low attenuation within the opacities. **C,** Printout of CT numbers of pixels through the abnormal area in the right lower lobe show values equal to fat attenuation (–50 to –150 HU).

with cyclosporine use after transplantation. The lymph node disorders include giant lymph node hyperplasia (i.e., Castleman's disease) and angioblastic lymphadenopathy.

Plasma Cell Granuloma

Plasma cell granuloma (i.e., inflammatory myelofibroblastic tumor) of the lung consists of a localized, benign proliferation of a variety of cells, with a predominance of mature plasma cells (Box 9-19). Pathogenesis of this lesion is uncertain, and it is sometimes referred to as a *postinflammatory pseudotumor*. However, in most cases, there is no evidence of prior inflammation or infection. Histologically, myofibroblasts, fibroblasts, and histiocytes often comprise the bulk of this tumor. In recognition of the fact that myelofibroblasts are the primary spindle cell type associated with this lesion, the term *inflammatory myelofibroblastic tumor* has also been used to describe this entity.

The disease affects women slightly more often than men, and it may occur at any age, although most patients are younger than 30 years. Patients are usually asymptomatic, and the lesion is discovered as a solitary pulmonary nodule on an incidental chest radiograph (Fig. 9-28). The nodule may range from 1 to 12 cm in diameter and occasionally may cavitate or calcify. It usually grows slowly in a matter of months to years. CT may show heterogeneous attenuation and enhancement of the nodule. Complete surgical resection with as little removal of adjacent lung as possible is the treatment of choice.

Pseudolymphoma

Although most patients are asymptomatic, pseudolymphoma (i.e., nodular lymphoid hyperplasia) may be seen in patients with a variety of autoimmune diseases (e.g., Sjögren's syndrome) or dysgammaglobulinemias (Box 9-20). Patients are usually of middle aged.

Pseudolymphoma usually manifests as a localized area of parenchymal consolidation (Fig. 9-29). It is caused by lymphoid interstitial proliferation, which compresses the

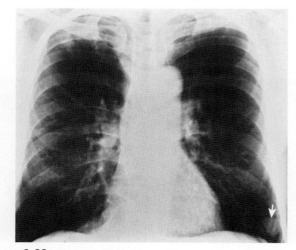

FIGURE 9-28. Plasma cell granuloma. The posteroanterior chest radiograph shows a well-defined, approximately 2-cm nodule near the left costophrenic angle *(arrow)*.

Box 9-19. Plasma Cell Granuloma

CHARACTERISTICS
Postinflammatory pseudotumor
Women affected more than men
Young, less than 30 years old
Asymptomatic

RADIOGRAPHIC FEATURES
Solitary nodule 1 to 12 cm in diameter
Slow growth with or without calcification and cavitation

COMPUTED TOMOGRAPHY FEATURES
Heterogenous attenuation and enhancement

Box 9-20. Pseudolymphoma (Nodular lymphoid hyperplasia)

CHARACTERISTICS
Asymptomatic
Associated with autoimmune diseases (e.g., Sjögren's syndrome) or dysgammaglobulinemias

RADIOGRAPHIC FEATURES
Chronic consolidation
Single or multiple focal areas
Air bronchograms

---

airspaces and creates air bronchograms. The consolidation is usually between 2 and 5 cm in diameter, and it may be scattered randomly throughout the lung. Lymphadenopathy and pleural effusions are absent. Differentiation from lymphocytic lymphoma is difficult, and malignant transformation is reported in 15% to 80% of cases.

Lymphocytic Interstitial Pneumonitis

LIP is a diffuse interstitial infiltration of the lung characterized predominantly by lymphocytes with various admixtures of plasma cells and other elements (Box 9-21). In pseudolymphoma, the lymphocytic infiltration is localized. In LIP the involvement is diffuse. Although the cause is unknown, it may be associated with abnormalities in the immune system, such as Sjögren's syndrome, pernicious anemia, chronic active hepatitis, and myasthenia gravis, or it may result from a viral infection. The disease may occur with some frequency in children with acquired immunodeficiency syndrome (AIDS).

The radiographic appearance varies, but it often consists of a bilateral, linear or reticulonodular pattern with basilar predominance (Fig. 9-30). Coarse flamelike opacities or diffuse, confluent lesions have been described. If a nodular pattern is present, the nodules tend to be smaller than those seen in lymphoma. In later stages, honeycombing may be seen. Pleural effusion occasionally occurs, but hilar and mediastinal adenopathy is rare. CT often shows a characteristic pattern of extensive ground-glass attenuation and scattered, thin-walled cysts. The cysts are thought to arise from overdistended airspaces distal to areas of bronchiolar stenosis. Other CT findings include centrilobular nodules and thickening of interlobular septa and bronchovascular bundles.

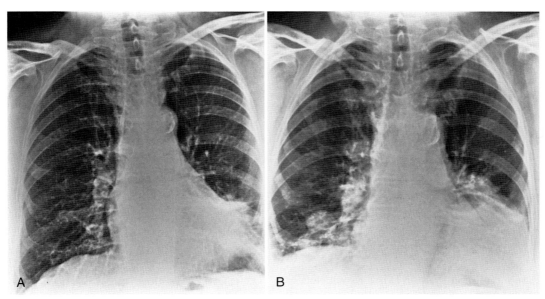

FIGURE 9-29. Pseudolymphoma in a patient with Sjögren's syndrome. **A,** The posteroanterior radiograph shows an ill-defined opacity with faint air bronchograms in the lingula that obliterates the left heart border. **B,** Two years later, the area of opacification on the left has increased in size, and there are new nodules in the right base.

Box 9-21. **Lymphocytic Interstitial Pneumonitis**

CHARACTERISTICS
Diffuse lymphocytic infiltration of the lung
Associated autoimmune diseases, children with AIDS
Progression to lymphoma in some non-AIDS patients

RADIOGRAPHIC FEATURES
Bilateral, linear or reticular nodular opacities
Basilar
Coarse, flamelike opacities
Late honeycombing
Adenopathy rare

COMPUTED TOMOGRAPHY FEATURES
Ground-glass attenuation
Thin-walled cysts

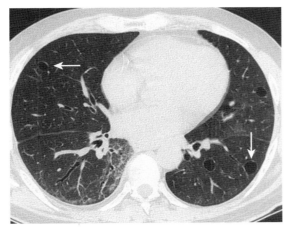

FIGURE 9-30. Lymphocytic interstitial pneumonitis in patient with Sjögren's syndrome. High-resolution CT shows scattered, thin-walled cysts *(arrows)* bilaterally and areas of ground-glass attenuation and reticulation, mostly in the right lower lobe.

Treatment of symptomatic cases consists of steroids and other immunosuppressive agents, but some cases show spontaneous remission without treatment. Neoplastic transformation may occur, and the reported incidence varies from a small percentage to 50% of cases.

Lymphomatoid Granulomatosis

Lymphomatoid granulomatosis is a pulmonary lymphoproliferative disorder, but it is discussed earlier in this chapter with other granulomatoses.

Follicular Bronchiolitis

Follicular bronchiolitis (Box 9-22) is defined as lymphoid hyperplasia of bronchus-associated lymphoid tissue (BALT). Its cause is unknown, but it most commonly arises in association with collagen vascular disorders, especially rheumatoid arthritis. CT commonly shows small centrilobular nodules, which correspond histologically to foci of lymphoid proliferation in the bronchiolar interstitium. CT also may show bronchial wall thickening, bronchial dilation, interlobular septal thickening, and ground-glass attenuation.

Box 9-22. **Follicular Bronchiolitis**

CHARACTERISTICS
Lymphoid hyperplasia of bronchus-associated lymphoid tissue
Associated with collagen vascular disorders, especially rheumatoid arthritis

RADIOGRAPHIC FEATURES
Centrilobular nodules on CT
Bronchial wall thickening and dilation
Interlobular septal thickening
Ground-glass attenuation

Box 9-23. Mucosa-Associated Lymphoid Tissue Lymphoma

CHARACTERISTICS

Extranodal, marginal zone B-cell lymphoma

Involves bronchus-associated lymphoid tissue

Associated with autoimmune disorders (e.g., Sjögren's syndrome

RADIOGRAPHIC FEATURES

Solitary or multiple, poorly defined nodules or foci of consolidation on CT

Air bronchograms

Ground-glass halos surrounding lesions

Mucosa-Associated Lymphoid Tissue Lymphoma

Mucosa-associated lymphoid tissue (MALT) specializes in mucosal defense and is present on the body's mucosal surfaces, including along the bronchi (BALT). MALT lymphoma is classified as an extranodal, marginal zone B-cell lymphoma (Box 9-23). Many patients have an underlying autoimmune disorder such as Sjögren's syndrome. The stomach is the most common site for MALT lymphoma.

CT features of thoracic MALT lymphoma include solitary or multiple, poorly defined nodules and foci of consolidation. Air bronchograms are frequently observed in the lesions, and peripheral ground-glass halos may be seen surrounding the lesions. These lesions may be cured with local treatment (i.e., surgery or radiation) and are associated with high remission rates and long survival times.

Posttransplantation Lymphoproliferative Disorders

Posttransplantation lymphoproliferative infiltration of the lung is usually associated with cyclosporine and can occur in up to 3% of posttransplantation patients. This entity represents a heterogeneous group of lymphoproliferative disorders ranging from benign polyclonal B-cell proliferation to a relatively malignant monoclonal lymphomatous lesion. It is closely related to the Epstein-Bar virus in most cases. It usually occurs 4 to 6 months after transplantation, but the time course varies.

The radiographic features include solitary masses, multiple nodules, and mediastinal and hilar adenopathy (see Fig. 9-25). There may also be involvement of gastrointestinal tract. Symptoms include fever, weight loss, and lethargy. The disorder usually regresses with a decrease of immunosuppression, but concomitant treatment with chemotherapy, irradiation (for localized disease), anti–B-cell monoclonal antibody therapy, or cell-based therapies may be employed for cases of monoclonal malignant lymphoma that do not respond to reduced immunosuppression.

▬ SUGGESTED READINGS

Aberle, D.R., Gamsu, G., Lynch, D., 1990. Thoracic manifestations of Wegener's granulomatosis. Radiology 174, 703–706.

Allen, J.N., Davis, W.B., 1994. Eosinophilic lung diseases. Am. J. Respir. Crit. Care Med. 150, 1423–1438.

Allen, J.N., Pacht, E.R., Gadek, J.E., Davis, W.B., 1989. Acute eosinophilic pneumonia as a reversible cause of noninfectious respiratory failure. N. Engl. J. Med. 321, 569–574.

Ansell, G., 1987. Radiology of Adverse Reactions to Drugs and Toxic Hazards, second ed. Chapman & Hall, London.

Badesch, D.B., King, T.E., Schwarz, M.I., 1989. Acute eosinophilic pneumonia: a hypersensitivity reaction? Am. Rev. Respir. Dis. 139, 249–252.

Boiselle, P.M., Morrin, M.M., Huberman, M.S., 2000. Gemcitabine pulmonary toxicity: CT features. J. Comput. Assist. Tomogr. 24, 977–980.

Bouros, D., Wells, A.U., Nicholson, A.G., 2002. Histopathologic subsets of fibrosing alveolitis in patients with systemic sclerosis and their relationship to outcome. Am. J. Respir. Crit. Care Med. 165, 1581–1586.

Buchheit, J., Eid, N., Rodgers Jr., F., et al., 1992. Acute eosinophilic pneumonia with respiratory failure: a new syndrome?. Am. Rev. Respir. Dis. 145, 716–718.

Camus, P., Fanton, A., Bonniaud, P., et al., 2004. Interstitial lung disease induced by drugs and radiation. Respiration 71, 301–326.

Carrington, C.B., Addington, W.W., Goff, A.M., et al., 1969. Chronic eosinophilic pneumonia. N. Engl. J. Med. 280, 787–790.

Churg, J., Strauss, L., 1951. Allergic granulomatosis, allergic angiitis, and periarteritis nodosa. Am. J. Pathol. 27, 277–283.

Collard, H.R., King, T.E., 2007. Pulmonary lymphomatoid granulomatosis. In: Rose, B.D. (Ed.), UpToDate (CD-ROM). UpToDate, Waltham, MA, Available at http://www.uptodate.com/patients/content/topic. do?topicKey=~0YxcId8bOPEFbH (accessed September 2009).

Collard, H.R., King, T.E., 2007. Bronchocentric granulomatosis. In: Rose, B.D. (Ed.), UpToDate (CD-ROM). UpToDate, Waltham, MA, Available at http://www. uptodate.com/patients/content/topic.do?topicKey=~O6DoD5MWX7eZWhb &selectedTitle=1~150&source=search_result (accessed September 2009).

Cooper, J.A. (Ed.), 1990. Drug-induced pulmonary disease. Clin. Chest Med. 11, 1–194.

Cooper, J.A., White, D.A., Matthay, R.A., 1986. Drug induced pulmonary disease. Part I. Cytotoxic drugs. Am. Rev. Respir. Dis. 133, 321–340.

Cooper, J.A., White, D.A., Matthay, R.A., 1986. Drug induced pulmonary disease. Part II. Noncytotoxic drugs. Am. Rev. Respir. Dis. 133, 488–505.

Desai, S.R., Veeraraghavan, S., Hansell, D.M., et al., 2004. CT features of lung disease in patients with systemic sclerosis: comparison with idiopathic pulmonary fibrosis and nonspecific interstitial pneumonitis. Radiology 232, 560–567.

Do, K.H., Lee, J.S., Seo, J.B., et al., 2005. Pulmonary parenchymal involvement of low-grade lymphoproliferative disorders. J. Comput. Assist. Tomogr. 29, 825–830.

Dreisin, R.B., 1982. Pulmonary vasculitis. Clin. Chest Med. 3, 607–618.

Fauci, A.S., Haynes, B.F., Katz, P., 1978. The spectrum of vasculitis: clinical, pathologic, immunologic, and therapeutic considerations. Ann. Intern. Med. 89, 660–664.

Franquet, T., 2001. High-resolution CT of lung disease related to collagen vascular disease. Radiol. Clin. North Am. 39, 1171–1187.

Fraser, R.S., Muller, N.L., Colman, N.L., Pare, P.D., 1999. Fraser and Pare's Diagnosis of Diseases of the Chest, 4th ed. Philadelphia, Elsevier.

Gaensler, E.A., Carrington, C.B., 1977. Peripheral opacities in chronic eosinophilic pneumonia: the photographic negative of pulmonary edema. AJR Am. J. Roentgenol. 128, 1–5.

Gefter, W.B., 1984. Drug induced disorders in the chest. In: Taveras, J.M., Ferrucci, J.T. (Eds.), Radiology: Diagnosis, Imaging, Intervention. JB Lippincott, Philadelphia.

Gimenez, A., Franquet, T., Prats, R., et al., 2002. Unusual primary lung tumors: a radiologic-pathologic overview. Radiographics 22, 601–619.

Hartman, T.E., Jensen, E., Tazelaar, H.D., et al., 2007. CT findings of granulomatous pneumonitis secondary to *Mycobacterium avium-intracellulare* inhalation: "hot tub lung.". AJR Am. J. Roentgenol. 188, 1050–1053.

Jeong, Y.J., Kim, K., Seo, I.J., et al., 2007. Eosinophilic lung diseases: a clinical, radiologic, and pathologic overview. Radiographics 27, 617–639.

Kim, E.A., Lee, K.S., Johkoh, T., et al., 2002. Interstitial lung diseases associated with collagen vascular diseases: radiologic and histopathologic findings. Radiographics 22, S151–S165.

Kuhlman, J.E., Hruban, R.H., Fishman, E.K., 1991. Wegener's granulomatosis: CT features of parenchymal lung disease. J. Comput. Assist. Tomogr. 15, 948–952.

Lake, F.R., 2007. Overview of lung diseases associated with rheumatoid arthritis. In: Rose, B.D. (Ed.), UpToDate (CD-ROM). UpToDate, Waltham, MA, Available at http://www.uptodateonline.com/patients/content/topic. do?topicKey=~fcc5y6DqbRXDkI (accessed September 2009).

Liebow, A.A., 1973. The J Burns Amberson Lecture: pulmonary angiitis and granulomatosis. Am. Rev. Respir. Dis. 108, 1–5.

Liebow, A.A., Carrington, C.B., Friedman, P.J., 1972. Lymphomatoid granulomatosis. Hum. Pathol. 3, 457–461.

Lohrmann, C., Uhl, M., Kotter, E., et al., 2005. Pulmonary manifestations of Wegener granulomatosis: CT findings in 57 patients and review of the literature. Eur. J. Radiol. 53, 471–477.

Malo, J., Pepys, J., Simon, G., 1977. Studies in chronic allergic bronchopulmonary aspergillosis. 2. Radiological findings. Thorax 32, 262–265.

Matthay, R.A., Putman, C.E., 1981. Pulmonary-renal syndromes. In: Putman, C.E. (Ed.), Pulmonary Diagnosis: Imaging and Other Techniques. Appleton Communications, New York.

Matthay, R.A., Schwartz, M., Petty, T.L., 1977. Pleuro-pulmonary manifestations of connective tissue diseases. Clin. Notes Respir. Dis. 16, 3–6.

Matthay, R.A., Schwartz, M.I., Petty, T.L., et al., 1975. Pulmonary manifestations of systemic lupus erythematosus: review of 12 cases of acute lupus pneumonitis. Medicine (Baltimore) 54, 397–401.

Mayberry, J.P., Primack, S.L., Müller, N.L., 2000. Thoracic manifestations of systemic autoimmune diseases: radiographic and high-resolution CT findings. Radiographics 20, 1623–1635.

McCarthy, D.S., Pepys, J., 1971. Allergic bronchopulmonary aspergillosis: clinical immunology. I. Clinical features. Clin. Allergy 1, 261–264.

McLoud, T.C., Carrington, C.B., Gaensler, E.A., 1983. A new scheme for description of diffuse infiltrative lung disease. Radiology 149, 353–357.

Mino, M., Noma, S., Taguchi, Y., et al., 1997. Pulmonary involvement in polymyositis and dermatomyositis: sequential evaluation with CT. AJR Am. J. Roentgenol. 169, 83–87.

Müller, N.L., Miller, R., 1990. Computed tomography of chronic diffuse infiltrative lung disease. Part I. Am Rev. Respir. Dis. 142, 1206–1210.

Müller, N.L., Miller, R., 1990. Computed tomography of chronic diffuse infiltrative lung disease. Part II. Am Rev. Respir. Dis. 142, 1440–1445.

Noth, I., Strek, M.E., Leff, A.R., 2003. Churg-Strauss syndrome. Lancet 361, 587–594.

Pepys, J., 1969. Hypersensitivity disease of the lungs due to fungi and organic dusts. In: Monographs in Allergy. Karger, Basel.

Pepys, J., 1966. Pulmonary hypersensitivity disease due to inhaled organic antigens. Ann. Intern. Med. 64, 943–946.

Remy-Jardin, M., Remy, J., Cortet, B., et al., 1994. Lung changes in rheumatoid arthritis: CT findings. Radiology 193, 375–382.

Schwartz, M.I., Matthay, R.A., Lahn, S.A., et al., 1976. Interstitial lung disease in polymyositis, dermatomyositis. Analysis of six cases and a review of the literature. Medicine (Baltimore) 55, 89–95.

Symposium, 1991. Lung and heart disease associated with drug therapy and abuse. J. Thorac. Imaging 6: 1–84.

Tanaka, N., Kim, J.S., Newell, J.D., et al., 2004. Rheumatoid arthritis–related lung diseases: CT findings. Radiology 232, 81–91.

Wechsler, R.J., Steiner, R.M., Spirn, P.W., et al., 1996. The relationship of thoracic lymphadenopathy to pulmonary interstitial disease in diffuse and limited systemic sclerosis: CT findings. AJR Am. J. Roentgenol. 167, 101–104.

CHAPTER 10

Chronic Obstructive Pulmonary Disease and Asthma

Theresa C. McLoud and Phillip M. Boiselle

▬ CHRONIC OBSTRUCTIVE PULMONARY DISEASE

Chronic obstructive pulmonary disease (COPD) consists of disorders characterized by airway obstruction leading to decreased expiratory flow rates and increased airways resistance with decreased intrapulmonary diameters. COPD includes chronic bronchitis, which is defined in clinical terms, and emphysema, which is defined anatomically (Box 10-1). Although asthma is also characterized by airflow obstruction, it differs from COPD in its pathogenic and therapeutic responses. Asthma is therefore considered a separate clinical entity from COPD, and it is discussed at the end of the chapter. However, there is some overlap between these conditions, and some patients have COPD and asthma. COPD is predominantly a disease of smokers, although only about 15% of smokers develop disabling airflow obstruction.

The chest radiograph is an important imaging modality in the assessment of patients with COPD. However, it has limitations in the detection and differential diagnosis of obstructive airways disease. It is relatively insensitive in the detection of early emphysema, and it is frequently normal for patients with pure chronic bronchitis and asthma. High-resolution CT has significantly improved our ability to image morphologic abnormalities associated with chronic airflow obstruction, particularly in emphysema, bronchiectasis, and bronchiolitis. CT also can delineate functional abnormalities such as air trapping and decreased perfusion.

▬ EMPHYSEMA

Emphysema is a condition of the lung characterized by abnormal, permanent enlargement of the airspaces distal to the terminal bronchiole, accompanied by destruction of their walls without obvious fibrosis (Box 10-2).

Pathology

The four anatomically defined types of emphysema are centrilobular or centriacinar, panlobular or panacinar, paraseptal or distal acinar, and paracicatricial or irregular emphysema. The acinus is the air-exchanging unit of the lung, and it is located distal to the terminal bronchiole. It includes the respiratory bronchioles, alveolar ducts, alveolar sacs, and alveoli (Fig. 10-1). Although this classification relies on the relationship of emphysema to the acinus, acini cannot be resolved on high-resolution CT,

and it may be more useful for the radiologist to consider the types of emphysema relative to their location at the lobular level (i.e., centrilobular, panlobular, and paraseptal). Centrilobular, panlobular, and paraseptal emphysema often can be distinguished morphologically, but as emphysema becomes severe, distinction among the three types becomes more difficult.

Centrilobular emphysema (e.g., proximal acinar emphysema, centriacinar emphysema) affects predominately the respiratory bronchioles in the central portion of the secondary pulmonary lobule (Fig. 10-2). It is usually identified in the upper lung zones, and it is associated with cigarette smoking.

Panlobular (panacinar) emphysema involves all of the components of the acinus and therefore involves the entire lobule (Fig. 10-3). It is classically associated with α_1-protease inhibitor (α_1-antitrypsin) deficiency, although it may be seen without protease deficiency in smokers, in the elderly, and distal to bronchial and bronchiolar obstruction. Thurlbeck described this entity as a "diffuse simplification of the lung structure with progressive loss of tissue until little remains but the supporting framework of vessels, septa, and bronchi."

Paraseptal emphysema (i.e., distal acinar emphysema) is characterized by involvement of the distal part of the secondary lobule (i.e., alveolar ducts and sacs), and it therefore occurs in a subpleural location (Fig. 10-4). It can be seen in the periphery of the lung adjacent to the chest wall and along the interlobular septa and the fissures. Paraseptal emphysema, which can be an isolated phenomenon in young adults, is associated with spontaneous pneumothorax without other evidence of restriction in lung function. However, it can also be seen in older patients with centrilobular emphysema.

Paracicatricial or irregular emphysema refers to abnormal airspace enlargement associated with pulmonary fibrosis. This is most frequently a localized phenomenon.

Box 10-1. Chronic Obstructive Pulmonary Diseases

Emphysema
Chronic bronchitis
Asthma
Cystic fibrosis and other causes of diffuse
  bronchiectasis
Bronchiolitis obliterans

Box 10-2. Emphysema

PATHOLOGY
Centrilobular (central lobule)
Panlobular (entire lobule)
Paraseptal (distal lobule, subpleural)
Paracicatricial (around scars)

CLINICAL FEATURES
Cigarette smoking
Dyspnea
Chronic airflow obstruction (DLco, FEV₁, RV, TLC)

STANDARD RADIOGRAPHY
Overinflation
Low, flat diaphragm
Increased retrosternal clear space
Vascular deficiency shown by areas of irregular lucency
Bullae

DLco, diffusing capacity for carbon monoxide; FEV₁, forced expiratory volume in 1 second; RV, residual volume; TLC, total lung capacity.

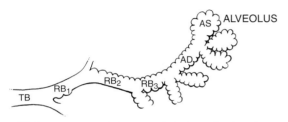

FIGURE 10-1. The acinus is the part of the lung distal to the terminal bronchiole (TB). AD, alveolar duct; AS, alveolar sac; RB, respiratory bronchiole. (From Thurlbeck WM: Chronic Airflow Obstruction in Lung Disease. Philadelphia, WB Saunders, 1976.)

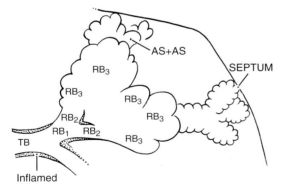

FIGURE 10-2. Centrilobular emphysema. The respiratory bronchioles are selectively and dominantly involved. AD, alveolar duct; AS, alveolar sac; RB, respiratory bronchiole; TB, terminal bronchiole. (From Thurlbeck WM: Chronic Airflow Obstruction in Lung Disease. Philadelphia, WB Saunders, 1976.)

Clinical Features

Emphysema is defined anatomically and pathologically. Emphysema may occur without detectable chronic airway obstruction. Mild degrees of emphysema are frequently found in smokers at autopsy. Widespread and severe emphysema is usually associated with a history of cigarette smoking, chronic airflow obstruction, and dyspnea. The airflow obstruction can be measured with pulmonary function

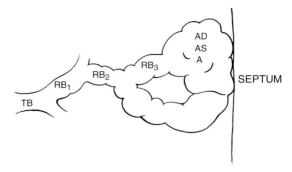

FIGURE 10-3. Panlobular emphysema. The enlargement and destruction of airspaces (A) involve the acinus more or less uniformly. AD, alveolar duct; AS, alveolar sac; RB, respiratory bronchiole; TB, terminal bronchiole. (From Thurlbeck WM: Chronic Airflow Obstruction in Lung Disease. Philadelphia, WB Saunders, 1976.)

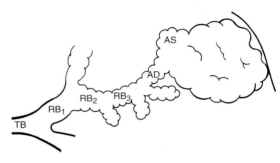

FIGURE 10-4. Paraseptal emphysema. The peripheral part of the acinus (alveolar ducts and sacs) is dominantly and selectively involved. (From Thurlbeck WM: Chronic airflow obstruction in lung disease. Philadelphia, 1976, WB Saunders.)

tests by a diminution of the forced expiratory volume in 1 second (FEV₁) or the ratio of the FEV₁ to the forced vital capacity (FVC). Lung volumes increase in emphysema as a result of hyperinflation with increases in the total lung capacity, functional residual capacity, and residual volume, with a concomitant decrease in vital capacity as the emphysema becomes more severe. The loss of the internal surface area of the lung and of the alveolar capillary bed, two components of emphysema, is reflected in a decrease in the diffusing capacity of carbon monoxide.

Radiographic Features

Standard Radiography
Emphysema can be diagnosed by standard radiography when the disease is severe. If the lungs are mildly affected by emphysema, the chest radiograph is usually normal. Only about one half of cases of moderately severe emphysema are diagnosed radiologically. The standard radiograph is not considered a reliable tool for diagnosing and quantitating emphysema. However, certain radiographic signs are accurate in the diagnosis of emphysema (Fig. 10-5). The first sign is overinflation of the lungs. Hyperinflation is characterized by a low, flat diaphragm, particularly on the lateral view. The diaphragm is considered to be flattened when the highest level of the dome is less than 1.5 cm above a straight line drawn between the costophrenic junction and the vertebral phrenic

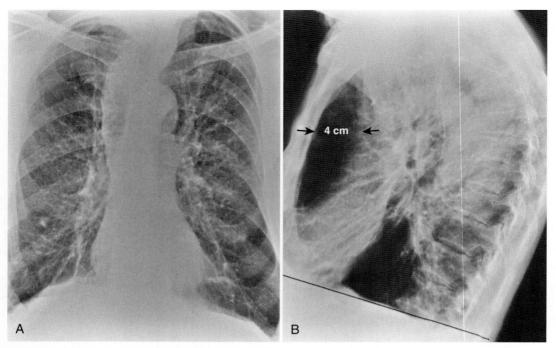

FIGURE 10-5. Emphysema. Standard posteroanterior (**A**) and lateral (**B**) radiographs demonstrate low, flat hemidiaphragms and a retrosternal clear space *(arrows)* that is 4 cm wide. The highest level of the dome of the diaphragm abuts a line drawn between the costophrenic junction and the vertebral phrenic junction. The heart is long and narrow.

junction. The angle formed by the diaphragm and the anterior chest wall is often 90 degrees or greater compared with the acute angle seen with a normal upwardly curved diaphragm. Another criterion of overinflation is a widened retrosternal air space greater than 2.5 cm in diameter. The cardiac silhouette tends to be long and narrow. Similar radiographic findings are seen in patients with severe asthma, but the signs of overexpansion abate with clinical improvement. In emphysema, they persist. The second major sign of emphysema is a rapid tapering and attenuation of pulmonary vessels accompanied by irregular radiolucency of affected areas (Fig. 10-6). Although this is an important radiographic finding, it is subjective and difficult to detect before the disease is severe. Localized lucent areas, particularly if they are surrounded by consolidation, may be apparent in the periphery of the lungs.

Bullae may occur in emphysema (see Fig. 10-6). A bulla is a sharply demarcated area of emphysema that is 1 cm or more in diameter and that has a wall less than 1 mm thick. Evidence of bullae should be sought on standard radiographs to support the diagnosis of emphysema. Bullae reflect only locally severe involvement and do not necessarily mean that the disease is widespread.

High-Resolution Computed Tomography
Computed tomography (CT) is superior to chest radiography in showing the presence, extent, and severity of emphysema. High-resolution CT (HRCT) has elevated sensitivity and has high specificity for emphysema. It is also possible with HRCT to distinguish among the anatomic types of emphysema (Box 10-3).

Centrilobular emphysema is characterized on HRCT by the presence of multiple, small, round areas of abnormally low attenuation that are several millimeters to 1 cm in diameter and distributed throughout the lung, usually with

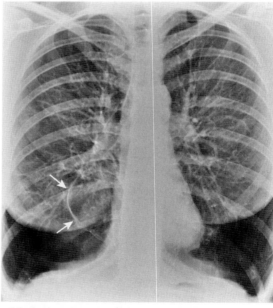

FIGURE 10-6. Emphysema in a patient with α_1-antitrypsin deficiency. This disorder is characterized by panlobular emphysema that is most marked at the bases. Notice the attenuation of pulmonary vessels and increased lucency at the lung bases. There is a bulla in the right lower lobe *(arrows)*.

an upper lobe predominance (Fig. 10-7). The centrilobular location of these lucencies can sometimes be recognized. The lucencies tend to be multiple, small, and "spotty." Classically, the areas of low attenuation of centrilobular emphysema lack visible walls. As the disease becomes more severe, the areas of lung destruction become more confluent, and the centrilobular distribution may no longer

Box 10-3. Emphysema as Seen on High-Resolution Computed Tomography

TYPES
Centrilobular
  Multiple, small areas of low attenuation
  No walls
  Upper lobes
Panlobular
  Fewer and smaller vessels
  Lower lobes
  Low attenuation parenchyma
Paraseptal
  Subpleural and along fissures
  Thin walls
  Single row
Paracicatricial
  Usually focal
  Associated with scars

DIFFERENTIAL DIAGNOSIS
Honeycombing
Pneumatoceles
Cystic lung disease
Bronchiolitis obliterans

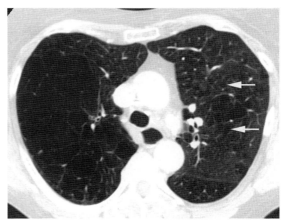

FIGURE 10-8 Severe centrilobular emphysema in a heavy smoker. Confluent areas of lung destruction are indicated by marked attenuation of the pulmonary vasculature in the right lung. The centrilobular distribution is not apparent. In regions of the left lung that are less severely involved, the centrilobular distribution can be recognized *(arrows)*.

be recognizable (Fig. 10-8). The HRCT appearance can then closely simulate panlobular emphysema.

Panlobular emphysema is characterized on HRCT by the presence of fewer and smaller-than-normal pulmonary vessels (Fig. 10-9). It is almost always more severe in the lower lobes but may appear diffuse. When it is advanced, extensive lung destruction can be identified, and the associated paucity of vessels is readily detectable. However, in moderate disease, increased lucency of the lung parenchyma and a limited, slight decrease in the caliber of the pulmonary vessels may be more difficult to recognize.

Mild paraseptal emphysema (Fig. 10-10) is easily detected by HRCT. The appearance is that of multiple areas of subpleural emphysema, often with visible thin walls that correspond to interlobular septa. The emphysema is localized in the subpleural zones and along the interlobar fissures. When larger than 1 cm, areas of paraseptal emphysema are most appropriately called *bullae*. Subpleural bullae are manifestations of paraseptal emphysema, although they may be seen in all types of emphysema. They are often associated with spontaneous pneumothorax in young adults.

Paracicatricial or irregular emphysema (Fig. 10-11) is focal emphysema that is usually found adjacent to parenchymal scars, in diffuse pulmonary fibrosis, and in the pneumoconioses, particularly when progressive, massive fibrosis is present. It is usually recognized on CT when the associated fibrosis is identified.

Clinical Indications

HRCT is infrequently used as a diagnostic tool in emphysema. The diagnosis is usually based on a combination of clinical features, a smoking history, and compatible pulmonary function abnormalities. However, HRCT may be useful in diagnosing patients whose clinical findings suggest another disease process, such as interstitial lung disease or pulmonary vascular disease: shortness of breath and a low diffusing capacity without evidence of airway obstruction on pulmonary function tests. For these patients, HRCT can be valuable in detecting the presence of emphysema and in excluding other abnormalities in the chest.

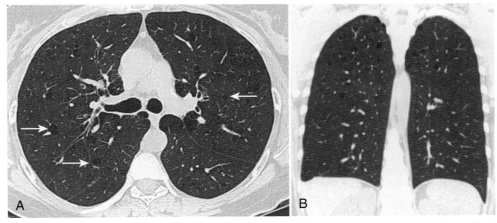

FIGURE 10-7. Centrilobular emphysema. **A**, Axial CT image shows multiple, round areas of low attenuation without visible walls. A centrilobular location can be recognized for several of the focal lucencies *(arrows)*. **B**, Coronal reformation image shows that the emphysema predominates in the upper lobes.

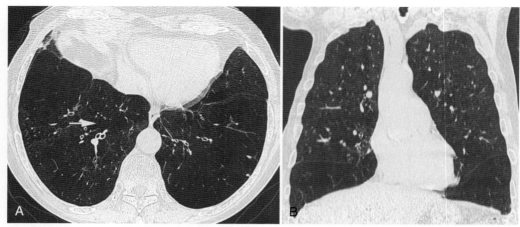

FIGURE 10-9. Panlobular emphysema in a patient with α_1-antitrypsin deficiency and a history of cigarette smoking. **A**, Axial CT image shows a pronounced paucity of vessels in both lower lobes, sometimes referred to as a *simplification of lung architecture*. "Empty" secondary pulmonary lobules nearly devoid of vessels can be identified *(arrow)*. **B**, Coronal reformation image shows the lower lobe predominance of panlobular emphysema and less severe centrilobular emphysema in the upper lobes.

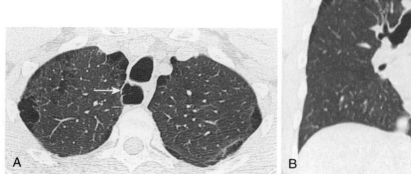

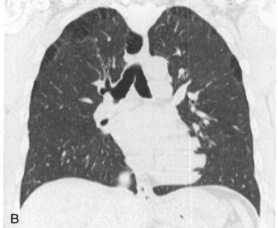

FIGURE 10-10. Paraseptal emphysema. **A**, Axial CT image shows many areas of emphysema localized to the subpleural regions bilaterally and a bulla is noted on the right medially *(arrow)*. **B**, Coronal reformation image shows upper lobe distribution of emphysema.

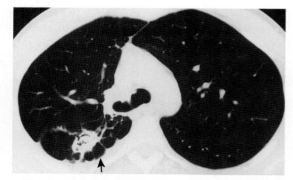

FIGURE 10-11. Paracicatricial emphysema. Focal emphysema *(arrow)* surrounds an old tuberculous cavity with an intracavitary fungus ball.

Several HRCT methods are available to quantitate the degree and severity of emphysema. The most common quantitative method is lung densitometry analysis. This technique provides histograms of lung attenuation values and calculates the area of lung occupied by pixels within a predetermined range of attenuation values. The threshold value for emphysema is usually set between −900 and −950 Hounsfield units. By applying this technique to a volumetric CT data set, the volume of lung tissue that is involved by emphysema can be determined compared with the total lung volume (Fig 10-12). Previous studies have shown that visual and quantitative CT methods for estimating severity of emphysema correlate well with findings on pathologic specimens of emphysematous lungs. However, quantitative methods have been shown to provide more objective and reliable assessment than visual scoring.

Although not routinely employed, postprocessing of CT data using a minimum-intensity projection (minIP) technique, which highlights the lowest-attenuation voxels on CT, has been shown to enhance the detection of mild emphysema (Fig 10-13). This method may help to improve the detection of mild emphysema when conventional HRCT images are equivocal.

Differential Diagnosis
Several entities should be considered in the differential diagnosis of emphysema on HRCT. The first is honeycombing, which occurs in pulmonary fibrosis and is characterized

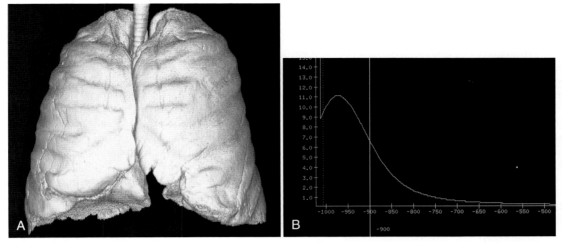

FIGURE 10-12. CT densitometry technique for quantification of emphysema. **A,** Three-dimensional shaded surface display of the lungs represents the model from which attenuation and volume measurements are obtained. **B,** Histogram shows the percentage of lung volume below –900 HU [*y* axis = % volume of lung, *x* axis = lung attenuation in Hounsfield units]. (Images courtesy of Diana Litmanovich, MD, and Shezhang Lin, MD, Beth Israel Deaconess Medical Center, Boston, MA.)

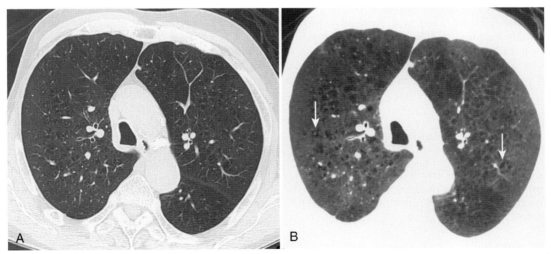

FIGURE 10-13. Minimum intensity projection method for enhanced detection of emphysema. **A,** Axial CT image demonstrates subtle foci of low attenuation that are consistent with centrilobular emphysema. **B,** Minimum intensity projection CT image at same level shows enhanced conspicuity of emphysema *(arrows).*

by areas of subpleural cystic lesions that somewhat mimic the appearance of paraseptal emphysema. However, honeycomb cysts are usually smaller; they occur in several layers along the pleural surface, are localized in the lung bases, and are associated with other findings of fibrosis. Paraseptal emphysema is often associated with bullae, and the areas of emphysema are larger and occur in a single layer. They predominate in the upper lobes without evidence of fibrosis.

The second feature to be considered in the differential diagnosis of emphysema is pneumatoceles. A pneumatocele is a thin-walled, gas-filled space within the lung that usually is associated with acute pneumonia or more chronic infections, such as *Pneumocystis jiroveci* (formerly *P. carinii*) pneumonia. They are usually transient and can be identical to bullae on HRCT. However, the association with current or previous infection should suggest the diagnosis.

The third entity is cystic lung disease. Multiple, thin-walled lung cysts can be seen in a variety of disorders, particularly the infiltrative lung diseases, such as lymphangioleiomyomatosis and Langerhans cell histiocytosis. These cysts usually can be differentiated from centrilobular emphysema because the walls are more distinct and lung cysts appear larger. When the lucency can be clearly identified as within the center of the pulmonary lobule, it is diagnostic of centrilobular emphysema. Cystic bronchiectasis can be readily differentiated from lung cysts and emphysema based on connectivity with the proximal airways and a constant relationship with its accompanying pulmonary artery.

The fourth possibility is bronchiolitis obliterans. Bronchiolitis obliterans, a disease of the small airways, can result in increased lung volume and oligemia that is similar to that of panlobular emphysema. However, it usually has a patchy distribution, which is an important distinguishing feature. Some dilation of the central airways with mild bronchiectasis is more common in patients with bronchiolitis obliterans than in patients with panlobular emphysema.

Other Features

Other features of emphysema are summarized in Box 10-4. Bullous emphysema does not represent a specific pathologic entity but refers to the presence of emphysema associated with large bullae. Bullae can develop in association with any type of emphysema, but they are most common in paraseptal emphysema and centrilobular emphysema. A bulla is a sharply demarcated area of emphysema that is more than 1 cm in diameter and that possesses a well-defined wall less than 1 mm thick. Bullae occasionally can become quite large and may be rather focal; occasionally, they are not associated with diffuse emphysema. Large bullae may result in compromised respiratory function. This syndrome has been referred to as bullous emphysema, vanishing lung syndrome, and primary bullous disease of the lung (Fig. 10-14). This entity may occur in young men and is characterized by large progressive upper lobe bullae. Most are smokers, but the entity may occur in nonsmokers. CT, particularly HRCT, may be helpful in delineating the volume, location, and number of bullae and in determining the degree of compression of the underlying lung and the severity of emphysema in the remainder of the lung parenchyma (see Fig. 10-14). The assessment is often helpful because the bullae can be resected, with marked improvement in pulmonary function. CT is of value in the preoperative assessment of these patients.

HRCT plays an important role in the preoperative evaluation of patients with severe emphysema who are selected for lung volume–reduction surgery (LVRS). This surgery typically involves the bilateral resection of target areas of emphysema to reduce lung volume, restore elastic recoil, and improve ventilation-perfusion matching. In selected patients, this procedure has improved respiratory mechanics, diminished oxygen requirement, reduced dyspnea, increased exercise capacity, improved the quality of life, and extended survival. Based on the results of the National Emphysema Treatment Trial, which randomized patients to LVRS or to maximal medical therapy, patients with upper lobe–predominant emphysema are candidates for this procedure.

Various bronchoscopic techniques have been introduced as an alternative to LVRS. Most of these methods attempt to occlude the conducting airways to regions of severe emphysema by using a variety of techniques, including endobronchial airway sealants, plugs, one-way valves, and radiofrequency ablation. The goal of most of these approaches is to achieve atelectasis of the targeted lung segments, resulting in nonsurgical volume reduction. Similar to LVRS, these methods are designed to treat patients with heterogenous distribution of emphysema rather than diffuse disease. In contrast, *airway bypass* is a new bronchoscopic technique under investigation for treating patients with homogenous distribution of emphysema. This method aims to decrease hyperinflation by placing shunts between the lung parenchyma and central airways, creating new conducting expiratory airways to bypass high-resistance, collapsing airway segments. These methods are undergoing assessment in clinical trials and are not yet routinely performed in clinical practice. It is anticipated that one or more of these bronchoscopic methods will confer benefits similar to those of surgery for selected patients but with less morbidity and mortality.

About 5% of patients evaluated by CT prior to LVRS had incidentally detected lung cancer. When evaluating patients with emphysema, it is important to obtain a volumetric data set to enhance the detection of lung nodules, which may be overlooked with traditional, noncontiguous HRCT techniques. Multidetector-row CT scanners provide the ability to create thin-section (HRCT) and thick-section CT images from the same data set. This is the method of choice for imaging patients with emphysema because it enhances the ability to detect lung nodules and provides volumetric data that can be used for three-dimensional, quantitative CT densitometry of emphysema.

Box 10-4. Other Features of Emphysema

BULLAE
Paraseptal and centrilobular emphysema
   Lesions more than 1 cm in diameter
   Well-defined wall, less than 1 mm thick
Vanishing lung syndrome (i.e., bullous emphysema)
   Young men
   Upper lobe giant bullae
   Preoperative detection with CT

MANAGEMENT
Evaluation with CT
Lung volume–reduction surgery for selected areas of emphysema

---

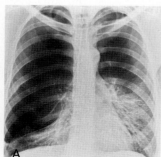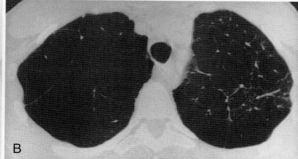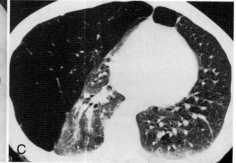

FIGURE 10-14. Vanishing lung syndrome in a 30-year-old man. **A,** The posteroanterior chest radiograph shows bilateral upper lobe bullae with compression of the basilar lung. The minor fissure is depressed. **B,** HRCT through the upper lobes shows bilateral bullae, with the right side more severely affected. **C,** HRCT at the bases demonstrates compression of the middle and lower lobes, which are relatively free of emphysema.

CHRONIC BRONCHITIS

Clinical and Pathologic Features

Chronic bronchitis (Box 10-5), unlike emphysema, is defined in clinical rather than pathologic terms. It is defined as a productive cough occurring on most days for at least 3 consecutive months and for not less than 2 consecutive years. Other causes of chronic productive cough, including bronchiectasis, tuberculosis, and other chronic infections, must be excluded before the diagnosis of chronic bronchitis can be made. Most patients with chronic bronchitis are smokers, and they often have emphysema.

Pathologically, the hallmark of chronic bronchitis is hyperplasia of mucous glands. They have increased volumes, which can be assessed by the ratio of the bronchial gland to the bronchial wall, called the *Reid index*.

Radiographic Features

The radiographic features are nonspecific, and the chest radiograph is most frequently normal. Described features include thickened bronchial walls seen end-on in cross section or in profile (i.e., tram lines) and hyperinflation of the lungs (Fig. 10-15). Bronchial wall thickening is a nonspecific finding that may be seen in patients with interstitial pulmonary edema or other interstitial diseases, asthma, and bronchiectasis, and it is occasionally seen in healthy subjects. On

HRCT, the most prominent finding is usually emphysema, although some bronchial wall thickening and mild dilation can be observed. The diagnosis of chronic bronchitis is based on clinical rather than radiographic findings.

ASTHMA

Clinical Features

Asthma is a chronic illness that causes widespread narrowing of the tracheobronchial tree (Box 10-6). It is characterized by reversible bronchospasm that may be provoked by a variety of stimuli. Acute exacerbations often resolve spontaneously or with therapy. It is a common disease, estimated to affect 3% to 5% of the population of the United States. At least two thirds of patients are atopic, and the pathogenesis of asthma in these individuals is related to a reaction to different types of allergens. Although death is rare, the mortality rates have been increasing for several

---

Box 10-5. Chronic Bronchitis

CLINICAL AND PATHOLOGIC FEATURES
Defined clinically (long-term, productive cough)
Pathology: mucous gland hyperplasia

RADIOGRAPHIC FEATURES
Normal
Thickened bronchial walls
    End-on ring shadows
    Tram lines (in profile)
Overinflation

Box 10-6. Asthma

CLINICAL AND PATHOLOGIC FEATURES
Reversible bronchospasm
Two thirds of cases atopic
Active inflammation of the airways

RADIOGRAPHIC FEATURES
Uncomplicated
    Normal in most patients
    Signs of hyperinflation
    Bronchial wall thickening
    Bronchial wall thickening and mild dilation of
        bronchi on HRCT
Complicated
    Pneumonia
    Lobar or segmental atelectasis
    Mucoid impaction (allergic bronchopulmonary
        aspergillosis)
    Pneumomediastinum
    Pneumothorax

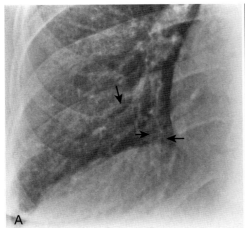 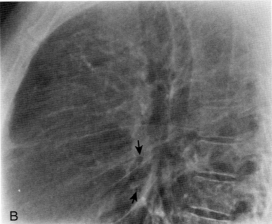

FIGURE 10-15. Chronic bronchitis. **A,** The posteroanterior radiograph demonstrates bronchial wall thickening (i.e., tram tracking) in profile *(arrows)*. Bronchi are seen more peripherally in the lung than is normally the case. **B,** The lateral radiograph shows thickened end-on bronchi peripheral to the hilar areas.

years. Pathologically, the disease is characterized by an active inflammatory process in the airways, even when patients are asymptomatic. Other features include edema of the bronchial mucosa and excessive mucus production.

Radiographic Features

Uncomplicated Asthma

There is some controversy regarding the indications for a chest radiograph in asthma. For adults, a chest radiograph should be obtained when asthma is first suspected and when conventional treatment is ineffective to exclude other causes of wheezing, such as neoplasm, congestive heart failure, bronchiectasis, and foreign bodies. For pediatric patients, chest radiographs are seldom abnormal and should be obtained only when there is no improvement or there is worsening of symptoms despite conventional therapy; when there is fever associated with auscultatory findings that persist after treatment; and when there is a clinical suspicion of a complication such as pneumothorax.

For most patients with asthma, the chest radiograph is normal. Radiographic changes, more common in children than in adults, usually consist of signs of hyperinflation, flattening of the hemidiaphragms (best identified on the lateral radiograph), and increase in the retrosternal airspace. Another radiographic feature of asthma is that of bronchial wall thickening. In children, the walls of secondary bronchi are normally not discernible beyond the mediastinum and hila; when visualized more peripherally in the lung, they are considered abnormal. In adults and children, the thickening of the bronchial walls can best be detected in bronchi seen in cross section, most commonly in the perihilar areas. Bronchi seen in the longitudinal plane often appear as *tram lines*, which are paired parallel lines separated by lucency. Occasionally, the thickening of the bronchial walls may produce a perihilar haze or stringy linear opacities in the perihilar areas. Transient pulmonary hypertension during severe attacks of asthma increases the size of the central pulmonary arteries on standard radiographs. This effect is probably caused by alveolar hypoxia.

On HRCT, mild bronchial dilation has been reported in 15% to 77% of asthmatic patients, and more than 90% may have bronchial wall thickening. Less common HRCT

findings include branching or nodular centrilobular opacities and a mosaic perfusion pattern. Expiratory HRCT may detect areas of regional air trapping (Fig 10-16), even in the absence of inspiratory HRCT abnormalities. The severity of HRCT findings correlates with the severity of asthma as measured by pulmonary function tests. Hyperpolarized gas magnetic resonance imaging (MRI) techniques have been employed to assess regional ventilation in patients with asthma. Studies have shown that asthmatics have more ventilation defects than the general population and that the number of defects increases proportionately with the severity of asthma.

Complicated Asthma

The most frequent complication in asthma is pneumonia. In the pediatric age group, most exacerbations are caused by viral infections, particularly respiratory syncytial virus in infants and parainfluenza and rhinoviruses in older children. The radiographic appearance is similar to viral pneumonias in the nonasthmatic population. Lobar or segmental atelectasis can occur in cases of asthma, but it is unusual. It is seen more commonly in children and most frequently involves the right middle lobe because of retention of mucus in the large airways.

Allergic bronchopulmonary aspergillosis is discussed in more detail in the Chapter 13. The most characteristic finding is the presence of central bronchiectasis, which frequently involves or predominates in the upper lobes. The ectatic bronchi are often filled with mucoid material that contains *Aspergillus* organisms. Radiographic findings of mucoid impaction include a bandlike opacity that appears like a gloved finger; it can also be V-shaped, Y-shaped, or round (Fig. 10-17). Mucous plugs are typically located centrally in the perihilar areas and upper lobes (see Chapter 13).

Pneumomediastinum is a complication of asthma that occurs in approximately 1% to 5% of asthma cases. It has a bimodal distribution that peaks at ages 4 to 6 and 13 to 18 years. The postulated mechanism is a mucous plug or infection that causes a check-valve obstruction that increases intra-alveolar pressure. With deep inspiration or cough, the alveolar wall may rupture, with tracking of interstitial air toward the hilum and eventual extension into the mediastinum along the perivascular sheaths. Patients usually have

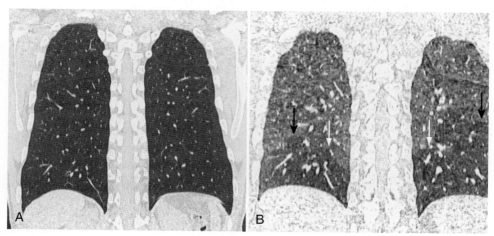

FIGURE 10-16. Air trapping in an asthmatic patient. **A,** Inspiratory coronal reformation image of lungs is normal. **B,** Expiratory coronal reformation image demonstrates many areas of air trapping *(arrows)* that are manifested by areas of abnormal low attenuation in the lungs at expiration.

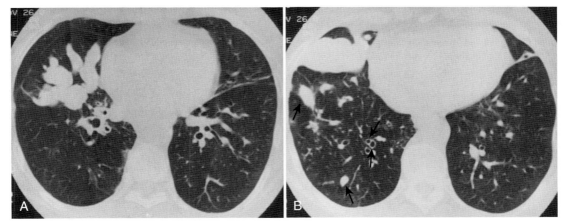

FIGURE 10-17. Mucoid impaction with allergic bronchopulmonary aspergillosis (ABPA) in an asthmatic patient. **A,** Branching, V-shaped, mucus-filled, dilated bronchi are identified in the right lung anteriorly. **B,** The mucous plugs in the lower lobes are oval or round *(arrows)*. Bronchi are slightly dilated with wall thickening *(arrows)*.

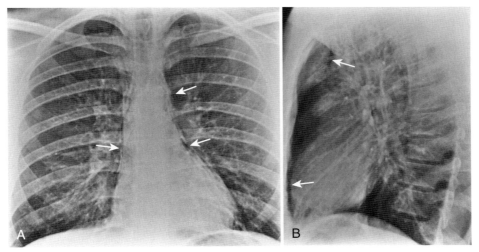

FIGURE 10-18. Pneumomediastinum in 19-year-old man with asthma. **A,** Streaks of air outline the heart, aorta, and superior vena cava *(arrows)*. **B,** On the lateral view, air is seen behind the sternum and outlining the thymus *(arrows)*.

symptoms of chest or neck pain. Radiographic findings are described in Chapter 5. The findings are often subtle (Fig. 10-18). Air encircling major bronchi and hilar vessels and outlining the trachea and the esophagus, the aorta, and the heart is characteristic. It may be observed more easily on the lateral view. Air eventually dissects into the neck, and examination should include a careful search of the soft tissues of the neck for evidence of air, which can often be more easily detected than air in the mediastinum. Occasionally, inferior dissection of air may result in a pneumoperitoneum or an extraperitoneal air collection.

Pneumothorax may occur in conjunction with pneumomediastinum, and although rare, it may be fatal. It can be caused by barotrauma in intubated asthmatic patients. It usually occurs with long-standing disease. A small pneumothorax may be important in patients who are intubated and maintained on intermittent positive-pressure breathing. The chest radiograph is diagnostic, and expiratory films may increase the visibility of a small pneumothorax.

■ **SUGGESTED READINGS**

Altes, T.A., Powers, P.L., Knight-Scott, J., et al., 2001. Hyperpolarized ³He MR lung ventilation imaging in asthmatics: preliminary findings. J. Magn. Reson. Imaging 13, 378–384.

Bankier, A.A., De Maertelaer, V., Keyzer, C., Gevenois, P.A., 1999. Pulmonary emphysema: subjective visual grading versus objective quantification with macroscopic morphometry and thin-section CT densitometry. Radiology 211, 851–858.

Bergin, C.J., Müller, N.L., Nichols, D.M., et al., 1986. The diagnosis of emphysema: a computed tomographic-pathologic correlation. Am. Rev. Respir. Dis. 133, 541–546.

Blair, D.N., Coppage, L., Shaw, C., 1986. Medical imaging in asthma. J. Thorac. Imaging 1, 23–35.

Brenner, M., Hanna, N.M., Mina-Araghi, R., et al., 2004. Innovative approaches to lung volume reduction for emphysema. Chest 126, 238–248.

Burrows, B., 1990. Airways obstructive diseases: pathogenetic mechanisms and natural history of the disorders. Med. Clin. North Am. 74, 547–559.

Cardoso, W.V., Thurlbeck, W.M., 1994. Pathogenesis and terminology of emphysema. Am. J. Respir. Crit. Care Med. 149, 1383.

Carr, D.H., Pride, N.B., 1984. Computed tomography in pre-operative assessment of bullous emphysema. Clin. Radiol. 35, 43–45.

de Lange, E.E., Altes, T.A., Patrie, J.T., et al., 2006. Evaluation of asthma with hyperpolarized helium-3 MRI: correlation with clinical severity and spirometry. Chest 130, 1055–1062.

Fishman, A., Martinez, F., Naunheim, K., et al., 2003. A randomized trial comparing lung-volume-reduction surgery with medical therapy for severe emphysema. N. Engl. J. Med. 348, 2059–2073.

Foster Jr., W.L., Gimenez, E.I., Roubidoux, M.A., et al., 1993. The emphysemas: radiologic-pathologic correlations. Radiographics 13, 311–328.

Foster Jr., W.L., Pratt, P.C., Roggli, V.L., et al., 1986. Centrilobular emphysema: CT-pathologic correlation. Radiology 159, 27–32.

Fraser, R.G., Fraser, R.S., Renner, J.W., et al., 1976. The roentgenologic diagnosis of chronic bronchitis: a reassessment with emphasis on parahilar bronchi seen end-on. Radiology 120, 1–9.

Fraser, R.S., Muller, N.L., Colman, N.C., Pare, R.D., 1999. Fraser and Pare's Diagnosis of Diseases of the Chest, 4th ed. Philadelphia, Elsevier.

Harmanci, E., Kebapci, M., Metintas, M., Ozkan, R., 2002. High-resolution computed tomography findings are correlated with disease severity in asthma. Respiration 69, 420–426.

Heitzman, R.B. (Ed.), 1984. Chronic Obstructive Pulmonary Disease. second ed. Mosby–Year Book, St. Louis, pp. 429–456.

Hodson, M.E., Simon, G., Batten, J.C., 1974. Radiology of uncomplicated asthma. Thorax 29, 296–303.

Kim, J.S., Müller, N.L., 1997. Obstructive lung disease. In: Freundlich, I.M., Bragg, D.G. (Eds.), A Radiologic Approach to Diseases of the Chest. second ed. Williams & Wilkins, Baltimore, pp. 709–722.

Kinsella, M., Müller, N.L., Abboud, R.T., et al., 1990. Quantitation of emphysema by computed tomography using a "density mask" program and correlation with pulmonary function test. Chest 97, 315–321.

Klein, J., Gamsu, G., Webb, W.R., et al., 1992. High-resolution CT diagnosis of emphysema in symptomatic patients with normal chest radiographs and isolated low diffusing capacity. Radiology 182, 817–821.

Lynch, D.A., Newell, J.D., Tschomper, B.A., et al., 1993. Uncomplicated asthma in adults: comparison of CT appearance of the lungs in asthmatic and healthy subjects. Radiology 188, 829–833.

McFadden, E.R., Gilbert, I.A., 1992. Asthma. N. Engl. J. Med. 327, 1928–1937.

Miller, R.R., Müller, N.L., Vedal, S., et al., 1989. Limitations of computed tomography in the assessment of emphysema. Am. Rev. Respir. Dis. 139, 980–983.

Miniati, M., Filippi, E., Falaschi, F., et al., 1995. Radiographic evaluation of emphysema in patients with chronic obstructive pulmonary disease. Am. J. Respir. Crit. Care Med. 151, 1359–1367.

Müller, N.L., Staples, C.A., Miller, R.R., Abboud, R.T., 1988. "Density mask": an objective method to quantitate emphysema using computed tomography. Chest 94, 782–787.

Neeld, D.A., Goodman, L.R., Gurney, J.W., et al., 1990. Computerized tomography in the evaluation of allergic bronchopulmonary aspergillosis. Am. Rev. Respir. Dis. 142, 1200–1206.

Pawels, R., Sonia Buist, A., Calverley, P., et al., 2001. Global strategy for the diagnosis, management and prevention of chronic obstructive pulmonary disease. NHLBI/WHO Global Initiative for Chronic Obstructive Lung Disease (GOLD). Workshop summary. Am. J. Respir. Crit. Care Med. 163, 1256–1276.

Park, K.J., Bergin, C.J., Clausen, J.L., 2001. Quantification of emphysema with three-dimensional CT densitometry: comparison with two-dimensional analysis, visual emphysema scores and pulmonary function test results. Radiology 211, 541–547.

Pratt, P.G., 1987. Role of conventional chest radiography in diagnosis and exclusion of emphysema. Am. J. Med. 82, 998–1006.

Remy-Jardin, M., Remy, J., Gosselin, B., et al., 1996. Sliding thin slab, minimum intensity projection technique in the diagnosis of emphysema: histopathologic-CT correlation. Radiology 200, 665–671.

Snider, G.L., 1992. Emphysema: the first two centuries—and beyond. A historical overview, with suggestions for future research. Part 1. Am. Rev. Respir. Dis. 146, 1334–1344.

Snider, G.L., 1992. Emphysema: the first two centuries—and beyond. A historical overview, with suggestions for future research. Part 2. Am. Rev. Respir. Dis. 146, 1615–1622.

Snider, G.L., Kleinerman, J., Thurlbeck, W.M., Bengali, Z.H., 1985. The definition of emphysema. Report of a National Heart, Lung, and Blood Institute, Division of Lung Diseases Workshop. Am. Rev. Respir. Dis. 132, 182–185.

Spouge, D., Mayo, J.R., Cardoso, W., Müller, N.L., 1993. Panacinar emphysema: CT and pathologic correlation. J. Comput. Assist. Tomogr. 17, 710–713.

Stern, E.J., Webb, W.R., Weinacker, A., Müller, N.L., 1994. Idiopathic giant bullous emphysema (vanishing lung syndrome): imaging findings in nine patients. AJR Am. J. Roentgenol. 162, 279–282.

Thurlbeck, W.M., 1976. Chronic airflow obstruction in lung disease. WB Saunders, Philadelphia, pp. 12–30.

Thurlbeck, W.M., Henderson, J.A., Fraser, R.G., Bates, D.V., 1970. Comparison between clinical, roentgenologic, functional and morphologic criteria in chronic bronchitis, emphysema, asthma, and bronchiectasis. Medicine (Baltimore) 48, 82–145.

Thurlbeck, W.M., Müller, N.L., 1994. Emphysema: definition, imaging, and quantification. AJR Am. J. Roentgenol. 163, 1017–1025.

Thurlbeck, W.M., Simon, G., 1978. Radiographic appearance of the chest in emphysema. AJR Am. J. Roentgenol. 130, 429–440.

Webb, W.R., 1994. High-resolution computed tomography of obstructive lung disease. Radiol. Clin. North Am. 32, 745–755.

Webb, W.R., Müller, N.L., Naidich, D.P., 1996. High Resolution CT of the Lung. second ed. Lippincott-Raven, Philadelphia, pp. 227–265.

CHAPTER 11

Pulmonary Neoplasms

Theresa C. McLoud and Subba R. Digumarthy

The most important neoplasm involving the lung is lung cancer (i.e., bronchogenic carcinoma), the leading cause of cancer mortality in the United States. It accounts for more than 150,000 deaths each year. In addition to lung cancer, there are other primary malignant neoplasms, benign neoplasms, and other tumoral processes that originate in the lung. The lungs are a common site of metastases from extrathoracic malignancies.

▬ BENIGN NEOPLASMS AND OTHER NONNEOPLASTIC TUMORS

A wide variety of benign tumoral lesions can occur in the lung. Some are true neoplasms, and others are of uncertain nature or origin. Benign neoplasms may arise in the tracheobronchial glands, soft tissue, bone, and cartilage, or they may be from mixed mesenchymal origin. Nonneoplastic tumors include hamartomas and inflammatory pseudotumors.

Hamartoma

Characteristics

Hamartomas (Box 11-1) are acquired lesions composed of tissues normally found within the organ, but they demonstrate disorganized growth. Hamartomas, the most common benign tumors of the lung, account for 5% to 8% of solitary pulmonary nodules.

Clinical Features

The peak incidence occurs in the sixth decade of life, with an age range of 30 to 70 years. The lesions are slightly more predominant in women. Most patients are asymptomatic, and the hamartoma is discovered on a routine chest radiograph as a solitary pulmonary nodule. Occasionally, hamartomas can occur endobronchially and may produce obstructive symptoms (see Chapter 13).

Pathologic Features

These tumors contain nests of cartilage surrounded by fibrous tissue and mature fat cells. Other mesenchymal components, such as bone, vessels, and smooth muscle, may be present.

Radiographic Features

Characteristically, hamartomas appear as well-defined, solitary, spherical nodules or masses. They are usually less than 4 cm in diameter, and they have well-defined margins. Calcification is seen in 10% to 15% of cases on standard radiographs, although it is more frequently identified on CT. The calcification has a characteristic morphology that produces a popcorn appearance (Fig. 11-1). Hamartomas typically grow slowly, and in rare cases, they can be multiple.

Thin-collimation CT can be valuable in diagnosing pulmonary hamartomas. The presence of focal deposits of fat (–50 to –150 HU) is most helpful in making this diagnosis (Fig. 11-2). In approximately 25% of cases, calcification can be identified.

Amyloid

Characteristics

Amyloid, a waxy pink material that stains with Congo red, has a typical birefringence with polarization microscopy (Box 11-2). It occurs in two major forms: primary and secondary. Lung involvement in primary amyloidosis is estimated to occur in 30% to 90% of cases. Secondary amyloidosis is usually associated with rheumatoid arthritis, suppurative disease such as osteomyelitis, and malignant neoplasms. Amyloidosis may also be associated with multiple myeloma. In the thorax, amyloid occurs in two locations. The first is the tracheobronchial tree. Airway amyloidosis is discussed in Chapter 12. Amyloidosis may also involve the lung parenchyma in a nodular form or as a diffuse, infiltrative process.

Clinical Features

Nodular disease usually occurs late in life (i.e., seventh decade), and it has an equal sex prevalence. Patients are usually asymptomatic, and the prognosis is excellent. The diffuse, infiltrative form is less common and usually occurs in the sixth decade. Patients with the diffuse form are symptomatic. Diffuse infiltration of amyloid material associated with giant cells and plasma cells involves the vascular walls and interstitial compartments of the lung.

Box 11-1. Hamartomas

CHARACTERISTICS
Acquired lesion
Composed of tissues normally found within the organ
Disorganized growth of tissues
Account for 5% to 8% of solitary pulmonary nodules

CLINICAL FEATURES
Patients 30 to 70 years old
Patients asymptomatic

PATHOLOGIC FEATURES
Nests of cartilage surrounded by fibrous tissue and
  mature fat cells
May contain bone, vessels, and smooth muscle

RADIOLOGIC FEATURES
Solitary, well-defined pulmonary nodule
Calcification in 10% to 15%
Fat and calcium (25%) seen on CT

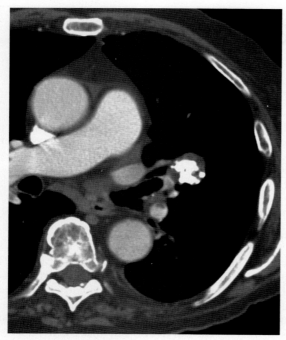

FIGURE 11-1. Hamartoma. A well-defined, 3-cm, spherical nodule in the left perihilar area in lung parenchyma has a classic popcorn pattern of calcification.

Box 11-2. Amyloid

CHARACTERISTICS
Waxy, pink material that stains with Congo red
Forms
  Primary
  Secondary
Thoracic involvement
  Airway
  Parenchyma
    Nodules
    Diffuse infiltration

CLINICAL FEATURES
Nodular type
  Occurs in seventh decade of life
  Asymptomatic
Infiltrative type
  Occurs in sixth decade of life
  Symptomatic

RADIOLOGIC FEATURES
Nodular type
  Solitary or multiple masses
  Calcification in 30% to 50%
  Slow growth
Infiltrative type
  Linear or nodular pattern

The disease is accompanied by symptoms of progressive dyspnea, which leads to eventual death from respiratory insufficiency.

Radiographic Features

The radiologic appearance of the nodular form consists of solitary or multiple nodules and masses (Fig. 11-3). Calcification is common, occurring in 30% to 50% of patients, but cavitation is rare. The lower lobes are more frequently involved, often in a subpleural distribution. These nodules may exhibit slow growth.

In the diffuse, infiltrative form, bilateral and fine linear, nodular, or reticulonodular patterns may be present (Fig. 11-4). There is no specific distribution in the lung parenchyma. Associated nodal calcification may be identified.

Laryngotracheal Papillomatosis

Laryngotracheal papillomatosis is discussed in Chapter12.

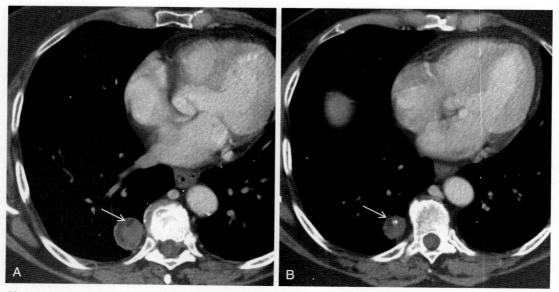

FIGURE 11-2. Hamartoma. **A,** CT shows a well-defined, 3-cm, spherical nodule in the right lower lobe that contains fat *(arrow).* **B,** A small, focal calcification is seen inferiorly in the nodule *(arrow).*

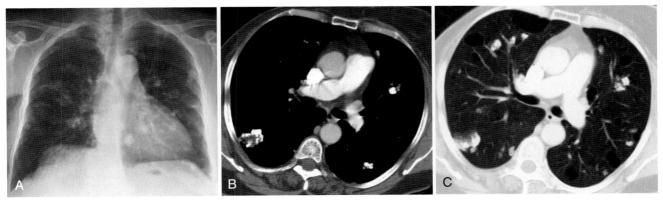

FIGURE 11-3. Amyloidosis, nodular form. **A,** Frontal radiograph shows multiple pulmonary nodules. **B** and **C,** CT using mediastinal and lung windows shows several calcified and noncalcified nodules. Notice the cysts in the lungs.

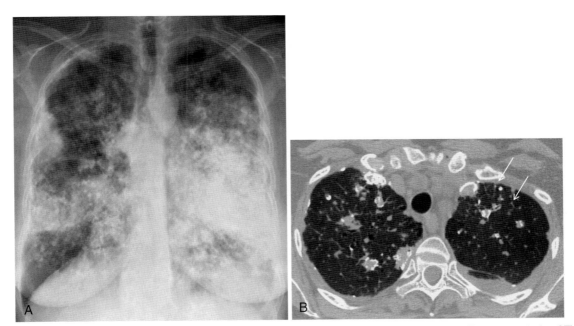

FIGURE 11-4. Amyloidosis, diffuse infiltrative form. **A,** Frontal radiograph shows a diffuse reticulonodular pattern. **B,** High-resolution CT shows linear and nodular opacities with septal thickening *(arrows)*. Note also presence of calcification.

Leiomyoma

Neoplasms of smooth muscle are among the most common primary soft tissue tumors of the lung. A leiomyoma usually manifests as a solitary, well-circumscribed nodule; it is peripheral and occasionally may calcify.

Other Benign Soft Tissue Tumors of the Lung

Lipomas, chondromas, and fibromas may represent a one-dimensional histologic expression of hamartomas. They typically manifest as solitary, peripheral pulmonary nodules. The chondromas are frequently calcified.

Pulmonary Pseudotumor

Characteristics

Pulmonary pseudotumors include a number of histologic entities, such as plasma cell granuloma, inflammatory pseudotumor, histiocytoma, xanthoma, and mast cell granuloma (Box 11-3). The cause of pulmonary pseudotumors

Box 11-3. Pulmonary Pseudotumors

CHARACTERISTICS
Types
 Plasma cell granuloma
 Inflammatory pseudotumor
 Histiocytoma
 Xanthoma
 Mast cell granuloma
Cause
 May be sequela of organized pneumonia

CLINICAL FEATURES
Wide age range
Asymptomatic

RADIOGRAPHIC FEATURES
Solitary, well-defined nodules
Calcification in 20%

is unknown, although they were thought to represent a localized form of organizing pneumonia in patients with subclinical infection. Plasma cell granuloma is discussed more extensively in Chapter 9. Pulmonary pseudotumors occur slightly more frequently in males than in females over a wide age range. Patients are often asymptomatic, and antecedent infection can be documented in less than one fifth of cases.

Pathologic Features

These tumors usually consist of a mixture of spindle cells, plasma cells, lymphocytes, and histiocytes. Plasma cells predominate in the plasma cell granuloma form.

Radiographic Features

Pulmonary pseudotumors manifest as solitary, peripheral pulmonary nodules that are well marginated (Fig. 11-5). Calcification occurs in about one fifth of cases, and airway involvement is uncommon. Rarely, particularly in children, these tumors may invade adjacent structures. Airway involvement is unusual.

■ LUNG CANCER

Bronchogenic carcinoma is the leading cause of cancer mortality in the United States, with more than 160,000 individuals diagnosed each year and more than 140,000 succumbing to the disease. It is the most common cancer in men worldwide, and it has surpassed breast cancer as the leading cause of cancer death in women. Lung cancer is one of the most common lung diseases that radiologists in practice encounter. Computed tomography (CT), positron emission tomography (PET), magnetic resonance imaging (MRI), and standard radiography play important roles in the diagnosis and staging of patients with lung cancer.

Clinical Features

Between 85% and 90% of lung cancer deaths are directly attributable to cigarette smoking. The risk is related to the number of cigarettes smoked, the duration of smoking years, the age at which smoking began, and the depth of

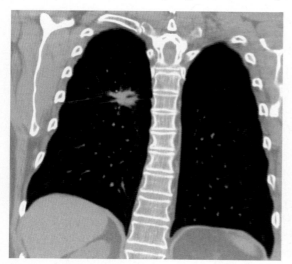

FIGURE 11-5. Inflammatory pseudotumor. Coronal CT shows a spiculated nodule in the right upper lobe and adjacent to the major fissure that mimics malignancy.

inhalation. The risk decreases with cessation of smoking but never completely disappears. Other etiologic factors may play a role in the development of bronchogenic carcinoma, including genetic profiles, occupational exposures, and concomitant disease in the lungs.

Certain occupational agents may increase the risk of lung cancer, and they are listed in Box 11-4. The most important of these is asbestos. A combination of asbestos exposure and cigarette smoking is multiplicative and results in a marked increased risk of lung cancer, particularly if asbestosis is present in the parenchyma of the lungs. Most of the concomitant lung diseases associated with bronchogenic carcinoma reflect the presence of fibrosis in the lungs (Box 11-5), including any cause of end-stage lung disease, such as idiopathic pulmonary fibrosis, and localized fibrosing disease, such as tuberculosis.

Only 10% of patients with lung carcinoma are asymptomatic (Box 11-6). Most often, symptoms are caused by

---

Box 11-4. Occupational and Environmental Agents Associated with Lung Cancer

Asbestos
Arsenic
Chromium
Chloromethyl ether
Mustard gas

Box 11-5. Diseases Associated with Lung Cancer

Asbestosis
Idiopathic pulmonary fibrosis
Scleroderma

Box 11-6. Symptoms of Lung Carcinoma

NO SYMPTOMS
10% of patients

CENTRAL TUMORS
Hemoptysis
Cough
Fever

LOCAL INFILTRATION OF THORACIC STRUCTURES
Pleuritic and chest wall pain
Pancoast syndrome
Superior vena cava obstruction

PARANEOPLASTIC SYNDROMES
Clubbing
Hypertrophic pulmonary osteoarthropathy
Migratory thrombophlebitis
Ectopic hormone production
  Adrenocorticotropic hormone (ACTH)
  Antidiuretic hormone (ADH)
  Parathormone
  Neurologic symptoms

central tumors that result in obstruction of a major bronchus. This leads to cough, wheezing, hemoptysis, and postobstructive pneumonia. Local intrathoracic spread may result in related symptoms, such as pleuritic or chest wall pain, Pancoast syndrome, and symptoms related to obstruction of the superior vena cava. Occasionally, patients may have symptoms that result from distant metastases (i.e., a seizure related to metastases to the brain).

Several paraneoplastic syndromes are associated with lung carcinoma, including clubbing and hypertrophic pulmonary osteoarthropathy, which consists of periosteal new bone formation that usually involves the bones of the lower arms and legs (Fig. 11-6). These lesions are usually associated with pain. Other paraneoplastic syndromes include migratory thrombophlebitis and ectopic hormone production, including Cushing's syndrome from adrenocorticotropic hormone (ACTH) production, hyponatremia associated with inappropriate secretion of antidiuretic hormone (ADH), and hypercalcemia due to excessive parahormone production. There are also a variety of neurologic paraneoplastic syndromes.

Radiologic-Pathologic Correlation

Lung cancer is broadly divided in to small cell lung cancer (SCLC) and non–small cell lung cancer (NSCLC) based on histologic features and differences in treatment approach. SCLC is considered to be a systemic disease and is treated with a combination of chemotherapy and radiotherapy. NSCLC in the early stages can be treated with surgery. NSCLC is broadly further subclassified as adenocarcinoma, squamous cell carcinoma, and large cell carcinoma (Box 11-7).

Adenocarcinoma
Clinical Features
Adenocarcinoma (Box 11-8) has been increasing in incidence; it is now the most common cell type, accounting for approximately 50% of lung cancer cases. It is the most common cell type in women and in nonsmokers. Because these lesions are typically peripheral in the lung, they may not produce symptoms, and they are found incidentally on a routine chest radiograph.

Pathologic Features
Adenocarcinomas typically grow slowly. However, they tend to metastasize early, and they are associated with focal and diffuse pulmonary fibrosis. Pathologically, adenocarcinomas are characterized by the formation of glands or papillary structures, and they can have intracellular or extracellular mucin. They are most frequently peripheral and subpleural in location, and they show evidence of expansile growth. Occasionally, they may occur endobronchially.

Radiographic Features
These neoplasms are typically peripheral in location. They manifest as a solitary nodule or mass, often with lobulated, spiculated, and ill-defined borders (Fig. 11-7).

Bronchioloalveolar Carcinoma
Bronchioloalveolar carcinoma is a subtype of adenocarcinoma. It may manifest with one of three distinct radiologic patterns (Box 11-9). The most common is a solitary nodule. The nodules share the same appearance as adenocarcinoma, although they are often rather hazy and ill defined (Fig. 11-8). They are located peripherally and

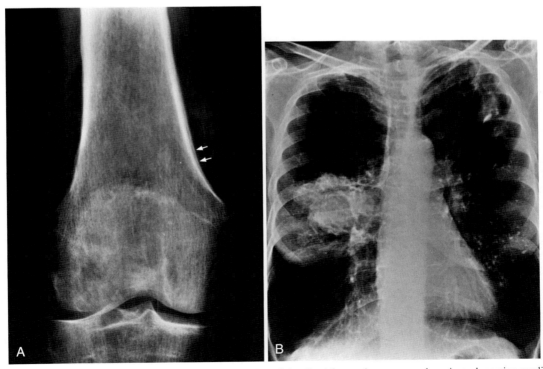

FIGURE 11-6. Hypertrophic pulmonary osteoarthropathy. **A,** Frontal view of the distal femur shows a smooth periosteal reaction medially *(arrows).* **B,** A large mass in the right lung proved to be lung cancer.

Box 11-7. **Histologic Classification of Lung Cancer**

SMALL CELL LUNG CARCINOMA
Combined small cell carcinoma (variant)

NON–SMALL CELL LUNG CARCINOMA
Squamous cell carcinoma
  Papillary
  Clear cell
  Small cell
  Basaloid
Adenocarcinoma
  Acinar
  Papillary
  Bronchioloalveolar carcinoma
    Nonmucinous (Clara or pneumocyte
      type II)
    Mucinous
    Mixed mucinous and nonmucinous or
      intermediate cell type
  Solid adenocarcinoma with mucin
  Adenocarcinoma with mixed subtypes
  Variants
    Well-differentiated fetal adenocarcinoma
    Mucinous ("colloid") adenocarcinoma
    Mucinous cystadenocarcinoma
    Signet ring adenocarcinoma
    Clear cell adenocarcinoma

Large cell carcinoma
  Variants
    Large cell neuroendocrine carcinoma
    Combined large cell neuroendocrine carcinoma
    Basaloid carcinoma
    Lymphoepithelioma-like carcinoma
    Clear cell carcinoma
    Large cell carcinoma with rhabdoid phenotype
Adenosquamous carcinoma

CARCINOMAS WITH PLEOMORPHIC, SARCOMATOID, OR SARCOMATOUS ELEMENTS
Carcinomas with spindle or giant cells
Spindle cell carcinoma
Giant cell carcinoma
Carcinosarcoma
Pulmonary blastoma

CARCINOID TUMOR
Typical carcinoid
Atypical carcinoid

CARCINOMAS OF SALIVARY GLAND TYPE
Mucoepidermoid carcinoma
Adenoid cystic carcinoma

UNCLASSIFIED CARCINOMA

Modified from the 1999 World Health Organization/International Association for the Study of Lung Cancer Histological Classification of Lung and Pleural Tumours.

---

exhibit lipidic growth, and the growth along the alveolar walls probably accounts for the relatively low density on standard radiographs. On CT, they may exhibit ground-glass opacification, particularly around the periphery of the nodule (see Fig. 11-8). The solitary nodule is associated with an excellent prognosis when it is resected at this stage. An air bronchogram may be identified on standard x-ray films and on CT. The second appearance is that of a pneumonia-like consolidation, which occurs in approximately 20% of cases (Fig. 11-9). This consolidation may be associated with nodules in the same lobe or in other lobes of either lung. This appearance reflects the presumed mode of dissemination of this tumor through the tracheobronchial tree. The third appearance is that of multiple nodules scattered throughout both lungs (Fig. 11-10). These nodules are typically 5 to 6 mm in diameter and tend to have very irregular borders. Very few patients present with this pattern of disease.

One of the classic clinical features of bronchioloalveolar carcinoma is the presence of bronchorrhea, which may be extreme and may lead to the expectoration of a large amount of mucus with severe morbidity.

Box 11-8. **Adenocarcinoma**

CLINICAL FEATURES
Most common cell type (50%)
Most often found in women
Occasionally asymptomatic

PATHOLOGIC FEATURES
Slow growing
Metastasize early
Associated with fibrosis
Peripheral, subpleural location
Mucin

RADIOGRAPHIC FEATURES
Peripheral location
Solitary nodule or mass
Spiculated, lobulated, or ill-defined border

Squamous Cell Carcinoma
Clinical Features

Squamous cell carcinoma represents about one third of all lung cancers. It is associated with relatively better prognosis (Box 11-10). Although it grows rapidly, distant metastases occur at a later phase than in adenocarcinoma. There is a strong association with cigarette smoking. Squamous cell carcinoma is the most common cause of Pancoast syndrome, and the cell type is most commonly associated with hypercalcemia due to ectopic parathormone production.

Superior sulcus tumors (i.e., Pancoast tumors) occur at the very apex of the lung in the superior sulcus (Box 11-11). They are typically characterized by pain, Horner's

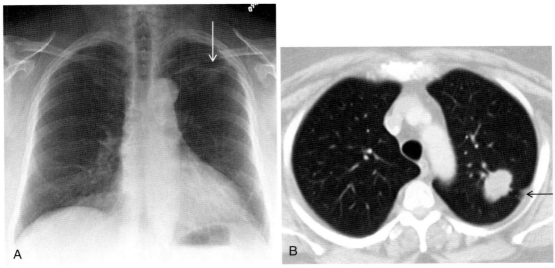

FIGURE 11-7. Adenocarcinoma. **A,** Frontal radiograph shows a small, irregular, spiculated lesion in the left upper lobe. **B,** Thin collimation CT of the lesion better illustrates the irregular margins. The tail *(arrow)* extends to the pleural surface and may represent a fibrous strand or local tumor extension.

Box 11-9. **Bronchioloalveolar Carcinoma**

CLINICAL FEATURES
Subtype of adenocarcinoma
Severe bronchorrhea

RADIOGRAPHIC FEATURES
Solitary nodule
　Most common
　Hazy, ill defined
　Ground-glass appearance on CT
　Air bronchogram
Consolidation
Multiple nodules

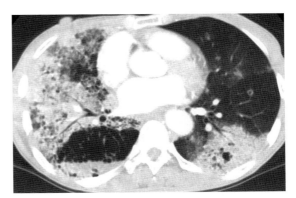

FIGURE 11-9. Bronchioloalveolar carcinoma, pneumonic form. The bilateral, multifocal consolidation results from a tumor that contains air bubbles and air bronchograms.

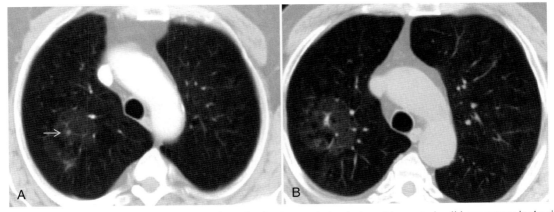

FIGURE 11-8. Bronchioloalveolar carcinoma. **A,** CT shows an irregular, focal, ground-glass lesion with a central, solid component in the right upper lobe *(arrow)*. **B,** CT after 8 months shows an increase in size.

syndrome, destruction of bone, and atrophy of hand muscles. These tumors typically invade the chest wall and extend into the neck. Local extension may result in involvement of the brachial plexus, spread to the spinal canal and vertebral bodies, involvement of the sympathetic ganglion, and anterior extension with invasion of the subclavian artery. If the local tumor is not extensive, it can be treated successfully with a combination of preoperative irradiation and chemotherapy, followed by lobectomy and chest wall resection.

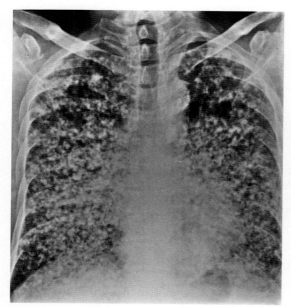

FIGURE 11-10. Bronchioloalveolar carcinoma, diffuse nodular form. In both lungs, multiple nodules of various sizes have fuzzy, irregular borders.

Box 11-10. Squamous Cell Carcinoma

CLINICAL FEATURES
Relatively better prognosis
One third of all lung cancers
Pancoast syndrome
Ectopic parathormone production

PATHOLOGIC FEATURES
Central, endobronchial location
Local metastases to lymph nodes
Central necrosis

RADIOGRAPHIC FEATURES
Two thirds in central location
    Endobronchial lesion best seen on CT
    Atelectasis of lung or lobe
    Postobstructive pneumonitis
One third in peripheral location
    Thick-walled, cavitary mass
    Solitary nodule

Pathologic Features

Squamous cell carcinomas often arise in areas of squamous metaplasia, and there appears to be an orderly progression of alterations in bronchial mucosa in cigarette smokers from squamous metaplasia to invasive carcinoma. Typically, these tumors occur in main, segmental, or subsegmental bronchi, and they grow endobronchially. Eventually, bronchial wall invasion occurs with proximal growth along the bronchial mucosa. Metastases to regional lymph nodes are common, and they may spread by direct extension. Central necrosis is a common feature. Histologic features typical for squamous cell carcinomas include the formation of keratin pearls and intercellular bridges.

Box 11-11. Superior Sulcus Carcinoma

CLINICAL FEATURES
Pain
Horner's syndrome
Bone destruction
Atrophy of hand muscles

PATHOLOGIC FEATURES
Most common: squamous cell
Invasion
    Chest wall
    Base of neck
    Brachial plexus
    Vertebral bodies and spinal canal
    Sympathetic ganglion
    Subclavian artery

RADIOGRAPHIC FEATURES
Apical mass or asymmetric thickening
Bone destruction
On MRI
    Multiplanar imaging
    Local extension

Radiographic Features

The radiologic presentation depends on the location of the carcinoma. The most common finding is that of a central endobronchial obstructing lesion, which produces a hilar or perihilar mass (Fig. 11-11). Involvement of the central bronchus may range from focal thickening to complete occlusion. When the lesion is small, the tumor may not be evident on the standard radiograph, but the bronchial wall abnormalities are well depicted on CT (Fig. 11-12). Atelectasis or obstructive pneumonitis is usually identified distal to the obstructed bronchus. Any patient presenting with atelectasis and signs of infection should be followed radiographically to complete resolution and reexpansion of the involved lobe. Failure of resolution strongly suggests a central lung carcinoma.

Approximately one third of squamous cell carcinomas occur in the lung periphery. The most characteristic appearance is a thick-walled, cavitary mass that usually does not have an air-fluid level. The diameter ranges from 2 to 10 cm (Fig. 11-13). The cavity may be indistinguishable radiographically from a primary lung abscess. A solitary nodule or mass without cavitation can occur in the periphery of the lung parenchyma.

On standard radiographs, a superior sulcus tumor usually appears as an apical mass or an asymmetric pleural thickening with irregularity that occasionally is associated with rib destruction. Apical thickening alone may be a normal finding; usually, its prevalence is related to age. Much more commonly seen in older individuals, it is usually bilateral, but it may be asymmetric. Any irregular apical thickening that is 5 mm or greater than that on the opposite side should be considered with suspicion. However, most patients with superior sulcus tumors do have clinical symptoms of chest pain. MRI is the preferred modality for evaluating superior sulcus tumors because of its ability to visualize structures at the apex of the thorax in multiple planes. Features of superior sulcus tumors on MRI are discussed later in the section on staging (see "Staging of Lung Cancer").

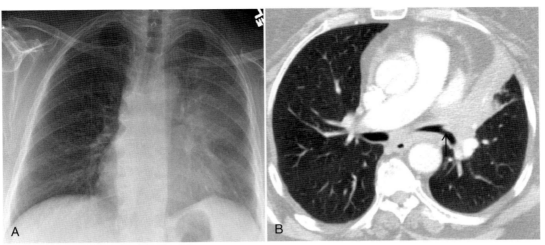

FIGURE 11-11. Squamous cell carcinoma **A,** Frontal radiograph shows a large, left hilar mass with atelectasis of the left upper lobe **B,** CT shows an endobronchial tumor occluding the left upper lobe bronchus *(arrow).*

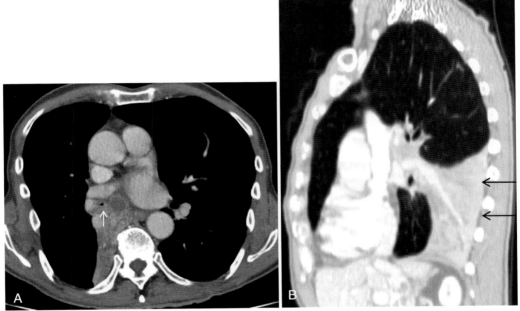

FIGURE 11-12. Squamous cell carcinoma. **A,** A tumor surrounds and narrows the right lower lobe bronchus *(arrow).* Notice the enlarged subcarinal lymph node. **B,** Sagittal reformatted image shows atelectasis of the right lower lobe *(arrows).*

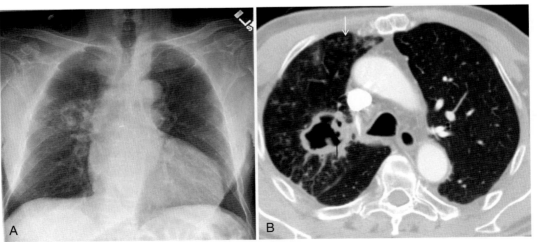

FIGURE 11-13. Cavitary squamous cell carcinoma. **A, The** frontal radiograph shows a thick-walled cavity in the right upper lobe. **B,** CT shows a cavity with a thick, irregular, and nodular wall. Notice the bronchi in the cavity *(black arrow)* and the tree-in-bud opacities in the right lower lobe due to postobstructive pneumonia *(white arrow).*

Small Cell Lung Carcinoma
Clinical Features
SCLC, the most aggressive form of lung cancer, is characterized by rapid growth and early metastases, which are present in two thirds of patients at the time of presentation (Box 11-12). It is associated with the poorest survival, and it has the strongest and most irrefutable association with cigarette smoking. It accounts for approximately 15% to 20% of all lung cancers. SCLC does not respond to surgical treatment, but it is often managed successfully with chemotherapy. However, long-term survival is extremely poor, and when treated, the median survival is 9 to 18 months. SCLC is staged into two groups: limited-stage disease and extensive disease. Limited-stage disease is limited to one hemithorax with regional nodes, including hilar, ipsilateral, and contralateral mediastinal and supraclavicular nodes. Patients with ipsilateral pleural effusion, irrespective of positive cytology for malignancy, are included under limited-stage disease. Extensive disease typically has extrathoracic disease or thoracic disease that cannot be encompassed in same radiation portal as the primary tumor. Tumor-node-metastasis (TNM) staging is not used, because this system historically relied on surgical confirmation for accuracy, and patients with SCLC are seldom candidates for surgery. However, the SCLC subcommittee of the International Association for the Study of Lung Cancer (IASLC) recommends that TNM staging be applied in SCLC and that stratification by TNM stage be incorporated into clinical trials. Patients with limited-stage disease (i.e., confined to the thorax) have a 2-year survival rate of approximately 25%.

SCLC is the most common cause of superior vena cava syndrome. It is also associated with Cushing's syndrome and inappropriate secretion of ADH.

Pathologic Features
SCLC most often occurs as a large, central mass that is associated with stenosis of a bronchial lumen, although an endobronchial lesion is seldom identified. It is characterized by extensive tumor necrosis and hemorrhage.

Radiographic Features
The radiographic features usually consist of a hilar or perihilar mass associated with massive, bilateral mediastinal adenopathy (Fig. 11-14). There may be associated lobar collapse. The primary tumor may not be readily evident because it is obscured by the extensive adenopathy. However, CT may show the primary tumor to better advantage. Occasionally, an SCLC manifests as a peripheral nodule that can be resected, and in these relatively uncommon cases, the prognosis is better (Fig 11-15).

Undifferentiated Large Cell Carcinoma
Clinical Features
Large cell carcinomas account for 2% to 5% of lung cancers, and they have a strong association with cigarette smoking (Box 11-13). They are characterized by rapid growth, early metastases, and a poor prognosis.

Pathologic Features
Typically, these tumors are peripherally located, although they may involve segmental or subsegmental bronchi by bronchial extension. They are characterized by large cells

---

Box 11-12. Small Cell Lung Carcinoma

CLINICAL FEATURES
Most aggressive type
Strongest association with smoking
Poorest survival
Accounts for 15% to 20% of cancers
Treated with chemotherapy
Inappropriate ADH production, ectopic ACTH

PATHOLOGIC FEATURES
Large central mass
Tumor necrosis

RADIOGRAPHIC FEATURES
Hilar or perihilar mass
Massive adenopathy, often bilateral
Lobar collapse
Peripheral nodule (rare)

ACTH, adrenocorticotropic hormone; ADH, antidiuretic hormone.

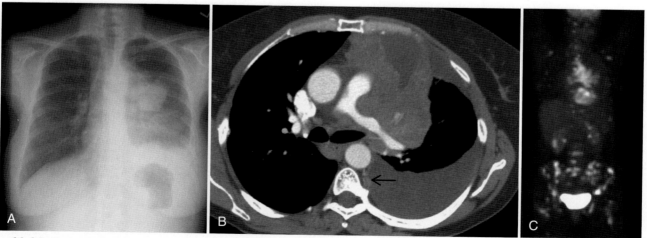

FIGURE 11-14. Extensive small cell carcinoma. **A,** The frontal radiograph shows a left hilar mass, widening of the mediastinum and a left pleural effusion. **B,** On CT, the large left hilar and mediastinal mass encases the left main pulmonary artery. Notice the left pleural effusion and a pleural nodule *(arrow)*. **C,** FDG-PET demonstrates diffuse metastases in the bones, liver, and right kidney. Notice the increased FDG uptake in the chest mass.

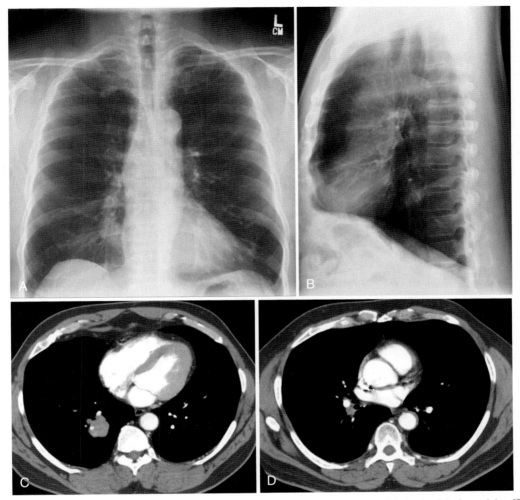

FIGURE 11-15. Limited small cell carcinoma. **A** and **B**, The frontal and lateral radiographs show a nodule in the right lower lobe. **C** and **D**, CT shows lobulated right lower lobe nodule and an enlarged right hilar node.

Box 11-13. Undifferentiated Large Cell Carcinoma

CHARACTERISTICS
Accounts for 2% to 5% of lung cancers
Strong association with cigarette smoking
Rapid growth
Early metastases
Poor prognosis

PATHOLOGIC FEATURES
Peripheral location
Large size (>4 cm in diameter)

RADIOLOGIC FEATURES
Peripheral location
Large size (>4 cm in diameter)

---

with large nuclei, and on gross inspection, they are large and bulky, often greater than 4 cm in diameter with areas of necrosis. Giant cell carcinoma, a subtype of large cell carcinoma, is characterized by the presence of multiple giant cells with bizarre shapes. It has a highly aggressive behavior and a poor prognosis.

Radiographic Features
The lesions are usually peripheral and quite large. More than 70% of the tumors are larger than 4 cm at presentation (Fig. 11-16).

Multidifferentiated Tumors
Adenosquamous carcinoma consists of malignant squamous and glandular components. It is typically peripherally located, and it is associated with early metastases and a poor prognosis.

Staging of Lung Cancer

TNM Classification
Staging of any tumor consists of the determination of the extent of the disease. The rationale for staging is to select patients who will benefit from surgical resection and to identify patients who benefit from adjuvant chemotherapy and radiotherapy. Staging also determines prognosis.

The TNM system is widely used to classify lung tumors. In the TNM classification, *T* indicates the features of the primary tumor, *N* indicates metastasis to regional lymph nodes, and *M* refers to the presence or

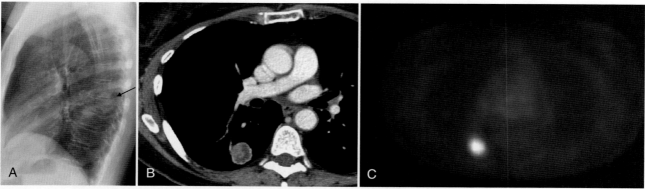

FIGURE 11-16. Large cell (giant cell) carcinoma. **A,** A lateral view shows a mass in the right lower lobe and overlying the spine *(arrow)*. **B,** CT shows a peripherally enhancing mass. **C,** There is increased uptake on the FDG-PET scan.

absence of distant metastasis. In 1997, the staging system was revised based on epidemiologic evidence of improved survival after surgical resection in patients who had previously been classified as having unresectable disease. However, these conclusions were derived from analysis of a relatively small database accumulated since 1975. Since then, there have many innovative changes in clinical staging with the routine use of CT and with PET imaging. The IASLC established a lung cancer staging project to analyze a much larger worldwide database of lung cancer. Following this extensive analysis, the Working Committee proposed changes to existing TNM staging system, which will be incorporated in the seventh TNM classification of malignant tumors (Tables 11-1 and 11-2).

The current system consists of four stages; stage IV includes only patients with evidence of distant metastasis (M1a and M1b). Stages I to III have been redefined and each subdivided into two substages: a and b. Of these six categories, stage IIIB is considered unresectable disease. Tumors with limited invasion of the chest wall and mediastinum are included in the operable category in this classification (IIIA). The designation T4 is used to describe lesions with extensive invasion of the mediastinum or diaphragm, which includes involvement of vital mediastinal structures such as the great vessels, heart, and aerodigestive tract. N1 disease refers to ipsilateral metastases to hilar nodes. The presence of ipsilateral hilar adenopathy alters the overall survival rate, but it does not alter the decision regarding surgery, and these patients are considered to have resectable disease. Patients with N2 disease (metastases to ipsilateral mediastinal nodes) are considered to have potentially resectable disease. However, most patients with N2 disease are usually entered into protocols that may consist of neoadjuvant chemotherapy that is sometimes combined with radiation therapy before surgery. The N3 category refers to contralateral mediastinal and hilar lymph node involvement or supraclavicular lymph node metastasis; it is considered unresectable disease.

Although the TNM system is used for the classification of NSCLC and SCLC, a more useful classification for SCLC includes two categories of disease: limited and extensive.

Computed Tomography, Positron Emission Tomography, and Magnetic Resonance Imaging

Several imaging modalities are used in staging lung cancer. These included standard and conventional tomography, CT, PET, and MRI. In some instances, accurate staging and the determination of appropriate treatment for patients with lung cancer can be made noninvasively with imaging modalities alone, although in most instances, some degree of surgical staging is necessary.

CT and PET have now become the preferred imaging modality for the evaluation of patients with lung carcinoma. These scans can be performed separately and interpreted together, or they can be performed together on the newer combined CT/PET scanners. CT/PET is useful for staging, as a guide to surgical management, and in the determination of appropriate methods for surgical staging. Several studies have established the improved accuracy of combined CT/PET in the staging of lung cancer.

Evaluation of the Primary Tumor: The T Factor

T3 tumors include tumors greater than 7 cm and tumors of any size with direct extension into the chest wall, diaphragm, mediastinal pleura, or pericardium without involvement of vital mediastinal structures. T4 tumors are tumors of any size with invasion of the mediastinum (i.e., heart, great vessels, trachea, and esophagus), vertebral body, or carina or with an associated malignant pleural effusion.

It is not always possible to distinguish T3 from T4 lesions with imaging studies. Lesions with chest wall invasion are classified as T3 lesions and are potentially resectable. Surgical treatment, however, requires en bloc resection of the pulmonary malignancy and the contiguous chest wall, and it is associated with an operative mortality rate in the range of 8% to 15%. In selecting patients as operative candidates, it is sometimes desirable to determine preoperatively if chest wall invasion is present.

The value of CT in the determination of chest wall invasion is somewhat limited. Although CT provides incremental information over standard films, many of the findings described in the literature that are said to be associated with chest wall invasion were later shown to be neither sensitive nor specific. These findings include pleural thickening adjacent to the tumor, encroachment

TABLE 11-1 Proposed Definitions for T, N, and M Descriptors

Stage	Description
Primary Tumor (T)	
TX	Primary tumor cannot be assessed, or tumor proven by the presence of malignant cells in sputum or bronchial washings but not visualized by imaging or bronchoscopy
T0	No evidence of primary tumor
Tis	Carcinoma in situ
T1	Tumor ≤ 3 cm in greatest dimension, surrounded by lung or visceral pleura, without bronchoscopic evidence of invasion more proximal than the lobar bronchus (i.e., not in the main bronchus)*
T1a	Tumor ≤ 2 cm in greatest dimension
T1b	Tumor > 2 cm but ≤ 3 cm in greatest dimension
T2	Tumor > 3 cm but ≤ 7 cm or tumor with any of the following features (T2 tumors with these features are classified T2a if ≤ 5 cm): involves main bronchus, ≥ 2 cm distal to the carina; invades visceral pleura; is associated with atelectasis or obstructive pneumonitis that extends to the hilar region but does not involve the entire lung
T2a	Tumor > 3 cm but ≤ 5 cm in greatest dimension
T2b	Tumor > 5 cm but ≤ 7 cm in greatest dimension
T3	Tumor > 7 cm or one that directly invades any of the following: chest wall (including superior sulcus tumors), diaphragm, phrenic nerve, mediastinal pleura, parietal pericardium; or tumor in the main bronchus ≤ 2 cm distal to the carina* but without involvement of the carina; or associated atelectasis or obstructive pneumonitis of the entire lung or separate tumor nodule(s) in the same lobe
T4	Tumor of any size that invades any of the following: mediastinum, heart, great vessels, trachea, recurrent laryngeal nerve, esophagus, vertebral body, carina; separate tumor nodule(s) in a different ipsilateral lobe
Nodal Involvement (N)	
NX	Regional lymph nodes cannot be assessed
N0	No regional lymph node metastasis
N1	Metastasis in ipsilateral peribronchial and/or ipsilateral hilar lymph nodes and intrapulmonary nodes, including involvement by direct extension
N2	Metastasis in ipsilateral mediastinal and/or subcarinal lymph node(s)
N3	Metastasis in contralateral mediastinal, contralateral hilar, ipsilateral or contralateral scalene, or supraclavicular lymph node(s)
Distant Metastasis (M)	
MX	Distant metastasis cannot be assessed
M0	No distant metastasis
M1	Distant metastasis
M1a	Separate tumor nodule(s) in a contralateral lobe; tumor with pleural nodules or malignant pleural (or pericardial) effusion†
M1b	Distant metastasis

* The uncommon superficial spreading tumor of any size with its invasive component limited to the bronchial wall, which may extend proximally to the main bronchus, is also classified as T1.
† Most pleural (and pericardial) effusions with lung cancer are caused by tumor. In a few patients, however, multiple cytopathologic examinations of pleural (pericardial) fluid are negative for tumor, and the fluid is not bloody and is not an exudate. When these elements and clinical judgment dictate that the effusion is not related to the tumor, the effusion should be excluded as a staging element, and the patient's disease should be classified as T1, T2, T3, or T4.
Modified from Goldstraw P, Crowley J, Chansky K, et al: The IASLC Lung Cancer Staging Project: proposals for revision of the TNM stage groupings in the forthcoming (seventh) edition of the TNM classification of malignant tumors. J Thorac Oncol 2:706-714, 2007.

on or increased density of extrapleural fat, or an obtuse angle between the pulmonary mass and the pleural surface (Fig 11-17). Only a mass in the chest wall and definite rib destruction are helpful indicators of chest wall invasion (Fig. 11-18). MRI has a slight advantage over CT in the evaluation of chest wall invasion. T1- and T2-weighted, spin-echo sequences may show direct tumor extension into the chest wall, and the yield is improved with the use of gadolinium contrast (Fig. 11-19).

Superior sulcus carcinomas are defined as bronchogenic carcinomas occurring at the extreme apex of the lung. The tumors, which may be considered resectable, are usually managed with radiation therapy followed by surgery with chest wall resection if there is no evidence of mediastinal or distant metastases. However, accurate assessment of the local extent of disease is an important aspect in the staging of these lesions. MRI is useful in determining certain parameters of unresectability, such as invasion of the vertebral body and involvement of the subclavian artery and brachial plexus (Fig. 11-20). Sagittal and coronal images are particularly useful in imaging these lesions. T2-weighted images help to differentiate apical tumor from surrounding muscle and to define the extension of the tumor into the base of the neck.

TABLE 11-2 Descriptors, Proposed T and M Categories, and Proposed Stage Groupings

Proposed T/M	N0	N1	N2	N3
T1a	IA	IIA	IIIA	IIIB
T1b	IA	IIA	IIIA	IIIB
T2a	IB	IIA*	IIIA	IIIB
T2b	IIA*	IIB	IIIA	IIIB
T3	IIB*	IIIA*	IIIA	IIIB
T4	IIIA*	IIIA*	IIIB	IIIB
M1a	IV*	IV*	IV*	IV*
M1b	IV	IV	IV	IV

* This is a change from the sixth edition for the particular TNM category.
Modified from Goldstraw P, Crowley J, Chansky K, et al: The IASLC Lung Cancer Staging Project: proposals for revision of the TNM stage groupings in the forthcoming (seventh) edition of the TNM classification of malignant tumors. J Thorac Oncol 2:706-714, 2007.

CT may be useful when extensive mediastinal invasion is present. Contrast-enhanced images may show vascular encasement and involvement of major mediastinal organs (Fig. 11-21). However, CT in some instances is unable to distinguish contiguity of tumor with the mediastinum from actual invasion of the walls of vital mediastinal structures. MRI has been more accurate than CT in delineating the extent of malignant invasion. Findings consistent with invasion include encasement or distortion of major mediastinal organs (Fig. 11-22). However, the decision regarding resectability of lung cancers with suspected mediastinal invasion often is made at the operating table.

Evaluation of Nodal Metastases: The N Factor
CT has become the method of choice for the assessment of mediastinal nodes in bronchogenic carcinoma. Previously, patients with mediastinal nodal metastases from bronchogenic carcinoma were not considered to benefit from surgical therapy. However, several studies have consistently documented improved survival of selected patients after resection of limited mediastinal nodal disease combined with adjuvant radiation therapy. The new cancer staging system considers patients with ipsilateral mediastinal lymph node metastases (N2) as having potentially surgically resectable stage IIIA disease. Included in this group are patients with intracapsular rather than extracapsular involvement and with positive nodes identified at thoracotomy after a negative mediastinoscopy result. Current reports indicate that even patients with gross and bulky ipsilateral nodal metastases (N2) may benefit from surgery if this treatment is combined with neoadjuvant chemotherapy and radiation therapy. However, patients with contralateral mediastinal nodal involvement (N3) are considered to have nonoperable stage IIIB disease.

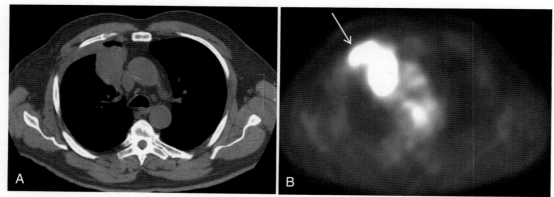

FIGURE 11-17. Lung cancer with indeterminate chest wall invasion. **A,** CT shows broad contact with the pleura without rib destruction or a chest wall mass. **B,** PET scan shows increased FDG uptake in the chest wall muscles *(arrow).*

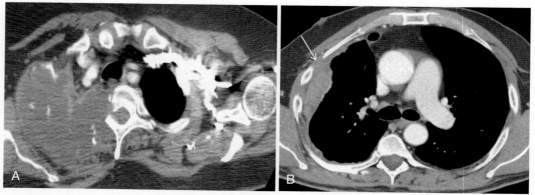

FIGURE 11-18. Lung cancer with definite chest wall invasion. **A,** CT shows rib destruction and extension of the mass into the soft tissues of the chest wall. **B,** In another patient, CT shows thickening of the chest wall muscles *(arrow).*

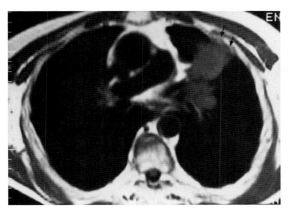

FIGURE 11-19. Chest wall invasion. T1-weighted MRI sequence shows tongues of tumor *(arrows)* extending into the subcostal fat.

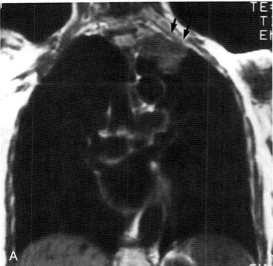

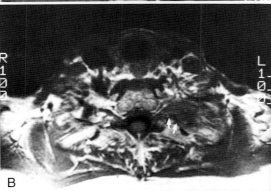

FIGURE 11-20. Superior sulcus (Pancoast) tumor. **A,** Coronal MRI demonstrates a mass impinging on the lowest branch of the brachial plexus *(arrows)*. **B,** Surface-coil, axial, T1-weighted image shows tumor extending into the intervertebral foramen *(arrows)*. Compare with the bright signal intensity of epidural fat on the opposite side. (From Choplin RH, MacMahon H, McLoud TC, et al: ACR professional self-evaluation program. In Siegel BA, Proto AC [eds]: Chest Disease, 5th series. Test and Syllabus. Reston, VA, American College of Radiology, 1996.)

Several studies have addressed the accuracy of CT in the staging of mediastinal nodal metastases in lung cancer. In most studies, nodes larger than 1 cm in the short axis are considered abnormal and should cause suspicion

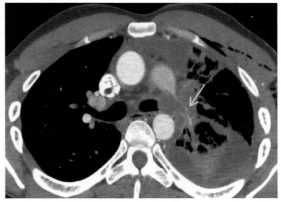

FIGURE 11-21. Mediastinal invasion of the left upper lobe by lung cancer. CT performed with contrast shows encasement and narrowing of left main pulmonary artery *(arrow)*.

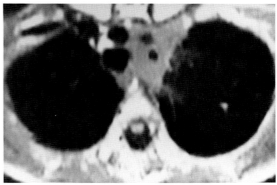

FIGURE 11-22. Mediastinal invasion by lung carcinoma. Axial, T1-weighted MRI shows tumor replacing mediastinal fat and encasing the left common carotid and subclavian arteries.

concerning nodal metastases. Some early investigations reported a high sensitivity—88% to 94%—values that are equivalent to the sensitivity of mediastinoscopy. Opinions based on these data suggested that mediastinoscopy was unnecessary in cases in which the CT scan showed no evidence of enlarged nodes. Subsequent studies that have employed total nodal sampling and the American Thoracic Society (ATS) lymph node classification have shown a lower sensitivity for CT in the detection of nodal metastases—in the range of 60% to 79% with specificities of 60% to 80%. The limitations of CT in the identification of N2 and N3 disease have become well accepted. MRI is constrained by similar limitations, and there appears to be no clear advantage to MRI over CT in identifying lymph node involvement by tumor. PET imaging is superior to CT in determining the nodal involvement, with a sensitivity and specificity of 80% and 90%, respectively (Fig. 11-23).

Despite the limitations of CT in staging mediastinal lymph nodes, it does provide important information concerning the nodal status of patients with lung cancer. Identification and localization of enlarged lymph nodes aids in the selection of the appropriate invasive procedure for surgical staging. Mediastinoscopy, performed in the pretracheal plane, allows an adequate approach to paratracheal and anterior subcarinal lymph nodes. However, nodes in the aortopulmonary window and anterior mediastinal nodes

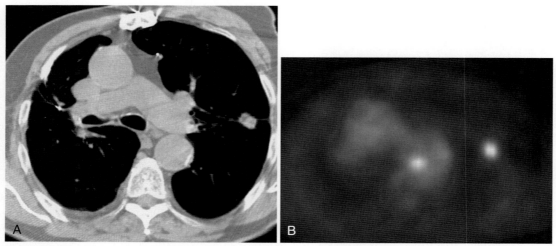

Figure 11-23. FDG-PET used for nodal assessment. **A,** CT shows a lung cancer in the left upper lobe and a subcentimeter lymph node adjacent to the aorta. **B,** PET shows increased FDG uptake in the lung cancer and in the lymph node, indicative of metastasis.

cannot be biopsied with this procedure. These nodes may require a small anterior thoracotomy (i.e., Chamberlain procedure), percutaneous transthoracic needle biopsy, or video-assisted thoracoscopic biopsy. Evidence of extensive lymphadenopathy with secondary signs, such as obstruction of the superior vena cava or destruction of the vertebral bodies, may preclude further need for staging procedures if the histologic characteristics of the primary lesion are known.

A negative CT scan for mediastinal adenopathy is a more controversial issue. We think that these patients still merit mediastinoscopy because of the limitations of CT. However, in some institutions, mediastinoscopy may not be available or preferred. If patients are selected immediately for thoracotomy without precedent mediastinoscopy, careful nodal sampling must be done at the time of surgery. Because of the low specificity of CT, enlarged lymph nodes require biopsy before surgery. Enlarged hyperplastic nodes occur frequently in the setting of central tumors associated with obstructive pneumonitis (Fig. 11-24). Various procedures are available for sampling,

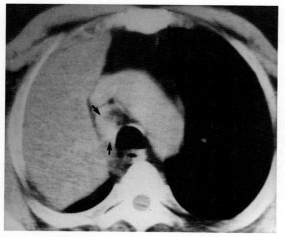

Figure 11-24. Enlarged hyperplastic nodes. CT shows an enlarged, 2-cm, right paratracheal lymph node *(arrows)*. Obstructive pneumonitis involves the right upper lobe. Histologic examination of the node showed only reactive changes, with no evidence of metastatic cancer.

including mediastinoscopy, Wang needle biopsy, and percutaneous needle biopsy.

The issue of CT staging of the mediastinum for T1 lesions is controversial. T1 tumors are defined as lesions 3 cm or smaller in the greatest diameter, surrounded by lung or visceral pleura without evidence of invasion proximal to the lobar bronchus. Several studies have suggested a low prevalence of mediastinal nodal metastatic disease with T1 cancers (5% to 15%). Because of such a low prevalence, it has been suggested that CT may not be necessary for these patients and that the preoperative staging should be limited to plain chest radiographs. However, Seely and others, in a study of 104 patients with T1 lesions, found a higher prevalence of nodal metastases (21%). The sensitivity of CT in this study was 77%. The high prevalence of metastases to the mediastinum suggests the need for further careful preoperative staging in these patients, which includes CT scanning.

Evaluation of Distant Metastases: The M Factor

The probability for metastases increases with advanced stage lung cancer. Most patients routinely undergo CT/PET for staging, and unsuspected distant metastases are detected in up to 25% of patients. There is some controversy regarding evaluation for metastases in patients with stage I NSCLC due to the unlikely finding of distant metastases in this population. The adrenal glands are one of the most common sites for extrathoracic metastases. The prevalence of adrenal metastases at the time of presentation ranges from 5% to 10%. Examination of the adrenal glands and the liver can be done easily at the time of the CT examination of the chest. However, two thirds of adrenal masses identified by CT in patients with lung carcinoma are not malignant. Adrenal adenomas are quite common. The CT characteristics of adrenal adenomas include a diameter less than 3 cm and low attenuation (<10 HU) because of the fat content (Fig. 11-25). However, in lesions not meeting these criteria, dedicated adrenal protocol CT, PET, or chemical shift MRI may be helpful in distinguishing adenomas from metastatic disease. Patients with a higher stage of NSCLC and all patients with SCLC require brain imaging.

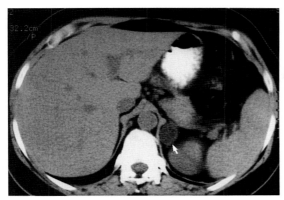

Figure 11-25. Adrenal adenoma. CT of the abdomen shows a well-defined, 2-cm, low-attenuation mass (–5 HU) in the left adrenal *(arrow)*.

▄ OTHER PRIMARY MALIGNANT NEOPLASMS

Other primary malignant neoplasms of the lungs are listed in Box 11-14. Most of these tumors are uncommon. The most frequently encountered is the carcinoid tumor. Carcinoid tumors were previously classified with adenoid cystic carcinomas and mucoid epidermoid carcinomas as types of *bronchial adenoma*, a term no longer in use. These tumors are not adenomas but are instead low-grade malignancies. Adenoid cystic carcinomas and mucoepidermoid carcino-mas, which occur almost exclusively in the trachea and central bronchi, are discussed in Chapters 12 and 13.

Carcinoid Tumors

Carcinoid tumors are among a group of neoplasms that arise from pulmonary neuroendocrine cells (Box 11-15). Neuroendocrine tumors are classified as type 1, typical carcinoid tumor; type 2, atypical carcinoid tumor; and type 3, small cell lung cancer. Carcinoid tumors are low-grade malignant neoplasms that represent between 0.6% and 2.5% of all primary pulmonary neoplasms. They usually have a good prognosis, with a 5-year survival rate of approximately 90%, and there is no association with cigarette smoking.

Clinical Features
Males and females are equally affected over a wide age range. The median age is 50 years. Patients may present with cough and hemoptysis.

Carcinoid tumors may be associated with ectopic hormone production, specifically ACTH. However, these tumors do not produce the clinical carcinoid syndrome unless liver metastases are present.

Pathologic Features
Carcinoid tumors are composed of small cells that are arranged in nests or trabeculae with a vascular stroma. Electron microscopy studies show an ultrastructure consisting of

---

Box 11-14. Other Malignant Neoplasms of the Lung

PULMONARY NEUROENDOCRINE CELL ORIGIN
Carcinoid tumor

TRACHEOBRONCHIAL GLANDS ORIGIN
Adenoid cystic carcinoma
Mucoepidermoid carcinoma

LYMPHORETICULAR NEOPLASMS AND LEUKEMIA
Hodgkin's disease
Non-Hodgkin's lymphoma
Leukemia

NEOPLASMS OF SOFT TISSUE, BONE, AND CARTILAGE
Muscle
　Leiomyosarcoma
Vascular tissue
　Kaposi's sarcoma
　Intravascular bronchioloalveolar tumor
　Angiosarcoma
Bone and cartilage
　Chondrosarcoma
　Osteosarcoma
Adipose tissue
　Liposarcoma
Fibrous tissue
　Malignant fibrous histiocytoma

MISCELLANEOUS TYPES
Pulmonary blastoma
Carcinosarcoma

Box 11-15. Carcinoid Tumors

CHARACTERISTICS
Arise from neuroendocrine cells
Type 1, typical carcinoid
Type 2, atypical carcinoid
Low-grade malignancy in type 1
Good prognosis

CLINICAL FEATURES
Median age at diagnosis: 50 years
Men and women equally affected
Cough, hemoptysis
Cushing's syndrome (rare)

PATHOLOGIC FEATURES
Small cells
Neurosecretory granules
Atypical carcinoids
　Peripheral
　10% of cases
　Metastasis in 40% to 50% of cases

RADIOGRAPHIC FEATURES
Central location
　80% of cases
　　Lobar, segmental, subsegmental bronchi
　　Hilar mass
　　Obstructive pneumonia and atelectasis
Peripheral location
　20% of cases
　Slow growth if typical
　Large and faster growth if atypical
　Calcification seen on CT

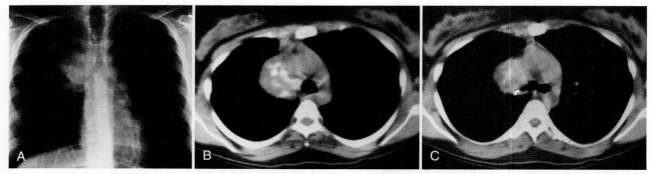

FIGURE 11-26. Central carcinoid tumor. **A,** Frontal radiograph of the chest shows a hilar mass with partial atelectasis of the right upper lobe. **B,** CT scan demonstrates a calcified central mass. **C,** This obstructs the origin of the right upper lobe bronchus *(arrow).*

neurosecretory granules. Typical carcinoid tumors rarely metastasize, but atypical carcinoid tumors metastasize in 40% to 50% of patients. Atypical carcinoids account for 10% of cases, and they tend to be peripheral in location. They may be associated with early metastases, particularly osteoblastic bone metastases.

Radiographic Features

Carcinoid tumors may be centrally or peripherally located. The central tumors account for most cases in 80% of patients and are discussed in more detail in Chapter 13. They originate in the lobar, segmental, or subsegmental bronchi (Fig. 11-26). They may appear as a small endobronchial nodule or a hilar or perihilar mass with associated postobstructive pneumonia and atelectasis. Because they are slow growing, they may produce low-grade infection with bronchiectasis in the involved lobe. Approximately 20% of cases occur as a solitary pulmonary nodule in the periphery of the lung (Fig. 11-27). Typical carcinoids in the periphery grow at a slow rate, and carcinoid tumors should be considered in the differential diagnosis of slow-growing solitary pulmonary nodules. Atypical carcinoids also occur in the periphery and are usually large. In pathologic studies, up to 30% of carcinoid tumors contain calcification or ossification. Although such calcification is usually not identified on standard radiographs, it can be identified on CT scans. Most carcinoid tumors also show vigorous enhancement after contrast administration because of their vascular nature.

Intravascular Bronchoalveolar Tumor

Intravascular bronchoalveolar tumor is an uncommon, multifocal pulmonary neoplasm that arises from endothelial cells, and it is characterized by extensive intravascular spread. The radiographic features consist of multiple, well-defined or ill-defined nodules measuring up to 2 cm in diameter. They show little or no growth on serial studies.

Carcinosarcoma

Carcinosarcomas are rare tumors that occur mainly in middle-aged and elderly men. They carry a poor prognosis because of their aggressive nature and are characterized by local invasion of surrounding structures and widespread metastases. These tumors consist of an epithelial component of squamous cell carcinoma or adenocarcinoma and a mesenchymal component, most commonly of the spindle cell type. These tumors may occur centrally with endobronchial growth or peripherally as a large mass.

The radiographic features correspond to the location and may consist of a large, peripheral, sharply circumscribed mass or a central lesion with atelectasis and obstructive pneumonitis. There is an upper lobe predominance. Disease may extend to the pleura, chest wall, and mediastinum.

Pulmonary Blastoma

Pulmonary blastoma is an uncommon primary lung tumor with a mixture of immature epithelial and mesenchymal components. It morphologically mimics embryonal lung. The tumor occurs predominantly in men in the first and seventh decades of life, and it has a biphasic age distribution. It is associated with a generally poor prognosis. The radiologic findings usually consist of a well-circumscribed, large, peripheral mass (Fig. 11-28) with occasional pleural invasion and metastases.

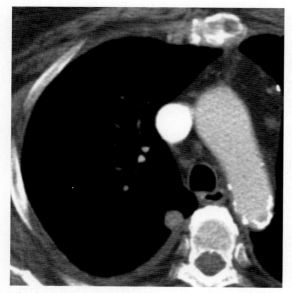

FIGURE 11-27. Carcinoid tumor. CT scan shows a well-defined, enhancing nodule in the right lower lobe.

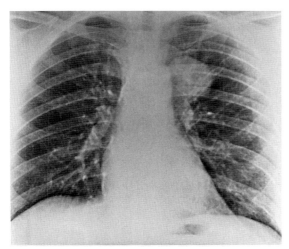

FIGURE 11-28. Pulmonary blastoma. The frontal view demonstrates a well-defined, 3-cm mass in the left upper lobe.

Other Malignant Mesenchymal Tumors

Malignant tumors of mesenchymal origin are rare in the lung. They include neoplasms arising from muscle, vascular tissue, bone and cartilage, and neural and adipose tissue, as well as from fibrohistiocytic tissue. Examples include fibrosarcoma, leiomyosarcoma, and osteogenic sarcoma.

Lymphoma

Lymphomas account for about 4% of malignancies diagnosed every year. Lymphomas are traditionally classified as Hodgkin's or non-Hodgkin's disease (Table 11-3). Hodgkin's and non-Hodgkin's lymphoma frequently involve the thorax. Although the most common sites are the mediastinal and hilar lymph nodes, the chest wall, lung parenchyma, and pleura may also be involved.

Hodgkin's Disease
Pathologic Classification
The pathologic classification for Hodgkin's disease is given in Tables 11-4 and 11-5. The pathologic diagnosis is based on the recognition of typical Reed-Sternberg cells. The nodular sclerosing form is associated with abundant fibrous tissue stroma.

Clinical Features
In Hodgkin's disease, there is a bimodal age peak of presentation (Box 11-16). The disease is most commonly seen in young adults in their late teens and 20s. A second peak

TABLE 11-3 WHO Classification of Lymphoma 2008

Class	Examples
Precursor lymphoid neoplasms	B lymphoblastic leukemia/lymphoma not otherwise specified (NOS) B lymphoblastic leukemia/lymphoma with recurrent genetic abnormalities B lymphoblastic leukemia/lymphoma with t(9;22); BCR-ABL1 B lymphoblastic leukemia/lymphoma with t(v;11q23); MLL rearranged B lymphoblastic leukemia/lymphoma with t(12;21); TEL-AML1 and ETV6-RUNX1 B lymphoblastic leukemia/lymphoma with hyperploidy B lymphoblastic leukemia/lymphoma with hypodiploidy B lymphoblastic leukemia/lymphoma with t(5;14); IL3-IGH B lymphoblastic leukemia/lymphoma with t(1;19); E2A-PBX1 and TCF3-PBX1 T lymphoblastic leukemia/lymphoma
Mature B-cell neoplasms	Chronic lymphocytic leukemia/small lymphocytic lymphoma B-cell prolymphocytic leukemia Splenic marginal zone lymphoma Hairy cell leukemia Lymphoplasmacytic lymphoma/Waldenström macroglobulinemia Heavy chain disease Plasma cell myeloma Solitary plasmacytoma of bone Extraosseous plasmacytoma Extranodal marginal zone B-cell lymphoma of mucosa-associated lymphoid tissue (MALT) type Nodal marginal zone lymphoma Follicular lymphoma Primary cutaneous follicular lymphoma Mantle cell lymphoma Diffuse large B-cell lymphoma, NOS (T-cell/histiocyte-rich type; primary CNS type; primary leg skin type and Epstein-Barr virus–positive (EBV[+]) elderly type) Diffuse large B-cell lymphoma with chronic inflammation Lymphomatoid granulomatosis Primary mediastinal large B-cell lymphoma Intravascular large B-cell lymphoma ALK[+] large B-cell lymphoma Plasmablastic lymphoma Large B-cell lymphoma associated with HHV8[+] Castleman disease Primary effusion lymphoma Burkitt lymphoma B cell lymphoma, unclassifiable, Burkitt-like B cell lymphoma, unclassifiable, Hodgkin's lymphoma-like

(Continued)

TABLE 11-3 WHO Classification of Lymphoma 2008—cont'd

Class	Examples
Mature T-cell and natural killer (NK) cell neoplasms	T-cell prolymphocytic leukemia T-cell large granular lymphocytic leukemia Chronic lymphoproliferative disorder of NK cells Aggressive NK-cell leukemia Systemic T-cell lymphoproliferative disorder of childhood Hydroa vacciniforme-like lymphoma Adult T-cell lymphoma/leukemia Extranodal T-cell/NK-cell lymphoma, nasal type Enteropathy-associated T-cell lymphoma Hepatosplenic T-cell lymphoma Subcutaneous panniculitis-like T-cell lymphoma Mycosis fungoides Sézary syndrome Primary cutaneous CD30+ T-cell lymphoproliferative disorder Primary cutaneous gamma-delta T-cell lymphoma Peripheral T-cell lymphoma, NOS Angioimmunoblastic T-cell lymphoma Anaplastic large cell lymphoma, ALK+ type Anaplastic large cell lymphoma, ALK- type
Hodgkin's lymphoma (Hodgkin's disease)	Nodular lymphocyte-predominant Hodgkin's lymphomas Classic Hodgkin's lymphomas Nodular sclerosis Hodgkin's lymphoma Lymphocyte-rich classic Hodgkin's lymphoma Mixed-cellularity Hodgkin's lymphoma Lymphocyte-depletion Hodgkin's lymphoma
Posttransplantation lymphoproliferative disorders (PTLD)	Plasmacytic hyperplasia Infectious mononucleosis–like PTLD Polymorphic PTLD Monomorphic PTLD (B and T/NK cell types) Classic Hodgkin's disease–type PTLD
Histiocytic and dendritic cell neoplasms	Histiocytic sarcoma Langerhans cell histiocytosis Langerhans cell sarcoma Interdigitating dendritic cell sarcoma Follicular dendritic cell sarcoma Fibroblastic reticular cell tumor Indeterminate dendritic cell sarcoma Disseminated juvenile xanthogranuloma

Modified from Swerdlow SH, Campo, E., Harris, N.L., Jaffe, E.S., Pileri, S., Stein, H., Thiele, J., Vardiman, J., ed. WHO Classification of Tumours of Haematopoietic and Lymphoid Systems. 4th ed. Lyon: IARC; 2008.

TABLE 11-4 Hodgkin's Disease Classification: Rye Modification of the Lukes and Butler System

Subtype	Frequency	Prognosis	Involvement	Comment
Lymphocyte predominance (LP)	Less than 5% (young patients)	Most favorable	Early-stage disease	Nodular and diffuse forms
Nodular sclerosis (NS)	Most common (<75%)	Less favorable than LP	Mediastinum usually involved	Large fibrotic component, few cells (infrequent RS cells)
Mixed cellularity	Second most frequent (older patients)	Less favorable than NS	More advanced stage at presentation than NS	Frequent RS cells
Lymphocytic depletion	Uncommon (<5%)	Worst prognosis	Advanced disease, older patients, systemic symptoms	Frequent RS cells

RS cells, Reed-Sternberg cells.
From Bragg DG: Hodgkin disease and non-Hodgkin lymphoma of the thorax. In Freundlich IM, Bragg DG (eds): A Radiologic Approach to Diseases of the Chest. Baltimore, Williams & Wilkins, 1997.

occurs later, in elderly men. The original Ann Arbor Staging System has been expanded to the currently accepted system, called the Cotswold's Staging Classification (see Table 11-5). Patients may seek treatment because of an enlarging, painless mass in the neck or groin. The presence of systemic symptoms such as fever, weight loss, or pruritus is classified by the modifier *B* in the staging system, and these symptoms are often associated with extensive intra-abdominal disease. Most Hodgkin's patients have localized stage I or stage II disease at presentation. Long-term survival approximating 75% can be achieved with radiotherapy alone. The addition of chemotherapy reduces the rate of recurrence.

TABLE 11-5 Cotswold's Staging Classification of Hodgkin's Disease

Classification	Description
Stage I	Involvement of a single lymph node region or lymphoid structure
Stage II	Involvement of two or more lymph node regions on the same side of the diaphragm (the mediastinum is considered a single site, whereas hilar lymph nodes are considered bilaterally); the number of anatomic sites should be indicated by a subscript (e.g., II$_3$).
Stage III	Involvement of lymph node regions or structures on both sides of the diaphragm
III$_1$	With or without involvement of splenic, hilar, celiac, or portal nodes
III$_2$	With involvement of para-aortic, iliac, and mesenteric nodes
Stage IV	Involvement of one or more extranodal sites in addition to a site for which the designation E has been applied
Designations Applicable to Any Disease Stage	
A	No symptoms
B	Fever (>38 °C), drenching night sweats, unexplained loss of > 10% of body weight within the preceding 6 months
X	Bulky disease (i.e., widening of the mediastinum by more than one third or the presence of a nodal mass with a maximum dimension > 10 cm)
E	Involvement of a single extranodal site that is contiguous or proximal to the known nodal site
CS	Clinical stage
PS	Pathologic stage (determined by laparotomy)

Modified from Urba WJ, Longo DL: Hodgkin disease in adults. Invest Radiol 28:737-752, 1993.

Box 11-16. Hodgkin's Disease

CLINICAL FEATURES
Bimodal age distribution
  Young adults
  Elderly men
Mass in neck or groin
Systemic symptoms: B classification
Survival rate of 75% for stage I and II with
  radiotherapy alone

RADIOGRAPHIC FEATURES
CT used for staging
Thoracic involvement in 85% of cases
Hilar and mediastinal adenopathy
Multiple lymph node groups
Anterior mediastinum most common
Lung involvement
  Primary Hodgkin's rare in lung
  Nodules, masses
    Perihilar
    Cavitation
    Air bronchograms
Follow-up
  Recurrence adjacent to radiation portal
  Pericardial nodes
On T2-weighted MRI
  Differentiation of residual from recurrent tumor
    from fibrosis
    Fibrosis: low signal intensity
    Tumor: bright signal intensity
Eggshell calcification in nodes
PET is superior for staging and assessment of
  response to therapy

Combination treatment with chemotherapy and irradiation is usually reserved for the patient who has massive mediastinal involvement and advanced-stage disease.

Radiographic Features
CT is usually required for the staging evaluation of patients with Hodgkin's disease. Approximately 85% of cases have intrathoracic involvement. The most common location in the thorax is the mediastinal and hilar nodes (Fig. 11-29). Hodgkin's disease usually produces involvement of multiple lymph node groups, but the anterior mediastinal compartment is the most frequently involved. Mediastinal involvement is seen most commonly in the nodular sclerosing type. Bulky and massive mediastinal adenopathy may produce superior vena caval syndrome or life-threatening compression of the trachea. Between 80% and 85% of patients with Hodgkin's disease have mediastinal lymph node involvement. CT is necessary to define the extent of Hodgkin's disease within the thorax. MRI has no advantage over CT in staging, but it may be useful for patient follow-up.

The lung parenchyma may be involved with Hodgkin's disease. Primary pulmonary Hodgkin's disease is extremely uncommon. More frequently, the lung is involved when the disease is widespread, and there is abundant bulky mediastinal and hilar adenopathy (Fig. 11-30). The pattern is usually that of ill-defined masses and nodules that spread out from the hila in an axial distribution along the bronchovascular bundles (Fig. 11-31). The appearance may simulate that seen in sarcoidosis or Kaposi's sarcoma, particularly on high-resolution CT (HRCT). Cavitation may occur, and air bronchograms are a conspicuous feature of parenchymal Hodgkin's disease.

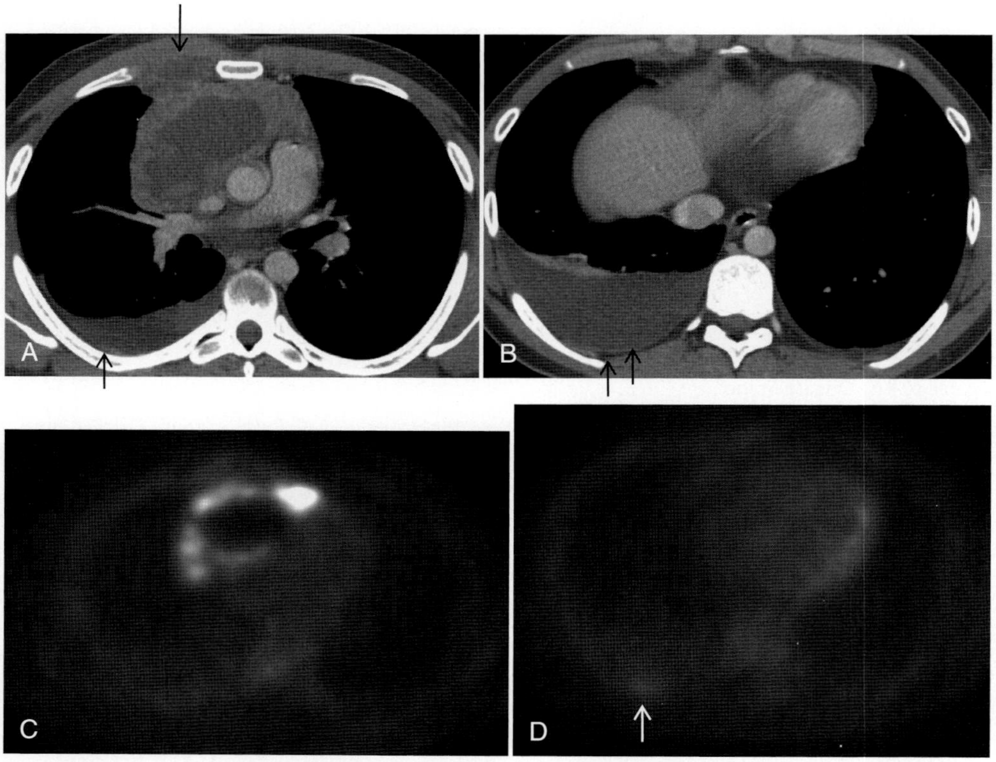

FIGURE 11-29. Hodgkin's lymphoma chest wall and pleural involvement. **A** and **B**, CT shows a necrotic, large mass in the anterior mediastinum with invasion of the right anterior chest wall *(arrow)* and pleura *(arrow)*. Notice the pleural effusion, thickening, and nodularity *(arrows)*. **C** and **D**, PET scan shows increased FDG uptake in the centrally necrotic mediastinal mass and in the pleura.

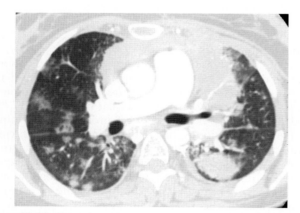

FIGURE 11-30. Parenchymal involvement by Hodgkin's disease. Notice the bilateral lung nodules and the large, anterior mediastinal and left hilar mass.

If Hodgkin's disease recurs, it is often within the thorax. Recurrence is typically seen close to the radiation treatment port margins in the adjacent untreated areas of the lung. The recurrences may appear as nodular or mass lesions in the lung or as perihilar, ill-defined opacities. Involvement of pericardial or diaphragmatic nodes that are not included in the mantle radiation treatment portal may be seen; they appear initially as a mass in the cardiophrenic angle (Fig. 11-32). Patients should be evaluated with CT, which can demonstrate the nature of the cardiophrenic angle mass.

In some patients with Hodgkin's disease, particularly those with a nodular sclerosing histologic subtype, a mediastinal mass may persist after treatment. It is difficult using CT alone to differentiate residual masses due to fibrosis from active or recurrent disease. MRI may make the

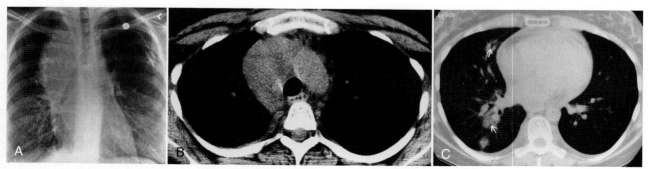

FIGURE 11-31. Hodgkin's disease. **A**, The frontal view demonstrates a large mediastinal mass. **B**, CT shows a large, anterior and paratracheal mass caused by enlarged lymph nodes. **C**, Lung windows demonstrate pulmonary parenchymal involvement. Ill-defined nodules are distributed axially along the bronchovascular bundles. Air bronchograms can be identified in the nodules *(arrows)*.

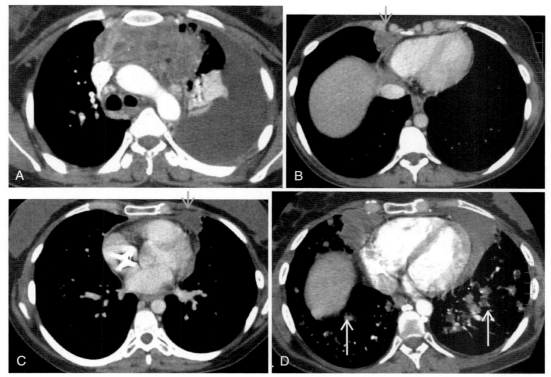

Figure 11-32. Recurrent Hodgkin's disease involving pericardial nodes. **A,** On the initial pretreatment CT scan, there is an anterior mediastinal mass and left pleural effusion. After treatment, the adenopathy and effusion resolved. **B** and **C,** Follow-up CT scans 12 months later show enlarged pericardial lymph nodes *(arrows)* caused by recurrent tumor. **D,** CT scan after 16 months exhibits further enlargement of nodes. Notice the multiple lung nodules *(arrows)*.

differentiation more accurately. On T2-weighted images, a node replaced by fibrosis has low signal intensity compared with a node that contains active tumor; the latter has bright signal intensity. Gadolinium may demonstrate enhancing lymph nodes if active tumor is present.

Calcification may occur in mediastinal lymph node sites after treatment with irradiation or chemotherapy (Fig. 11-33). Typically, these nodes are calcified in an eggshell distribution.

PET and PET/CT imaging is superior to CT alone and provides information that can change treatment. PET imaging can detect more foci of disease and potentially upstage disease; examples include detection of increased ^{18}F-fluorodeoxy-D-glucose (FDG) uptake in small-sized nodes, detection of disease in extranodal sites such as bone marrow, cortical bone, liver, and spleen. Pretreatment and posttreatment PET imaging is used to assess response to treatment and to detect early recurrence, and it can differentiate posttreatment fibrosis from residual or recurrent tumor (Fig. 11-34).

Non-Hodgkin's Lymphoma
Pathologic Classification

The histologic classification of non-Hodgkin's lymphoma has undergone many changes over the past 4 decades (Box 11-17). The earlier Rappaport and Working Formulation for Clinical Usage classifications were largely replaced by Revised European-American

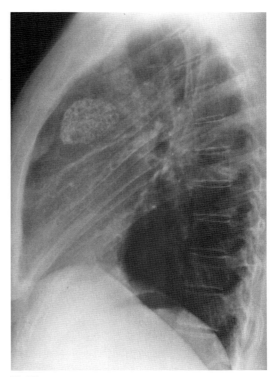

Figure 11-33. Hodgkin's disease with calcified nodules after treatment. The lateral view shows a large area of calcification in the area of a treated anterior mediastinal mass.

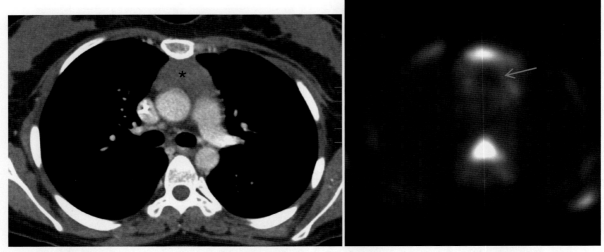

FIGURE 11-34. Posttreatment fibrosis. A, CT reveals a residual mass in the anterior mediastinum after treatment *(asterisk).* B. On FDG-PET, there is no uptake in the mass, suggesting no residual tumor *(arrow).* Notice the increased uptake in the bone marrow due to use of granulocyte colony-stimulating factor during chemotherapy.

Box 11-17. Non-Hodgkin's Lymphoma

CLINICAL FEATURES

Low grade
 Older patients
 Generalized lymphadenopathy
 Asymptomatic
Intermediate and high grade
 Younger patients
 Treatment with aggressive chemotherapy
Immunocompromised hosts
 AIDS patients
 Transplant recipients
Intrathoracic involvement in less than 50%

RADIOGRAPHIC FEATURES

Similar to Hodgkin's disease
Chest wall involvement
 More common
 Direct extension or primary site
Pleural involvement
 Direct extension
 Localized plaquelike seeding
 Pleural effusions (lymphatic obstruction)
Lung parenchyma involvement
 Primary extranodal site
 Mass with air bronchogram
 Multiple masses or consolidation
Follow-up
 Localized recurrence
 Recurs within 2 years

RADIATION PNEUMONITIS AND FIBROSIS

Occurs 6 to 8 weeks after treatment
Conforms to portal
Consolidation with air bronchograms
Fibrosis
 Loss of volume
 Linear opacities
 Traction bronchiectasis

Lymphoma Classification (REAL) based on histology, immunophenotyping, and cytogenetics. It was further modified by the World Health Organization (WHO) in 2008 (see Table 11-3).

Clinical Features

Older patients with fairly generalized lymphadenopathy and low-grade non-Hodgkin's lymphoma may not complain of any symptoms. They may not undergo treatment unless they develop symptoms of a more aggressive high-grade lymphoma. However, younger patients with intermediate- or high-grade non-Hodgkin's lymphoma are treated with aggressive chemotherapy.

Non-Hodgkin's lymphomas may occur in immuno-compromised patients, particularly transplant recipients and patients with acquired immunodeficiency syndrome (AIDS). These lymphomas tend to be aggressive and typically involve the central nervous system. Posttransplantation lymphoproliferative disorder is associated with Ebstein-Barr virus infection.

Most low-grade lymphomas are defined as stage III or stage IV on initial presentation, whereas the intermediate- and high-grade lymphomas usually are localized stage I tumors. Intrathoracic disease is found with non-Hodgkin's lymphoma at presentation in less than 50% of adult cases.

Radiographic Features

Less than 50% of non-Hodgkin's lymphoma patients have thoracic involvement on initial presentation. The appearance usually is similar to that of Hodgkin's disease.

Chest wall involvement is much more common in non-Hodgkin's lymphoma as a result of direct extension of disease from the mediastinum (Fig. 11-35). Occasionally, the chest wall is involved as a primary site of extranodal lymphoma. It usually appears as a destructive lesion of a rib with a surrounding soft tissue mass.

The pleura may be involved by a direct extension from a contiguous chest wall mass or parenchymal lung disease. Occasionally, localized plaquelike opacities may be observed on the pleural surface, and these represent direct

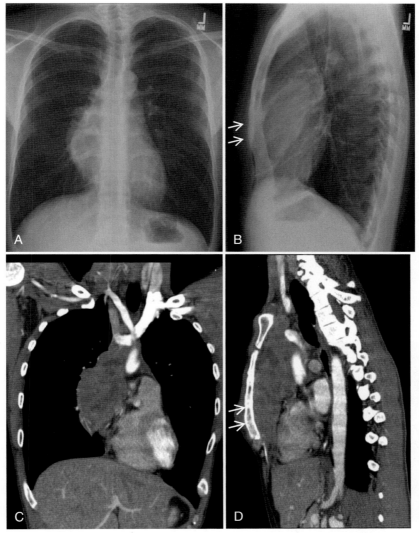

FIGURE 11-35. Diffuse large B-cell lymphoma (i.e., non-Hodgkin's lymphoma). **A** and **B**, The frontal and lateral radiographs demonstrate a large, anterior mediastinal mass. Notice the extension into the anterior chest wall *(arrows)* of the mediastinal mass. **C** and **D**, Coronal and sagittal reconstruction CT scans demonstrate the anterior mediastinal mass and the soft tissue extension into the anterior chest wall *(arrows)*. Notice the posterior displacement of mediastinal vessels and the heart in the sagittal reconstruction.

seeding of the pleura from known lymphoma (Fig. 11-36). Pleural involvement is best evaluated with CT. Most patients with lymphoma who have pleural effusions have no direct involvement of the pleura by the lymphomatous process. The effusion most likely is caused by lymphatic obstruction from enlarged hilar and mediastinal nodes.

The lung parenchyma is a common site of involvement by extranodal non-Hodgkin's lymphoma. This condition is sometimes referred to as *primary pulmonary lymphoma*. It usually appears as a mass lesion, frequently with an air bronchogram (Fig. 11-37). Multiple masses or areas simulating airspace consolidation can be seen. Other patterns are identical to those described earlier for Hodgkin's disease.

Posttransplantation lymphoproliferative disorder manifests as multiple lung nodules. There may be lymphadenopathy and pleural effusions (Fig. 11-38).

FDG-PET or PET/CT is superior to CT alone and has significant impact in treatment of patients. In one study, PET imaging resulted in a change of staging for 44%

patients and a change of treatment for 66% (Fig. 11-39). PET imaging can also reliably differentiate viable tumor from fibrosis in the posttreatment setting (Fig. 11-40).

Follow-up
As in Hodgkin's disease, most patients with high-grade non-Hodgkin's lymphomas usually experience recurrences within 2 years after completion of treatment. With the intermediate- and high-grade tumors of non-Hodgkin's lymphoma, tumor tends to recur at the initial localized disease site.

Radiation pneumonitis and fibrosis can be observed in most patients who have received mantle radiation therapy for Hodgkin's or non-Hodgkin's lymphoma. Classically, radiation pneumonitis can be identified within 6 to 8 weeks after the completion of treatment on standard radiographs, but it often becomes demonstrable on CT at an earlier time (Fig. 11-41). The consolidative process is limited by the radiation portals, and it usually has a sharp lateral margin.

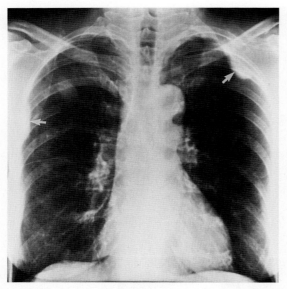

FIGURE 11-36. Pleural involvement by non-Hodgkin's lymphoma. Plaquelike and more rounded areas of pleural involvement can be seen bilaterally *(arrows)*.

Air bronchograms are common. Fibrosis usually develops within 6 to 12 months after radiation therapy. Volume loss can be identified in the paramediastinal lung; this involves the upper lobes with dilated air bronchograms as a result of traction bronchiectasis.

METASTATIC DISEASE

Pulmonary metastases represent the most common lung neoplasms. The most common sites of primary malignancies include breast, colon, pancreas, stomach, skin (i.e., melanoma), head and neck, and kidney. The probability of lung metastasis increases with advanced tumor stage.

Mechanisms of Spread

Tumors may spread by direct extension or seeding of body cavities such as the pleura. However, true metastatic disease to the lungs occurs by one of three mechanisms and through one or more of three pathways: hematogenous, lymphatic, and endobronchial. Hematogenous spread is the most common, and it reaches the lungs through the

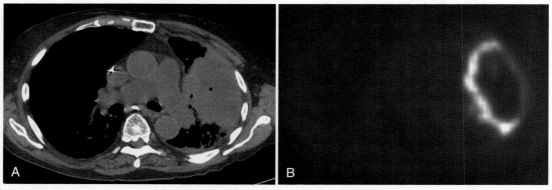

FIGURE 11-37. Primary pulmonary lymphoma by non-Hodgkin's disease. **A,** CT shows large mass in the left lung with a small, central cavity. **B,** The FDG-PET scan shows only peripheral FDG uptake due to central necrosis.

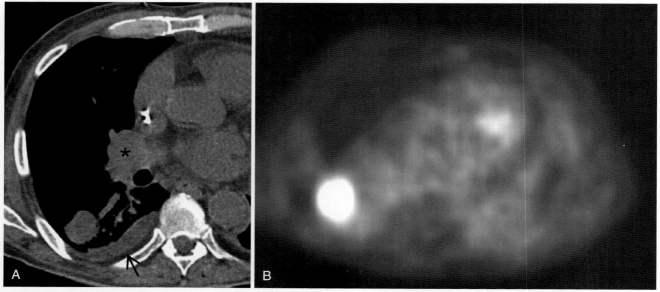

FIGURE 11-38. Lymphoproliferative disorder after bone marrow transplantation. **A,** Peripheral nodule in the right lower lobe. Notice the enlarged right hilar node *(asterisk)* and small pleural effusion *(arrow)*. **B,** The PET scan shows increased FDG uptake in the lung nodule.

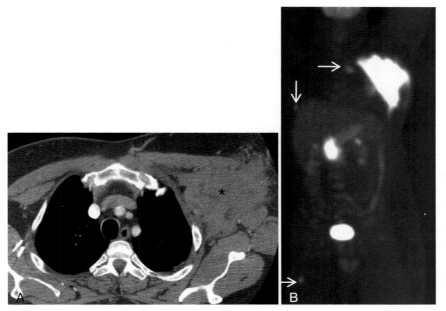

FIGURE 11-39. Burkitt's lymphoma. **A**, CT shows a large mass in the left axilla *(asterisk)*. **B**, PET shows increased FDG uptake in the axillary mass and in unsuspected lesions in the ribs and right femur *(arrows)*. No bony abnormality was seen on CT.

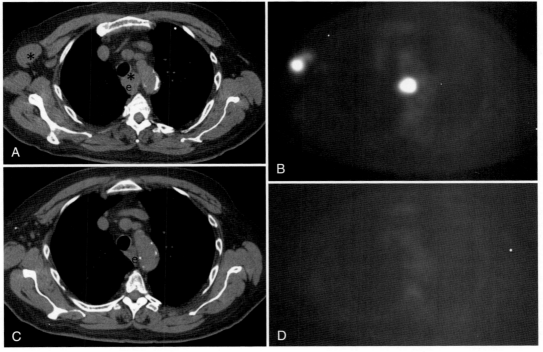

FIGURE 11-40. Posttreatment fibrosis in diffuse B-cell lymphoma (i.e., non-Hodgkin's disease). **A** and **B**, CT and PET scans show enlarged and metabolically active lymphoma nodes in the right axilla and middle mediastinum *(asterisk)*. **C** and **D**, The residual middle mediastinal node without increased FDG uptake represents fibrosis. The esophagus is labeled (e).

arterial system. Lymphangitic spread of carcinoma may result from bloodborne metastases extending from capillaries into the lymphatics. Retrograde lymphatic spread from the hilar disease and the upper abdomen may also occur. Endobronchial spread occurs rarely and is seen in cases of bronchioloalveolar carcinoma of the lung and in malignancies that involve the upper airways or paranasal sinuses.

Radiographic Features

CT is much more sensitive than standard radiography for the detection of metastases. However, increased sensitivity also significantly limits its specificity. Many small nodules detected on CT are frequently benign. In a study done by Chalmers, 80% of nodules detected by CT in patients with malignancies were benign.

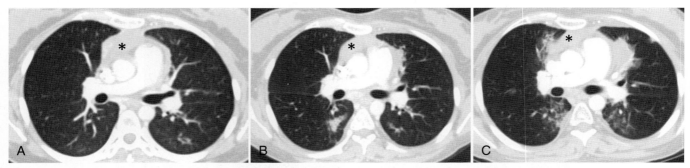

FIGURE 11-41. Radiation pneumonitis in a patient treated for Hodgkin's disease. A–C, CT shows progressive development of ground-glass opacities in the paramediastinal upper and lower lobes over a period of 4 months. Notice the well-defined lateral border and the anterior mediastinal mass *(asterisk)*.

Hematogenous Metastases

Patients most often present with bilateral, multiple nodules (Box 11-18). The bases of the lungs are more frequently involved than the apices (Fig. 11-42). Between 80% and 90% of metastases occur in the periphery, and most lie close to the pleura (Fig. 11-43). The mass-vessel sign consists of a vessel that leads to and terminates in a nodule, and it is considered a sign of hematogenous metastasis. The pulmonary arterial branches may be thickened and show beaded appearance due to tumor emboli growing within walls and lumen (Fig. 11-44). The incidence of pulmonary metastases manifesting as a solitary nodule is less than 10%. However, solitary metastasis can occur in several primary tumors, including carcinoma of the colon, sarcoma, and carcinomas of the breast, bladder, kidney, and testicle. A solitary nodule in an adult with an extrathoracic primary squamous cell carcinoma is more likely to represent a primary lung cancer than a metastatic tumor. If the primary tumor is an adenocarcinoma, the likelihood of the nodule in the lung representing a solitary metasta-

sis is equal to the incidence of a second primary tumor. However, with melanoma or sarcoma, a solitary metastasis is more likely. Granulomas and subpleural intraparenchymal lymph nodes, both of which tend to be less than 5 mm in diameter, can be indistinguishable from metastases.

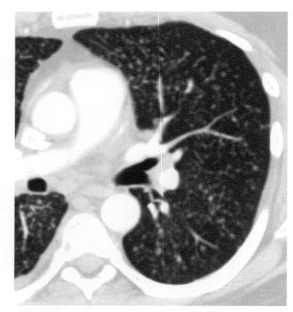

FIGURE 11-42. Metastases from thyroid cancer. CT shows multiple, small nodules in the lungs that represent hematogenous metastases. This pattern is typical for thyroid cancer.

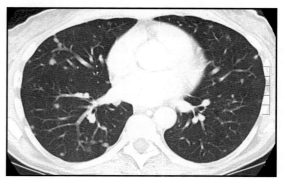

FIGURE 11-43. Multiple hematogenous metastases from colon carcinoma. CT demonstrates the typical peripheral and subpleural location of metastases, which are smooth and well defined.

Box 11-18. Metastatic Disease: Hematogenous Spread

CHARACTERISTICS
Round, well-marginated lesions
  Variable doubling times and growth rates
  May cause hemorrhage

RADIOGRAPHIC FEATURES
Bilateral, multiple nodules between 1 mm and 5 cm or larger
Lung bases more frequently involved than apices
80% to 90% of metastases in periphery
Calcification
  Primary bone and cartilage tumors
  Mucinous adenocarcinomas
Cavitation
  Metastatic squamous cell
Solitary pulmonary nodule
  Occurs in less than 10% of cases
  If squamous cell type, likely a lung primary
Diagnosis with CT
  High sensitivity, low specificity
  False positives because of intraparenchymal lymph nodes and granulomas

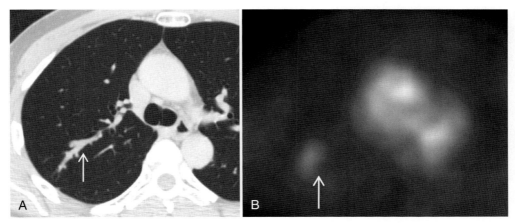

FIGURE 11-44. Tumor emboli metastasized to the right upper lobe segmental artery from hepatocellular carcinoma. **A,** There are beaded, thickened pulmonary arteries in the posterior segment of right upper lobe *(arrow).* **B,** There is increased FDG uptake on the PET scan *(arrow).*

Most metastases tend to be round and very sharply marginated, and they can vary from 1 mm to 5 cm or larger. Small miliary nodules are seen in metastases from thyroid cancer, kidney cancer, and melanoma. Based on density, metastatic nodules can be classified as solid, ground-glass, and mixed solid and ground-glass nodules. Solid nodules are the most common. Ground-glass nodules and mixed solid and ground-glass nodules result from surrounding hemorrhage or airspace involvement. Hemorrhage is seen in metastases from vascular tumors such as choriocarcinoma, angiosarcoma, melanoma, and renal cell carcinoma (Fig. 11-45). Involvement of the alveolar walls occurs in bronchoalveolar carcinoma (Fig. 11-46). Irregular margins are usually attributable to hemorrhage around the periphery of the metastatic nodule, and irregularity can occur in other types of metastases after therapy. Calcification may occur in several metastatic lesions (Fig. 11-47), including primary bone and cartilage tumors, such as osteosarcoma and chondrosarcoma, and papillary and mucinous adenocarcinomas. Dystrophic calcification occurs in areas of necrosis after therapy. Cavitation is uncommon and occurs most often in squamous cell carcinomas that are metastatic from the head and neck in men, from the cervix in women, and from transitional carcinoma (Fig. 11-48). The cavities are typically thick walled. Cavities can also occur after treatment of metastases. Occasionally, pneumothorax may be

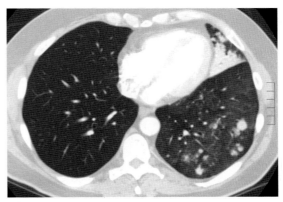

FIGURE 11-46. Bronchoalveolar carcinoma with metastases. CT shows ground-glass and nodular opacities in the left lower lobe due to lepidic spread of bronchoalveolar carcinoma. Notice the primary tumor in the lingula.

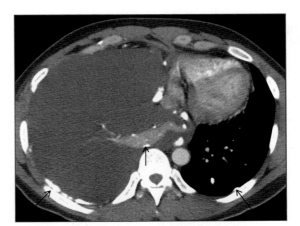

FIGURE 11-47. Osteosarcoma metastases. Ossified metastases can be seen in the subpleural zones of both lungs *(arrows).* There is also a large malignant right pleural effusion with ossified pleural nodules.

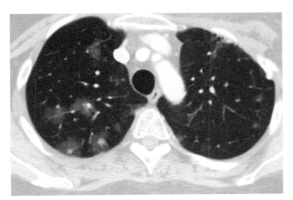

FIGURE 11-45. Typical pattern for hemorrhagic metastases. CT shows multiple nodules with surrounding ground-glass opacity in a patient with angiosarcoma.

associated with cavitation of a subpleural metastatic focus, particularly in osteosarcoma.

The growth rates of hematogenous metastases vary broadly. The tumor doubling time is the time required for a nodule to double in volume or increase 25% in diameter. Carcinoma of the thyroid is an example of an extremely

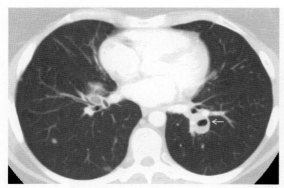

FIGURE 11-48. Cavitary metastases from vulvar squamous cell carcinoma. CT shows solid and cavitary nodules *(arrow)*.

slow-growing tumor that may take months to double in volume. Most sarcomas, melanomas, and germ cell tumors have rapid doubling times, which may even approach 1 to 2 weeks.

After chemotherapy, many metastatic lesions decrease in size or completely resolve. However, some metastatic lesions initially respond to therapy and then become stable in size. These nodules may only contain necrotic or fibrous tissue without viable tumor. Occasionally, biologic markers may distinguish viable tumor from residual fibrotic disease.

Lymphangitic Metastases

Most lymphangitic metastases are thought to result from hematogenous spread (Box 11-19). In these cases, tumor involves pulmonary capillaries, lymphatics, and surrounding interstitium. Primary sites of origin of lymphangitic spread of tumor include carcinomas of the lung and breast and upper abdominal malignancies, such as those of the stomach and pancreas. The spread may be unilateral or bilateral, although unilateral involvement is less common. Lymphangitic spread of primary lung cancer can occur to other areas of the same lung or to the opposite side.

Box 11-19. Metastatic Disease: Lymphangitic Spread

CHARACTERISTICS
May result from hematogenous spread
Primary sites
   Lung
   Breast
   Upper abdominal malignancy
More commonly bilateral

RADIOGRAPHIC FEATURES
Standard radiography
   Reticulonodular pattern
   Kerley B lines
   Pleural effusion (60%)
   Adenopathy (25%)
High-resolution CT
   Nodular thickening of bronchovascular bundles
   Polygonal arcades
   Beaded septal thickening

The standard radiograph may be normal, but there is often a mixed reticulonodular pattern (Fig. 11-49). This may be associated with prominent thickening of the interlobular septa (i.e., Kerley B and Kerley A lines). The pattern is usually bilateral; it is associated with pleural effusion in 60% of cases and with hilar adenopathy in less than 25% of cases. CT is more sensitive than conventional chest radiographs in the diagnosis of lymphangitic carcinomatosis. CT should be performed using a high-resolution technique, as described in Chapter 7. The typical findings include nodular thickening of the bronchovascular bundles centrally and the interlobular septa (Fig. 11-50). The septal thickening is usually beaded (i.e., beaded septum sign), and it produces a pattern of polygonal arcades. These arcades represent secondary pulmonary lobules. In the center of the arcade is a prominent dot that represents the centrilobular core, which consists of the pulmonary artery surrounded by infiltrating tumor.

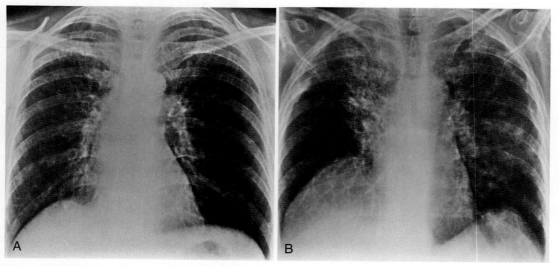

FIGURE 11-49. Lymphangitic metastases in a woman who had bilateral mastectomies for breast carcinoma. The frontal views (**A** and **B**) obtained several weeks apart show a reticulonodular pattern, which becomes more confluent over time. There is bilateral hilar adenopathy.

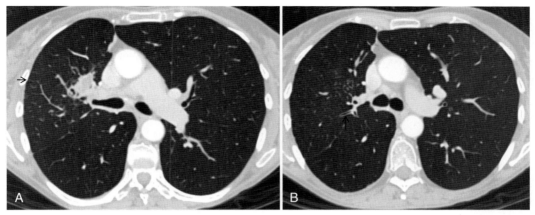

FIGURE 11-50. Lymphangitic spread of tumor from a lung primary in the right upper lobe. **A,** Nodular septal thickening creates polygonal arcades *(arrow)*. **B,** There is nodular thickening along bronchovascular bundles *(arrow)*.

The pattern is usually diffuse, although it may be focal in less than one half of cases. Small, isolated nodules and pleural effusions may be identified. Lymphadenopathy is more commonly identified on CT than on standard radiographs. The differential diagnosis includes sarcoidosis and lymphoma.

Endobronchial Metastases

Metastases to major bronchi are uncommon and occur in less than 5% of patients at autopsy (Box 11-20). Common sites of primary tumors include the kidney, skin (i.e., melanoma), thyroid, breast, and colon. Patients often present with cough and hemoptysis. The radiographic findings consist of lobar, segmental, or subsegmental atelectasis sometimes associated with postobstructive pneumonitis (Fig. 11-51). A hilar or central mass may be present. This appearance must be differentiated from that of a primary bronchogenic carcinoma.

Intrathoracic Adenopathy

Extrathoracic primary tumors may metastasize to mediastinal and hilar lymph nodes alone or in combination with parenchymal metastases (Fig. 11-52 and Box 11-21). The most common sites of origin include genitourinary neoplasms, those arising in the head and neck, breast carcinoma, and skin cancer (i.e., melanoma). Concomitant parenchymal metastases are present in 40% of cases.

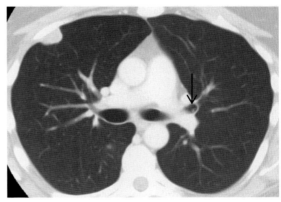

FIGURE 11-51. Endobronchial metastases from metastatic melanoma. There is a nodule in the left upper lobe bronchus *(arrow)*. Notice the parenchymal nodules in the right lung.

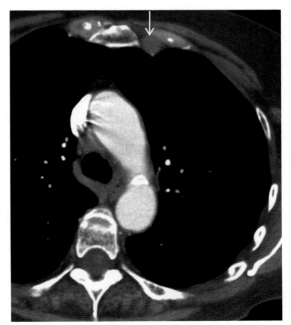

FIGURE 11-52. Nodal metastasis from ovarian cancer. CT shows an enlarged left internal mammary node *(arrow)*.

Box 11-20. **Metastatic Disease: Endobronchial Metastases**

SITES OF PRIMARY MALIGNANCY
Kidney
Skin (melanoma)
Thyroid
Breast
Colon

RADIOGRAPHIC FEATURES
Atelectasis
Hilar mass

Box 11-21. Metastatic Disease: Intrathoracic Adenopathy

SITES OF PRIMARY MALIGNANCY
Genitourinary tract
Head and neck
Breast
Skin (melanoma)

RADIOGRAPHIC FEATURES
Adenopathy
Parenchymal metastases (with or without)

Diagnostic Workup

The diagnosis of pulmonary metastases can often be made on standard chest radiographs, and comparison with previous examinations is important. CT has markedly higher sensitivity compared with standard radiographs, but it has lower specificity because of the inability to differentiate granulomas and intraparenchymal lymph nodes from small metastases. PET imaging when combined with CT is even more sensitive for detecting metastases in the chest. However, PET imaging is limited by size and may not detect metabolic activity in lesions less than 10 mm in diameter. PET imaging also lacks specificity, because inflammatory and infectious lesions can show increased metabolic activity. Despite these limitations, PET/CT is superior to other modalities in the assessment of metastatic disease.

Approximately 3% to 4% of all cancers manifest with metastatic carcinoma to the lung without a known primary. These are typically adenocarcinomas. The average survival from diagnosis is 3 to 7 months. An extensive imaging search for a primary tumor in these situations is somewhat controversial. Needle aspiration biopsy of a lung metastasis may establish the diagnosis and identify the types of adenocarcinoma that may be likely to respond to specific treatments (i.e., hormone therapy in prostate and breast carcinoma).

◼ SOLITARY PULMONARY NODULE

The solitary pulmonary nodule represents a common clinical problem. In series in which these *coin lesions* have been resected, approximately one half are found to be benign, about 40% represent primary lung cancer, and 10% are solitary metastases. A solitary pulmonary nodule can be defined as a well-circumscribed, round or oval lesion measuring less than 3 cm in diameter.

Several clinical indicators may be helpful in distinguishing benign from malignant solitary nodules (see Table 11-3). Unfortunately, they are only indicators and are not sufficiently specific to be helpful in individual cases. However, solitary pulmonary nodules in patients younger than 35 years with no history of an extrathoracic malignancy usually are considered to be benign and may not require further diagnostic workup.

Standard Radiographs

Criteria have been described to help separate benign from malignant solitary nodules, such as size, shape, contour, location, edge definition, the presence of satellite lesions,

and cavitation. However, none of these findings is specific. The only specific and reliable signs of the benign nature of a solitary nodule include the identification of certain benign types of calcification and the absolute absence of growth over a 2-year period. Benign types of calcification (Fig. 11-53 and see Fig. 11-1) include those with a central nidus, popcorn, or laminated pattern. Stippled or eccentric calcification may be identified in 7% to 15% of malignant lung carcinomas. The growth rate or doubling time is an indicator, but it is not a useful discriminant between benign and malignant lesions. Benign lesions typically have a doubling time of less than 1 month or more than 16 months. However, there is significant overlap of growth rates among rapidly growing nodules. Only nodules that are stable over a 2-year period can be considered benign. Occasionally, certain acute processes such as infarcts or focal pneumonias may produce a solitary nodule. However, there are important clinical clues such as fever and chest pain. The lesions should be followed for a 2- to 6-week period to ensure that they resolve and do not represent coincidental carcinoma.

Computed Tomography

CT is helpful and often diagnostic in the workup of solitary pulmonary nodules. In some cases, the morphologic characteristics of a solitary lesion on CT can establish a specific diagnosis, and CT densitometry may allow the identification of benign lesions such as hamartomas and granulomas. CT can be performed with a conventional scanner that obtains 1- to 2-mm-thick sections (HRCT) or a helical scanner with a single breath hold and 1-mm sections through the nodule.

Certain lesions in the lung may produce the appearance of a nonspecific, solitary pulmonary nodule or lesion on standard studies. However, CT may identify specific diagnostic features, including arteriovenous fistulas, rounded atelectasis, fungus balls, mucoid impaction, and infarcts. Arteriovenous fistulas can be diagnosed because of the presence of a feeding artery and draining vein, as well as

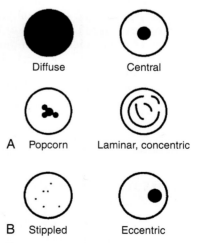

FIGURE 11-53. Patterns of calcification in benign (**A**) and malignant (**B**) nodules. A benign nodule must be less than 3 cm in diameter and have smooth borders, and benign types of calcification include those with a central nidus, popcorn, or laminated pattern. Stippled or eccentric calcification may be identified in up to 15% of malignant lung carcinomas. (From Webb WR: Radiologic evaluation of the solitary pulmonary nodule. AJR Am J Roentgenol 154:701-708, 1990.)

intense enhancement after the administration of contrast material (Fig. 11-54). The features of rounded atelectasis include a peripheral rounded lesion in the lung abutting pleural thickening associated with a classic comet tail sign, consisting of a crowding of pulmonary vessels and bronchi leading to the mass (see Chapter 1). A fungus ball within a preexisting cavity may appear as a solitary pulmonary nodule on standard films, but CT can clearly identify the presence of a nodule within a cavity (see Chapters 3 and 4). Mucoid impaction on CT can be diagnosed because of the classic features of branching opacities located endobronchially that are often associated with bronchiectasis (Fig. 11-55). Infarcts on CT may have a classic appearance.

They abut the pleura and are round or wedge shaped, and they often contain pseudocavities or air bronchograms.

CT densitometry is useful in detecting the presence and distribution of calcification and fat within solitary nodules. CT is more sensitive than standard radiographic studies in the detection of calcification. Between 22% and 38% of uncalcified nodules on standard studies appear calcified on CT. The presence of calcification can often be confirmed visually by direct examination of the image, or a pixelgram can be obtained by placing a cursor over the lesion (Fig. 11-56). A printout of each of the CT numbers in every pixel through the lesion is required. Values greater than +200 indicate a calcification.

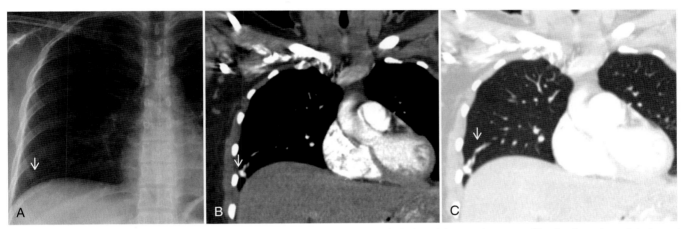

FIGURE 11-54. Arteriovenous malformation. **A,** The frontal radiograph shows a nodular lesion with a prominent vessel leading in to the nodule *(arrow)*. **B** and **C,** CT shows the nodular lesion with feeding and draining vessels (arrow).

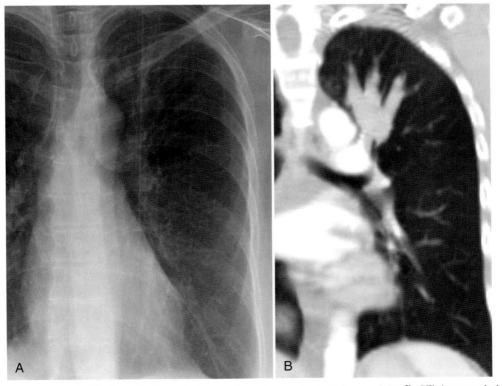

FIGURE 11-55. Mucoid impaction. **A,** The frontal radiograph shows an irregular mass in the left upper lobe. **B,** CT shows a tubular branching opacity in the left upper lobe.

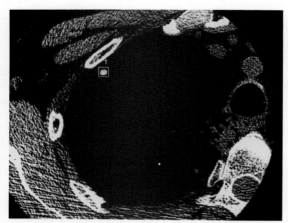

FIGURE 11-56. Calcified granuloma identified by CT densitometry. A thin-collimation image of a solitary nodule in the right lung shows a dense calcification. CT numbers throughout the lesion showed values greater than + 1200.

Fat may be present in hamartomas. Fat appears as an area of low attenuation and measures between approximately –50 to –150 HU (see Fig. 11-2). In a study of 47 hamartomas, 30 were correctly diagnosed on CT by the presence of fat alone (focal or diffuse); by a combination of fat and calcification; or by the presence of popcorn calcification alone.

Other Imaging Techniques

There are some promising imaging techniques for the evaluation of solitary pulmonary nodules. It has been shown that malignant pulmonary nodules enhance to a greater degree than benign lesions after the administration of contrast. Enhancement of greater than 20 HU is highly sensitive for the presence of malignancy, although the specificity is slightly lower because active inflammatory lesions occasionally may enhance. PET-FDG may also be used to distinguish benign from malignant lesions. High sensitivities for detecting malignancy have been reported. FDG is an analog of glucose and is taken up avidly by malignant tumors because of their increased metabolism.

Diagnostic Workup

A scheme for the proposed diagnostic workup of a solitary pulmonary nodule is presented in Fig. 11-57.

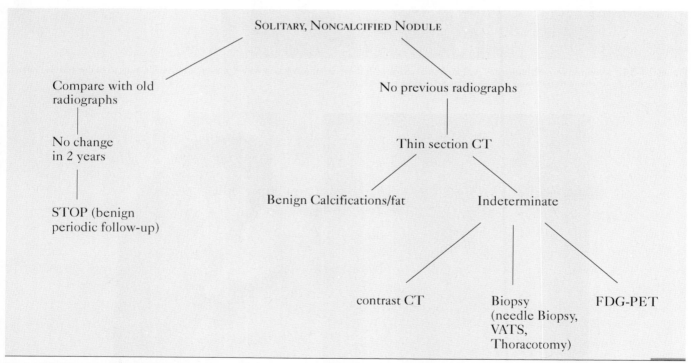

FIGURE 11-57. Diagnosis of a Solitary, Noncalcified Nodule in Patients Older Than 35 Years. FDG-PET, ^{18}F-fluorodeoxyglucose positron emission tomography; VATS, video-assisted thoracoscopy.

▬ SUGGESTED READINGS

Aquino, S., 2005. Imaging of metastatic disease to the thorax. Radiol. Clin. North Am. 43, 481–495.

Balakrishnan, J., Meziane, M.A., Siegelman, S.S., Fishman, E.K., 1989. Pulmonary infarction: CT appearance with pathologic correlation. J. Comput. Assist. Tomogr. 13, 941–945.

Bragg, D., 1997. Hodgkin disease and non-Hodgkin lymphoma of the thorax. In: Freundlich, I.M., Bragg, D.G. (Eds.), A radiologic approach to diseases of the chest. Williams and Wilkins, Baltimore, pp. 597–608.

Braman, S.S., Whitcomb, M.E., 1975. Endobronchial metastasis. Arch. Intern. Med. 135, 543–547.

Brambilla, E., Travis, W.D., Colby, T.V., et al., 2001. The new World Health Organization classification of lung tumours. Eur. Respir. J. 18, 1059–1068.

Chalmers, N., Best, J.J.K., 1991. The significance of pulmonary nodules detected by CT but not by chest radiography in tumor staging. Clin. Radiol. 44, 410–412.

Chang, A.E., Schaner, E.G., Conkle, D.M., et al., 1979. Evaluation of computed tomography in detection of pulmonary metastases: a prospective study. Cancer 43, 913–916.

Coppage, L., Shaw, C., Curtis, A., 1987. Metastatic disease to the chest in patients with extrathoracic malignancy [review]. J. Thorac. Imaging 2, 24–37.

Crow, J., Slavin, G., Kreel, L., 1981. Pulmonary metastases: a pathologic and radiologic study. Cancer 47, 2595–2602.

Cummings, S.R., Lillington, G.A., Richard, R.J., 1986. Estimating the probability of malignancy in solitary pulmonary nodules: a Bayesian approach. Am. Rev. Respir. Dis. 134, 449–452.

D'Angio, G.J., Iannaccone, G., 1961. Spontaneous pneumothorax as a complication of pulmonary metastases in malignant tumors of childhood. AJR Am. J. Roentgenol. 86, 1092–1102.

Edwards, W.M., Cox, R.S., Garland, L.H., 1962. The solitary nodule (coin lesion) of the lung: an analysis of 52 consecutive cases treated by thoracotomy and a study of prospective diagnostic accuracy. AJR Am. J. Roentgenol. 88, 1020–1042.

Faling, L.J., Pugatch, R.D., Jung-Legg, Y., 1981. Computed tomography scanning of the mediastinum in the staging of bronchogenic carcinoma. Am. Rev. Respir. Dis. 124, 690–695.

Filderman, A.E., Shaw, C., Matthay, R.A., 1986. Lung cancer. Part I. Etiology, pathology, natural history, manifestations, and diagnostic techniques. Invest. Radiol. 21, 80–90.

Forster, B.B., Müller, N.L., Miller, R.R., et al., 1989. Neuroendocrine carcinomas of the lung: Clinical, radiologic, and pathologic correlation. Radiology 170, 441–445.

Fraser, R.G., Paré, J.A.P., 1989. Diagnosis of Diseases of the Chest, vol. 2, third ed. WB Saunders, Philadelphia, pp. 1327–1699.

Glazer, G.M., Orringer, M.B., Gross, B.H., Quint, L.E., 1984. The mediastinum in non-small cell lung cancer: CT-surgical correlation. AJR Am. J. Roentgenol. 142, 1101–1105.

Goldstraw, P., Crowley, J., Chansky, K., et al., 2007. The IASLC Lung Cancer Staging Project: proposals for revision of the TNM stage groupings in the forthcoming (seventh) edition of the TNM classification of malignant tumors. J. Thorac. Oncol. 2, 706–714.

Gurney, J.W., Lyddon, D.M., McKay, J.A., 1993. Determining the likelihood of malignancy in solitary pulmonary nodules with Bayesian analysis. Part II. Application. Radiology 186, 415–422.

Gurney, J.W., 1993. Determining the likelihood of malignancy in solitary pulmonary nodules with Bayesian analysis. Part I. Theory. Radiology 186, 405–413.

Haggar, A.M., Perlberg, J.L., Froelich, J.W., et al., 1987. Chest wall invasion by carcinoma of the lung: detection by MR imaging. AJR Am. J. Roentgenol. 148, 1075–1078.

Hill, C.A., 1984. Bronchioloalveolar carcinoma: a review. Radiology 150, 15–20.

Janower, M.L., Blennerhassett, J.B., 1971. Lymphangitic spread of metastatic cancer to the lung. Radiology 101, 267–273.

Kumar, R., Millard, I., Schuster, S.J., et al., 2004. Utility of fluorodeoxyglucose-PET imaging in the management of patients with Hodgkin's and non-Hodgkin's lymphomas. Radiol. Clin. North Am. 42, 1083–1100.

Kuriyama, K., Tateishi, R., Doi, O., et al., 1987. CT-pathologic correlation in small peripheral lung cancers. AJR Am. J. Roentgenol. 149, 1139–1143.

Libshitz, H.I., Jing, B.S., Wallace, S., et al., 1983. Sterilized metastases: a diagnostic and therapeutic dilemma. AJR Am. J. Roentgenol. 140, 15–19.

Libshitz, H.I., McKenna, R.J., Haynie, T.P., et al., 1984. Mediastinal evaluation in lung cancer. Radiology 151, 295–299.

Libshitz, H.I., McKenna, R.J., 1984. Mediastinal lymph node size in lung cancer. AJR Am. J. Roentgenol. 143, 715–718.

Libshitz, H.I., 1997. Pulmonary metastatic disease. In: Freundlich, I.M., Bragg, D.G. (Eds.), A Radiologic Approach to Diseases of the Chest. Williams and Wilkins, Baltimore, pp. 561–576.

Mayo, J.R., Webb, W.R., Gould, R., et al., 1987. High-resolution CT of the lungs: an optimal approach. Radiology 163, 507–510.

McHugh, K., Blaquiere, R.M., 1989. CT features of rounded atelectasis. AJR Am. J. Roentgenol. 153, 257–260.

McLoud, T.C., Bourgouin, P.M., Greenberg, R.W., et al., 1992. Bronchogenic carcinoma: analysis of staging in the mediastinum with CT by correlative lymph node mapping and sampling. Radiology 182, 319–323.

McLoud, T.C., Filion, R.B., Edelman, R.R., Shepard, J.O., 1989. MR imaging of superior sulcus carcinoma. J. Comput. Assist. Tomogr. 13, 233–239.

Mountain, C., 1986. A new international staging system for lung cancer. Chest 89 (Suppl.), 225–233.

Mountain, C.F., 1989. Value of the new TNM staging system for lung cancer. Chest 96, 47–49.

Munk, P.L., Müller, N.L., Miller, R.R., et al., 1988. Pulmonary lymphangitic carcinomatosis: CT and pathologic findings. Radiology 166, 705–709.

O'Connell, R.S., McLoud, T.C., Wilkins, E.W., 1983. Superior sulcus tumor: radiographic diagnosis and workup, AJR Am. J. Roentgenol. 140, 25–30.

Pancoast, H.K., 1932. Superior pulmonary sulcus tumor: tumor characterized by pain, Horner's syndrome, destruction of bone and atrophy of hand muscles. JAMA 99, 1391–1396.

Patz, E.F., Lowe, V.J., Hoffman, J.M., et al., 1993. Focal pulmonary abnormalities: evaluation with F-18 fluorodeoxyglucose PET scanning. Radiology 188, 487–290.

Pennes, D.R., Glazer, G.M., Wimbish, K.J., et al., 1985. Chest wall invasion by lung cancer: limitations by CT evaluation. AJR Am. J. Roentgenol. 144, 507–511.

Pugatch, R.D., Munden, R.F., 1997. Primary pulmonary neoplasm. In: Freundlich, I.M., Bragg, D.G. (Eds.), A Radiologic Approach to Diseases of the Chest. Williams and Wilkins, Baltimore, pp. 543–560.

Remy, J., Remy-Jardin, M., Wattinne, L., et al., 1992. Pulmonary arteriovenous malformations: evaluation with CT of the chest before and after treatment. Radiology 182, 809–816.

Remy-Jardin, M., Remy, J., Giraud, F., et al., 1993. Pulmonary nodules: detection with thick-section spiral CT versus conventional CT. Radiology 187, 513–520.

Schaner, E.G., Chang, A.E., Doppman, J.L., et al., 1978. Comparison of computed and conventional whole lung tomography in detecting pulmonary nodules: a prospective radiology-pathology study. AJR Am. J. Roentgenol. 131, 51–54.

Schoder, H., Meta, J., Yap, C., et al., 2001. Effect of whole body 18 F-FDG PET on clinical staging and management of patients with malignant lymphoma. J. Nucl. Med. 42, 1139–1143.

Seely, J., Mayo, J.R., Miller, R.R., Mauuller, N.L., 1993. T1 lung cancer: prevalence of mediastinal nodal metastases (diagnostic accuracy of CT). Radiology 186, 129–132.

Shuman, L.S., Libshitz, H.I., 1984. Solid pleural manifestations of lymphoma. AJR Am. J. Roentgenol. 142, 269–273.

Siegelman, S.S., Khouri, N.F., Leo, F.P., et al., 1986. Solitary pulmonary nodules: CT assessment. Radiology 160, 307–312.

Siegelman, S.S., Khouri, N.F., Scott, W.W., et al., 1986. Pulmonary hamartoma: CT findings. Radiology 160, 313–317.

Shepherd, F.A., Crowley, J., Van Houtte, P., et al., 2007. for the International Association for the Study of Lung Cancer: Lung cancer staging project: proposals regarding the clinical staging of small cell lung cancer in the forthcoming (seventh) edition of the tumor, node, metastasis classification for lung Cancer. J. Thorac. Oncol. 2, 1067–1077.

Skarin, A., Jochelson, M., Sheldon, F., et al., 1989. Neoadjuvant chemotherapy in marginally resectable stage III MO non-small cell lung cancer: long-term follow-up in 41 patients. J. Surg. Oncol. 40, 266–274.

Staples, C.A., Müller, N.L., Miller, R.R., et al., 1988. Mediastinal nodes in bronchogenic carcinoma: comparison between CT and mediastinoscopy. Radiology 167, 367–372.

Swensen, S.J., Brown, L.R., Colby, T.V., Weaver, A.L., 1995. Pulmonary nodules: CT evaluation of enhancement with iodinated contrast material. Radiology 194, 393–398.

Swensen, S.J., Morin, R.L., Schueler, B.A., et al., 1992. Solitary pulmonary nodule: CT evaluation of enhancement with iodinated contrast material—a preliminary report. Radiology 182, 343–347.

Swerdlow, SH, Campo, E., Harris, N.L., Jaffe, E.S., Pileri, S., Stein, H., Thiele, J., Vardiman, J., ed. WHO Classification of Tumours of Haematopoietic and Lymphoid Systems. 4th ed. Lyon: IARC; 2008.

Theros, E.G., 1977. The 1976 Caldwell lecture. Varying manifestations of peripheral pulmonary neoplasms: a radiologic-pathologic correlative study. AJR Am. J. Roentgenol. 128, 893–914.

Tisi, G.M., Friedman, P.H., Peters, R.M., et al., 1983. for the American Thoracic Society: Clinical staging of primary lung cancer. Am. Rev. Respir. Dis. 127, 659–664.

Travis, W.D., Colby, T.V., Corrin, B., Shimosato, Y., Brambilla, E. In Collaboration with Sobin LH and Pathologists from 14 Countries. 1999 World Health Organization International Histological Classification of Tumours. Histological Typing of Lung and Pleural Tumours, Springer-Verlag 3rd ed.

Webb, W.R., Gatsonis, C., Zerhouni, E., et al., 1991. CT and MR imaging in staging non-small cell bronchogenic carcinoma: report of the Radiology Diagnostic Oncology Group. Radiology 178, 705–713.

Webb, W.R., 1990. Radiologic evaluation of the solitary pulmonary nodule. AJR Am. J. Roentgenol. 154, 701–708.

Webb, W.R., 1997. The solitary pulmonary nodule. In: Freundlich, I.M., Bragg, D.G. (Eds.), A Radiologic Approach to Diseases of the Chest. Williams and Wilkins, Baltimore, pp. 101–108.

Zerhouni, E.A., Stitik, F.P., Siegelman, S.S., et al., 1986. CT of the pulmonary nodule: a cooperative study. Radiology 160, 319–327.

Zwiebel, B.R., Austin, J.H.M., Grines, M.M., 1991. Bronchial carcinoid tumors: assessment with CT of location and intratumoral calcification in 31 patients. Radiology 179, 483–486.

Zwirewich, C.V., Vedal, S., Miller, R.R., Müller, N.R., 1991. Solitary pulmonary nodule: high-resolution CT and radiologic-pathologic correlation. Radiology 179, 469–476.

CHAPTER 12

The Trachea

Subba R. Digumarthy and Jo-Anne O. Shepard

ANATOMY

The trachea is a cartilaginous and membranous tube that extends from the cricoids cartilage to the carina, and it is approximately 11 cm long. The trachea is almost cylindrical, with slight flattening posteriorly. Its diameter from side to side is approximately 2 to 2.5 cm. The trachea is divided in to a shorter extrathoracic and a longer intrathoracic segment at the upper border of manubrium. The trachea and extrapulmonary bronchi are composed of hyaline cartilage, fibrous tissue, muscular fibers, mucous membrane, and glands. The tracheal cartilages form incomplete C-shaped rings that occupy the anterior two thirds of the trachea. The bronchial cartilages are shorter and narrower than those of the trachea, but they have the same shape and arrangement. Calcification of cartilage is seen in older people, more so in women. Posteriorly, the membranous wall of the trachea and main bronchi is completed by fibrous tissue and nonstriated muscular fibers.

RADIOGRAPHIC EVALUATION

Plain Films

Several radiographic studies are used to evaluate the trachea and main bronchi (Table 12-1). The plain chest radiograph in the posteroanterior and lateral projections is the most frequently used screening study. A high-kilovoltage (140-kVp) technique is preferred because it reduces the visibility of the bony thorax and improves imaging of the various mediastinal interfaces. However, it is easy to miss a tracheal or main bronchial lesion on standard posteroanterior and lateral chest radiographs because there is considerable overlap of the trachea with the mediastinum and bony thorax. Bilateral, oblique chest radiographs improve visibility of the trachea and main bronchi by rotating the spine so that it is not superimposed on the central airways (Fig. 12-1). In most cases, additional imaging is usually indicated.

Computed Tomography

Computed tomography (CT) has become the imaging modality of choice for most tracheobronchial lesions. Because of the clarity of anatomic detail on cross-sectional imaging, there is a direct display of tracheobronchial anatomy. The superior contrast resolution compared with conventional radiography permits evaluation of adjacent mediastinal soft tissues. This is particularly important in cases of tracheal neoplasms, which may invade the adjacent mediastinum, or in cases of mediastinal masses such as goiters or vascular rings, which may compress the trachea. CT can identify calcific and fatty densities and vascular enhancement of tumors and aneurysms after intravenous contrast administration. Paired inspiratory and expiratory CT scans can identify abnormal collapsibility of the

trachea and main bronchi in cases of tracheobronchomalacia. High-resolution computed tomography (HRCT) can be obtained with the use of thin (1- to 1.5-mm) sections and a bone reconstruction algorithm. The major disadvantage of conventional CT is that craniocaudally oriented trachea and bronchi are not imaged in the long axis. Although images may be reconstructed in sagittal and coronal planes, the resolution is limited by the inherent scan thickness on conventional CT scans.

Multidetector CT (MDCT) has significantly improved the way the trachea is imaged. MDCT increases the capacity to register data and significantly shortens the scan time. The entire trachea and major bronchi can be imaged in a single breath hold of a few seconds. The isometric data set obtained with MDCT has equal resolution in all the imaging planes, and artifacts seen with multiplanar reformats in conventional CT can be avoided. High-quality, multiplanar images are possible if thin sections (1 to 2.5 mm) and an overlapping image reconstruction algorithm are used (Fig. 12-2). The image reconstruction thickness can be selected prospectively or retrospectively after raw data set is acquired. The same data can be transferred to a dedicated workstation to obtain three-dimensional images. The two commonly used three-dimensional techniques are external volume rendering of the airways (Fig. 12-3A) and internal rendering or virtual bronchoscopic views (see Fig. 12-3B). These imaging techniques supplement but do not replace conventional axial images. There are several advantages of using these techniques. The craniocaudal extent and shape of the lesion is better displayed, complex and subtle lesions can be better demonstrated (Fig. 12-4), and simulated bronchoscopic views can be used as a guide in planning interventional procedures.

Because of high temporal resolution, MDCT allows dynamic CT imaging during expiration and coughing. These techniques are more sensitive in demonstrating malacia than paired inspiratory and expiratory images.

Historically, conventional tomography in the anteroposterior, lateral, and oblique projections was routinely used to evaluate the trachea and central bronchi. With refinements in CT scanning, conventional airway tomography is no longer routinely employed. However, it does permit an accurate assessment of patency or the degree of obstruction in the central airways and provides a direct image of the airways in the long axis. Conventional tomograms can determine accurately the length of tracheal lesions relative to the larynx or carina. The major disadvantage of conventional tomography is the inability to visualize adjacent mediastinal structures.

Magnetic Resonance Imaging

The role of magnetic resonance imaging (MRI) in the evaluation of the trachea and bronchi is limited. The trachea,

TABLE 12-1 Approach to Diagnostic Imaging of the Trachea

Study	Clinical Indications
Chest radiographs (posteroanterior, lateral, oblique projections)	Screening study
Conventional tomography (anteroposterior, lateral, 55-degree posterior oblique projections)	Postintubation tracheal stenosis Preoperative assessment of length of lesion Postoperative assessment of bronchial anastomosis
Computed tomography	Tracheobronchial tumor location and extent Density determination Vascularity of tumor Airway diameter Wall thickness Tracheomalacia Compression of airway by mediastinal mass or vessel Tracheobronchial rupture Tracheobronchial dehiscence
Magnetic resonance imaging	Multiplanar imaging Mediastinal invasion by airway, neoplasm Airway obstruction by vascular rings
Fluoroscopy	Tracheomalacia Air trapping due to bronchial obstruction

main bronchi, and lobar bronchi are well demonstrated on spin echo images, but the spatial resolution of MRI permits observation of only an occasional segmental bronchus. MRI offers the advantages of multiplanar imaging, high-contrast resolution without the use of intravenous contrast agents, and absence of ionizing radiation. MRI

is particularly useful in patients with vascular rings or tracheal compression by vascular anomalies and other mediastinal masses (Fig. 12-5).

■ TRACHEAL DIVERTICULA

Tracheal diverticula are outpouchings from the tracheal wall. They are seen in up to 1% of population. They can be congenital or acquired. The congenital diverticula are single, located 4 to 5 cm below the vocal cords or just above

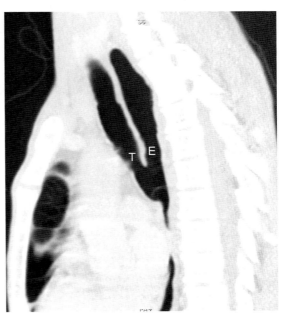

FIGURE 12-2. Tracheoesophageal fistula. High-resolution, multiplanar reconstruction with multidetector CT in the sagittal plane demonstrates communication between the lower trachea (T) and the esophagus (E).

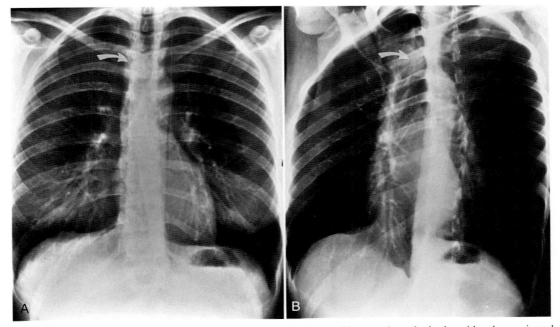

FIGURE 12-1. Tracheal tumor. **A,** Posteroanterior view of the chest reveals a focal area of increased opacity in the midtrachea projected over the spine *(arrow)*. **B,** A left anterior oblique projection shows the trachea to the right of the spine. A focal, well-defined, intraluminal mass *(arrow)*, which is better characterized in the midtrachea, represents an adenoid cystic carcinoma.

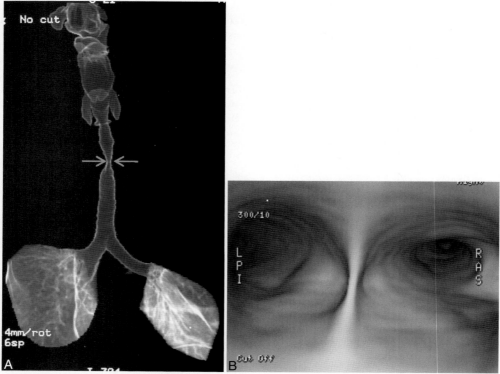

FIGURE 12-3. Three-dimensional imaging techniques. **A,** The technique of external volume rendering shows subtle tracheal stenosis *(arrow)* due to a tracheostomy injury. **B,** Virtual bronchoscopic view at the level of carina shows the normal carina and main bronchi.

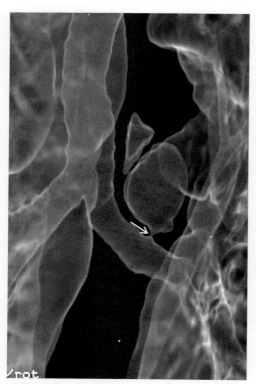

FIGURE 12-4. Left bronchial diverticulum. **A,** The technique of three-dimensional external volume rendering shows outpouching from left main bronchus with a narrow neck *(arrows).*

the carina, and contain all the layers of tracheal wall. The acquired diverticula are outpouchings from a weak posterior wall and are lined by respiratory epithelium. They lack other layers of the tracheal wall, such as smooth muscle and cartilage. The acquired diverticula may be single or multiple and are thought to be associated with increased intraluminal pressure and chronic cough.

Most tracheal diverticula are asymptomatic and are discovered incidentally. They can manifest with recurrent episodes of airway infection and chronic cough because the diverticula may act as reservoirs of infection.

On standard radiographs, small diverticula are often missed. Thin-section CT with multiplanar and three-dimensional reconstructions establishes the relation to the trachea, and further imaging is usually not required (Fig. 12-6; see Fig. 12-4).

The differential diagnosis of a paratracheal air collection includes laryngocele, pharyngocele, Zenker's diverticula, and apical paraseptal blebs or bullae. These entities can be easily distinguished by CT and barium swallow occasionally is required.

■ TRACHEAL STENOSIS

Diffuse tracheal narrowing is seen in several conditions, including chronic obstructive pulmonary disease (COPD); after tracheal trauma; as the result of viral, fungal, tuberculous, or bacterial infections; and in other diseases, such as sarcoidosis, Wegener's granulomatosis, relapsing

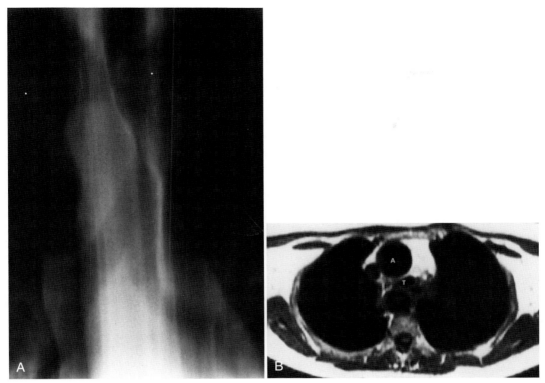

FIGURE 12-5. Tracheal compression by a right aortic arch. **A,** The anteroposterior tomogram demonstrates extrinsic compression and smooth narrowing of the midtrachea by a right paratracheal mass. **B,** Axial, T1-weighted MRI shows a slightly dilated ascending aorta (A), which extrinsically compresses and narrows the tracheal lumen (T).

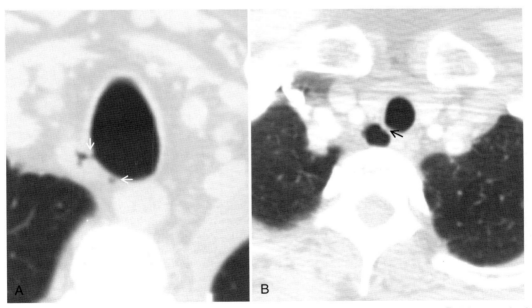

FIGURE 12-6. Tracheal diverticula. **A,** Two small tracheal diverticula arise from the posterior tracheal wall *(arrows)*. **B,** A large tracheal diverticulum has a narrow neck *(arrow)*.

polychondritis, amyloidosis, and tracheobronchopathia osteochondroplastica. The narrowing may be idiopathic and may involve the larynx (Table 12-2).

Idiopathic Laryngotracheal Stenosis

Idiopathic laryngotracheal stenosis is an uncommon cause of narrowing in the larynx and subglottic trachea. It typically

affects middle-aged women who have no history of intubation, trauma, infection, or other underlying systemic disease. Clinically, patients experience progressive shortness of breath accompanied by wheezing, stridor, or hoarseness. The average duration of symptoms is approximately 2 years.

The radiologic appearance of idiopathic laryngotracheal stenosis varies, including lesions that may be smooth and

TABLE 12-2 Diffuse Tracheal Stenosis

Causative Conditions	Tracheobronchial Findings	Other Findings
Idiopathic	Smooth, tapered, irregular, lobulated, or eccentric morphology 2-4 cm long, usually subglottic	±Laryngeal involvement
Postintubation cuff injury	Smooth narrowing with hourglass configuration	
Posttraumatic	Smooth narrowing with hourglass configuration	±Upper rib and sternal fractures
Saber-sheath trachea	Smooth narrowing of intrathoracic trachea Coronal diameter ≤ one half of sagittal diameter	Hyperinflated lungs
Tracheopathia osteochondroplastica	Submucosal nodularity of anterolateral walls of trachea and main bronchi with ossification Membranous wall is spared	
Relapsing polychondritis	Diffusely thickened tracheobronchial walls with diffuse narrowing of trachea and main bronchi ±Calcification of wall ±Tracheobronchomalacia	Auricular and nasal chondritis, arthritis
Wegener's granulomatosis	Focal or diffuse tracheobronchial wall thickening and narrowing ±Enlarged calcified cartilages	Renal involvement
Amyloidosis	Diffuse tracheobronchial wall-thickening and narrowing Focal nodular masses ±Calcification Contrast enhancement of masses on CT or MRI Slowly progressive	±Lymphadenopathy, may calcify
Sarcoidosis	Smooth, irregular, or nodular stenosis Tracheobronchial wall thickening Bronchial compression by lymph node	±Lymphadenopathy, ±calcification ±Reticular/nodular interstitial lung disease
Infectious		
Tracheobronchial papillomatosis	Diffuse nodules or masses in trachea and bronchi	Laryngeal involvement ±Multiple pulmonary nodules, may cavitate Complicated by squamous cell carcinoma
Rhinosclerosis	Nodular masses or diffuse, symmetric narrowing of trachea and bronchi Slowly progressive	
Tuberculosis		
Hyperplastic stage	Irregular tracheobronchial wall thickening and narrowing	Hilar/mediastinal lymphadenopathy Parenchymal cavitation and consolidation
Fibrostenotic stage	Smooth tracheobronchial narrowing	Atelectasis and scarring Bronchiectasis Calcified lymph nodes

tapered (Fig. 12-7) or irregular, lobulated, and eccentric (Fig. 12-8). The stenosis is 2 to 4 cm long, with severe compromise of the lumen measuring no more than 5 mm at the narrowest point.

Histologically, the stenotic areas show dense keloid fibrosis involving the adventitia and the lamina propria and sparing the mucosa, muscularis propria, and the cartilage. Small areas of spindle cell proliferation are similar to fibrosing mediastinitis or retroperitoneal fibrosis. The mucosa may show squamous metaplasia without dysplastic changes. The lesions may be treated surgically or conservatively with dilation, intubation, stenting, steroid injection, cryotherapy, or electrocoagulation.

Postintubation Injuries

Most long-term complications of intubation are related to cuff injury. Cuffed endotracheal tubes became common-

place only after the introduction of intermittent positive-pressure breathing for the treatment of respiratory failure during the poliomyelitis epidemic of 1952. As patients survived for longer periods with respiratory assistance, new long-term complications arose, including tracheal stenosis, tracheoesophageal fistula, and tracheoinnominate artery fistula (Box 12-1).

A *stenosis* may occur at the level of the tracheostomy stoma or rarely where the tip of the tube impinges on the tracheal mucosa. However, pressure necrosis at the cuff site is responsible for most long-term postintubation complications. If the cuff pressure exceeds capillary pressure, blood supply to the mucosa is compromised, leading to ischemic necrosis. Initially, the mucosa becomes inflamed, followed by ulceration in the mucosa overlying the cartilaginous rings. As the ulcers enlarge, there is increasing exposure of the cartilage, which becomes colonized with bacteria. With further pressure on the wall, necrosis develops, and softening and

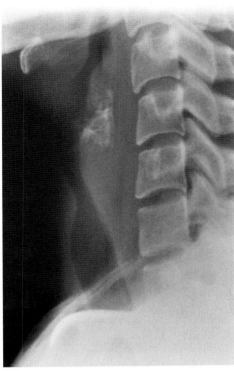

FIGURE 12-7. Idiopathic laryngotracheal stenosis. A lateral view of the soft tissue of the neck reveals a smooth and tapered stenosis of the subglottic larynx and proximal trachea.

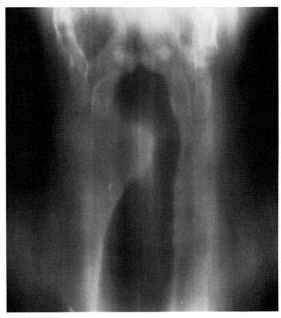

FIGURE 12-8. Idiopathic tracheal stenosis. An anteroposterior tomogram of the larynx and proximal trachea reveals a focal, eccentric, and lobulated stenosis of the proximal trachea.

dissolution of the cartilage lead to tracheomalacia or to scarring and stenosis formation. Radiographically, the stenosis has a smooth, gradual narrowing with an hourglass configuration (Fig. 12-9). Typically, symptoms of stenosis develop in 2 to 6 weeks after extubation and, in some patients, months later. Most stenoses are appropriately treated with resection of the damaged segment and end-to-end anastomosis. In the past 20 years, most tracheostomy and endotracheal tubes have been designed with large-volume, low-pressure cuffs, which has dramatically reduced the incidence of tracheal stricture. Postintubation tracheal strictures continue to occur but at a much reduced rate.

Box 12-1. **Postintubation Injury**

Tracheal stenosis
  At stomal level
  At cuff site (most frequent)
  At tube tip
Tracheoesophageal fistula
Tracheoarterial fistula

Tracheoesophageal fistula may result from ventilation with a cuffed tube, occurring more often when an indwelling esophageal tube is also being used in neurologically impaired patients who are ventilated for a long time. The mechanism of injury is pressure necrosis resulting from pressure exerted by the cuff on the tracheal wall against

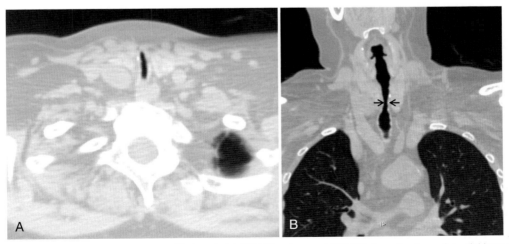

FIGURE 12-9. Postintubation tracheal stenosis due to cuff injury. Axial CT (**A**) and coronal CT (**B**) show the circumferential hour-glass stenosis at the site of tracheostomy.

a foreign body in the esophagus. The injury occurs most often from the cuff on a tracheostomy tube rather than that on an endotracheal tube. The marked inflammatory reaction that ensues causes fusion of the tissue planes. As a result, the fistula enters the esophagus directly, without communication with the mediastinum. The fistula often results in recurrent aspiration pneumonias, which are manifested as patchy parenchymal consolidations (Fig. 12-10) (see Chapter 13).

Most *tracheoarterial fistulas* occur from erosion by the angle of the tube itself. Rarely does the cuff erode the vessel directly.

Posttraumatic Tracheal Stenosis

Tracheal injury is seen in patients with penetrating injuries, in cases of strangulation, and in motor vehicular accidents. Tracheal injury may also occur during surgery and bronchoscopic procedures. If a tracheal tear is incomplete and there is preservation of the peritracheal connective tissue, or if the tear is occluded by a cuff or fibrin deposition, pneumothorax or pneumomediastinum may not be present. Tears that manifest in this fashion may be missed initially and have delayed recognition. If healing ensues, an untreated partial laceration will develop a stenosis with the typical hourglass configuration (Figs. 12-11 and 12-12).

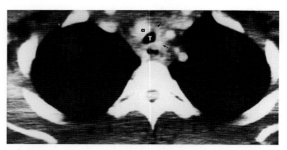

FIGURE 12-11. Posttraumatic tracheal stenosis in a patient with tracheal laceration. Axial CT through the superior mediastinum reveals a narrowed and misshapen tracheal lumen (T). The wall of the trachea is thickened and irregular in its interface with the mediastinum, representing fibrous tissue at the site of laceration *(arrows)*. The innominate artery (a) is closely applied to the tracheal lumen and was found to occlude part of the anterior wall of the trachea at the time of tracheal repair.

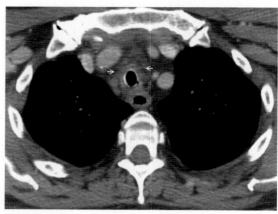

FIGURE 12-12. Posttraumatic tracheal stenosis in a patient who suffered thermal injury during carbon dioxide laser treatment. Axial CT reveals circumferential wall thickening of the trachea with extensive fibrosis and mediastinal fat stranding *(arrows)*.

Saber-Sheath Trachea

Saber-sheath trachea is an abnormality of the intrathoracic trachea that affects men who smoke and have COPD. Typically, there is an abrupt change in the tracheal caliber that begins at the thoracic inlet and that may extend the entire intrathoracic length of the trachea. The trachea is narrowed in the coronal diameter, such that it is no more than one half of the corresponding sagittal diameter (Fig. 12-13). Changes in the configuration of the trachea result from abnormal intrathoracic transmural pressures and chronic cough. The tracheal wall thickness and the main bronchi are normal.

Tracheopathia Osteochondroplastica

Tracheopathia osteochondroplastica is a condition of unknown origin seen in men past the sixth decade of life. Multiple, submucosal osteocartilaginous nodules are deposited along the anterolateral walls of the trachea and cartilage bearing bronchi. The posterior membranous wall is typically spared because of the absence of cartilage in this area, a distinguishing feature in many other diffuse tracheal diseases. The submucosal deposits may cause distortion and narrowing of the airways. Radiographically, the tracheobronchial cartilages are thickened and nodular in appearance, with resultant narrowing of the lumen.

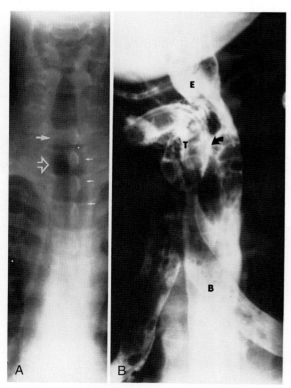

FIGURE 12-10. Tracheoesophageal fistula in a neurologically impaired patient after prolonged mechanical intubation and an indwelling nasogastric tube. **A,** An anteroposterior radiograph of the trachea reveals a tracheal stenosis *(upper arrow)* proximal to a tracheostomy stoma *(open arrow)*. The proximal esophagus is distended with air *(three arrows)* close to the tracheoesophageal fistula. **B,** A contrast esophagram demonstrates filling of the tracheoesophageal fistula *(arrow)* and aspiration of contrast from the esophagus (E) into the trachea (T) and main bronchi (B).

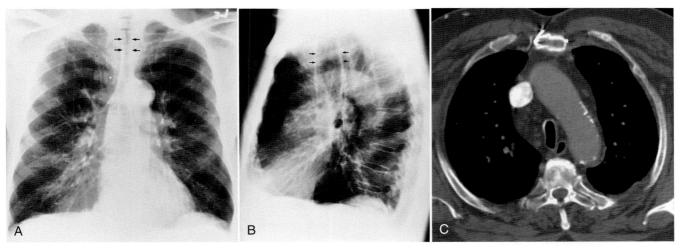

FIGURE 12-13. Saber-sheath trachea. The posteroanterior (**A**) and lateral (**B**) views of the chest reveal hyperinflated lungs. The trachea is narrowed in the coronal plane but increased in diameter in the sagittal plane *(arrows)*. Notice the point of transition from a normal cervical trachea to a narrowed intrathoracic trachea at the thoracic inlet. Axial CT (**C**) in another patient demonstrates decreased transverse and increased anteroposterior diameters.

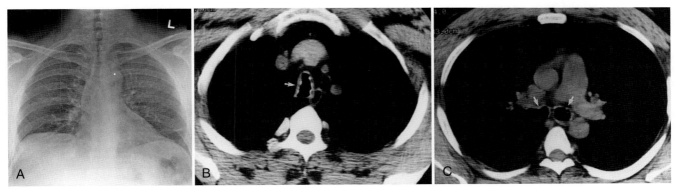

FIGURE 12-14. Tracheopathia osteochondroplastica. A posteroanterior radiograph (**A**) reveals diffuse, irregular narrowing of the cervical and thoracic trachea. CT scans through the trachea (**B**) and main bronchi (**C**) demonstrate nodularity of the anterior and lateral cartilaginous walls of these structures *(arrows)*. Notice the smooth, normal-appearing posterior membranous wall.

Ossification within the nodules can be detected by CT. The membranous wall maintains a normal thin appearance (Fig. 12-14). This condition is usually asymptomatic, but it can cause wheezing, cough, and hemoptysis. There is no associated tracheomalacia.

Relapsing Polychondritis

Relapsing polychondritis is a rare inflammatory disease of unknown origin that affects the cartilages of the ears, nose, upper respiratory tract, and joints. An autoimmune cause is suspected, and there is an association with other connective tissue diseases. Antibodies directed against type 2 collagen have been reported. There is no gender or age predilection, but it is seen commonly between the fifth and sixth decades of life. Recurrent episodes of cartilaginous inflammation result in fragmentation of the cartilages, which are replaced by fibrosis. Auricular chondritis is the most common manifestation. The respiratory tract is affected in approximately 50% of patients, and airway obstruction is the major cause of death.

A spectrum of changes affects the airways. Early in the disease, when mucosal edema is present, the airways become narrowed. As the cartilage dissolves, the airways become more collapsible, and as the destroyed cartilages are replaced by fibrous tissue, fixed stenosis of the airway develops.

The radiographic appearance is that of a diffusely thickened tracheobronchial wall with diffuse, smooth narrowing of the trachea and main bronchi. In addition to the tracheal and main bronchial narrowing, CT demonstrates stenoses involving the segmental and subsegmental bronchi in some cases, and the tracheobronchial walls are thickened (Fig. 12-15). Calcification occasionally develops within the tracheobronchial wall. It is treated with corticosteroids and immunosuppressive therapy.

Wegener's Granulomatosis

Wegener's granulomatosis is an autoimmune, systemic vasculitis diagnosed by demonstrating serum levels of cytoplasmic antineutrophil cytoplasmic antibodies (c-ANCAs). The upper and lower respiratory tracts are most often involved in conjunction with renal and other organ involvement. Laryngeal and subglottic tracheal involvement is characteristic. Diffuse tracheobronchial involvement is rare and usually occurs late in the disease process. Radiographic findings include tracheobronchial luminal narrowing and thickening, as well as an irregularity of the wall that may

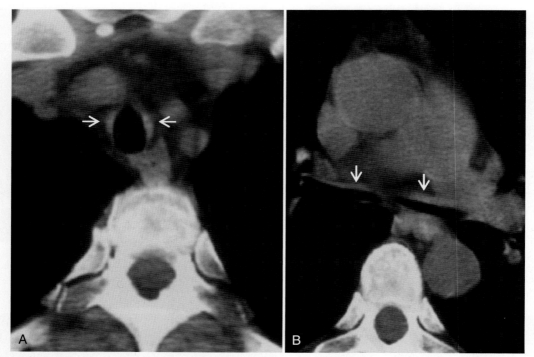

FIGURE 12-15. Relapsing polychondritis. CT scans of the trachea (**A**) and main bronchi (**B**) reveal diffuse, smooth thickening of the cartilaginous wall *(arrows)*. Notice the sparing of the membranous posterior wall.

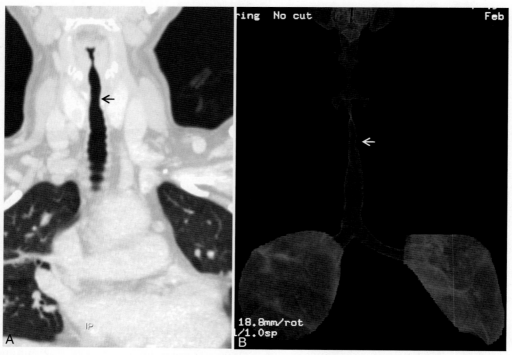

FIGURE 12-16. Wegener's granulomatosis. The coronal CT image (**A**) and three-dimensional external volume-rendering image (**B**) show circumferential stenosis of the subglottic trachea *(arrows)*.

be focal or diffuse (Fig. 12-16). Granulomatous tissue may obstruct a bronchus and cause atelectasis. Associated mediastinal adenopathy often is seen on CT. Enlarged, calcified tracheal cartilages have also been reported. Tracheobronchomalacia is not a feature. The treatment consists of corticosteroids and immunosuppression.

Amyloidosis

Amyloidosis is manifested by the extracellular deposition of an insoluble protein that stains with Congo red. Involvement of the respiratory tract is more commonly seen in the primary form of the disease. Amyloidosis may involve any portion of the respiratory tract in a diffuse or

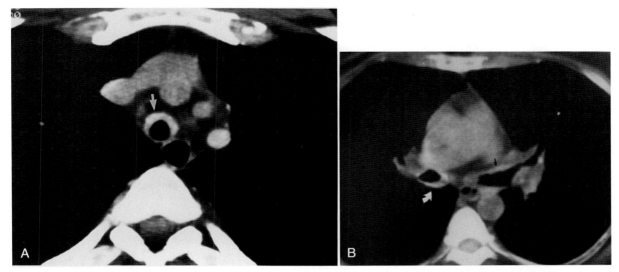

FIGURE 12-17. Diffuse tracheobronchial amyloidosis. CT scans of the trachea (**A**) and bronchi (**B**) at the hilar level reveal diffuse thickening of the trachea and bronchi with slight nodularity of the walls *(black arrow)*. Notice the involvement of the posterior wall of the bronchus intermedius *(white arrow)*.

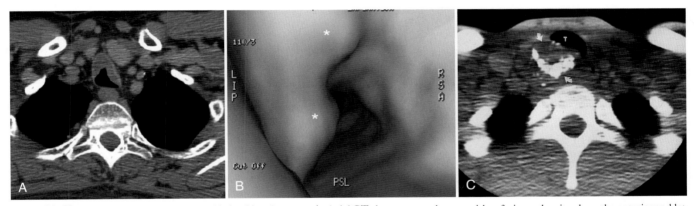

FIGURE 12-18. Amyloidosis of the trachea with focal involvement. **A,** Axial CT shows a smooth mass with soft tissue density along the anterior and lateral walls of the proximal trachea, causing significant luminal narrowing. **B,** The three-dimensional virtual bronchoscopic image reveals protrusion of the submucosal mass *(asterisk)* in to the tracheal lumen, causing stenosis **C,** A large, calcified, soft tissue mass *(arrows)* arising from the right posterolateral wall of the trachea (T) in a different patient is causing stenosis.

focal fashion. Any level of airway can be involved, but distal tracheal and central bronchial involvement is the most common.

Radiographs and CT demonstrate diffuse (Fig. 12-17) or focal (Fig. 12-18) narrowing of the trachea and bronchi by the submucosal amyloid deposits that protrude into and narrow the lumen. The tracheobronchial walls appear thickened (see Fig. 12-18A and B), and there may be calcification or ossification in some lesions (see Fig. 12-18C). Typically, amyloid lesions grow slowly over many years. Associated adenopathy is sometimes present. Focal lesions may enhance with intravenous iodinated contrast on CT or with gadolinium on MRI.

Sarcoidosis

Sarcoidosis is a systemic granulomatous disease of unknown origin. Noncaseous epithelioid granulomas are seen on

biopsy specimens. Airway abnormalities include tracheobronchial mural thickening, which may be smooth, irregular, or nodular; luminal narrowing (Fig. 12-19); and airway compression by lymphadenopathy. Tracheobronchial wall thickening represents granulomas in the bronchial mucosa and along the peribronchovascular interstitium (Fig. 12-20). This accounts for the high diagnostic success of transbronchial biopsy.

Tracheobronchial Papillomatosis

Laryngeal and tracheobronchial papillomatosis is caused by the human papillomavirus types 6 and 11. Histologically, papillomas in the airway are polypoid or sessile masses with central fibrovascular cores and layers of well-differentiated squamous epithelium. Juvenile laryngeal papillomatosis is probably caused by transmission of virus from mother during vaginal delivery, and multiple papillomas are usually

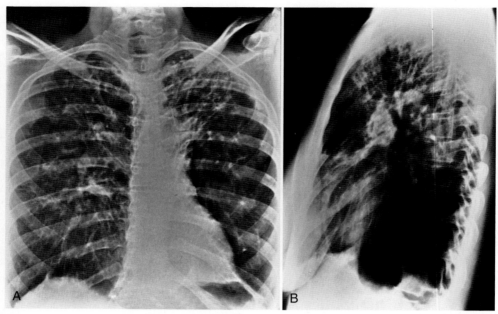

FIGURE 12-19. Tracheal stenosis in sarcoidosis. Posteroanterior (**A**) and lateral (**B**) chest films reveal stenosis of the intrathoracic trachea. Notice the coarse reticular opacities throughout the lungs, particularly in the upper lung zones. There is distortion of the lung parenchyma with upper lobe volume loss and traction bronchiectasis. The lower lobes are hyperinflated.

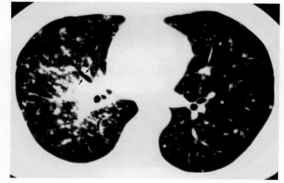

FIGURE 12-20. Sarcoidosis. CT through the lower lung reveals peripheral reticulonodular opacities and pronounced axial interstitial involvement along the bronchovascular interstitium. Notice the irregularity of the bronchi *(arrows)*.

confined to the larynx and upper trachea. In adults, the papillomas may be solitary or multiple and suggests a variable host response to the human papillomavirus. Rarely, papillomas may spread distally to the trachea, bronchi, and lung. Distal disease in the absence of laryngeal disease is more common in adults than in children.

Laryngeal disease manifests with hoarseness and stridor. Patients with disseminated airway disease present with wheezing, atelectasis, or recurrent pneumonia. In the lung, sheets of squamous cells proliferate within alveoli. Central necrosis leads to cavitation. The lesions can transform into invasive squamous cell carcinoma.

Radiographically, diffuse papillomatosis manifests as diffuse nodularity of the involved airway (Fig. 12-21A and B). When the lung is involved, cavitary nodules are typically seen posteriorly in the lower lobes, and they

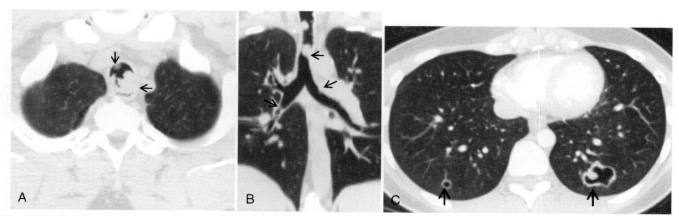

FIGURE 12-21. Diffuse tracheobronchial papillomatosis. Axial (**A**) and coronal (**B**) CT scans of the trachea and bronchi reveal polypoid and sessile masses within the trachea and left main bronchus *(arrows)*; the patient had obstructive symptoms. The axial CT scan (**C**) reveals cavitary nodules in the lower lobes that represent lung involvement *(arrows)*.

may result from aerial dissemination from interventional procedures performed on papillomas (see Fig. 12-21C). Treatment consists of repeated laser or surgical resections of obstructing papillomas in the trachea and proximal bronchi.

Rhinosclerosis

Rhinosclerosis is a chronic granulomatous disorder of the upper respiratory tract that is associated with *Klebsiella rhinoscleromatis*, a gram-negative bacterium. This disease primarily affects the nose, paranasal sinuses, and pharynx. It involves the proximal trachea in less than 10% of patients, but it may involve the entire trachea and bronchi in some patients.

Nodular masses or diffuse, symmetric narrowing may develop and slowly progress over a period of 20 years. An initial catarrhal stage is followed by a nodular stage and a healing stage in which dense fibrous tissue and subsequent stenosis develop.

Tuberculous Tracheobronchial Stenosis

Tuberculous tracheobronchial stenosis may be caused by granulomatous changes in the airway wall or by extrinsic compression by peribronchial and paratracheal lymph nodes. The histopathologic changes include a hyperplastic stage in which tubercles form in the submucosal layer and there is ulceration and necrosis of the wall. Stenosis forms in the fibrostenotic stage that follows. Bronchial involvement may result from contact of the mucosa with infected secretions, especially when parenchymal cavitation is present, or it may result from the submucosal spread of infection through the lymphatics from infected lymph nodes or lung. There is a high prevalence of lymphadenopathy with tuberculous bronchial lesions; this supports the concept of lymphatic spread of infection.

In the hyperplastic stage, the tracheobronchial walls are irregularly thickened with various degrees of luminal narrowing seen on radiographs. Associated hilar or mediastinal lymphadenopathy may demonstrate some contrast enhancement. Thick, irregular cavities may be seen in lobes drained by the affected bronchi (Fig. 12-22).

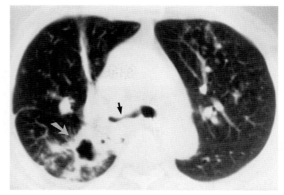

FIGURE 12-22. Bronchial stenosis, hyperplastic stage. CT demonstrates an irregular stenosis of the left upper lobe bronchus *(thin arrow)* with endobronchial granuloma *(arrowhead)*. There is consolidation and cavitation in the left upper lobe *(thick arrow)*.

In the fibrostenotic stage, the stenotic trachea and bronchi may remain thickened, but they have a smooth appearance and associated luminal stenosis (Fig. 12-23). Scarring, calcification, bronchiectasis, and atelectasis are often observed in the lung parenchyma. If the stenosis obstructs, the associated lobe or lung will completely collapse (Fig. 12-24).

■ TRACHEOBRONCHOMEGALY: MOUNIER-KUHN SYNDROME

Mounier-Kuhn syndrome (i.e., tracheobronchomegaly) is a rare condition in which there is diffuse dilation of the trachea and main bronchi. Characteristically, there is an abrupt transition to normal-appearing peripheral airways at the segmental level. The disease occurs primarily in men in their third or fourth decade. The associations with cutis laxis in children and Ehlers-Danlos syndrome and Marfan syndrome in adults suggest an underlying defect in elastic tissue. Thin, atrophied, muscular and elastic tissue is found in the trachea and main bronchi. Forced expiration or cough reveals increased flaccidity and collapsibility. Most patients present in early childhood with recurrent respiratory infections.

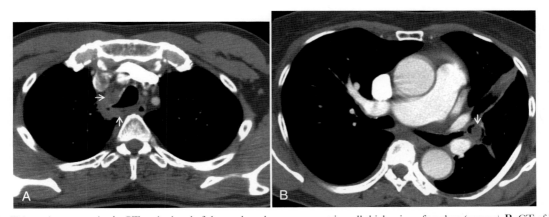

FIGURE 12-23. Tuberculous stenosis. **A,** CT at the level of the trachea shows asymmetric wall thickening of trachea *(arrows)*. **B,** CT of left upper lobe bronchus shows stenosis with an endobronchial granuloma represented by a soft tissue density *(arrow)*. Notice the parenchymal changes in the left upper lobe.

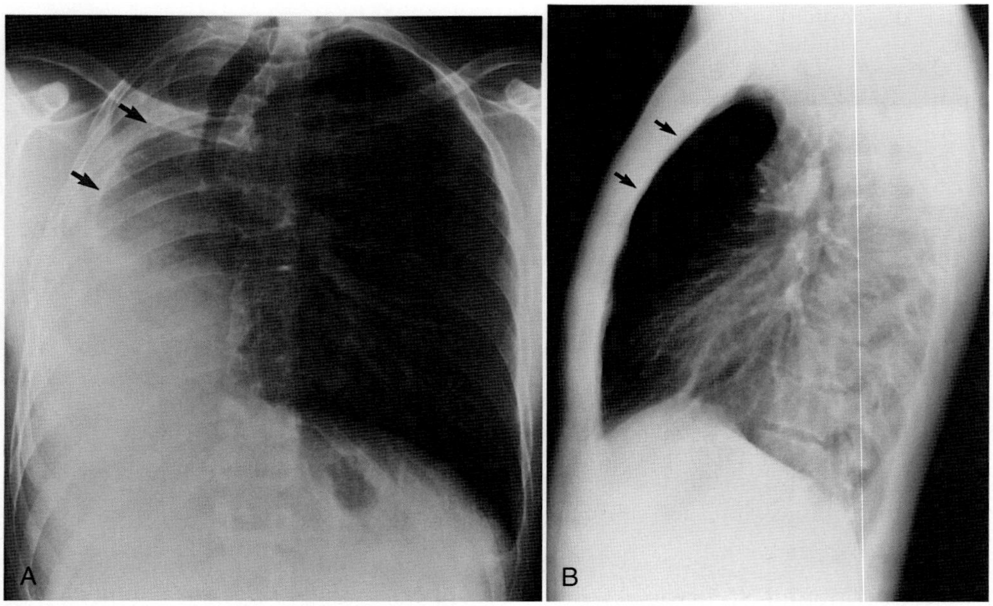

FIGURE 12-24. Tuberculous tracheal stenosis, fibrotic stage. Posteroanterior (**A**) and lateral (**B**) chest radiographs demonstrate a diffuse, smooth stenosis of the trachea and resultant collapse of the right lung. There is compensatory hyperinflation of the left lung and shift of the mediastinum to the right. Notice the herniated left lung into the right hemithorax and anteriorly in the retrosternal space *(arrows)*.

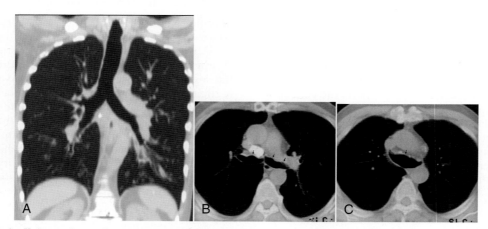

FIGURE 12-25. Mounier-Kuhn syndrome. Coronal, multiplanar reformation CT (**A**) reveals diffuse dilation of the trachea and bronchi, with an abrupt change in caliber at segmental bronchi. Diffuse, cylindrical bronchiectasis and tree-in-bud opacities are also seen. Axial CT scans in a different patient through the trachea (**B**) and main bronchi (**C**) demonstrate pronounced dilation of the trachea and main bronchi and a scalloped appearance of the airway wall due to protrusion of the mucosa *(arrows)* between cartilaginous rings.

The diagnosis of tracheobronchomegaly is usually apparent on chest radiographs, which demonstrate diffuse dilation of the trachea and main bronchi. Typically, the mucosa protrudes through the trachealis muscle between the cartilaginous rings. This finding, which can be detected on conventional tomograms, CT, or MRI, produces a scalloped or corrugated appearance of the trachea and main bronchi. Because patients may have repeated respiratory infections, bronchiectasis also may be present (Fig. 12-25 and Box 12-2).

Box 12-2. Radiographic Findings in Mounier-Kuhn Syndrome

Increased flaccidity and collapsibility of the trachea and bronchi
Diffuse dilation of the trachea and main and lobar bronchi
Protrusion of mucosa between cartilaginous rings
Bronchiectasis

■ TRACHEAL TUMORS

Primary tracheal tumors are approximately one hundred times less common than bronchial tumors. Primary tracheal tumors manifest with equal frequency in men and women, predominately between the ages of 30 and 50 years.

The clinical manifestations of tracheal tumors include shortness of breath and wheezing. These symptoms usually do not appear until the lumen has been reduced to one third of its width or less, because the luminal narrowing is a gradual process. Approximately one third of patients with tracheal tumors are initially mistakenly treated for asthmatic bronchitis or bronchial asthma. Patients with a dyspnea that cannot be unequivocally attributed to cardiac or pulmonary disorders should be evaluated to exclude upper airway obstruction.

Tumors of the trachea can be classified as epithelial, mesenchymal, or lymphomatous. Although 90% of tracheal tumors in children are benign, malignant tumors predominate in adults. The most common benign tracheal tumors include hemangioma, papilloma (see "Tracheobronchial Papillomatosis"), and hamartoma (see Chapter 13). The most common primary malignant tracheal tumors are adenoid cystic carcinoma and squamous cell carcinoma. The most common secondary malignant tumors include esophageal carcinoma and thyroid neoplasms, both of which may cause direct tracheal invasion (Fig. 12-26 and Box 12-3).

Squamous Cell Carcinoma

Squamous cell carcinoma of the trachea accounts for approximately one half of all primary tracheal malignant tumors (Box 12-4). It predominates in male smokers older than 40 years, and it tends to grow slowly and exophytically and commonly ulcerates. Squamous cell carcinoma has a tendency to invade the mediastinum. Synchronous

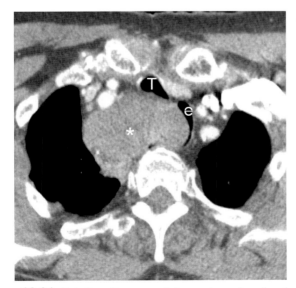

FIGURE 12-26. Spindle cell sarcoma of the esophagus invading the trachea. Axial CT shows a large mass (asterisk) arising from the right lateral wall of esophagus (e) and invading the posterior wall of trachea (T).

Box 12-3. Tracheal Tumors

MOST COMMON BENIGN TUMORS
Hemangioma
Papilloma
Hamartoma

MOST COMMON MALIGNANT TUMORS
Primary
    Squamous cell carcinoma
    Adenoid cystic carcinoma
Secondary
    Esophageal carcinoma
    Thyroid carcinoma

Box 12-4. Squamous Cell Carcinoma of the Trachea

Male smokers older than 40 years
Slow-growing tumors
Exophytic growth
Ulceration
Mediastinal invasion
Synchronous or metachronous tumors of the larynx, lungs, or esophagus

---

and metachronous squamous cell carcinomas of the trachea, larynx, lungs, and esophagus are found in some patients.

Radiographically, the tracheal wall appears focally and circumferentially thickened and irregular. The lumen is secondarily narrowed by the tumor, which may be nodular in appearance and have ulceration. CT is valuable in demonstrating the primary tumor and extension into the adjacent mediastinal fat. Direct extension manifests as an irregular soft tissue opacity within the mediastinal fat or surrounding adjacent mediastinal vessels, bronchi, and esophagus. Lymph nodes that measure 1 cm or more in the short axis should be assessed for metastasis. Localized tumors are best treated with resection. Irradiation is offered for inoperable tumors. Treated patients should be followed with CT to detect recurrences and new tumors in the trachea and lungs (Fig. 12-27).

Adenoid Cystic Carcinoma

Adenoid cystic carcinoma accounts for approximately one third of all primary tracheal malignant tumors (Box 12-5). Adenoid cystic carcinoma is unrelated to smoking, has no gender predilection, and is usually seen in the fifth decade. This tumor arises from mucous glands and usually grows slowly, with endophytic spread extending in the submucosal plane of the trachea and bronchi. On radiographs, the trachea typically has a thickened and smooth or nodular appearance, with associated luminal narrowing (Fig. 12-28). Adenoid cystic carcinoma may spread into the surrounding tissues of the neck and mediastinum; it is seen on CT as a soft tissue extension into the adjacent

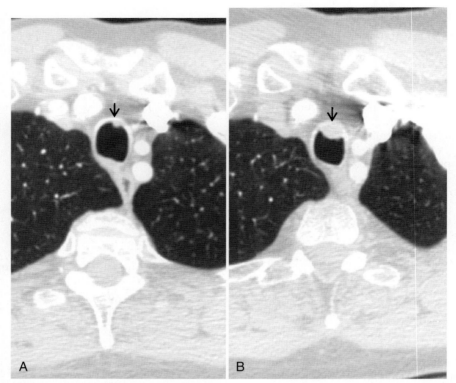

Figure 12-27. Early squamous cell carcinoma of the trachea in a patient with previous squamous cell lung cancer. **A,** Axial CT reveals a small mucosal nodule *(arrow)* in the anterior wall trachea. **B,** Follow-up CT 7 months later shows significant increase in the nodule's size. No extratracheal extension or lymph nodal metastasis was found.

Box 12-5. Adenoid Cystic Carcinoma

Not smoking related
Male and female incidences equal
Peak occurrence in fifth decade
Slow-growing tumors
Endophytic growth with submucosal spread
Mediastinal extension

---

mediastinal fat. Cervical and mediastinal lymph nodes are the first to be involved by metastases. Distant hematogenous metastases to lungs, liver, and bone occur. When the tumor is localized, surgical resection and reconstruction is potentially curative. Adenoid cystic carcinoma is radiosensitive. Radiation therapy is indicated for unresectable tumor. In such cases, the tumor typically recurs several years later.

Benign Tracheal Tumors

Radiographically, a benign tracheal tumor is visualized as a focal, well-defined, smooth or lobulated mass without evidence of contiguous tracheal or mediastinal invasion (Fig. 12-29 and Box 12-6). Benign lesions, such as hamartomas and lipomas, contain fat-density areas. Hamartomas, carcinoids, and chondromas may demonstrate calcification.

In contrast, invasive malignant tracheal tumors may demonstrate contiguous circumferential tracheal wall thickening, direct invasion of adjacent mediastinal fat planes, and lymphadenopathy. Although a more advanced tumor may be readily apparent on chest radiographs as an intraluminal mass or a stenosis, early tracheal tumors are often initially missed on chest x-ray films. Chest CT is ideal for identifying the endoluminal and mediastinal extent of tracheal neoplasms.

TRACHEOBRONCHOMALACIA

Tracheobronchomalacia refers to a weakness in the tracheal or bronchial walls and supporting cartilages, with resultant collapsibility. The flaccidity of the trachea or bronchi is usually most apparent during coughing or forced expiration. Primary malacia is associated with a congenital deficiency of the cartilage. Acquired malacia is caused by intubation, COPD, trauma, infection, and relapsing polychondritis. Focal areas of malacia can develop as a result of large goiters or mediastinal masses, aneurysms, or aberrant pulmonary vessels that compress the trachea or bronchus. Acquired malacia also can be idiopathic (Box 12-7).

The increased flaccidity of the airways results in an inefficient cough mechanism, retained mucus, infection, and bronchiectasis. Fluoroscopy (Fig. 12-30), dynamic CT, or inspiration and expiration CT scans (Fig. 12-31) are the preferred imaging modalities for evaluation. The normal

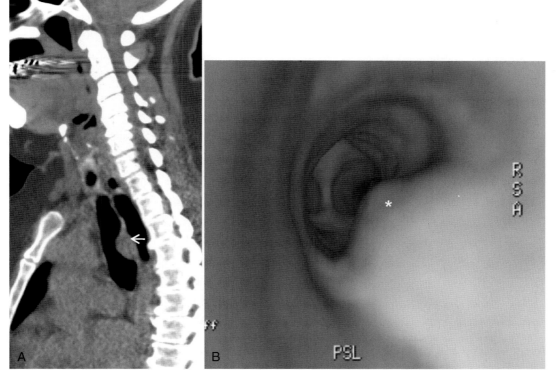

FIGURE 12-28. Adenoid cystic carcinoma of the trachea. **A,** Sagittal CT reveals a lobulated mass in the posterior wall of the trachea *(arrow).* **B,** The three-dimensional bronchoscopic view shows a lobulated surface and luminal narrowing *(asterisk).*

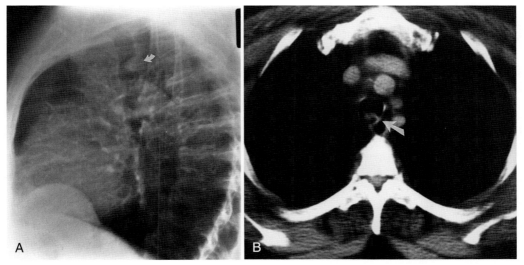

FIGURE 12-29. Solitary benign papilloma of trachea. **A,** The lateral chest radiograph reveals a focal, well-defined, nodular mass *(arrow)* arising from the posterior wall of the trachea. The mass was not apparent on the posteroanterior view. **B,** CT scan through the upper trachea reveals a nodular mass arising from the tracheal wall on a pedicle *(arrow).* There is no evidence for mediastinal invasion.

Box 12-6. **Benign Tracheal Tumors**

Focal mass
Smooth and well-defined margins
No mediastinal invasion

Box 12-7. **Causes of Tracheobronchomalacia**

PRIMARY CAUSE
Congenital deficiency of cartilage

SECONDARY OR ACQUIRED CAUSES
Intubation
Chronic obstructive pulmonary disease
Trauma
Infection
Relapsing polychondritis
Adjacent compression by mediastinal mass or vessel
Idiopathic condition

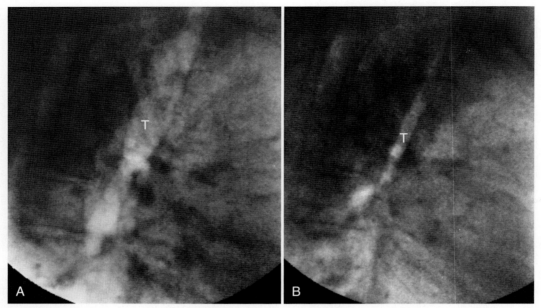

FIGURE 12-30. Tracheobronchomalacia. Lateral views of the trachea during fluoroscopy on inspiration (**A**) and expiration (**B**) reveal collapse of the trachea on forced expiration.

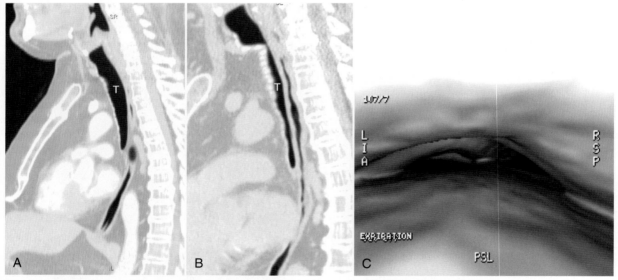

FIGURE 12-31. Tracheobronchomalacia. Sagittal CT scans through the tracheal lumen on inspiration (**A**) and on expiration (**B**) reveal abnormal collapse of the tracheal wall and a pronounced decrease in the tracheal lumen on expiration. The three-dimensional bronchoscopic view (**C**) reveals increased collapsibility of the trachea and main bronchi and a narrowed anteroposterior diameter.

tracheobronchial lumen decreases approximately 10% to 30% with expiration or coughing because of normal invagination of the posterior membranous tracheal wall. A lumen that decreases by more than 50% should be considered abnormal. The treatment options for severe tracheomalacia include stent placement, tracheostomy to bypass the abnormal segment, and tracheoplasty.

▬ SUGGESTED READINGS

Boiselle, P.A., Lee, K.S., Ernst, A., 2005. Multidetector CT of the central airways. J. Thorac. Imaging 20, 186–195.
Buterbaugh, J.E., Erly, W.K., 2008. Paratracheal cysts: A common finding on routine CT examinations of the cervical spine and neck that may mimic pneumomediastinum in patients with traumatic injuries. Am. J. Neuroradiol. 29, 1218–1221.
Case Records of the Massachusetts General Hospital, 1995. Case 1-1995. N. Engl. J. Med. 332, 110–115.
Case Records of the Massachusetts General Hospital, 1992. Case 3-1992. N. Engl. J. Med. 326, 184–191.
Case Records of the Massachusetts General Hospital, 1992. Case 46-1992. N. Engl. J. Med. 327 (21), 1512–1518.
Choe, K.O., Jeong, H.J., Sohn, H.Y., 1990. Tuberculous bronchial stenosis: CT findings in 28 cases. AJR Am. J. Roentgenol. 155, 971–976.
Choplin, R.H., Wehunt, W.D., Theros, E.G., 1983. Diffuse lesions of the trachea. Semin. Roentgenol. 18, 38–50.
Cordier, J.F., Loire, R., Breene, J., 1986. Amyloidosis of the lower respiratory tract. Chest 90, 827–831.
Davis, S.D., Berkmen, Y.M., King, T., 1989. Peripheral bronchial involvement in relapsing polychondritis: demonstration by thin-section CT. AJR Am. J. Roentgenol. 153, 953–954.
Di Benedetto, R.J., Ribaudo, C., 1966. Bronchopulmonary sarcoidosis. Am. Rev. Respir. Dis. 94, 952–958.
Dolan, D.L., Lemmon, G.D., Teitelbaum, S.L., 1966. Relapsing polychondritis. Am. J. Med. 41, 285–299.

Dunne, M.G., Reiner, B., 1988. CT features of tracheobronchomegaly. J. Comput. Assist. Tomogr. 12, 388–391.

Feldman, F., Seaman, W.B., Baker, D.C., 1967. The roentgen manifestations of scleroma. AJR Am. J. Roentgenol. 101, 807–813.

Ferretti, G.R., Vining, D.J., Knoplioch, J., et al., 1996. Tracheobronchial tree: three-dimensional spiral CT with bronchoscopic perspective. J. Comput. Assist. Tomogr. 20, 777–781.

Fraser, R.G., Paré, J.A.P., Paré, P.D., et al. (Eds.), 1990. Diagnosis of Diseases of the Chest, vol. 3. WB Saunders, Philadelphia.

Grillo, H.C., 1983. Tracheal tumors. In: Choi, N.C., Grillo, H.C. (Eds.), Thoracic Oncology. Lippincott-Raven, New York.

Handousa, P., Elivi, A.M., 1958. Some clinicopathological observations on scleroma. J. Laryngol. Otol. 72, 32–47.

Im, J.G., Chung, J.W., Han, S.K., et al., 1988. CT manifestations of tracheobronchial involvement in relapsing polychondritis. J. Comput. Assist. Tomogr. 12, 792–793.

Jokinen, K., Palva, T., Nuutinen, J., 1977. Bronchial findings in pulmonary tuberculosis. Clin. Otolaryngol. 2, 139–148.

Katz, M., Konen, E., Rozenman, J., et al., 1995. Spiral CT and 3D image reconstruction of vascular rings and associated tracheobronchial anomalies. J. Comput. Assist. Tomogr. 19, 564–568.

Katz, I., LeVine, M., Herman, P., 1962. Tracheobroncheomegaly: the Mounier-Kuhn syndrome. Am J. Roentgenol. Radium. Ther. Nucl. Med. 88, 1084–1094.

Kauczor, H.U., Wolcke, B., Fischer, B., et al., 1996. Three-dimensional helical CT of the tracheobronchial tree: evaluation of imaging protocols and assessment of suspected stenoses with bronchoscopic correlation. AJR Am. J. Roentgenol. 167, 419–424.

Kwong, J.S., Müller, N.L., Miller, R.R., 1992. Diseases of the trachea and mainstem bronchi: correlation of CT with pathologic findings. Radiographics 12, 645–657.

Lenique, F., Brauner, M.W., Grenier, P., et al., 1995. CT assessment of bronchi in sarcoidosis: endoscopic and pathologic correlations. Radiology 194, 419–423.

McAdam, L.P., O'Hanlan, M.A., Bluestone, R., Pearson, C.M., 1976. Relapsing polychondritis: prospective study of 23 patients and a review of the literature. Medicine (Baltimore) 55, 193–215.

Mendelson, D.S., Norton, K., Cohen, B.A., et al., 1983. Bronchial compression: an unusual manifestation of sarcoidosis. J. Comput. Assist. Tomogr. 7, 892–894.

Mendelson, D.S., Som, P.M., Crane, R., et al., 1985. Relapsing polychondritis studied by computed tomography. Radiology 157, 489–490.

Miller, R.H., Shulman, J.B., Canalis, R.F., et al., 1979. Klebsiella rhinoscleromatis: a clinical and pathogenic enigma. Otolaryngol. Head Neck Surg. 87, 212–221.

Mounier-Khun, P., 1932. Dilatation de la trachee: constellations radiographiques et bronchosopiques. Lyon Med. 150, 106–109.

Newmark, G.M., Conces Jr., D.J., Kopecky, K.K., 1994. Spiral CT evaluation of the trachea and bronchi. J. Comput. Assist. Tomogr. 18, 552–554.

Onitsuka, H., Hirose, N., Watanabe, K., 1983. Computed tomography of tracheopathia osteoplastica. AJR Am. J. Roentgenol. 140, 268–270.

Poe, R.H., Utell, M.J., Israel, R.H., et al., 1979. Sensitivity and specificity of the nonspecific transbronchial lung biopsy. Am. Rev. Respir. Dis. 119, 25–31.

Quint, L.E., Whyte, R.I., Kazerooni, E.A., et al., 1995. Stenosis of the central airways: evaluation by using helical CT with multiplanar reconstructions. Radiology 194, 871–877.

Salkin, D., Cadden, A.V., Edson, R.C., 1943. The natural history of tuberculous tracheobronchitis. Am. Rev. Respir. Dis. 47, 351–369.

Sharma, O.P., 1978. Airway obstruction in sarcoidosis. Chest 73, 6–7.

Shepard, J.O., Grillo, H.C., Bhalla, M., et al., 1994. Inspiratory-expiratory chest CT in evaluation of large airway disease. Paper presented at the Radiological Society of North America Meeting, Chicago, Ill. Radiology 193(P), 181.

Shin, M.S., Jackson, R.M., Ho, K.J., 1988. Tracheobronchomegaly (Mounier-Kuhn syndrome): CT diagnosis. AJR Am. J. Roentgenol. 150, 777–779.

Spizarny, D.L., Shepard, J.O., McLoud, T.C., et al., 1986. CT of adenoid cystic carcinoma of the trachea. AJR Am. J. Roentgenol. 146, 1129–1132.

Stern, M.G., Gamsu, G., Webb, W.R., Stulbarg, M.S., 1986. Computed tomography of diffuse tracheal stenosis in Wegener granulomatosis. J. Comput. Assist. Tomogr. 10, 868–870.

Unger, J.M., Schuchman, G.G., Grossman, J.E., Pellett, J.R., 1989. Tears of the trachea and main bronchi caused by blunt trauma: radiologic findings. AJR Am. J. Roentgenol. 153, 1175–1180.

Urban, B.A., Fishman, E.K., Goldman, S.M., et al., 1993. CT evaluation of amyloidosis: spectrum of disease. Radiographics 13, 1295–1308.

Whyte, R.I., Quint, L.E., Kazerooni, E.A., et al., 1995. Helical computed tomography for the evaluation of tracheal stenosis [abstract]. Radiology 197 (883).

Zeiberg, A.S., Silverman, P.M., Sessions, R.B., et al., 1996. Helical (spiral) CT of the upper airway with three-dimensional imaging: technique and clinical assessment. AJR Am. J. Roentgenol. 166, 293–299.

CHAPTER 13

The Bronchi

Subba R. Digumarthy and Jo-Anne O. Shepard

ANATOMY AND TERMINOLOGY

The airways are categorized as purely conducting and gas-exchanging regions, with a transitional zone in between. Air reaches the gas-exchanging units of lungs from nasal and oral cavities through the conducting tracheobronchial airways. The *trachea* divides into two primary or *main bronchi*, which divide into the *lobar bronchi*, which branch further to become the *segmental* and *intrapulmonary bronchi* and *bronchioles*. There are about 23 divisions from the trachea to the alveoli. The bronchioles are seen after 6 to 20 divisions from the segmental bronchus. The bronchi contain cartilage in their walls, whereas the bronchioles lack cartilage. The last generation of purely conducting airways is the *terminal bronchiole*. The *respiratory bronchioles* are the transitional branches that lead to gas-exchanging *alveolar ducts*, *alveolar sacs*, and *alveoli*. An *acinus* is lung parenchyma distal to a terminal bronchiole, and it is composed of two to five generations of respiratory bronchioles, alveolar ducts, alveolar sacs, and alveoli. Airways that are less than 2 mm in diameter are called *small airways*.

The *secondary pulmonary lobule* is the smallest portion of the lung that is surrounded by connective tissue septa. It contains three to five acini, has a polyhedral shape, and is 10 to 25 mm in diameter. It is most visible in the subpleural portion of the lung on computed tomography (CT) and is best seen at the lung apices and lung bases. A lobular bronchiole and a pulmonary artery branch are found in the center of the lobule. Pulmonary veins and lymphatics are found in the peripheral interlobular septa. The limit of CT visibility for a small bronchus is 2 mm. Lobular bronchioles are beyond the limit of CT visibility because they are less than 1 mm in diameter and their walls are less than 0.1 mm thick. Lobular bronchioles branch into three or more terminal bronchioles. Each terminal bronchiole supplies one acinus.

EVALUATION

Computed Tomography Technique

The best CT technique for evaluating the central bronchi is to obtain 1- to 2.5-mm multiplanar images using multidetector CT. The isotropic data set obtained with multidetector CT has the same resolution in all imaging planes, and artifacts seen with image reconstruction using single-row detector CT can be avoided. Multiplanar images are important because they allow visualization of the full length of the bronchi in a single plane. If single-row detector CT is used, contiguous, overlapping, 2.5- to 5-mm scans through the hilar regions should be obtained. All of the normal lobar and segmental bronchi should be identified routinely by this technique. Occasionally, evaluation of small and obliquely oriented bronchi, such as the lingular bronchus, may necessitate scanning with angling of the gantry in the plane of the bronchus.

High-resolution CT (HRCT) is the preferred technique for the evaluation of bronchiectasis and bronchiolitis. For HRCT, 1- to 1.5-mm collimation, 10-mm intervals, and reconstruction with an edge-enhancing algorithm (i.e., bone) should be used. A window level of 700 Hounsfield units (HU) and window width of 1000 to 1500 HU is recommended. Modern CT scanners allow retrospective reconstruction of HRCT images from data acquired for regular chest CT. Paired inspiratory and expiratory scans performed at identical table levels are used to evaluate bronchomalacia and air trapping in patients with small airways disease, such as obliterative bronchiolitis. Measurement of attenuation values is useful in identifying fat in hamartomas and calcification in endobronchial hamartomas, chondromas, carcinoid tumors, and broncholiths. CT pixel histogram analysis allows measurement of fat not seen macroscopically.

Magnetic Resonance Imaging Technique

Magnetic resonance imaging (MRI) of the bronchi is not routinely performed because the spatial and temporal resolution is inferior to that of CT. The MR signal, which depends on the proton density, is also weak in the lungs due to the low density of air. The weak signal also decays rapidly because of magnetic susceptibility artifacts from air-tissue interfaces, and the lungs appear dark. However, MRI does not involve ionizing radiation and has better contrast resolution compared with CT. Interest has developed in functional imaging using hyperpolarized gas. Gases such as helium (He) are hyperpolarized using a process called optical pumping. This brings the nuclear spins of the gas atoms in to significant alignment, and when inhaled during scanning, the hyperpolarized gas causes a strong MR signal. Despite the low density of gas, the lungs appear bright. This method has shown ventilation defects in patients with obstructive airway disease even when pulmonary function tests were normal. These techniques are available in only few centers and continue to be evaluated.

Bronchial Anomalies

Bronchial anomalies include abnormal origin, supernumerary bronchi, bronchial atresia, and bronchial isomerism. A cardiac bronchus is a supernumerary bronchus that is seen in 0.1% of population (Box 13-1). The bronchus arises from the medial aspect of the bronchus intermedius and extends medially toward the heart (Fig. 13-1). The bronchus may end in a blind stump or supply a segment of lung; this is mostly an incidental finding. However, the blind ending bronchus may be a potential reservoir of infection and lead to recurrent infections and hemoptysis. If the patient is symptomatic, surgical resection is the treatment. Other bronchial anomalies are discussed in Chapter 2.

Box 13-1. **Cardiac Bronchus**

Supernumerary bronchus from the medial aspect of
the bronchus intermedius
Incidence of 0.1% to 0.5%
May end blindly or supply a segment of lung
Blind pouch may predispose to recurrent infection
and hemoptysis

ENDOBRONCHIAL LESIONS

Broncholithiasis

Broncholithiasis is a condition in which calcified material within a bronchus or adjacent to a bronchus distorts
the lumen. Broncholiths usually arise from calcified peribronchial lymph nodes that erode in to the adjacent bronchi. Most are caused by *Histoplasma capsulatum* infection.
However, other fungal infections, tuberculosis, sarcoidosis,
or silicosis may predispose the patient to broncholithiasis. Rarely, a neglected endobronchial foreign body may
calcify.

Patients present with hemoptysis, wheezing, and cough.
Coughing up stones (i.e., lithoptysis) is a rare but diagnostic sign.

Radiographically, the key finding is a calcified endobronchial lesion or peribronchial lymph node without associated soft tissue, which may be associated with findings of
bronchial obstruction such as atelectasis, postobstructive
pneumonia, and air trapping (Box 13-2 and Fig. 13-2).

Aspiration of a Solid Foreign Body

Most aspirated foreign bodies occur in children younger
than 10 years, and 50% occur in children younger than 3
years. Aspirated foreign bodies in adults are often seen in
patients with altered mental status or poor dentition. Most
are of vegetable origin, such as peanuts, or result from bro-
ken teeth or dental fixtures. Foreign bodies are usually

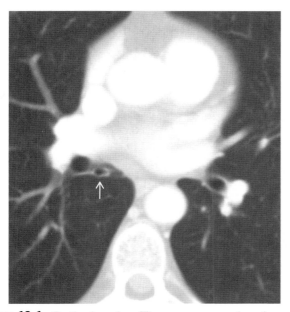

FIGURE 13-1. Cardiac bronchus. The supernumerary bronchus arises from the medial aspect of the bronchus intermedius *(arrow)* and courses toward the heart.

Box 13-2. **Findings for Broncholithiasis**

Calcified lymph node with peribronchial location
or erosion into the bronchus
Secondary findings of obstruction
No soft tissue mass

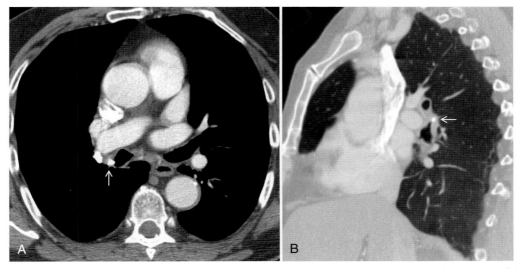

FIGURE 13-2. Broncholithiasis. Axial CT (**A**) and sagittal CT (**B**) scans show a calcified broncholith in the superior segment of the right lower lobe *(arrow)*. Notice the calcified right hilar node.

aspirated into the lower lobe bronchi. Aspirations into the right side are more common because of the more direct angle of the right main bronchus with the trachea.

Air trapping is the most common finding after acute aspiration of a foreign body because of a check-valve mechanism of bronchial obstruction. Air trapping may not be apparent on inspiration, but it is apparent on expiratory radiographs, expiratory CT scans, and decubitus chest radiographs. On expiration, the lung becomes more opaque. Similarly, on decubitus radiographs, the dependent lung is hypoinflated and therefore more opaque. If air trapping is present, the obstructed lobe or lung will remain lucent and not decrease in volume on expiration, or if the affected lung is in a more dependent position, the mediastinum will shift away from the side of air trapping

(Fig. 13-3). Hypoxic vasoconstriction may develop within an obstructed lobe or lung; it manifests radiographically as a hyperlucency of the lung and attenuation of the pulmonary vessels (Fig. 13-4). In adults, aspirated foreign bodies may remain clinically silent. In cases of chronic obstruction, atelectasis, recurrent pneumonia, intrabronchial mass, hemoptysis, or bronchiectasis may develop (Box 13-3). CT can identify the endobronchial site of an aspirated foreign body and demonstrate air trapping. A high-density foreign body suggests bone, metallic foreign body, or a tooth (Fig. 13-5). Vegetable material has soft tissue density and occasionally has fat density (Fig. 13-6). MRI may be helpful in identifying aspirated peanuts, which characteristically have a high-intensity signal on T1-weighted images.

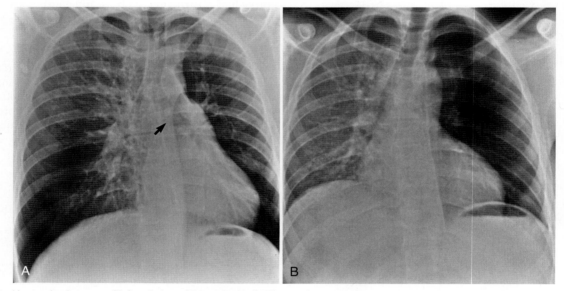

Figure 13-3. Air trapping in a case of left main bronchial carcinoid. **A,** The inspiratory chest radiograph reveals an oval lesion obstructing the left main bronchus *(arrow)*, hyperlucency of the left lung, and attenuation of the left pulmonary vasculature due to hypoxic vasoconstriction. There is slight volume loss in the left lung, with a shift of the mediastinum to the left. **B,** The expiratory chest radiograph demonstrates a normal decrease in right lung volume, elevation of the right diaphragm, shift of the mediastinum to the right, and crowding of right pulmonary vessels. There is hyperlucency and diffuse air trapping in the left lung without a change in lung volume.

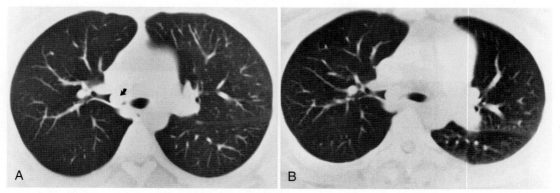

Figure 13-4. Air trapping in a case of carcinoid tumor. **A,** The inspiratory CT scan demonstrates an obstructing carcinoid tumor in the right upper lobe bronchus *(arrow)*. The right lung is more lucent than the left lung due to vascular attenuation from hypoxic vasoconstriction. **B,** The expiratory CT scan demonstrates a normal decrease in the left lung volume and increased attenuation of the left lung. The right lung remains inflated and lucent.

Box 13-3. Findings for Bronchial Obstruction

Air trapping
Hypoxic vasoconstriction with oligemia
Atelectasis
Pneumonia
Bronchiectasis

Bronchial Neoplasms

Hamartoma

Hamartoma is the most common benign tumor of the lung, accounting for 77% of tumors in a series by Arrigoni. Approximately 3% to 10% of these tumors arise within the bronchi. Bronchial hamartomas are slow-growing tumors seen within large bronchi. They contain normal components

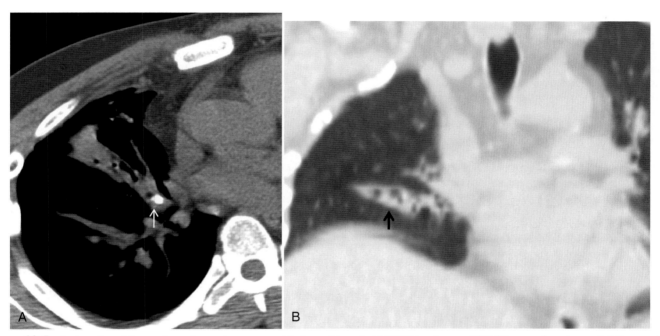

FIGURE 13-5. Aspirated tooth in a patient who was in a motor vehicular accident. Axial CT (**A**) and coronal CT (**B**) scans show the tooth *(thin arrow)* in the right middle lobe bronchus that is causing middle lobe atelectasis *(thick arrow)*.

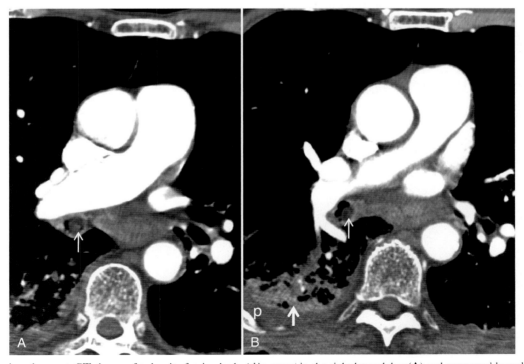

FIGURE 13-6. Aspirated peanut. CT shows a fat-density foreign body *(thin arrow)* in the right lower lobar (**A**) and segmental bronchi (**B**). Notice the distal pneumonia *(thick arrow)* and pleural effusion (p).

of bronchi, such as cartilage, fat, fibrous tissue, and epithelium, arranged in a disorganized fashion. The appearance of fat or characteristic popcorn calcification on CT suggests the diagnosis. Calcification is present in approximately 25% of hamartomas and is more common in larger lesions. Signs of bronchial obstruction such as collapse or recurrent pneumonia may be seen (Box 13-4 and Fig, 13-7).

Carcinoid Tumors

Carcinoid tumors originate from bronchial Kulchitsky (argentaffin) cells and are classified as neuroendocrine tumors of the lung. The Kulchitsky cell contains neurosecretory granules capable of producing serotonin, adrenocorticotropic hormone, bradykinin, and others substances. Based on the aggressiveness, these tumors are classified as typical (classic) carcinoid, atypical carcinoid, and small cell carcinoma.

The main clinical differences among typical carcinoid, atypical carcinoid, and small cell carcinoma lie in the prevalence of metastases and in the prognosis (Box 13-5). *Typical carcinoids* manifest in patients at an earlier age, usually 40 to 50 years. They are usually smooth, round, well-defined, small (<2.5 cm) masses that arise in the central bronchi (Fig. 13-8). There is a predilection for women, and they are not associated with smoking. Most carcinoids arise with the main, lobar, or segmental bronchi. Only 10% of carcinoids are seen in the periphery of the lung (Fig. 13-9). These tumors have an excellent prognosis, with 5-year survival rates of 90% to 95%. *Atypical carcinoids* are diagnosed in patients between 50 and 60 years old and are more common in men and smokers. They tend to be larger at diagnosis, may be centrally or peripherally located, and have a tendency to metastasize to hilar or mediastinal lymph nodes (Fig. 13-10). The 5-year survival rate is between 50% and 70%. *Small cell carcinoma* manifests in patients between 60 and 70 years old and is four times more common in men. The tumors commonly metastasize and have a strong association with smoking. These extremely malig-

---

Box 13-4. Bronchial Hamartomas

Slow-growing lesions
Most in the lung periphery; a few found within large bronchi
CT identification of fat aids diagnosis
Calcification seen in 25%

Box 13-5. Neuroendocrine Tumors of the Lung

TYPICAL CARCINOID
Affects women more than men
Peak occurrence between 40 and 50 years of age
Not associated with smoking
Round, smooth, well-defined nodule
Location: 90% in central bronchi, 10% in lung periphery
No tendency to metastasize
Five-year survival rate of 90% to 95%

ATYPICAL CARCINOID
Affects men more than women
Peak occurrence between 50 and 60 years of age
Associated with smoking
Larger nodule than the typical carcinoid
Central or peripheral location
Metastasis to hilar and mediastinal nodes
Five-year survival rate of 50% to 70%

SMALL CELL CARCINOMA
Affects men much more than women
Peak occurrence between 60 and 70 years of age
Strong association with smoking
Small, peripheral lung nodule often seen on CT
Bulky hilar and mediastinal adenopathy
Extrathoracic metastases common
Five-year survival rate of 5%

---

nant tumors are most often associated with bulky hilar and mediastinal adenopathy. A small, peripheral nodule representing the primary tumor is often found on CT. These tumors carry a poor prognosis.

Imaging studies may identify several distinguishing features of carcinoid tumors (Box 13-6). They are well-defined endobronchial tumors that may have extrabronchial extension. Calcification is seen in up to 40% of these tumors on CT (see Fig. 13-8). These highly vascular tumors demonstrate marked contrast enhancement with iodinated contrast on CT (see Fig. 13-9) and with gadolinium on MRI. Somatostatin receptors have been identified in a wide variety of human tumors with neuroendocrine characteristics, including carcinoid tumors. ^{123}I-Tyr$_3$-octreotide and ^{111}In-octreotide are radionuclide-coupled somatostatin analogues that can be used to visualize somatostatin

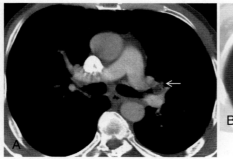
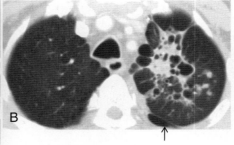

FIGURE 13-7. Endobronchial hamartoma. CT shows a fat-density lesion *(arrow)* in the left upper lobe bronchus (**A**) and postobstructive pneumonia (**B**) with cavities, bronchiectasis and loss of volume. Notice the displaced and elevated major fissure *(arrow)*.

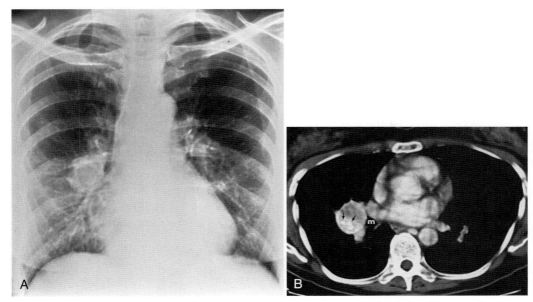

FIGURE 13-8. Right middle lobe typical carcinoid tumor. **A,** The radiograph shows a round, well-defined, right hilar mass. **B,** On contrast-enhanced CT, the mass obstructs the right middle lobe bronchus (m). The tumor demonstrates heterogeneous enhancement and calcification *(arrows)*.

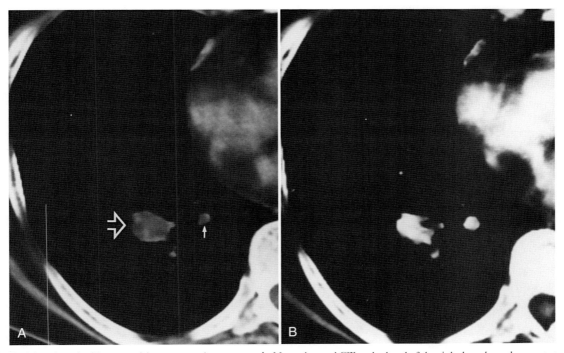

FIGURE 13-9. Peripheral carcinoid tumor with contrast enhancement. **A,** Nonenhanced CT at the level of the right lung base demonstrates a soft tissue nodule *(open arrow)* lateral to a small lower lobe pulmonary artery *(small arrow)*. **B,** After contrast administration, there is dense, uniform enhancement of the carcinoid tumor.

receptor–bearing tumors (Fig. 13-11). Known tumor sites have been visualized in 86% of patients in whom histologically confirmed carcinoids were present.

Endobronchial carcinoids often manifest with distal pneumonia, atelectasis, or bronchiectasis. Hemoptysis also is a common finding because of the increased vascularity of these tumors. Several clinical syndromes are associated with secreted neuroendocrine substances. The carcinoid and Cushing syndromes are most common, but they still are seen in only a minority of patients, accounting for about

5% of tumors. Other conditions such as Zollinger-Ellison syndrome and acromegaly are rare.

Mucoepidermoid Tumors

Mucoepidermoid tumors are uncommon, representing 0.2% of all lung tumors and 1% to 5% of bronchial tumors. These tumors resemble salivary gland tumors, and as the name implies, they contain squamous and mucus-secreting columnar cells. The mean age of patients at presentation is 36 years. There is no sex predilection, and smoking is

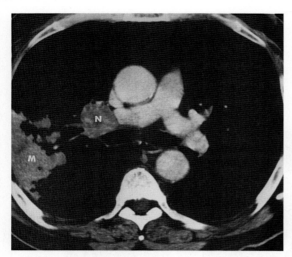

FIGURE 13-10. Atypical carcinoid tumor. A contrast-enhanced CT scan demonstrates an irregular, peripheral mass (M) in the right upper lobe and abutting the pleura. There is a partially enhancing metastatic right hilar lymph node mass (N).

Box 13-6. **Imaging Features of Carcinoid Tumors**

Slow-growing tumors
Calcification
Marked contrast enhancement
Octreotide uptake
Nodule or mass within a central bronchus associated
  with atelectasis, pneumonia, or bronchiectasis
Occur as a peripheral, solitary pulmonary nodule in
  10% of patients

---

not a risk factor. Mucoepidermoid tumors of the central airways may be high- or low-grade malignancies. The radiograph usually shows a focal endobronchial mass within a large central airway, and it may be associated with bronchial obstruction (Fig. 13-12).

FIBROSING MEDIASTINITIS

Fibrosing mediastinitis is a rare disorder of the mediastinum characterized by an exuberant proliferation of fibrous tissue that replaces mediastinal fat. It is most commonly a complication of a granulomatous mediastinitis resulting from infection by *H. capsulatum* or *Mycobacterium tuberculosis*. It is also associated with the use of drugs such as methysergide, with autoimmune disorders, and with idiopathic conditions. The mediastinal structures, such as the trachea, main bronchi, esophagus, superior vena cava, and pulmonary veins and arteries, are encased, invaded, and narrowed by the fibrous tissue. Structures with thin walls and long mediastinal courses are affected the most. Complications may include tracheobronchial stenosis, superior vena caval obstruction, esophageal obstruction, pulmonary artery occlusion, and obstruction of the pulmonary veins and thoracic duct.

Patients with fibrosing mediastinitis most often have cough, dyspnea, and hemoptysis. The most common radiologic finding is widening of the mediastinum and replacement of mediastinal fat by soft tissue density (Box 13-7). Calcification or calcified nodes may be identified within the mediastinal fibrosis, particularly on CT (Fig. 13-13). The mediastinal fibrosis typically encases and narrows affected mediastinal and hilar structures, including the bronchi. Contrast-enhanced CT or MRI is necessary to assess the vascular patency of the superior vena cava and the pulmonary veins and arteries.

If tracheobronchial obstruction is localized, surgical resection and reconstruction may be curative. In most cases, the obstruction is diffuse, and there is no effective treatment.

ESOPHAGOTRACHEOBRONCHIAL FISTULAS

Esophagotracheobronchial fistulas may be congenital or acquired (Box 13-8). Congenital esophagotracheobronchial fistulas are discussed in Chapter 2. Most acquired fistulas result from tumors of the esophagus, tracheobronchial tree,

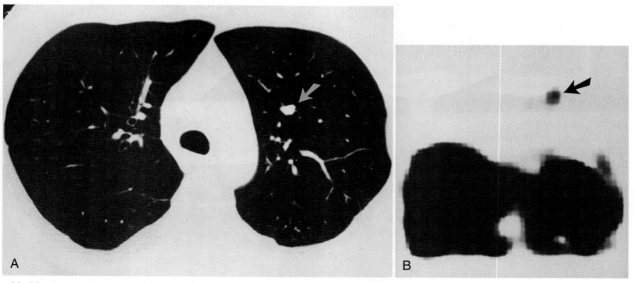

FIGURE 13-11. Octreotide uptake within a carcinoid tumor. **A,** CT demonstrates a 6-mm, left upper lobe nodule *(arrow)*. **B,** Octreotide uptake occurs within the carcinoid tumor in the left upper lobe *(arrow)*.

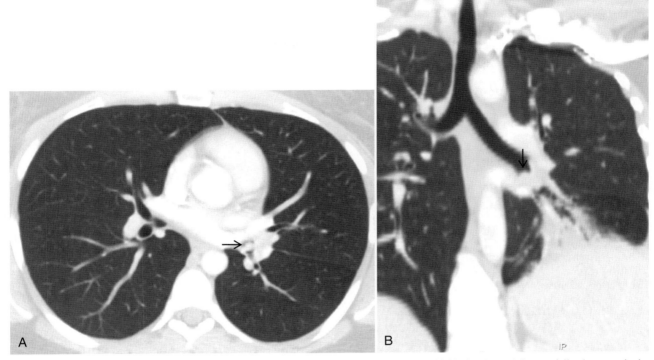

FIGURE 13-12. Mucoepidermoid tumor in a 37-year-old woman. **A,** Axial CT shows an endobronchial lesion *(arrow)* that partially obstructs the lumen. **B,** Coronal CT shows a nodular lesion that obstructs the left lower lobe bronchus *(arrow)*, distal obstructive pneumonia, and atelectasis. Notice the elevation of the left hemidiaphragm and downward displacement of the major fissure.

Box 13-7. Radiographic Features of Fibrosing Mediastinitis

Widened mediastinum
Replacement of mediastinal fat with soft tissue
  density of fibrosis
Calcification within mediastinal fibrosis and nodes
Encasement and narrowing of hilar and mediastinal
  structures

---

thyroid gland, and mediastinal nodes. Infection, trauma, and radiation are the chief causes of nonmalignant esophagotracheobronchial fistulas. Infections include histoplasmosis, tuberculosis, actinomycosis, and syphilis. Esophageal Crohn's disease is also a cause of fistula. Erosion of calcareous particles from peribronchial lymph nodes in which the infectious process is no longer active can also lead a fistula, particularly in cases of histoplasmosis.

The typical complaint of these patients is a strangulating sensation occurring immediately after ingestion

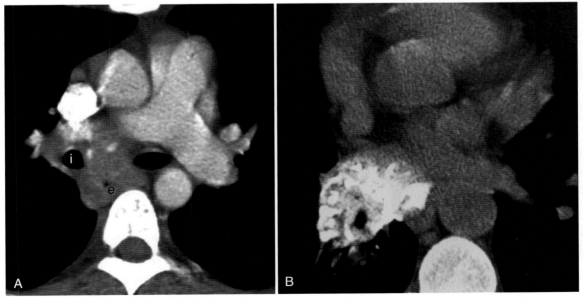

FIGURE 13-13. Fibrosing mediastinitis due to histoplasmosis in two patients. **A,** Calcified right paratracheal and subcarinal mediastinal tissue encases the right bronchus intermedius (i) and esophagus (e). **B,** Calcified right hilar mass encases and narrows the right lower lobe bronchus.

Box 13-8. **Esophagotracheobronchial Fistula**

CONGENITAL FISTULAS

ACQUIRED FISTULAS

Malignant tumors
    Esophageal
    Tracheobronchial
    Thyroid
    Lymph node
Infectious causes
    Histoplasmosis (most common)
    Tuberculosis
    Actinomycosis
    Syphilis
    HIV-related esophagitis
Traumatic injury
    Penetrating
    Long-standing endotracheal and nasogastric tubes
Radiation injury
Miscellaneous causes
    Crohn's disease

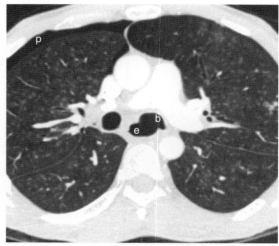

FIGURE 13-15. Esophagobronchial fistula in a patient with human immunodeficiency virus (HIV) infection after esophagitis and instrumentation. The large fistula lies between the esophagus (e) and left main bronchus (b). Notice the diffuse centrilobular and tree-in-bud nodules due to aspiration-related bronchiolitis. There is also a small pneumothorax (p).

of solids or liquids. Routine chest radiography does not disclose the presence of the fistula, but may reveal pneumonia or bronchiectasis related to recurrent aspiration pneumonias, particularly in the lower lobes. Occasionally, a nasogastric tube entering the tracheobronchial tree through the esophageal orifice is seen. Early diagnosis can be established with the judicious use of a contrast esophagogram (Fig. 13-14). High-osmolar contrast should be avoided because of the risk of pulmonary edema if contrast reaches the lungs. CT scan is useful in demonstrating the fistula and in evaluating

causative pathology and associated findings and complications (Fig. 13-15). Bronchoscopy and esophagoscopy can confirm the presence and site of fistulous communication and enable histologic, cytologic, and bacteriologic studies. The instillation of methylene blue in the esophagus during bronchoscopy may help to identify small fistulas.

The treatment of choice is direct surgical isolation of the fistula with diversion and closure. Esophageal stent placement is performed for malignancies.

BRONCHIECTASIS

Bronchiectasis is defined as abnormal dilation of the bronchi. It is not a single disease entity but an anatomic abnormality that may be the result of many underlying conditions (Box 13-9). Infection is the most common cause of bronchiectasis, particularly childhood viral illnesses such as respiratory syncytial virus (RSV) pneumonia. Tuberculosis is a common cause of upper lobe bronchiectasis. Causes of diffuse bronchiectasis include deficiencies in host defense, congenital abnormalities in bronchial structure, abnormal mucus production, and abnormal ciliary clearance. More focal bronchiectasis, for example, in a lobe may be the result of long-standing central bronchial obstruction. In patients with allergic bronchopulmonary aspergillosis (ABPA), central mucous plugging produces a characteristic pattern of central bronchiectasis. Inhalation of noxious fumes may result in the formation of bronchiectasis. Traction bronchiectasis is a secondary phenomenon that is the result of pulmonary fibrosis, which commonly is seen in radiation fibrosis and sarcoidosis (Fig. 13-16). The cause of bronchiectasis may not be identified in up to 50% of cases.

Various terms are used to further describe bronchiectasis. *Wet bronchiectasis* refers to active infection in bronchiectatic lung, whereas *dry bronchiectasis* refers to bronchiectasis without active infection. *Reversible bronchiectasis* is seen in the setting of an acute pneumonia,

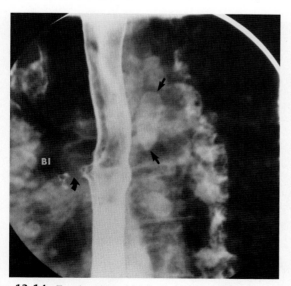

FIGURE 13-14. Esophagobronchial fistula in a patient with silicosis. The esophagogram shows filling of a fistula *(curved arrow)* between the esophagus and the bronchus intermedius (BI) in a patient with extensive calcified mediastinal nodes due to silicosis *(arrows).*

THORACIC RADIOLOGY: THE REQUISITES **315**

Box 13-9. Causes of Bronchiectasis

Infection unassociated with underlying disease
  Viral (respiratory syncytial virus, adenovirus)
  Bacterial *(Bordetella pertussis, Mycoplasma)*
  Tuberculosis and atypical mycobacteria
  Chronic or recurrent bacterial infections
  Recurrent aspiration pneumonia
Deficiency in host defense
  Agammaglobulinemia
  Granulomatous disease of childhood
  Acquired immunodeficiency syndrome (AIDS)
Abnormalities of cartilaginous structure
  Williams-Campbell syndrome
Abnormal mucus production
  Cystic fibrosis
Abnormal ciliary clearance
  Dyskinetic cilia syndrome
  Kartagener's syndrome
Bronchial obstruction
Allergic bronchopulmonary aspergillosis (ABPA)
Noxious fume inhalation
Traction bronchiectasis
  Radiation fibrosis
  Sarcoidosis
  Idiopathic interstitial pneumonias

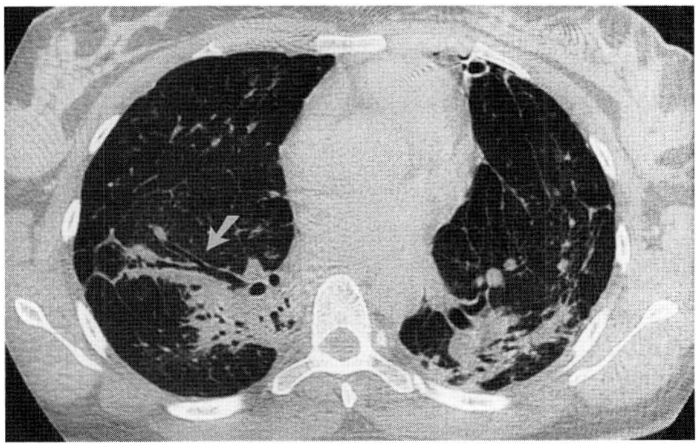

and it may persist as long as 4 to 6 months before resolving (Fig. 13-17).

The definitive pathologic description of bronchiectasis was reported by Reid (Box 13-10). In pathologic specimens and on bronchograms, fewer subdivisions of the bronchial tree between the hilum and the periphery of the lung are found in bronchiectatic lungs than in normal lungs.

The classification of bronchiectasis is based on the morphology of the bronchi and on the number of bronchial subdivisions that are present. Bronchiectasis can be classified in three groups. In *cylindrical bronchiectasis*, the bronchi are minimally dilated; have a straight, regular outline; and end squarely and abruptly. The average number of bronchial subdivisions is 16 on microscopic sections. In *varicose bronchiectasis*, the bronchi are dilated, have sites of relative constriction, and have a bulbous appearance similar to that of varicose veins. The average number of bronchial subdivisions is eight. In *saccular or cystic bronchiectasis*, the bronchi have a ballooned appearance, and the average number of bronchial subdivisions from the hilum to the pleura is four.

Although the chest radiograph may demonstrate more severe forms of bronchiectasis, it is frequently normal. In milder cases of bronchiectasis, streaky linear opacities occur in the distribution of the bronchi, representing thickened bronchial walls. Parallel, thickened walls in cylindrical bronchiectasis produce a tram-track appearance (Fig. 13-18A). In cystic bronchiectasis, clusters of air-filled cysts may be seen. When superinfection is present, the bronchial

FIGURE 13-16. Traction bronchiectasis in a patient with sarcoidosis. CT demonstrates bilateral parahilar fibrosis and pronounced distortion of the lung architecture. The hila are displaced posteriorly. The small, central lucencies within the fibrosis represent traction bronchiectasis. Notice the dilated medial and lateral segmental bronchi in the right middle lobe *(arrow)*, which represent traction bronchiectasis. The wall of the right middle lobe bronchus is irregular because of the granulomatous changes of sarcoidosis.

Box 13-10. Classification of Bronchiectasis

CYLINDRICAL
Bronchi are minimally dilated, have straight regular outlines, and end squarely and abruptly.
Average number of bronchial divisions seen microscopically is 16 (17 to 20 bronchial divisions normally).

VARICOSE
Dilation of bronchus with sites of relative constriction; bulbous appearance
Average number of bronchial divisions: 8

CYSTIC OR SACCULAR
Ballooned appearance, air-fluid levels
Average number of bronchial divisions: 4

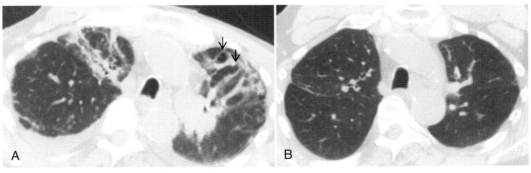

FIGURE 13-17. Reversible bronchiectasis in pneumonia. **A,** CT scan demonstrates bilateral upper lobe consolidation and bronchiectasis in the left upper lobe *(arrows).* **B,** Bronchiectasis has completely resolved 1 year later.

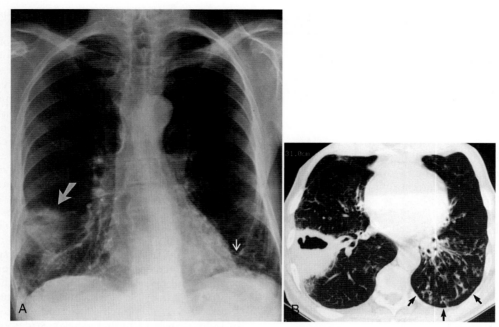

Figure 13-18. Bronchiectasis. **A,** The chest radiograph of a patient with a history of recurrent aspirations shows streaky, linear opacities at the lung bases, particularly in the left lower lobe, representing cylindrical bronchiectasis *(arrow)*. An irregular cavitary mass containing an air-fluid level is visualized in the right lower lobe *(arrow)* and is consistent with an abscess. **B,** The CT scan through the lung bases demonstrates bilateral cylindrical bronchiectasis that is most prominent in the left lower lobe and a thick-walled abscess in the right lower lobe. Notice the dilated bronchi and tree-in-bud opacities in the periphery of the left lower lobe *(arrows)* compared to the right lower lobe.

walls become thicker, and air-fluid levels may form within the cysts (Fig. 13-19). Focal bronchiectasis produces volume loss in the affected lobe or segment and, if severe, complete collapse.

CT, which is highly accurate in the diagnosis of bronchiectasis, has completely replaced bronchography. HRCT has become the examination of choice for the evaluation of bronchiectasis (Box 13-11). Using 1- to 1.5-mm collimation and 10-mm intervals, HRCT has a sensitivity of 96% and a specificity of 93%.

The predominant feature of bronchiectasis is a bronchial luminal diameter greater than that of the adjacent pulmonary artery (Box 13-12). Cylindrical bronchiectasis causes smooth dilation of the bronchi with lack of tapering, seen as tram-track lines when the bronchus is in the plane of the scan (Fig. 13-20) and as a signet ring sign when seen in cross section (Fig. 13-21). The signet ring sign refers to the thickened and dilated bronchus accompanied by a smaller pulmonary artery branch seen in cross section. Varicose bronchiectasis has a beaded appearance when seen in the plane of the bronchus, but it may mimic cylindrical bronchiectasis in cross section (Fig. 13-22). Cystic bronchiectasis demonstrates a string or cluster of cysts (Fig. 13-23). Retained secretions may create air-fluid levels within the cysts (Fig. 13-24). Cystic bronchiectasis must be distinguished from emphysema. In contrast to emphysema, the cysts occur in a linear array. They have discernible walls, accompany a pulmonary artery, and collapse on expiratory scans.

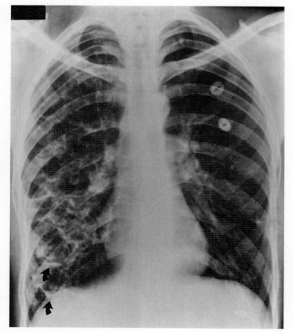

Figure 13-19. Bronchiectasis. The radiograph reveals multiple cystic lesions throughout the right lung that represent cystic bronchiectasis. The right lower lobe bronchi are thickened and contain some air-fluid levels *(arrows)*, indicating superinfection, or *wet bronchiectasis*.

***Box 13-11.* High-Resolution Computed Tomography Technique for Evaluation of Bronchiectasis**

Use of 1- to 1.5-mm collimation and multiplanar reformats
Bone algorithm
Selected expiratory scans at same levels as inspiratory scans to evaluate air trapping

Box 13-12. Radiographic Features of Bronchiectasis

Thick-walled bronchus larger in diameter than
  accompanying pulmonary artery
Dilated and thick-walled bronchi in the periphery of
  the lung
Cylindrical bronchiectasis
  Smooth dilation of bronchus and lack of tapering
  Tram-track lines when seen in the plane of the scan
  Signet ring sign when seen in cross section
Varicose bronchiectasis
  Bulbous appearance of bronchus
  May mimic cylindrical bronchiectasis in cross section
Cystic bronchiectasis
  String or cluster of cysts with discernible walls
  Air-fluid levels within cysts

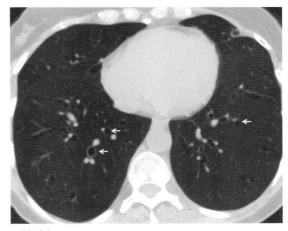

FIGURE 13-21. Bronchiectasis identified by the signet ring sign. CT scan through the lower lungs demonstrates bronchial wall thickening and dilation of the segmental bronchi in all visible lobes. The bronchi are larger in diameter than the accompanying pulmonary arteries, producing the signet ring sign *(arrows)*.

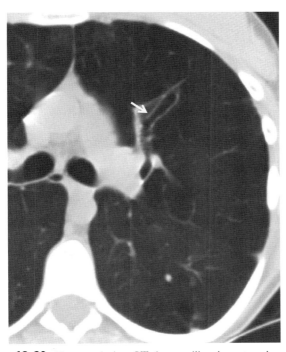

FIGURE 13-20. Tram-track sign. CT shows a dilated, nontapering, anterior segmental bronchus in the left upper lobe, with thickened walls *(arrow)* seen in the long-axis view.

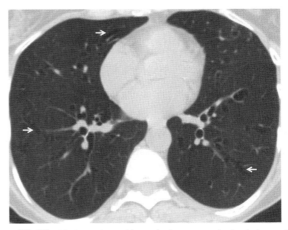

FIGURE 13-22. Varicose bronchiectasis is present in both lower lobes and the right middle lobe *(arrows)*.

A more subtle sign of bronchiectasis is the presence of dilated and thick-walled bronchi in the periphery of the lung (see Fig. 13-18B). On HRCT, normal bronchi can be seen only in the inner two thirds of the lung. Comparison with the normal contralateral lung can aid in the identification of minimally dilated bronchi.

There are a few pitfalls in the CT evaluation of bronchiectasis (Box 13-13). About 10% of asthmatic patients and some normal patients have bronchi slightly larger than the accompanying pulmonary artery. Occasionally, motion artifacts can simulate bronchiectasis, particularly adjacent to the heart. Bronchiectasis may be missed in areas of dense consolidation or collapse. Minimal cylindrical bronchiectasis may not be recognized in some cases.

MRI has limited role in imaging of bronchiectasis. It has inferior spatial resolution compared with CT.

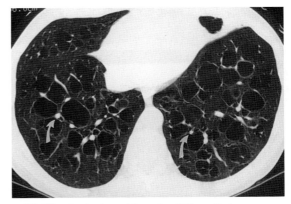

FIGURE 13-23. Cystic bronchiectasis. Thin-walled cysts are present in all visualized lobes. Notice the accompanying pulmonary artery branches *(arrows)*. The appearance is consistent with cystic bronchiectasis. Because of lack of secretions and thickening of the bronchi, this is called *dry bronchiectasis*.

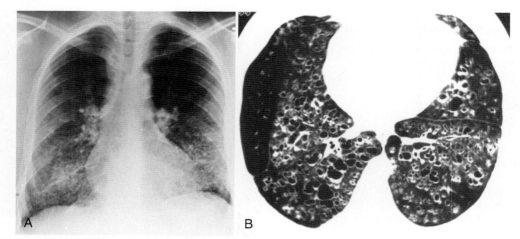

FIGURE 13-24. Cystic bronchiectasis resulting from childhood pertussis. **A,** Multiple, small, thick-walled cysts are present in both lung bases. **B,** CT through the lower lung zones demonstrates thick-walled cysts in clusters and some in a linear array, representing cystic bronchiectasis. Retained secretions are seen in the bronchi, and this is an example of wet bronchiectasis.

Box 13-13. Pitfalls in Evaluation of Bronchiectasis with Computed Tomography

Motion artifact may reduce accuracy.
Dense consolidation or atelectasis obscures findings.
Minimal cylindrical bronchiectasis can be missed.
Bronchial dilation can occur in asthmatic and some normal patients.

Box 13-14. Mucoid Impaction

Branching tubular opacities
Finger-in-glove appearance
V- or Y-shaped configuration
Occasional low attenuation of −5 to +20 HU
No enhancement with intravenous contrast

Mucoid Impaction

Mucoid impactions can complicate underlying bronchiectasis, particularly in cystic fibrosis (CF) and in ABPA. Inspissated secretions may also form distal to a bronchial obstruction.

Radiographic features of mucoid impactions include branching tubular opacities that emanate from larger central opacities in a finger-in-glove pattern (Box 13-14 and Fig. 13-25). The branching tubular opacities may have a V- or Y-shaped configuration. Occasionally, the mucoid impaction demonstrates a low attenuation of −5 to +20 HU, which suggests mucoid material. It may be necessary to distinguish a mucoid impaction from an arteriovenous

malformation. In a mucoid impaction, the normal bronchi are not discernible, but normal bronchi can be identified as separate from an arteriovenous malformation. In certain cases, contrast-enhanced CT or MRI may be necessary to make the distinction.

Cystic Fibrosis

Cystic fibrosis (CF) is the most common genetically transmitted abnormality in whites and occurs in 1 of 2000 to 3500 live births. CF is inherited by autosomal recessive transmission and affects both sexes equally. It is a multisystem disorder that affects the exocrine glands in the tracheobronchial tree, pancreas, large bowel, salivary glands, and

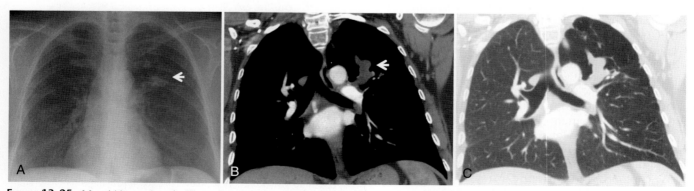

FIGURE 13-25. Mucoid impaction. **A,** The radiograph shows a large, branching mass in the left upper lobe that has nodular margins *(arrow)*. **B,** CT in mediastinal window demonstrates a branching tubular opacity in the left upper lobe with a finger-in-glove appearance, representing large mucoid impaction *(arrow)*. **C,** CT in lung windows demonstrates increased lucency in the left upper lobe.

sweat glands. Abnormal transport of chloride across epithelial cells in mucous surfaces is caused by a defect in the CF transmembrane regulator gene *(CFTR)*. Abnormal, thick, viscid secretions are produced by exocrine glands, leading to impaired mucociliary clearance. Characteristically, the sweat of CF patients contains elevated concentrations of sodium, chloride, and potassium, a basic requirement for the diagnosis. The major manifestations of CF are chronic obstructive pulmonary disease due to bronchiectasis and pancreatic insufficiency. Bronchiectasis is always present in adults with CF, and it is the leading cause of death. CF patients have a susceptibility to infections with *Staphylococcus aureus*, *Pseudomonas aeruginosa*, and *Haemophilus influenzae*, which are responsible for the development of bronchiectasis. *Pseudomonas cepacia* is a major cause of infection in the terminal stages of the disease.

Whereas the lungs of infants with CF appear normal on pathologic examination, older patients have a multitude of findings, including mucous plugging, pneumonia, abscess formation, obliterative bronchiolitis, bronchiectasis, focal atelectasis, and air trapping distal to obstructed segmental bronchi and pneumothorax (Fig. 13-26). There is predominant involvement of the upper lobes, and there is often associated hilar and mediastinal lymphadenopathy.

CT shows that bronchiectasis involves all lobes, but it is usually most severe in the upper lobes (Fig 13-27). The lungs usually are hyperinflated. Other findings related to obstruction of small- to medium-sized airways include air trapping, mucous plugging, tree-in-bud opacities, and atelectasis (Fig 13-28).

There is role for MRI in monitoring children with CF who need repeated imaging. MRI is useful in assessing the overall burden of disease, and it can demonstrate central bronchiectasis, bronchial wall thickening, mucous plug-

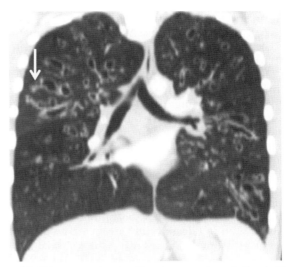

FIGURE 13-27. Cystic fibrosis. The lungs are hyperinflated. Diffuse bronchiectasis is present throughout but most severe in the upper lobes. Notice the cylindrical, varicoid, and cystic bronchiectasis; bronchial wall thickening; and mucus plugging *(arrow)*.

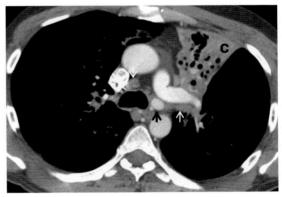

FIGURE 13-28. Cystic fibrosis. The scan shows complete left upper lobe collapse (c) with bronchiectasis. Notice the dilated bronchial artery *(thick arrow)* and hilar and mediastinal lymphadenopathy *(thin arrows)*.

ging, air-fluid levels, and consolidation. Distal bronchiectasis and bronchiolar disease cannot be assessed. MRI with hyperpolarized helium gas can show ventilation defects due to mucous plugging and bronchial wall inflammation.

Patients present with signs and symptoms of recurrent pulmonary infections. Hemoptysis and pneumothorax may occur. In the later stages of the disease, respiratory insufficiency and cor pulmonale develop. Treatment of these patients consists of physiotherapy, mucolytics, bronchodilators, antibiotics, and pancreatic enzyme supplements. For many patients with CF, lung transplantation has been a life-saving procedure.

Dyskinetic Cilia Syndrome

Dyskinetic cilia syndrome, or primary ciliary dyskinesia, is a group of inherited disorders transmitted in autosomal recessive pattern with a prevalence of 1 case in 16,000 births. The principal defect is in ciliary structure and function, leading to abnormal mucus clearance that predisposes to infection. Patients present with rhinitis, sinusitis, otitis media, bronchiectasis, and reduced fertility due to abnormal

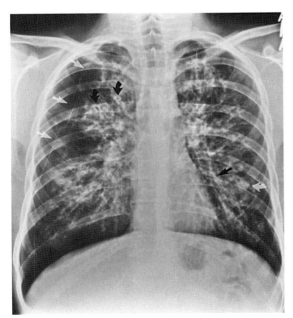

FIGURE 13-26. Cystic fibrosis. The lungs are hyperinflated. Diffuse bronchiectasis is present, with relative sparing of the lung bases. Ring shadows *(curved black arrows)* and tram tracks *(straight black arrow)* are present. Nodular opacities represent focal areas of mucoid impaction *(curved white arrow)*. A moderately large, right-sided pneumothorax can be seen *(white arrows)*.

motility of spermatozoa. Situs inversus or heterotaxy is seen in one half of these patients. A subset of dyskinetic cilia syndrome is Kartagener's syndrome, which is characterized by the triad of situs inversus, sinusitis, and bronchiectasis (Fig. 13-29). Diagnostic criteria include rhinitis and bronchial infections that start in early childhood and one or more of the following findings: situs inversus or dextrocardia in the patient or a sibling; living but immotile spermatozoa of abnormal appearance; absent or nearly absent tracheobronchial clearance; and nasal or bronchial biopsy demonstrating cilial ultrastructural defects.

Radiographic findings include bilateral bronchiectasis that is more severe in the lower lobes and bronchial wall thickening, hyperinflation, and focal areas of consolidation and atelectasis (Fig. 13-30). The findings are less severe than those seen in CF, and they are treated with repeated courses of antibiotics. Patients may have a normal life span.

Allergic Bronchopulmonary Aspergillosis

ABPA is a hypersensitivity response to the *Aspergillus* fungus in the airways. It is characterized by the presence of precipitating antibodies, immediate and often delayed skin sensitivity, the production of IgE, and bronchial wall and blood eosinophilia. Patients with asthma, atopy, or CF are susceptible to development of ABPA.

The disease is characterized by repeated exacerbations and is responsive to steroid treatment. The chronic inflammatory reaction results in damage to the bronchial walls. The lobar, segmental, and proximal subsegmental bronchi become dilated and result in central bronchiectasis with an upper lobe predominance. The dilated bronchi are filled with thick mucus that contains abundant eosinophils and fragments of fungal hyphae. Typically, radiographs and CT scans show branching, tubular opacities that emanate from the hilum in the distribution of the segmental and central

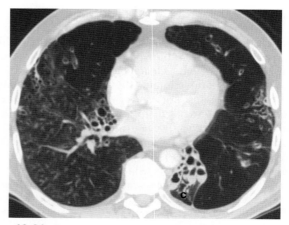

FIGURE 13-30. Primary ciliary dyskinesia. CT shows left lower lobe collapse (c), cystic bronchiectasis, and air-fluid levels. Diffuse bronchiectasis is most severe in the lower lobes. There are tree-in-bud opacities in the right lower lobe that are consistent with bronchiolitis. Notice the normal situs.

subsegmental bronchi, which is the typical finger-in-glove appearance (see Fig. 13-25). A particularly dilated mucus-filled bronchus is called a *mucocele.* The CT density of the mucocele may be lower or higher than that of soft tissue. The mucous plugs may stay unchanged for weeks, or they may clear by expectoration, leaving central, air-filled bronchiectasis (Fig. 13-31). During acute exacerbations, consolidation may be seen. Treatment consists of oral corticosteroids.

Other Causes of Bronchiectasis

A rare cause of bronchiectasis is *Williams-Campbell syndrome,* which is caused by a congenital deficiency of cartilage in subsegmental bronchi. *Young's syndrome,* or obstructive azoospermia, manifests as infertility and sinopulmonary infection. *Yellow nail syndrome* consists of a characteristic triad of

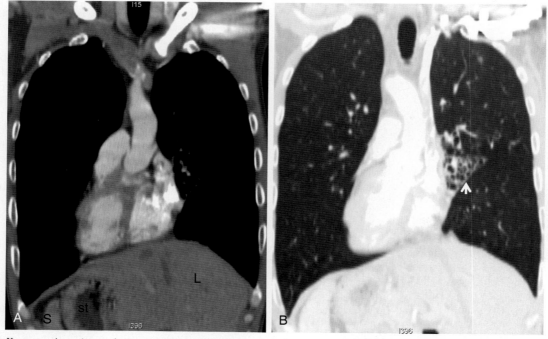

FIGURE 13-29. Kartagener's syndrome. **A,** Coronal CT using a mediastinal window demonstrates dextrocardia with the liver (L) on the left and the stomach (st) and spleen (S) on the right. **B,** Notice the bronchiectasis and collapse of the middle lobe *(arrow),* which is on the left (i.e., complete situs inversus).

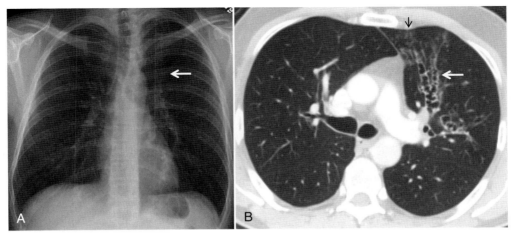

FIGURE 13-31. Allergic bronchopulmonary aspergillosis in an asthmatic patient with central bronchiectasis. **A,** The posteroanterior view of the left lung reveals central varicose bronchiectasis. **B,** CT demonstrates varicoid bronchiectasis of the left upper lobe segmental and subsegmental bronchi emanating from the left hilum *(white arrow).* Notice the tree-in-bud opacities and bronchial wall thickening *(black arrow).*

yellow nails, lymphedema, and pleural effusion. In *familial dysautonomia*, an autosomal recessive trait seen exclusively in those of Jewish descent, there is malfunction of the autonomic nervous system, with consequent hypersecretion by the mucous glands and obstruction of the bronchi. Patients have recurrent pneumonias. Radiographic findings resemble those of CF. Despite an extensive workup, no cause can be determined in up to 40% to 50% of patients with bronchiectasis, and these cases are called idiopathic (Fig. 13-32). Research suggests that some of these patients may have genetic defects in the epithelial sodium channel transport protein (SCNN, formerly designated ENaC).

DISEASES OF THE BRONCHIOLES

Bronchiolitis, or small airway disease, is a nonspecific term used to describe diseases affecting the airways that lack cartilage (airways < 2 mm). Because bronchioles do not have hyaline cartilage, which maintains patency, they rely on elastic fibers attached to the adjacent lung parenchyma

for support. The inner lining of bronchioles is surrounded by a layer of smooth muscle. The smallest structure routinely identified on HRCT is the lobular artery (1 mm) and its proximal intralobular branches (up to 0.5 mm) within the secondary pulmonary lobule. The normal lobular bronchiole with caliber of 1 mm and wall thickness of less than 0.1 mm is not seen.

Bronchiolitis can be classified based on cause and histologic features (Box 13-15). The two main types are cellular (proliferative) and obliterative (constrictive) bronchiolitis. These entities have similar or overlapping radiologic features. Because the normal bronchioles are not seen on imaging,

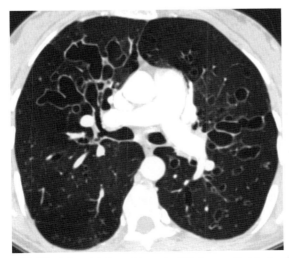

FIGURE 13-32. Idiopathic bronchiectasis. CT shows cylindrical and varicoid bronchiectasis in both upper lobes, affecting segmental and subsegmental bronchi.

Box 13-15. Classification of Bronchiolitis

CELLULAR (PROLIFERATIVE) BRONCHIOLITIS
Acute infectious and noninfectious bronchiolitis
  Associated with viruses, mycoplasma, mycobacteria, and other infectious organisms; aspiration; and toxic gas inhalation
Bronchiolitis associated with chronic large airway disease
  Associated with chronic obstructive pulmonary disease, bronchiectasis, asthma, and allergic bronchopulmonary aspergillosis
Subacute hypersensitivity pneumonitis
Smoking-related respiratory bronchiolitis
Follicular bronchiolitis
  Associated with connective tissue diseases, immunodeficiency diseases, and infection
Diffuse panbronchiolitis

ORGANIZING PNEUMONIA

OBLITERATIVE (CONSTRICTIVE) BRONCHIOLITIS
Associated with postinfection conditions, lung and bone marrow transplantation, connective tissue diseases, toxic fume inhalation, drugs, and idiopathic conditions

the diagnosis is based on signs that are often subtle and that are classified as direct or indirect (Box 13-16). The direct signs are related to presence of fluid, cells, inflammation, and fibrosis in or around the bronchioles, and indirect signs are related obliteration of the lumen by the fibrosis.

Plain Film Findings

The chest radiograph is usually normal in cases of bronchiolitis. Occasionally, small, ill-defined nodules may be seen in acute infective and noninfective bronchiolitis, subacute hypersensitivity pneumonitis, and smoking-related respiratory bronchiolitis. Large nodules and areas of increased opacity and consolidation are seen in organizing pneumonia and in some cases of infective bronchiolitis.

Air trapping, which is an indirect sign bronchiolitis, can be demonstrated by fluoroscopy and on standard chest radiographs obtained at full inspiration and maximum expiration. Findings of hyperinflation and air trapping are often subtle on plain chest radiographs. Generalized air trapping can manifest as a decrease in diaphragmatic excursion. Normally, the diaphragmatic excursion is 3 to 4 cm, but when air trapping is present, it may be decreased to 1 to 2 cm. In cases of unilateral air trapping, contiguous structures such as the mediastinum shift toward the contralateral side on expiration, and the diaphragm remains depressed on the side of air trapping (see Fig. 13-4). When a patient cannot cooperate fully for inspiration and expiration films, bilateral decubitus films may demonstrate similar findings. Normal lung deflates in the decubitus position.

If air trapping is present, the abnormal lung remains hyperinflated and lucent in the decubitus position.

Computed Tomography Findings

CT and particularly HRCT are much more sensitive examinations for bronchiolitis. Proper HRCT technique without breathing artifacts is important in imaging bronchiolitis. Multidetector CT with faster speed and high-quality multiplanar scans provides superior images. Expiratory scanning facilitates assessment of air trapping. At least six paired inspiratory and expiratory HRCT images should be obtained at identical levels. On expiratory CT scans, normal lung decreases in volume, and the attenuation increases (Fig. 13-33). In an area of air trapping, the abnormal lung remains lucent on expiration, and the volume of that portion of the lung remains constant. The caliber of vessels within the region of air trapping may be attenuated as a result of hypoxic vasoconstriction (see Fig. 13-4). The other major CT patterns of bronchiolitis include centrilobular nodules, branching linear opacities (i.e., tree-in-bud pattern), ground-glass attenuation and consolidation, and a mosaic pattern (Box 13-17). The first three patterns are found in cellular bronchiolitis, and the mosaic pattern with air trapping is identified in obliterative bronchiolitis.

Box 13-16. **Signs of Bronchiolitis**

Direct signs (cellular bronchiolitis)
  Centrilobular nodules
  Tree-in-bud opacities
  Bronchiolectasis
  Related to fluid, cells, inflammation, and fibrosis in bronchioles
Indirect signs
  Mosaic attenuation and air trapping (often the only finding in obliterative bronchiolitis)
  Related obliteration of the lumen by the fibrosis

Box 13-17. **Major Computed Tomography Patterns of Bronchiolitis**

Branching nodular opacities (tree-in-bud pattern)
  Acute infectious and noninfectious bronchiolitis
  Diffuse panbronchiolitis
  Chronic bronchial diseases such as allergic bronchopulmonary aspergillosis, chronic bronchitis and bronchiectasis
Centrilobular nodules
  Subacute hypersensitivity pneumonitis
  Respiratory bronchiolitis
  Follicular bronchiolitis
Nodules, ground-glass opacities, and consolidation
  Organizing pneumonia
Mosaic pattern
  Obliterative (constrictive) bronchiolitis

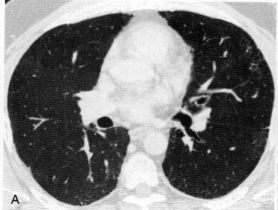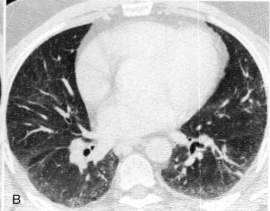

FIGURE 13-33. Inspiratory and expiratory HRCT. The inspiratory (**A**) and expiratory (**B**) images show a diffuse increase in the attenuation of the lungs on expiration. Notice the posterior displacement of the major fissures due to a decrease in lung volumes.

Centrilobular Nodules and Branching Linear Opacities

Centrilobular nodules and branching linear and nodular opacities (i.e., tree-in-bud pattern) are caused by inflammatory cells in the walls of the small airways and inflammatory exudate and mucus in the lumina. These findings are most often seen with *acute infectious bronchiolitis* caused by infection with RSV (Fig. 13-34), adenovirus, or typical and atypical mycobacteria and mycoplasma. However, any bronchopneumonia can result in this pattern if bronchioles are affected. Centrilobular nodular and linear opacities are seen in aspiration-related bronchiolitis (see Fig. 13-15) and after toxic gas inhalation. These findings are also seen in chronic inflammatory conditions of the bronchioles caused by *primary bronchial diseases*, such as asthma, ABPA, chronic bronchitis, and bronchiectasis (see Fig. 13-30).

Diffuse panbronchiolitis is a disease of unknown origin that is seen in Asians, particularly in Japanese men, and it is rare in North America. Patients usually present with a chronic productive cough and progressive dyspnea. Histologic examination reveals inflammation of the respiratory bronchioles and mononuclear cells and foamy macrophages in the bronchiolar lumina and alveoli. CT features include centrilobular nodules, branching linear opacities, bronchiolectasis, bronchiectasis, and air trapping. Although there may be a favorable initial response to treatment with erythromycin, the long-term prognosis is poor, with progression of bronchiectasis.

Follicular bronchiolitis may be a primary disease or more commonly associated with connective tissue disorders such as rheumatoid arthritis and Sjögren's syndrome, immunodeficiency diseases, and chronic airway infection, such as in bronchiectasis. Histologically, the disease is characterized by proliferation of lymphoid follicles in bronchiolar walls and surrounding interstitium. The predominant findings are nodules in a centrilobular distribution and, less commonly, a tree-in-bud pattern (Fig. 13-35). Primary follicular bronchiolitis is treated with corticosteroids.

Hypersensitivity pneumonitis is discussed in Chapter 9.

Ground-Glass Attenuation and Consolidation

Bronchiolar diseases with CT findings of ground-glass attenuation and consolidation include respiratory bronchiolitis and organizing pneumonia. *Respiratory bronchiolitis,*

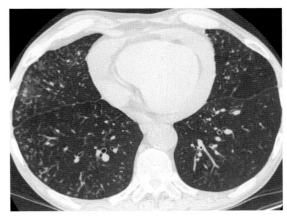

FIGURE 13-35. Follicular bronchiolitis in a patient with rheumatoid arthritis. Diffuse, centrilobular nodules have a tree-in-bud appearance in the right lung and lingula.

also known as smokers' bronchiolitis or smoker's lung, is a common incidental histologic finding in smokers, typically those 30 to 40 years old. Patients are usually asymptomatic, but they may complain of cough or shortness of breath. The respiratory bronchioles mainly are involved. Histologically, mild chronic inflammation of the bronchioles is associated with pigmented macrophages in respiratory bronchioles and adjacent alveoli. CT demonstrates ground-glass attenuation or centrilobular micronodules in the upper lung zones or in a diffuse distribution (Fig. 13-36). Organizing pneumonia is discussed in Chapter 7.

Mosaic Pattern

Low attenuation and a mosaic pattern on CT are seen with obliterative bronchiolitis, also known as constrictive bronchiolitis. Histologically, obliterative bronchiolitis is characterized by concentric narrowing of the bronchioles by submucosal and peribronchiolar fibrosis causing airflow obstruction. The distribution often is patchy. Diseases associated with obliterative bronchiolitis include childhood viral infections, toxic-fume inhalation, rheumatoid arthritis, bone marrow transplantation and a chronic graft-versus-host reaction, chronic rejection after lung transplantation, inflammatory bowel disease, and certain drugs, or the condition may be idiopathic (Box 13-18).

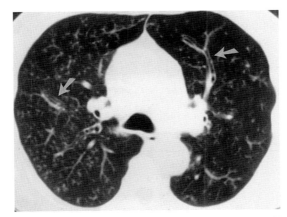

FIGURE 13-34. Viral pneumonia. Small, branching, linear opacities and nodular opacities occur throughout the right lung in a tree-in-bud pattern. Cylindrical bronchiectasis is present in both upper lobes *(arrows).*

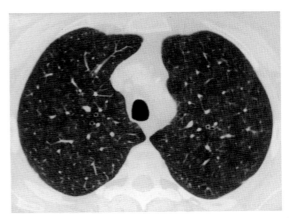

FIGURE 13-36. Respiratory bronchiolitis. CT through the upper lobes reveals diffuse, bilateral, small, ground-glass, nodular opacities in a peribronchiolar distribution.

Box 13-18. **Conditions Associated with Obliterative (Constrictive) Bronchiolitis**

Viral infections
Inhalation of toxic fumes
Connective tissue disorders
Bone marrow transplantation
Lung transplantation
Inflammatory bowel disease

The clinical symptoms include dry cough and progressive shortness of breath. In many instances, the disease is first diagnosed on CT in asymptomatic patients. Patients who are at high risk, such as after lung transplantation, undergo surveillance scans. Bronchiolitis obliterans is the leading cause of morbidity and mortality in this group of patients.

The radiographic features of obliterative bronchiolitis include various degrees of hyperinflation and peripheral attenuation of vessels. However, the radiograph is usually normal. The most common CT finding is air trapping, which is accentuated on expiratory scans (Fig. 13-37). A mosaic pattern of perfusion occurs as a result of hypoxic vasoconstriction in areas of bronchiolar obstruction, resulting in redistribution of blood flow to normal areas of the lung. Expiratory CT scanning allows differentiation of the mosaic pattern of attenuation due to air trapping from other causes, such as embolic or occlusive vascular disease and diffuse interstitial lung disease. When air trapping is present, the affected portion of the lung remains lucent during expiration. The pulmonary vessels are decreased in size in the low-attenuation areas when air trapping and vascular disease are present, but they have normal calibers in patients with diffuse infiltrative lung disease. Diffuse infiltrative lung disease may produce patchy areas of ground-glass attenuation and therefore a mosaic pattern. These areas are abnormal, whereas the ground-glass areas in vascular disease and bronchiolitis represent normally perfused lung (Table 13-1). Mild cylindrical bronchiectasis is often associated with obliterative bronchiolitis (Fig 13-38). Rarely, bronchiolar wall thickening and centrilobular branching are seen.

The *Swyer-James syndrome* is a variant of postinfectious obliterative bronchiolitis. It is related to an acute viral bronchiolitis in infancy or early childhood that prevents the normal development of the affected lung. It manifests as a unilateral, hyperlucent lung or lobe on standard radiographs, with normal or reduced volume during inspiration and air trapping on expiration. Typically, the ipsilateral hilum is small because of decreased blood flow on the affected side. On CT, the areas of bronchiolitis are usually not limited to a single lobe or lung, and patchy areas of air trapping can be observed bilaterally (Fig. 13-39).

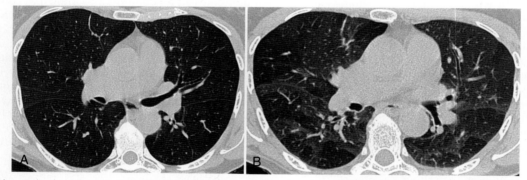

FIGURE 13-37. Air trapping in obliterative bronchiolitis. The inspiratory (**A**) and expiratory (**B**) CT scans show mosaic attenuation in the lungs. The regions of increased lucency during expiration represent air trapping.

TABLE 13-1 Causes of Mosaic Pattern

	Vessel Size	Inspiration/Expiration CT
Small airways disease	Decreased size and number in lucent lung	Air trapping
Vascular disease	Decreased size and number in lucent lung	No air trapping
Diffuse infiltrative disease	Similar size and number throughout the lung	No air trapping

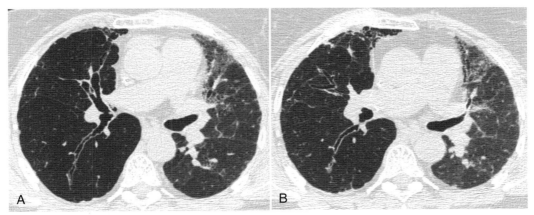

FIGURE 13-38. Obliterative bronchiolitis in a transplanted right lung. Inspiratory (**A**) and expiratory (**B**) HRCT shows uniform lucency in the transplanted right lung, indicating air trapping. Notice the bronchiectasis in the right lung. The native left lung has pulmonary fibrosis.

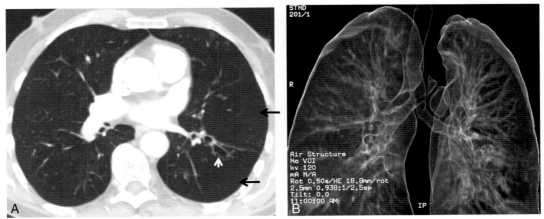

FIGURE 13-39. Postinfectious obliterative bronchiolitis in a patient with Swyer-James syndrome. **A,** Axial CT reveals that the left lung has a small volume. The scan shows bronchiectasis *(white arrow)* and areas of hyperlucency in which there is attenuation of vessels *(black arrows).* **B,** Three-dimensional external volume-rendering scan shows a lucent, small left lung and normal right lung.

■ SUGGESTED READINGS

Ahn, J.M., Im, J.-G., Seo, J.W., et al., 1994. Endobronchial hamartoma: CT findings in three patients. AJR Am. J. Roentgenol. 163, 49–50.

Akira, M., Higashihara, T., Sakatani, M., Hara, H., 1993. Diffuse panbronchiolitis: followup CT examination. Radiology 189, 559–562.

Akira, M., Kitatani, F., Yong-Sikl, et al., 1988. Diffuse panbronchiolitis: evaluation with high-resolution CT. Radiology 168, 433–438.

Altes, T.A., Eichinger, M., Puderbach, M., 2007. Magnetic resonance imaging of the lung in cystic fibrosis. Proc. Am. Thorac. Soc. 4, 321–327.

Altes, T., Salerno, M., 2004. Hyperpolarized gas MR imaging of the lung. J. Thorac. Imaging. 19, 250–258.

Arrigoni, M.G., Bernatz, P.E., Donoghue, F.E., 1971. Broncholithiasis. J. Thorac. Cardiovasc. Surg. 62, 231–237.

Arrigoni, M.G., Woolner, L.B., Bernatz, P.E., et al., 1970. Benign tumors of the lung: a ten-year surgical experience. J. Thorac. Cardiovasc. Surg. 60, 589–599.

Burke, C.M., Theodore, J., Dawking, K.D., et al., 1989. Post-transplant obliterative bronchiolitis and other later sequelae in human heart-lung transplantation. Chest 86, 824–825.

Choplin, R.H., Kowamoto, E.H., Dyer, R.B., et al., 1986. Atypical carcinoid of the lung: radiographic features. AJR Am. J. Roentgenol. 146, 665–668.

Conces, D.J., Tarver, R.D., Vix, V.A., 1991. Broncholithiasis: CT features in 15 patients. AJR Am. J. Roentgenol. 157, 249–253.

Dixon, G.F., Donnerberg, R.L., Schonfeld, S.A., Whitcomb, M.E., 1984. Advances in the diagnosis and treatment of broncholithiasis. Am. Rev. Respir. Dis. 129, 1028–1030.

Douek, P.C., Simoni, L., Revel, D., et al., 1994. Diagnosis of bronchial carcinoid tumor by ultrafast contrast-enhanced MR imaging. AJR Am. J. Roentgenol. 163, 563–564.

Eber, C.D., Stark, P., Bertozzi, P., 1993. Bronchiolitis obliterans on high-resolution CT. J. Comput. Assist. Tomogr. 17, 853–856.

Epler, G.R., Colby, T.V., 1983. The spectrum of bronchiolitis obliterans. Chest 83, 161–162.

Epler, G.R., Colby, T.V., McLoud, T.C., et al., 1985. Bronchiolitis obliterans organizing pneumonia. N. Engl. J. Med. 312, 152–158.

Fajac, I., Viel, M., Sublemontier, S., et al., 2008. Could a defective epithelial sodium channel lead to bronchiectasis?. Respir. Res. 9, 46.

Ferretti, G.R., Vining, D.J., Knoplioch, J., et al., 1996. Tracheobronchial tree: three-dimensional spiral CT with bronchoscopic perspective. J. Comput. Assist. Tomogr. 20, 777.

Garg, K., Lynch, D.A., Newell, J.D., King, T.E., 1994. Proliferative and constrictive bronchiolitis: classification and radiologic features. AJR Am. J. Roentgenol. 162, 803–808.

Glazer, H.S., Anderson, D.J., Sagel, S.S., 1989. Bronchial impaction in lobar collapse: CT demonstration and pathologic correlation. AJR Am. J. Roentgenol. 153, 485.

Grenier, P., Maurice, F., Musset, D., et al., 1986. Bronchiectasis: assessment by thin section CT. Radiology 161, 95–99.

Grote, T.H., Macon, W.R., Davis, B., et al., 1988. Atypical carcinoid of the lung: a distinct clinicopathologic entity. Chest 93, 370–375.

Gruden, J.F., Webb, W.R., 1993. CT findings in a proved case of respiratory bronchiolitis. AJR Am. J. Roentgenol. 161, 44–46.

Hansell, D.M., Wells, A.U., Rubens, M.B., Cole, P.J., 1994. Bronchiectasis: functional significance of areas of decreased attenuation at expiratory CT. Radiology 193, 369–374.

Heitmiller, R.F., Mathisen, D.J., Ferry, J.A., et al., 1989. Mucoepidermoid lung tumors. Ann. Thorac. Surg. 47, 394–399.

Katz, M., Konen, E., Rosenman, J., et al., 1995. Spiral CT and 3D image reconstruction of vascular rings and associated tracheobronchial anomalies. J. Comput. Assist. Tomogr. 19, 564–568.

Kauczor, H.U., Wolcke, B., Fischer, B., et al., 1996. Three-dimensional helical CT of the tracheobronchial tree: evaluation of imaging protocols and assessment of suspected stenoses with bronchoscopic correlation. AJR Am. J. Roentgenol. 167, 419–424.

Lentz, D., Bergin, C.J., Berry, G.J., et al., 1992. Diagnosis of bronchiolitis obliterans in heart-lung transplantation patients: importance of bronchial dilatation on CT. AJR Am. J. Roentgenol. 159, 463–467.

Loubeyre, P., Revel, D., Delignette, A., et al., 1995. Bronchiectasis detected with thin-section CT as a predictor of chronic lung allograft rejection. Radiology 194, 213–216.

Lynch, D.A., Newell, J.D., Tschomper, B.A., et al., 1993. Uncomplicated asthma in adults: comparison of CT appearance of the lungs in asthmatic and healthy subjects. Radiology 188, 829–833.

MacLeod, E.M., 1954. Abnormal transradiancy of one lung. Thorax 9, 147–153.

Marti-Bonati, L., Perales, R.F., Catala, F., et al., 1989. CT findings in Swyer-James syndrome. Radiology 172, 477–480.

Marti-Bonmati, L., Catala, F.J., Ruiz, P.F., 1991. Computed tomography differentiation between cystic bronchiectasis and bullae. J. Thorac. Imaging. 7, 83–85.

Martin, K.W., Sagel, S.S., Siegel, B.A., 1986. Mosaic oligemia simulating pulmonary infiltrates on CT. AJR Am. J. Roentgenol. 147, 670–673.

McGuinness, G., Naidich, D.P., Garay, S., et al., 1993. AIDS associated bronchiectasis: CT features. J. Comput. Assist. Tomogr. 17, 260–266.

McGuinness, G., Naidich, D.P., Garay, S.M., et al., 1993. Accessory cardiac bronchus: CT features and clinical significance. Radiology 189, 563–566.

McLoud, T.C., Epler, G.R., Colby, T.V., et al., 1986. Bronchiolitis obliterans. Radiology 159, 1–8.

Moore, A.D.A., Godwin, J.D., Dietrich, P.A., et al., 1992. Swyer-James syndrome: CT findings in eight patients. AJR Am. J. Roentgenol. 158, 1211–1215.

Morrish, W.F., Herman, S.J., Weisbrod, G.L., Chamberlain, D.W., 1991. Bronchiolitis obliterans after lung transplantation: findings at chest radiography and high resolution CT. Radiology 179, 487–490.

Müller, N.L., Bergin, C.J., Ostrow, D.N., Nichols, D.M., 1984. Role of computed tomography in the recognition of bronchiectasis. AJR Am. J. Roentgenol. 143, 971–976.

Müller, N.L., Miller, R.R., 1995. Diseases of the bronchioles: CT and histopathologic findings. Radiology 196:3–12.

Müller, N.L., Miller, R.R., 1990. Neuroendocrine carcinomas of the lung. Semin. Roentgenol. 25, 96–104.

Müller, N.L., Staples, C.A., Miller, R.R., 1990. Bronchiolitis obliterans organizing pneumonia: CT features in 14 patients. AJR Am. J. Roentgenol. 154, 983–987.

Müller, N.L., Thurlbeck, W.M., 1996. Thin-section CT, emphysema, air trapping, and airway obstruction. Radiology 199, 621–622.

Naidich, D.P., McCauley, D.I., Khouri, N.F., et al., 1982. Computed tomography of bronchiectasis. J. Comput. Assist. Tomogr. 6, 437–444.

Newmark, G.M., Conces Jr., D.J., Kopecky, K.K., 1994. Spiral CT evaluation of the trachea and bronchi. J. Comput. Assist. Tomogr. 18, 552–554.

O'Uchi, T., Tokumaru, A., Mikami, I., et al., 1992. Value of MR imaging in detecting a peanut causing bronchial obstruction. AJR Am. J. Roentgenol. 159, 481–482.

Pugatch, R.D., Gale, M.E., 1983. Obscure pulmonary masses: bronchial impaction revealed by CT. AJR Am. J. Roentgenol. 141, 909–914.

Reid, L.M., 1950. Reduction in bronchial subdivision in bronchiectasis. Thorax 5, 233–247.

Remy-Jardin, M., Remy, J., Boulenguez, C., et al., 1993. Morphologic effects of cigarette smoking on airways and pulmonary parenchyma in healthy adult volunteers: CT evaluation and correlation with pulmonary function tests. Radiology 186, 107–115.

Remy-Jardin, M., Remy, J., 1988. Comparison of vertical and oblique CT in evaluation of bronchial tree. J. Comput. Assist. Tomogr. 12, 956–962.

Sakai, F., Sone, S., Kujono, K., et al., 1994. MR of pulmonary hamartoma: pathologic correlation. J. Thorac. Imaging. 9, 51–55.

Schmidt, H.W., Clagett, O.T., McDonald, J.R., 1950. Broncholithiasis. J. Thorac. Cardiovasc. Surg. 62, 226–245.

Shin, M.S., Berland, L.L., Myers, J.L., et al., 1989. CT demonstration of an ossifying bronchial carcinoid simulating broncholithiasis. AJR Am. J. Roentgenol. 153, 51–52.

Silverman, P.M., Godwin, J.D., 1987. CT/bronchographic correlations in bronchiectasis. J. Comput. Assist. Tomgr. 11, 52–56.

Skeens, J.L., Fuhrman, C.R., Yousem, S.A., 1989. Bronchiolitis obliterans in heart-lung transplantation patients: radiologic findings in 11 patients. AJR Am. J. Roentgenol. 153, 253–256.

Stern, E.J., Frank, M.S., 1994. Small-airway diseases of the lungs: findings at expiratory CT. AJR Am. J. Roentgenol. 163, 37–41.

Sugiyama, Y., Tukeuchi, K., Yotsumoto, H., et al., 1986. A case of panbronchiolitis in a second generation Korean male. Jpn. J. Thorac. Dis. 24, 183–187.

Swyer, P.R., James, G.C.W., 1953. A case of unilateral pulmonary emphysema. Thorax 8, 133–136.

Tarver, R.D., Conces, D.J., Godwin, J.D., 1988. Motion artifacts on CT simulate bronchiectasis. AJR Am. J. Roentgenol. 151, 1117–1119.

Watanabe, Y., Nishiyama, Y., Kanayama, H., et al., 1987. Congenital bronchiectasis due to cartilage deficiency: CT demonstration. J. Comput. Assist. Tomogr. 11, 701–703.

Weissberg, D., Swartz, I., 1987. Foreign bodies in the tracheobronchial tree. Chest 91, 730–733.

Westcott, J.L., Cole, S.R., 1986. Traction bronchiectasis in end-stage pulmonary fibrosis. Radiology 161, 665–669.

Yousem, S.A., Burke, C.M., Billingham, M.E., 1985. Pathological pulmonary alterations in long-term human heart-lung transplantation. Human. Pathol. 16, 911–925.

Yousem, S.A., Hochholzer, L., 1987. Mucoepidermoid tumors of the lung. Cancer 60, 1346–1352.

Zwiebel, B.R., Austin, J.H., Grimes, M.M., 1991. Bronchial carcinoid tumors: assessment with CT of location and intratumoral calcification in 31 patients. Radiology 179, 483–486.

CHAPTER 14

Pulmonary Vascular Abnormalities

Phillip M. Boiselle and Conrad Wittram

The radiologic appearance of the pulmonary vessels depends on anatomic and physiologic parameters. In previous chapters, we have reviewed the normal pulmonary vascular anatomy on radiographs and on computed tomography (CT) scans. Knowledge of normal vascular anatomy should take into account the physiologic effects of gravity on the radiologic appearance of pulmonary vascularity. Gravitational differences in the lung are posturally dependent and are most striking in the erect position. Gravity has an important effect on the distribution of pulmonary blood flow, resulting in an increase in blood flow from the lung apices to the lung bases in an upright position. A gradual increase in the diameter of pulmonary vessels from the lung apices to the lung bases is seen on radiographs; this increase corresponds to the increasing distribution of pulmonary blood flow.

Gravitational effects are evident in other positions. In the supine position, there is a gradient between the anterior and posterior portions of the lung, which results in increased blood flow to the dependent, posterior portions. However, in contrast to the upright position, blood flow is fairly equivalent in the upper and lower lung zones. On supine chest radiographs, the caliber of vessels in the upper and lower lung zones are nearly equal. In the decubitus position, gravitational effects result in increased blood flow to the lung in the dependent position. A consequence of this phenomenon is unilateral pulmonary edema in the dependent lung of a patient who has been lying in a decubitus position.

In this chapter, we review the characteristic radiologic findings for several pulmonary vascular entities, including pulmonary artery hypertension, pulmonary venous hypertension, congestive heart failure, and pulmonary thromboembolism. When examining the pulmonary vasculature on a chest radiograph, the posturally dependent effect of gravity must always be considered. Subtle alterations in the pulmonary vasculature may be detectable only as a change in appearance from prior radiographs, and whenever possible, current radiographs should be compared with prior studies that were performed in the same position.

■ PULMONARY ARTERY HYPERTENSION

Definition

Pulmonary artery hypertension (PAH) is a condition of sustained elevation of pulmonary artery pressure. The diagnostic criterion for PAH is a systemic pulmonary artery pressure greater than 30 mm Hg or a mean pulmonary artery pressure greater than 20 mm Hg.

Causes

PAH may results from one of three basic mechanisms: increased flow of blood through the pulmonary vessels, decreased cross-sectional area of the pulmonary vasculature, and increased resistance to pulmonary venous drainage. These mechanisms provide a convenient framework for categorizing and understanding the large number of causes of PAH (Box 14-1). Another common way to categorize causes of PAH is to broadly divide them into precapillary causes (i.e., entities that result in increased blood flow or decreased cross-sectional area of the pulmonary vasculature) and postcapillary causes (i.e., entities that result in increased resistance to pulmonary venous drainage).

Most cases of PAH have a known cause; these cases are collectively referred to as *secondary PAH*. In a minority of cases, the cause remains unknown, and this is referred to as *primary PAH*. Primary PAH usually affects women younger than 40 years. A small percentage of patients with primary PAH have a familial form, which is inherited as an autosomal dominant trait. Affected patients usually present with symptoms of progressive dyspnea and easy fatigability. Approximately 10% of patients present with symptoms of Raynaud's phenomenon. Because of the nonspecific presenting symptoms and the subtlety of clinical findings early in the course of the disease, the diagnosis is often delayed.

Treatment of primary PAH consists of supportive medical therapy and transplantation (lung or combined heart and lung). Pulmonary vascular disease with clinical and radiologic manifestations similar to primary PAH has been described in association with portal hypertension, human immunodeficiency virus (HIV) infection, cocaine abuse, and appetite-suppressant drugs.

Radiographic Findings

Despite the wide variety of causes of PAH, the salient radiologic features are similar. There is usually marked enlargement of the main and hilar pulmonary arteries, which rapidly taper as they course distally (Fig. 14-1). The most striking feature of PAH is the disparity in size between the central and peripheral pulmonary arteries. Right-sided ventricular cardiac enlargement may occur and is best demonstrated on the lateral chest radiograph.

On chest radiographs, enlargement of the main pulmonary artery results in a prominent convex contour. However, the degree of pulmonary artery enlargement varies considerably among patients and conditions. A patient may have significant PAH despite a normal chest radiograph.

Box 14-1. **Causes of Pulmonary Artery Hypertension**

INCREASED PULMONARY BLOOD FLOW
Left-to-right shunts (atrial septal defect, patent ductus arteriosus, ventricular septal defect)
Increased total blood volume (thyrotoxicosis, anemia, pregnancy)

DECREASED CROSS-SECTIONAL AREA OF THE PULMONARY VASCULATURE

Resulting from Primary Disease in the Arterial Wall or Lumen
Chronic pulmonary embolism
Primary pulmonary hypertension
Peripheral pulmonary stenosis
Eisenmenger's syndrome
Pulmonary vasculitis

Resulting from Pulmonary or Pleural Disease
Emphysema
Diffuse lung disease
 Fibrosis
  Idiopathic pulmonary fibrosis
  Collagen vascular disease
  Sarcoidosis
  Pneumoconiosis
 Granulomatous infections

Bronchiectasis (cystic fibrosis)
Neoplasm
Postpneumonectomy
Fibrothorax
Chest wall deformity (thoracoplasty, kyphoscoliosis)

Resulting from Vasoconstriction Caused by Hypoventilation
Obesity-hypoventilation syndrome
Upper airway obstruction
High altitude
Neuromuscular disorders

INCREASED RESISTANCE TO PULMONARY VENOUS DRAINAGE
Pulmonary vein abnormalities
 Pulmonary venoocclusive disease
 Congenital narrowing or anomalous drainage
Left atrial abnormalities
 Cor triatriatum
 Left atrial myxoma or thrombus
Mitral valve disease (stenosis or regurgitation)
Left ventricular failure
Constrictive pericarditis
Fibrosing mediastinitis

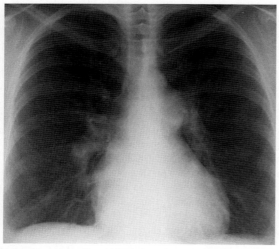

FIGURE 14-1. Primary pulmonary artery hypertension. A frontal chest radiograph demonstrates significant enlargement of the main and hilar pulmonary arteries, which rapidly taper as they course distally.

Compared with chest radiographs, CT scans allow a more accurate determination of the size of the main pulmonary artery, and a diameter greater than 3 cm on CT usually is considered abnormal (Fig. 14-2).

Evaluation of the hilar vessels on chest radiographs is usually a subjective assessment. An objective assessment of hilar vessel enlargement is the measurement of the diameter of the right interlobar artery. On posteroanterior, erect chest radiographs, the normal transverse diameter of the right interlobar artery as it descends adjacent to the bronchus intermedius is less than or equal to 16 mm.

In the setting of long-standing, severe PAH, the enlarged central pulmonary arteries may develop peripheral, atherosclerotic calcification. This is an unusual finding and is most frequently seen in patients with PAH caused by Eisenmenger's syndrome (Fig. 14-3), a condition characterized by a reversal in the direction of a long-standing, severe left-to-right shunt.

In cases of PAH caused by increased resistance to pulmonary venous return (i.e., postcapillary causes), radiographs show evidence of pulmonary venous hypertension. The most notable finding is cephalization of the pulmonary vasculature, also referred to as recruitment of upper lobe vessels. These terms refer to an increased caliber of the upper lobe vessels, which results from a diversion of blood flow. This is a reversal of the gravity-dependent increased caliber of lower lobe vessels seen on upright radiographs of normal individuals. Cephalization is best evaluated on upright radiographs.

An objective method for assessing cephalization is to examine the relative sizes of the anterior segment artery of either upper lobe and its adjacent bronchus, both of which are usually seen end-on on a posteroanterior, erect chest radiograph. In normal individuals, the diameter of the artery is about the same as that of the adjacent bronchus. Cephalization is diagnosed when the diameter of the artery is larger than that of the adjacent bronchus.

Cephalization of blood flow is not seen exclusively in postcapillary causes of PAH. It can be encountered in cases of PAH produced by precapillary causes. In precapillary PAH, recruitment of upper lobe vessels results from increased resistance in lower lobe pulmonary arteries.

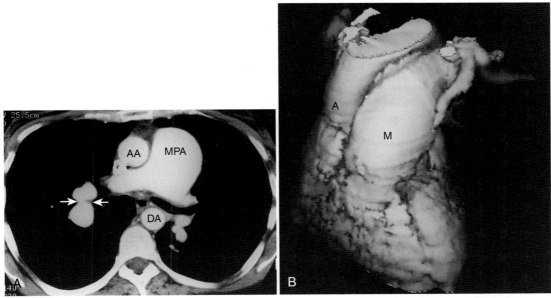

FIGURE 14-2. Pulmonary artery hypertension resulting from multiple, peripheral pulmonic stenoses. **A,** A contrast-enhanced, helical CT image of the chest reveals significant enlargement of the main pulmonary artery (MPA), which is approximately 4.5 cm in diameter. The weblike stenosis of the right interlobar pulmonary artery *(arrows)* is associated with poststenotic dilatation. Numerous additional sites of stenosis were evident on other images. AA, ascending aorta; DA, descending aorta. **B,** A three-dimensional, shaded-surface display image that was reconstructed from a helical CT acquisition shows the marked disparity in size between the enlarged main pulmonary artery (M) and the normal-caliber ascending aorta (A).

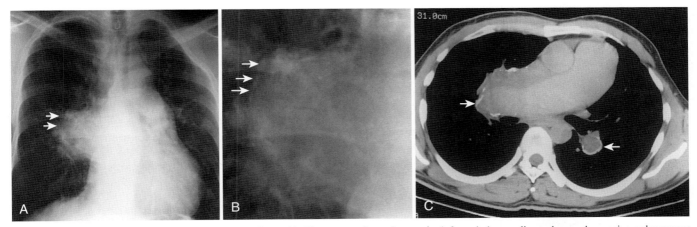

FIGURE 14-3. Pulmonary artery hypertension in a patient with Eisenmenger's syndrome. **A,** A frontal chest radiograph reveals massive enlargement of the main and hilar pulmonary arteries. Notice the presence of peripheral calcification *(arrows)* within the right interlobar pulmonary artery. **B,** The peripheral calcification *(arrows)* is seen in greater detail on the coned-down image of the right hilum. **C,** An axial image from unenhanced CT of the chest in the same patient demonstrates peripheral calcifications of both pulmonary arteries *(arrows)*. Atheromatous calcification is an unusual finding for pulmonary artery hypertension, and it is most frequently seen in patients with Eisenmenger's syndrome.

In addition to cephalization, several other radiographic findings may be associated with pulmonary venous hypertension, including interstitial edema (described later), hemosiderosis, and pulmonary fibrosis. Hemosiderosis is related to recurrent episodes of alveolar hemorrhage. When these episodes are severe, hemosiderosis may be detected on chest radiographs as tiny, punctate opacities in the middle and lower lung zones. Pulmonary fibrosis is related to recurrent episodes of pulmonary edema and hemorrhage. Radiographically, it is characterized by reticular opacities in the middle and lower lung zones.

It is important to identify the underlying cause of PAH, because each case has a different treatment regimen. For example, the treatment of patients with primary PAH may include a transplantation procedure, whereas the treatment for patients with secondary PAH from chronic thromboembolism is thromboendarterectomy. In some cases, a careful examination of the chest radiograph for ancillary cardiac, pulmonary, and pleural findings may provide clues to the underlying cause of PAH. In many cases, however, additional imaging studies such as echocardiography, ventilation-perfusion imaging, and pulmonary angiography are necessary to diagnose the precise cause of PAH. In cases of suspected chronic thromboembolic disease, CT and magnetic resonance imaging (MRI) can also be helpful (discussed later).

■ CONGESTIVE HEART FAILURE

Pulmonary edema refers to the presence of excess extravascular fluid within the interstitial and alveolar compartments of the lung. Under normal conditions, these compartments are kept relatively dry by two main factors: a balance between capillary pressure and plasma oncotic pressure and the maintenance of normal capillary wall permeability. Pulmonary edema usually occurs by means of one of two mechanisms: elevated pulmonary microvascular pressure or increased capillary membrane permeability. The former is referred to as cardiogenic or hydrostatic pulmonary edema, and the latter is referred to as noncardiogenic pulmonary edema.

We focus on cardiogenic pulmonary edema in this chapter. The most common cause of elevated pulmonary microvascular pressure is elevation of pulmonary venous pressure caused by diseases of the left side of the heart. Examples include left ventricular failure, diseases of the mitral valve, and left atrial abnormalities (see Box 14-1).

Interstitial Edema

Pulmonary edema usually follows a typical course. It begins in the interstitial compartment of the lung and extends into the alveolar compartment as it increases in severity. The first phase of pulmonary edema involves the interstitial compartment. It contains two major components: the peribronchovascular sheath and the interlobular septa. Fluid within the peribronchovascular sheath results in indistinctness of the pulmonary vessels and peribronchial cuffing (Fig. 14-4). Fluid within the interlobular septa results in Kerley lines (Table 14-1 and Fig. 14-5).

As interstitial edema progresses in severity, fluid may also accumulate within the subpleural space of the interlobar fissures. This subpleural edema results in thickening of the interlobar fissures on chest radiographs.

TABLE 14-1 Kerley A and B Lines

Type of Line	Location	Length
Kerley A lines	Central Radiate from hila	2-6 cm
Kerley B Lines	Peripheral Adjacent to costophrenic sulcus	<2 cm

Alveolar Edema

The second phase of pulmonary edema involves the extension of fluid into the alveolar spaces of the lung. Airspace involvement can be detected by identifying poorly defined nodular opacities, which represent fluid within the alveoli. As increasing amounts of fluid fill the alveoli, these opacities coalesce to produce airspace consolidation, which is usually most prominent in the central perihilar regions of the lungs.

Although the distribution of pulmonary edema is often bilateral and symmetric, there is considerable variability in its distribution. When asymmetric, pulmonary edema is usually more severe in the right lung (Fig. 14-6). An atypical pattern of pulmonary edema is often observed in patients with underlying lung disease. For example, patients with severe upper lobe emphysema often have a basilar predominance of pulmonary edema. Although the appearance of pulmonary edema may vary among patients, there is often a strikingly similar pattern in an individual patient from episode to episode. It is helpful to compare the current radiograph with one obtained during a prior episode of pulmonary edema, particularly for patients who present with an asymmetric or atypical distribution. Additional characteristic features of alveolar pulmonary edema include a fairly rapid onset, an often dramatic shift in distribution with various patient positions, and a relatively quick resolution in response to adequate therapy. These features can be helpful in differentiating asymmetric pulmonary edema from diffuse pneumonia.

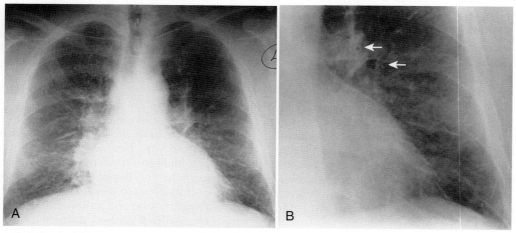

FIGURE 14-4. Interstitial pulmonary edema. **A,** A frontal chest radiograph reveals the presence of interstitial pulmonary edema, manifested by peribronchial cuffing, indistinctness of the pulmonary vessels, Kerley lines, and subpleural edema. **B,** The peribronchial cuffing *(arrows)* and Kerley lines are seen in greater detail on the coned-down image of the left lung.

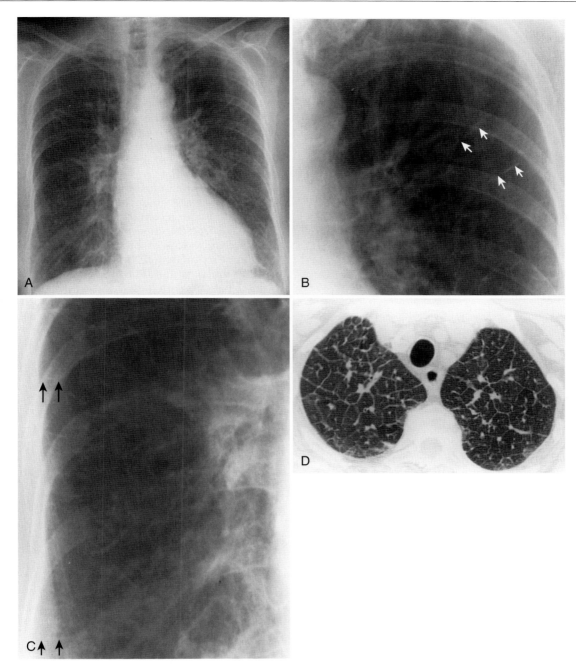

FIGURE 14-5. Interstitial pulmonary edema. **A,** A frontal chest radiograph reveals several linear opacities throughout both lungs. The linear opacities are referred to as Kerley lines, and they represent fluid-filled interlobular septa. **B,** A coned-down image of the left upper lobe demonstrates linear opacities radiating from the hila, consistent with Kerley A lines *(arrows)*. Notice that Kerley A lines do not extend to the pleural surface. **C,** A coned-down image of the right middle and lower lung zones reveals linear opacities in the lung periphery, consistent with Kerley B lines *(arrows)*. Notice that Kerley B lines extend to the pleural surface. **D,** A high-resolution CT scan image of the chest demonstrates smooth interlobular septal thickening, which outlines the secondary pulmonary lobules of the lungs. Interlobular septal thickening corresponds to the plain radiographic finding of Kerley lines. The ground-glass parenchymal opacities, peribronchovascular interstitial thickening, and increased vascular diameter are characteristic high-resolution CT findings of hydrostatic pulmonary edema.

Although we have presented the findings of interstitial and alveolar edema as separate entities, the radiographic findings for both often coexist. Because the interstitial compartment is affected first, interstitial edema may be present without alveolar edema. If alveolar edema is present, the interstitial compartment must also be edematous (even if it is not radiographically apparent).

Physiologic Correlation

The characteristic radiographic findings of pulmonary venous hypertension and congestive heart failure correlate with physiologic parameters such as pulmonary venous wedge pressures (PVWPs). The normal PVWP is less than 12 mm Hg. As the PVWP rises between 12 mm Hg

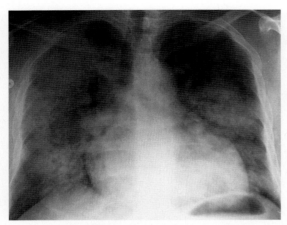

FIGURE 14-6. Alveolar edema. A frontal chest radiograph demonstrates the presence of bilateral airspace consolidation, which is more prominent in the right lung than in the left. When asymmetric, pulmonary edema is usually more severe in the right lung. Radiographs obtained during prior episodes of pulmonary edema demonstrated a similar pattern of asymmetric airspace consolidation.

and 17 mm Hg, cephalization of the pulmonary vessels is seen. At levels above 17 mm Hg, Kerley lines are seen. After the PVWP rises above 20 mm Hg, a pleural effusion may be seen, and it usually is right sided. At pressures greater than 25 mm Hg, airspace consolidation occurs. Keep in mind that these values are relative. For example, acinar opacities occasionally are seen at PVWP levels of 20 to 25 mm Hg. Moreover, as pulmonary edema resolves, the radiographic findings may lag behind the clinical improvement of the patient. Persistent radiographic evidence of pulmonary edema may exist despite the fact that hemodynamic measurements have returned to normal.

■ PULMONARY THROMBOEMBOLISM

Acute pulmonary embolism (PE) is the third most common acute cardiovascular disease, after myocardial infarction and stroke, causing hundreds of thousands of deaths each year in the United States because it often goes undetected. Prompt and accurate diagnosis is important because the mortality rate for untreated PE is high, and serious complications can occur with anticoagulation treatment. The clinical diagnosis of PE may be subtle, atypical, or obscured by a coexisting disease. The symptoms and signs of acute PE include dyspnea, pleuritic chest pain, tachypnea, and tachycardia; these findings indicate a need for further investigation. Initial imaging with contrast-enhanced CT has become the standard of care at many institutions.

The basic pathophysiology of PE and use of the D-dimer assay are reviewed in the next section, along with imaging manifestations of acute PE on the chest radiograph, ventilation-perfusion (V/Q) scintigrams, evaluation of the leg veins, and the use of CT, conventional MRI, and MR angiography.

Pathophysiology of Pulmonary Thromboembolism

In 1860, Virchow postulated that thrombus formation is caused by vessel injury, disturbance of blood flow, and hypercoagulability. The known risk factors for venous thromboembolism include recent surgery, prolonged immobilization, cerebrovascular accident, congestive heart failure, cancer, leg or pelvic bone fracture, obesity, pregnancy or recent delivery, estrogen therapy, inflammatory bowel disease, and genetic or acquired thrombophilia. Most thrombi arise within the deep venous system of the lower extremities. If thrombi dislodge and occlude the main, lobar, segmental, or subsegmental pulmonary arteries, they are referred to as *pulmonary thromboemboli*. Most have a predilection for the lower lobes of the lungs. Approximately 15% of pulmonary thromboemboli result in pulmonary infarction. Infarction occurs when the combined pulmonary and bronchial circulation is inadequate, often in patients with underlying cardiovascular disease. In most cases, lysis of thrombi results in the affected vessels returning to normal. However, in less than 1% of patients, recurrent thromboemboli and incomplete resolution of previous thromboemboli causes chronic thromboembolic pulmonary hypertension.

The measurement of the degradation products of cross-linked fibrin (D-dimer) within plasma is a highly sensitive but nonspecific test for suspected venous thromboembolism. Abnormal levels are also present in almost all patients with pulmonary thromboembolism. Elevated levels are found in patients with advancing age, during pregnancy, after trauma, during the postoperative period, in inflammatory states, and in cancer. Only a negative D-dimer test result is helpful in the evaluation of pulmonary thromboembolism.

Imaging Features of Acute Pulmonary Thromboembolism

Chest Radiography

Many episodes of PE do not result in radiographic abnormalities. The chest radiograph has two primary roles in the evaluation of a patient with suspected acute PE. The initial role is the detection of other abnormalities that may clinically mimic PE. For example, pleuritic chest pain and dyspnea may be the result of pneumothorax rather than PE. Second, the chest radiograph assists in the interpretation of the V/Q scintigram.

The chest radiographic signs of PE without infarction include focal oligemia (i.e., Westermark's sign (Fig.14-7), an increase in a central vessel size with abrupt tapering, and atelectasis. The chest radiographic signs of PE with infarction include peripheral consolidation with a convex border abutting the pleura (i.e., Hampton's hump), atelectasis, elevated hemidiaphragm, and pleural effusion. Atelectasis often manifests as linear parenchymal opacities that have a basilar distribution. The Prospective Investigation of Pulmonary Embolism Diagnosis (PIOPED) demonstrated that these radiographic signs do not provide sufficient information to accurately establish or exclude the diagnosis of acute PE.

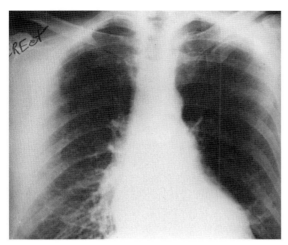

FIGURE 14-7. Westermark's sign. A frontal radiograph of the chest reveals asymmetry of the pulmonary vascularity of the two lungs, with diminished vascularity throughout the left lung. In this patient, the asymmetry is most apparent in the middle and lower lung zones because of the presence of bilateral upper lobe vascular attenuation caused by emphysema. A pulmonary angiogram demonstrated occlusive thrombus in the left main pulmonary artery.

Ventilation-Perfusion Scintigraphy

The V/Q scintigram relies on indirect radiologic signs for the diagnosis of PE. Xenon 133 is the usual inhaled ventilation agent, and technetium 99 m-macroaggregated human albumin is the perfusion agent that is injected intravenously. PE manifests as a ventilation-perfusion mismatch on the V/Q scintigram (Fig. 14-8). However, this pattern can also be caused by lung neoplasia, radiation effects, vasculitis, fat embolism, and pulmonary hypertension. When interpreting a V/Q scintigram, it is important to evaluate a current chest radiograph.

We recommend the use of the PIOPED study interpretative scheme. The V/Q scintigram is categorized as normal, low probability for PE, indeterminate probability for PE, or high probability for PE.

The PIOPED study results for V/Q scintigraphy demonstrated a sensitivity of 98% and a specificity of 10% for the diagnosis of acute PE. A normal V/Q scintigram virtually excludes the diagnosis of PE, and a high-probability V/Q scintigram is considered sufficient evidence to treat a patient with anticoagulation therapy. However, most patients fall between these two categories and therefore require further imaging. An in-depth discussion about V/Q scintigraphy can be found in *Nuclear Medicine: The Requisites.*

Evaluation of the Leg Veins

Clinicians faced with an indeterminate V/Q scintigram result and a high clinical suspicion for PE often search for the source of the emboli by imaging the deep veins of the legs. Studies have shown that ultrasound of the legs is positive in 10% to 20% of patients with suspected PE but without leg symptoms or signs, and it is positive in approximately 50% of patients with proven embolism. PE cannot be excluded on the basis of negative results on ultrasound. Contrast-enhanced CT of the veins of the pelvis and lower extremities is performed with the same contrast bolus used for chest CT. Multidetector CT venography is simple and accurate, and when combined with the lung CT angiography images, it provides a fast and comprehensive analysis of thromboembolic disease. However, because of radiation dose concerns, this method should not be used routinely in all patients. According to the Fleischner Society's recommendations, CT venography should be considered only when an expeditious complete vascular exam is desired clinically. In the setting of concerns for radiation exposure (such as in younger patients), they recommend substituting lower extremity ultrasound. When evaluation of the lower extremity veins is not important clinically, they recommend that CT venography may be omitted.

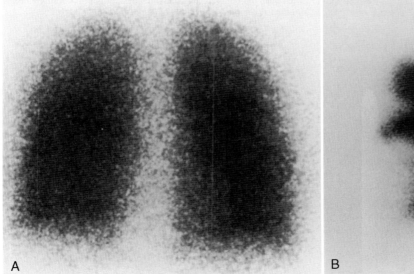
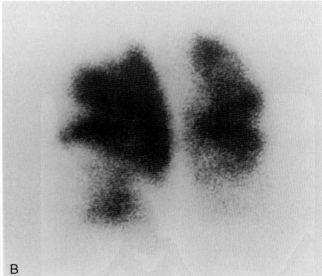

A   B

FIGURE 14-8. Multiple pulmonary emboli. **A,** A posterior image from the ventilation portion of a V/Q scan demonstrates homogenous ventilation to both lungs, without evidence of ventilation defects. **B,** A right anterior oblique image from the perfusion portion of a V/Q scan in the same patient reveals multiple subsegmental and segmental perfusion defects in both lungs consistent with multiple pulmonary emboli.

Computed Tomography

CT has provided a major advance in the diagnosis of PE. Multidetector CT can acquire contrast-enhanced images of the entire chest with a slice thickness of 1 mm in 8 seconds or less. The sensitivity and specificity of CT for the diagnosis of PE ranges from 53% to 100% and 83% to 100%, respectively. These wide ranges are explained by the evolution of CT technology. Multidetector scanners allow improved vascular resolution because of narrow slice thickness and less motion artifact due to faster scan times. CT accuracy is reported to have a sensitivity and specificity of more than 90%.

The diagnostic criteria for acute PE include (Box 14-2) the following:

- Intraluminal filling defects that have a sharp interface with the intravascular contrast
- Complete arterial occlusion with failure to opacify the entire lumen due to a large filling defect; the artery may enlarge compared with peers (Fig. 14-9)
- Partial filling defect surrounded by contrast; the "polo mint sign" seen on an image acquired perpendicular to long axis of vessel (Fig. 14-10) or the "railway track sign" demonstrated on a longitudinal image of the vessel (Fig. 14-11)
- A peripheral intraluminal defect; the eccentric filling defect makes an acute angle with the arterial wall (Fig. 14-12)

The ancillary findings of peripheral, wedge-shaped opacities and linear bands are indirect and nonspecific signs for PE.

Box 14-2. Computed Tomography Criteria for Acute Pulmonary Embolism

Intraluminal filling defect with a sharp interface
Complete arterial occlusion; the artery may enlarge at site of impaction
Partial filling defect; the "polo mint" or the "railway track" sign
Peripheral intraluminal defect that makes acute angles with the arterial wall

---

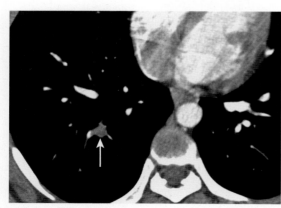

FIGURE 14-9. Acute occlusive pulmonary embolism on contrast-enhanced CT. The thrombus is seen within the posterior basal segment of the right lower lobe *(arrow)*. The artery is enlarged compared with its peers.

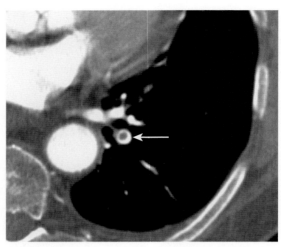

FIGURE 14-10. Acute pulmonary embolism affects the segmental artery of the posterior basal segment of the left lower lobe. This partial filling defect surrounded by contrast produces the polo mint sign *(arrow)*.

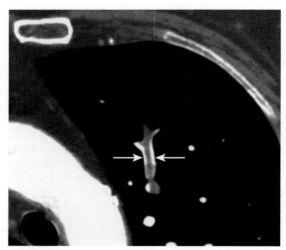

FIGURE 14-11. Acute pulmonary embolism causes a partial filling defect surrounded by contrast and the railway track sign affecting the anterior segment artery of the left upper lobe *(arrows)*.

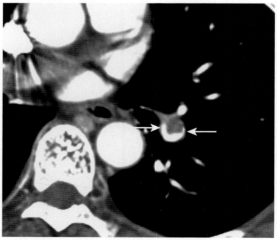

FIGURE 14-12. Acute pulmonary embolism results in a partial filling defect surrounded by contrast. The eccentrically located filling defect produces acute angles with the arterial wall *(arrows)*.

After an initial embolic event, a patient may be at risk for circulatory collapse because of right heart failure, and another embolism may be fatal. Right ventricular strain or failure is optimally evaluated by echocardiography. However, some morphologic abnormalities that can be quantified by CT pulmonary angiography (CTPA) suggest right ventricular failure. The CT signs include the following:

- Right ventricular dilation, in which the right ventricle cavity is wider than the left ventricle in the short axis (Fig. 14-13), with or without contrast reflux into hepatic veins
- Interventricular septum deviated toward the left ventricle (see Fig. 14-13)
- Occlusion of greater than 60% of the pulmonary arteries

Coincidental pulmonary emboli have been identified on 1.5% of contrast-enhanced CT scans performed for an indication other than PE evaluation. These are important observations because acute PE may be seen when it is not suspected clinically, and detection can determine further imaging needs and allow the timely initiation of appropriate therapy.

Most clinicians readily accept a positive CT scan in the diagnosis of PE. Follow-up studies of patient populations who have had a negative CTPA results suggest that it is safe to withhold anticoagulation in patients with a technically adequate negative CT pulmonary angiogram.

Several studies have demonstrated that CTPA provides an alternative diagnosis in most patients when the study is negative for PE. Abnormalities may be seen in the lung parenchyma, such as pneumonia, and in the cases that

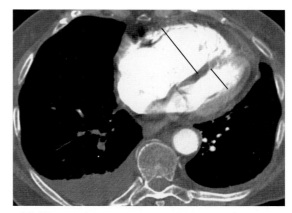

FIGURE 14-13. Right ventricle strain caused by acute pulmonary embolism. The short axis of the right ventricle *(longest line)* is wider than the short axis of the left ventricle.

are positive for PE, pulmonary infarcts may be identified. These typically appear as peripheral, wedge-shaped areas of consolidation with their bases abutting the visceral pleura (Fig. 14-14).

Angiography

Pulmonary angiography involves percutaneous advancement of a catheter through a femoral vein and through the right atrium and ventricle to the pulmonary arteries under fluoroscopic guidance. After the injection of intravascular contrast, images are acquired at a rapid rate. The angiographic signs of PE include a partial filling defect within a contrast-filled vessel and complete occlusion of the vessel, producing an abrupt vascular cutoff (Fig. 14-15).

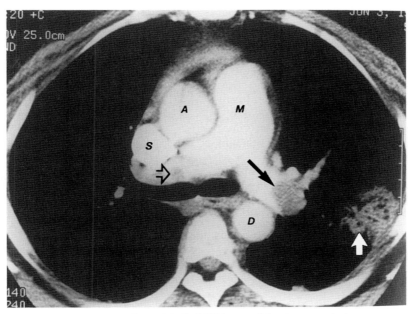

FIGURE 14-14. Acute pulmonary embolism. A contrast-enhanced, helical CT image of the chest reveals the presence of soft tissue attenuation thrombus within the distal left main pulmonary artery *(black arrow)* and the right pulmonary *(open arrow)*. Acute pulmonary emboli in these vessels were confirmed at angiography. Notice the peripheral consolidation in the left upper lobe *(white arrow)*, suggesting the pulmonary infarction. A, ascending aorta; D, descending aorta; M, main pulmonary artery; S, superior vena cava. (Case courtesy of Elizabeth Drucker, MD, Massachusetts General Hospital, Boston, MA.)

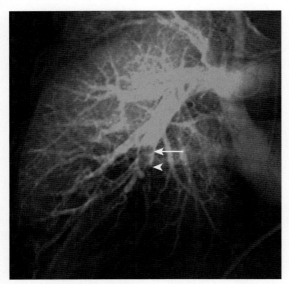

Figure 14-15. Pulmonary angiogram. Acute pulmonary embolism causes a partial filling defect *(arrow)* and the cut-off sign *(arrowhead)* within the posterior basal segment of the right lower lobe.

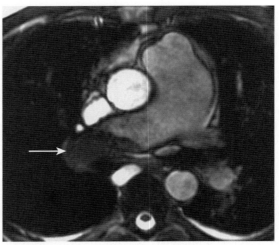

Figure 14-16. Large acute pulmonary embolism is demonstrated in the right pulmonary artery *(arrow)* on a magnetic resonance angiogram.

Traditionally, pulmonary angiography has been considered the gold standard for the diagnosis of PE. One study compared spiral CT angiography and pulmonary angiography against an independent gold standard in a porcine model of pulmonary emboli. CT and conventional angiography had a sensitivity of 87% in the detection of emboli. This study raised doubts about the status of conventional angiography as the undisputed gold standard in the diagnosis of PE. Pulmonary angiography should be reserved for solving difficult clinical problems. The decision to perform pulmonary angiography should be tempered by the quality of the CT pulmonary angiogram; if the CT is negative and the vessels are well demonstrated to the subsegmental level, a pulmonary angiogram is not required.

Magnetic Resonance Angiography

Similar to CT, pulmonary magnetic resonance angiography (MRA) can directly visualize emboli within arteries. MRA can be performed within a single, suspended inspiration (Fig. 14-16). Compared with CT, MRI does not require iodinated contrast media. MRA can be performed in patients with a history of iodinated contrast reaction and in those with poor renal function.

MRA has a high specificity but rather low sensitivity for the diagnosis of PE. A negative MRA result cannot exclude significant PE. A large outcome study is necessary to establish MRA's role in the evaluation of patients with suspected acute PE.

Chronic Pulmonary Thromboembolism

In a small number of patients, recurrent episodes of acute PE may result in chronic pulmonary thromboembolism and pulmonary arterial hypertension. Presenting clinical features include progressive dyspnea and fatigue. The treatment of choice for pulmonary arterial hypertension caused by chronic PE is thromboendarterectomy. Chest radiographic findings include enlargement of the main, right,

and left pulmonary arteries. V/Q scintigraphy findings of chronic PE are similar to those of acute PE (i.e. multiple segmental V/Q mismatches).

The diagnostic criteria for chronic PE on CT include the following (Box 14-3):

- Intraluminal filling defects that have a sharp interface with the intravascular contrast
- Complete occlusion of a vessel that is smaller than its peers (Fig. 14-17)
- A peripheral intraluminal defect; an eccentric crescentic filling defect that forms obtuse angles with the vessel wall (Fig. 14-18)
- Contrast flowing through thickened, often smaller, arteries due to recanalization (Fig. 14-19)
- Web or flap within a contrast filled artery (Fig. 14-20)
- Secondary signs: extensive bronchial or other systemic collateral vessels through the affected area, accompanying mosaic perfusion pattern, or calcification within eccentric vessel thickening

Ancillary findings of chronic PE may include the CT changes of pulmonary arterial hypertension with a pulmonary artery diameter greater than 3 cm and pericardial fluid.

Box 14-3. Computed Tomography Criteria for Chronic Pulmonary Embolism

Intraluminal filling defect with a sharp interface
Complete arterial occlusion; the artery is smaller than peers
Partial filling defect; band or web
Peripheral intraluminal defect that makes obtuse angles with the arterial wall
Recanalization may manifest as contrast flowing through a thickened small artery
Secondary signs include bronchial or other systemic collateral vessels, mosaic perfusion pattern, or pulmonary embolism calcification

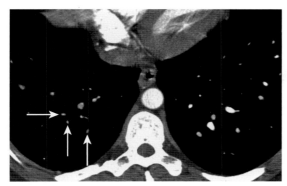

FIGURE 14-17. Chronic pulmonary embolism manifests as complete occlusion of vessels *(arrows)* that are smaller than their peers.

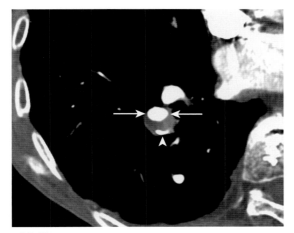

FIGURE 14-18. Chronic pulmonary embolism. The eccentrically located thrombus makes obtuse angles with the vessel wall *(arrows)*. Notice the dilated collateral bronchial artery *(arrowhead)*.

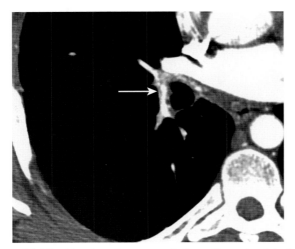

FIGURE 14-19. Chronic pulmonary embolism affects the right lower lobe pulmonary artery. It manifests as a small, recanalized vessel with a central lumen containing contrast *(arrow)*.

The characteristic features of chronic PE are also seen on conventional MRI and MRA. Angiographic recognition of residual thromboembolic material may be limited when chronic clot is incorporated concentrically in the vessel wall with new epithelial cells smoothing the internal contour.

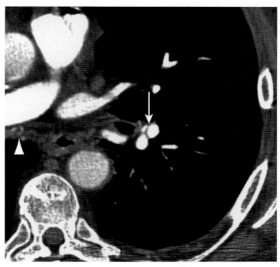

FIGURE 14-20. Chronic pulmonary embolism results in a flap *(arrow)* within the left lower lobe pulmonary artery. Notice the collateral bronchial artery dilatation *(arrowhead)*.

The sensitivity of MRI is limited by the spatial resolution needed to demonstrate crescentic thromboembolic material. Pulmonary angioscopy is invaluable in determining whether thromboembolic obstruction is accessible to surgical intervention. However, access to this technique is limited. The high spatial resolution of multidetector CT with three-dimensional volumetric imaging makes CT one of the methods of choice in the assessment of patients for potential surgical resection.

■ SUGGESTED READINGS

Baile, E.M., King, G.G., Muller, N.L., et al., 2000. Spiral computed tomography is comparable to angiography for the diagnosis of pulmonary embolism. Am. J. Respir. Crit. Care. Med. 161, 1010–1015.

Bergin, C.J., Hauschildt, J., Rios, G., et al., 1997. Accuracy of MR angiography compared with radionuclide scanning in identifying the cause of pulmonary artery hypertension. AJR Am. J. Roentgenol. 168, 1549–1555.

Contractor, S., Maldjian, P.D., Sharma, V.K., et al., 2002. Role of helical CT in detecting right ventricular dysfunction secondary to acute pulmonary embolism. J. Comput. Assist. Tomogr. 26, 587–591.

Fraser, R.G., Paré, J.A., Paré, P.D., et al., 1990. Pulmonary hypertension and edema. In: Fraser, R.G., Paré, J.A.P., Paré, P.D., et al. (Eds.), Diagnosis of Diseases of the Chest. WB Saunders, Philadelphia, pp. 1823–1968.

Goodman, L.R., Lipchik, R.J., Kuzo, R.S., et al., 2000. Subsequent pulmonary embolism: risk after a negative helical CT pulmonary angiogram—prospective comparison with scintigraphy. Radiology 215, 535–542.

Gosselin, M.V., Rubin, G.D., Leung, A.N., et al., 1998. Unsuspected pulmonary embolism: prospective detection on routine helical CT scans. Radiology 208, 209–215.

Gurney, J., 1992. Physiology. In: Freundlich, I.M., Bragg, D.G. (Eds.), A Radiologic Approach to Diseases of the Chest. Williams & Wilkins, Baltimore, pp. 8–25.

Hansell, D.M., Peters, A.M., 1995. Pulmonary vascular diseases and pulmonary edema. In: Armstrong, P., Wilson, A.G., Dee, P., et al. (Eds.), Imaging of Diseases of the Chest. second ed. Mosby, St. Louis, pp. 369–425.

Loud, P.A., Katz, D.S., Bruce, D.A., et al., 2001. Deep venous thrombosis with suspected pulmonary embolism: detection with combined CT venography and pulmonary angiography. Radiology 219, 498–502.

Mastora, I., Remy-Jardin, M., Masson, P., et al., 2003. Severity of acute pulmonary embolism: evaluation of a new spiral CT angiographic score in correlation with echocardiographic data. Eur. Radiol. 13, 29–35.

Meaney, J.F.M., Weg, J.G., Chenevert, T.L., et al., 1997. Diagnosis of pulmonary embolism with magnetic resonance angiography. N. Engl. J. Med. 336, 1422–1427.

Miller, S.W. The elements of cardiac imaging. In: Miller, S.W. (Ed.), Cardiac Radiology: The Requisites. St. Louis, Mosby, 1997, pp. 23–36.

Prospective Investigation of Pulmonary Embolism Diagnosis (PIOPED) Investigators, 1990. Value of the ventilation/perfusion scan in acute pulmonary embolism. Results of the Prospective Investigation of Pulmonary Embolism Diagnosis (PIOPED). JAMA 263, 2753–2759.

Randall, P.A., Heitzman, E.R., Groskin, S.A., Scalzetti, E.M., 1992. Pulmonary arterial hypertension. In: Freundlich, I.M., Bragg, D.G. (Eds.), A Radiologic Approach to Diseases of the Chest. Williams & Wilkins, Baltimore, pp. 151–162.

Rathburn, S.W., Raskob, G.E., Whitsett, T.L., 2000. Sensitivity and specificity of helical computed tomography in the diagnosis of pulmonary embolism: a systematic review. Ann. Intern. Med. 132, 227–232.

Remy-Jardin, M., Mastora, I., Remy, J., 2003. Pulmonary embolus imaging with multislice CT. Radiol. Clin. North Am. 41, 507–519.

Remy-Jardin, M., Pistolesi, M., Goodman, L.R., Gefter, W.B., Gottschalk, A., Mayo, J.R., Sostman, H.D., 2007. Management of suspected acute pulmonary embolism in the era of CT angiography: a statement from the Fleischner Society Radiology 245:315–329.

Rubin, L.J., 1997. Primary pulmonary hypertension. N. Engl. J. Med. 336, 111–117.

Thrall, J.H., Ziessman, H.A., 2001. Pulmonary system. In: Thrall, J.H., Ziessman, H.A., (Eds.), Nuclear Medicine: The Requisites. second ed. Mosby, St. Louis, pp. 145–166.

Washington, L., Goodman, L.R., Gonyo, M.B., 2002. CT for thromboembolic disease. Radiol. Clin. North Am. 40, 751–771.

Wittram, C., Maher, M., Yoo, A., et al., 2004. CT Angiography of pulmonary embolism: diagnostic criteria and causes of misdiagnosis. Radiographics 24, 1219–1239.

Wittram, C., Kalra, M.K., Maher, M.M., et al., 2006. Acute and chronic pulmonary emboli: angiographic-CT correlation. AJR Am. J. Roentgenol. 186 (Suppl. 2), S421–S429.

Worsley, L.F., Alavi, A., Aronchick, J.M., et al., 1993. Chest radiographic findings in patients with acute pulmonary embolism: observations from the PIOPED study. Radiology 189, 133–136.

CHAPTER 15

The Mediastinum: Anatomy

Phillip M. Boiselle

The mediastinum is an anatomic region bounded laterally by the two lungs, anteriorly by the sternum, posteriorly by the vertebrae, superiorly by the thoracic inlet, and inferiorly by the diaphragm. Many focal and diffuse abnormalities occur in the mediastinum. Computed tomography (CT) and magnetic resonance imaging (MRI) have improved our ability to detect, define, and characterize these abnormalities. In certain cases, the imaging features of a mediastinal mass allow a specific diagnosis to be made on the basis of imaging findings.

■ THE FOUR Ds OF MEDIASTINAL MASSES

The classic radiologic differential diagnosis of an anterior mediastinal mass (i.e., the four Ts) is one of the best known approaches among medical students and first-year radiology residents. However, before arriving at this seemingly simple differential diagnosis, several important observations and deductions must be made, including the four Ds of mediastinal masses: *detection* of an abnormality, *description* of the abnormality, placement of the abnormality into the appropriate anatomic *division* of the mediastinum, and generation of a limited *differential diagnosis* based on the descriptive features and anatomic location.

Chapters 16 and 17 address focal mediastinal masses and diffuse mediastinal abnormalities.

■ DETECTION: MEDIASTINAL LANDMARKS

To detect a mediastinal abnormality, the radiologist must be thoroughly familiar with the normal radiographic anatomy and with the characteristic changes produced by abnormalities within various portions of the mediastinum. The radiographic landmarks of normal mediastinal anatomy are the lines, stripes, and interfaces produced when the x-ray beam passes tangential to an edge formed between tissues of different attenuations (Box 15-1).

Lines

A *line* is a longitudinal opacity no greater than 2 mm wide. Examples include the anterior and posterior junction lines, which are formed by the close apposition of the visceral and parietal layers of pleura of both lungs as they approximate anteriorly and posteriorly to the mediastinum (Fig. 15-1). The anterior portion of the thorax begins at the thoracic inlet. The anterior junction line begins at the undersurface of the clavicles; it courses inferiorly toward the left in an oblique orientation to the level of the heart. Because the posterior portion of the thorax extends more superiorly than the anterior portion, the posterior junction line can be seen as it extends above the level of the clavicles. It frequently appears as a straight line and often projects through the tracheal air column. The anterior and posterior junction lines are not seen on all radiographic examinations. However, detection of a displaced junction line allows identification of a mediastinal abnormality and localization as anterior or posterior.

Two additional mediastinal lines are the right and left paraspinal lines, which are each about 1 mm wide. They are best seen on anteroposterior thoracic spine films. The left paraspinal line extends superiorly from the level of the aortic arch and inferiorly to the level of the diaphragm and parallels the lateral margin of the vertebral bodies. An important relationship is the one between the left paraspinal line and the descending aortic interface (see "Interfaces"). The left paraspinal line normally lies medial to the descending aortic interface. Displacement of the left paraspinal line lateral to the descending aortic interface signals the presence of a posterior mediastinal abnormality (Fig. 15-2). The right paraspinal line is less frequently visualized; when seen, it is often identified only over a portion of its course, usually between the 8th and 12th thoracic vertebral levels. Both paraspinal lines are normally straight and maintain a constant relationship with the adjacent vertebral bodies, except when displaced laterally by osteophytes. An ectatic aorta may displace the left paraspinal line laterally.

Box 15-1. **Detection: Mediastinal Landmarks**

LINES
Anterior junction line
Posterior junction line
Right and left paraspinal lines

STRIPES
Right paratracheal stripe

INTERFACES
Azygoesophageal interface
Descending aortic interface

Stripes

A *stripe* is a longitudinal composite opacity that is 2 to 5 mm wide. The right paratracheal stripe is formed by the apposition of the right upper lobe pleura and the right lateral tracheal wall. It can be identified on most chest radiographs. The normal right paratracheal stripe is identified as a smooth stripe adjacent to the right lateral border of the trachea air column, extending inferiorly to the level of the azygous vein (see Fig. 15-1). In normal individuals, it is seen as a smooth stripe of uniform width (≤3 mm). Widening of the right paratracheal stripe is a sign of middle mediastinal pathology, such as right paratracheal lymphadenopathy (Fig. 15-3).

Interfaces

An *interface* is the common boundary between the shadows of two juxtaposed tissues of different opacities, such as between the lungs and heart. Two interfaces that are important landmarks of normal mediastinal anatomy are the azygoesophageal interface and the descending aortic interface.

The azygoesophageal interface is formed by the juxtaposition of aerated lung within the right lower lobe or the soft tissue opacity of the right lateral margin of the azygous vein or esophagus, or both (see Fig. 15-1). The azygoesophageal recess of can be identified on well-penetrated posteroanterior chest radiographs as an interface beginning superiorly at the level of the azygous arch and extending inferiorly to the level of the diaphragm. The azygoesophageal interface normally produces a gentle concave slope as it curves slightly toward the left; a focal convexity of the azygoesophageal interface signals the presence of a mediastinal abnormality. Subcarinal masses such as bronchogenic cysts and esophageal abnormalities such as achalasia frequently produce abnormalities in the contour of the azygoesophageal interface (Fig. 15-4).

The descending aortic interface is formed by the juxtaposition of aerated lung and the soft tissue opacity of the left lateral margin of the descending thoracic aorta; it is usually visible from the top of the aortic arch to the level of the diaphragm inferiorly. Because the descending thoracic aorta is a posterior structure, abnormalities in the descending aortic interface imply pathology within the posterior mediastinum. A descending thoracic aortic aneurysm is a common cause for an abnormal contour of the descending aortic interface (Fig. 15-5).

In addition to a familiarity with the normal lines, stripes, and interfaces of the mediastinum, knowledge of the normal mediastinal contours on the frontal radiograph of the chest is essential (Fig. 15-6). The lateral chest radiograph also should be carefully assessed. There are normally two "clear" spaces: retrosternal, between the sternum and ascending aorta, and retrocardiac, between the heart and spine. Midline anterior mediastinal masses are often best visualized on lateral chest radiographs as opacification within the normally clear retrosternal space (Fig. 15-7).

A thorough knowledge of normal mediastinal anatomy and of the changes produced by abnormalities within various portions of the mediastinum is important for detection and localization of mediastinal abnormalities. A displaced mediastinal line, a widened stripe, and an abnormal contour of an interface are important signs of mediastinal pathology. Comparison of current and previous radiographs is necessary to detect subtle changes in the lines, stripes, and interfaces of the mediastinum on serial examinations.

DESCRIPTIVE FEATURES OF MEDIASTINAL MASSES

It is often difficult to determine whether a centrally located mass is mediastinal, pleural, or parenchymal in origin. Heitzman lists three primary descriptive features that are commonly seen in masses of mediastinal origin: intimate effect on mediastinal structures; smooth, sharp margins; and obtuse angles between the margins of the mass and adjacent lung.

The first feature, an intimate effect on mediastinal structures, is considered the most important for determining whether a centrally located mass is mediastinal in origin (Fig. 15-8). Displacement or compression of mediastinal structures, particularly a localized effect, strongly suggests that a mass has a mediastinal origin. The tracheal air column and esophagus must be inspected for signs of displacement or compression when evaluating a centrally located mass.

The second descriptive feature of mediastinal masses is smooth, sharp margins (Fig. 15-9). Smooth margins are created by displacement of the adjacent visceral and parietal layers of pleura, which surround the lateral margin of a mediastinal mass. If a mass demonstrates irregular margins, it is more likely to originate in the lung than in the mediastinum.

The third feature is the formation of obtuse angles between the margins of the mass and adjacent lung (see Fig. 15-9). Masses originating within the lung more often demonstrate acute angles. However, because there is considerable overlap between mediastinal and lung masses, it is better to combine criteria to determine whether a mass originates within the mediastinum or lung (Table 15-1).

Additional features that can help to determine whether a mass is mediastinal include an epicenter in the mediastinum, bilaterality, and movement with swallowing rather than movement with respiration.

DIVISIONS OF THE MEDIASTINUM

After an abnormality is detected and it has been determined to be is mediastinal in origin, localizing the abnormality within a specific anatomic division of the mediastinum is the next step in generating a limited differential diagnosis. Several classification systems of the mediastinum are based on landmarks on the lateral chest radiograph rather than true anatomic fascial planes. The classification described here, a modified classification proposed by Fraser and Paré, has been chosen for its simplicity and wide recognition (Table 15-2). In this classification system, the mediastinum is divided into three compartments: anterior, middle, and posterior (Fig. 15-10).

Some classification systems include a fourth compartment, the superior mediastinum, which is bounded inferiorly by a line drawn from the sternal angle to the fourth intervertebral disk. Rather than containing structures unique to one compartment, this compartment contains structures that are continuous with compartments below it.

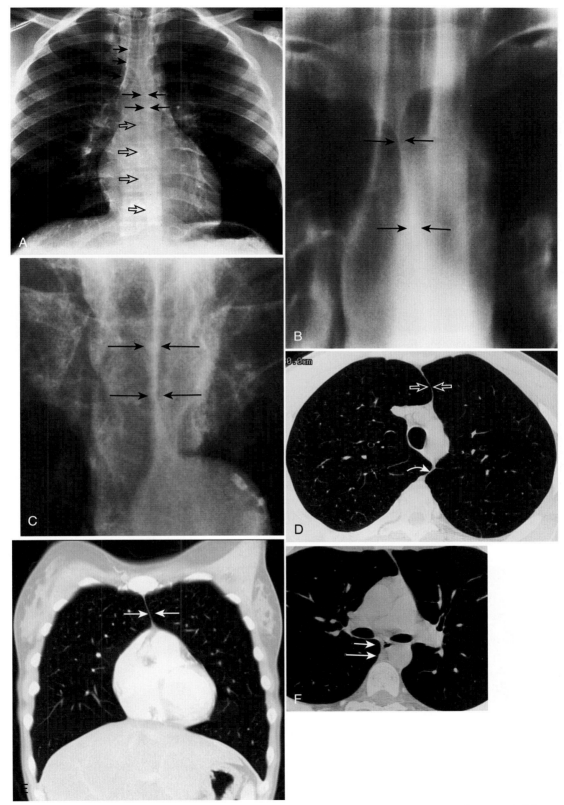

FIGURE 15-1. Mediastinal lines, stripes, and interfaces. **A,** Frontal chest radiograph shows the anterior junction line *(long arrows)*, right paratracheal stripe *(short arrows)*, and azygoesophageal interface *(open arrows)*. **B,** Anteroposterior tomogram shows the anterior junction line *(arrows)*. Notice that the anterior junction line begins below the level of the clavicles. **C,** Coned-down frontal chest radiograph shows the posterior junction line *(arrows)*. Notice that the posterior junction line extends superiorly above the level of the clavicles. **D,** Axial, high-resolution CT image shows the anterior *(open arrows)* and posterior *(curved arrow)* junction lines. **E,** Anterior coronal CT reformation image shows the anterior junction line *(arrows)*. **F,** Axial CT image shows the azygoesophageal interface, formed by the juxtaposition of aerated lung and the lateral walls of the azygous vein *(long arrow)* and esophagus *(short arrow)*.

DIFFERENTIAL DIAGNOSIS

Using a compartmental division of the mediastinum allows generation of a limited differential diagnosis for a focal mediastinal abnormality. Based on location, lesions that are likely to occur in a specific division can be considered, and abnormalities that are unlikely to occur within that division can be excluded.

First, abnormalities of the normal structures that reside in a given compartment are considered (see Table 15-2). For example, for a mass localized within the anterior mediastinum, abnormalities of the thymus gland, lymph nodes, anterior mediastinal fat, and internal mammary vessels should be considered. Abnormalities of the thymus gland, specifically thymoma, account for most anterior mediastinal masses in adults in most series. Abnormalities of the lymph nodes, especially Hodgkin's lymphoma, are also a common cause of anterior mediastinal masses. A knowledge of other common masses that occur within the anterior mediastinum, such as germ cell neoplasms, help to complete the list of diagnostic considerations in most cases.

Table 15-3 summarizes the common differential diagnoses for each of the three mediastinal compartments. Most diagnoses listed are related to abnormalities of structures normally located within each compartment. These differential diagnoses are based on the statistical likelihood of a mass occurring within a given compartment. Many of these entities can occur in any of the three compartments but are much more likely to occur in the one described. For example, although bronchogenic cysts have been described in all three mediastinal compartments, most occur in the middle mediastinum.

Careful analysis of imaging features and correlation with clinical data, such as patient age and symptoms, can effectively narrow the differential diagnosis, and in some cases, this process can lead to a specific diagnosis. Imaging

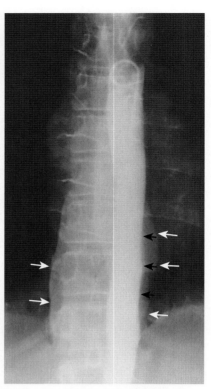

FIGURE 15-2. The anteroposterior radiograph from an aortographic study shows contrast opacification of the aorta and bilateral lateral displacement of the paraspinal lines *(two white arrows)* in a patient with posterior mediastinal lymphadenopathy from lymphoma. Notice that the left paraspinal line *(three white arrows)* is displaced lateral to the descending aortic interface *(black arrows)*.

features and demographic characteristics of common mediastinal masses in each compartment are described in Chapter 16.

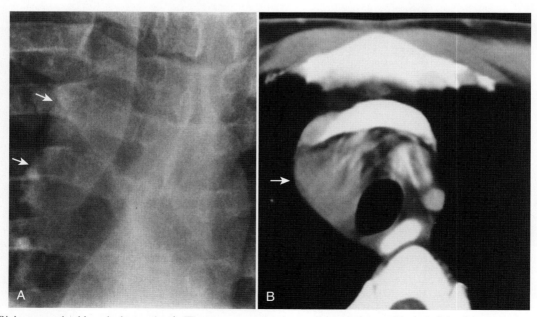

FIGURE 15-3. Right paratracheal lymphadenopathy. **A,** The posteroanterior chest radiograph shows widening of the right paratracheal stripe *(arrows)*. **B,** Axial, contrast-enhanced CT shows right paratracheal lymphadenopathy *(arrow)*.

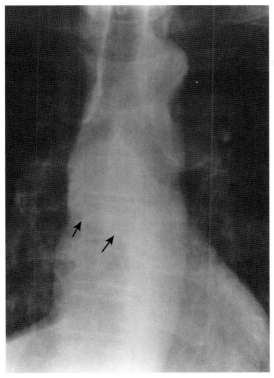

FIGURE 15-4. Bronchogenic cyst. The posteroanterior chest radiograph shows an abnormal convex contour of the azygoesophageal interface *(arrows)* caused by a subcarinal mass. Compare with the normal azygoesophageal interface in Figure 15-1A.

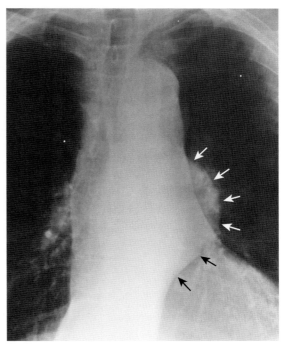

FIGURE 15-5. Descending thoracic aortic aneurysm. The posteroanterior chest radiograph reveals the convexity of the descending thoracic aortic interface *(white and black arrows)*, corresponding to the form of an aneurysm.

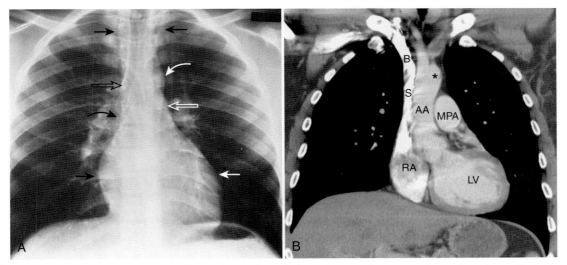

FIGURE 15-6. Normal mediastinal contours. **A,** The frontal chest radiograph shows the normal structures that produce the mediastinal contours (superior to inferior): left and right brachiocephalic vessels *(small black arrows)*; aortic arch *(curved white arrow)*; azygous arch *(open black arrow)*; main pulmonary artery *(open white arrow)*; ascending aorta *(curved black arrow)*; right atrium *(large, short black arrow)*; and left ventricle *(large, short white arrow)*. **B,** Coronal reformation CT shows the cardiovascular contents of the mediastinum (superior to inferior): brachiocephalic vein (B); aortic arch *(asterisk)*; superior vena cava (S); main pulmonary artery (MPA); ascending aorta (AA); right atrium (RA); and left ventricle (LV).

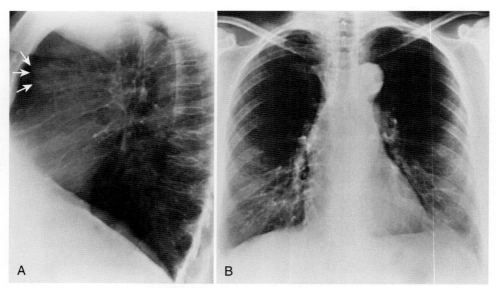

FIGURE 15-7. Thymoma. **A,** An anterior mediastinal mass is easily visualized on the lateral chest radiograph as a sharply defined, round opacity *(arrows)* in the retrosternal space, but it is difficult to identify on the frontal chest radiograph. **B,** Because the mass is not in direct contact with the structures that form the normal mediastinal contours on the frontal radiograph, it does not obliterate the margins of these structures.

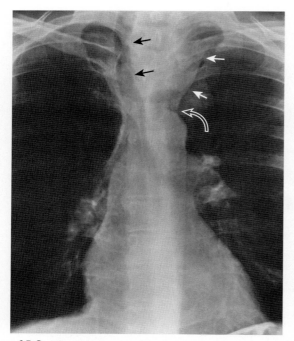

FIGURE 15-8. Thyroid adenoma. The frontal chest radiograph shows a large mass at the thoracic inlet that shows four features suggesting a mediastinal origin: smooth, sharp margins *(white arrows)*; obtuse angles with the adjacent lung *(curved open arrow)*; an epicenter in the mediastinum; and an intimate effect on mediastinal structures, such as displacement of the trachea *(black arrows)*.

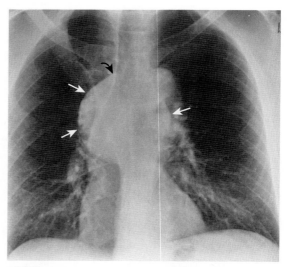

FIGURE 15-9. Posterior mediastinal mass. The frontal chest radiograph shows a large, centrally located, posterior mass. Three features suggest a mediastinal mass: smooth, sharp margins *(white arrows)*; obtuse angles with the adjacent lung *(black arrow)*; and an epicenter within the mediastinum.

TABLE 15-1 Mediastinal Mass versus Lung Mass

Mediastinal Mass	Lung Mass
Smooth, sharp margins	Usually irregular margins
Obtuse angles	Acute angles
Intimate effect on mediastinal structures	Does not usually produce an intimate effect on mediastinal structures

TABLE 15-2 Divisions of the Mediastinum

Division	Boundaries	Normal Structures
Anterior	Bounded anteriorly by the sternum and posteriorly by the anterior margins of the pericardium, aorta, and brachiocephalic vessels	Thymus gland Lymph nodes Fat Internal mammary vessels
Middle	Bounded by the posterior margin of the anterior division and anterior margin of the posterior division	Heart and pericardium Ascending and transverse aorta Brachiocephalic vessels Superior and inferior vena cava Main pulmonary vessels Trachea and main bronchi Lymph nodes Fat
Posterior	Bounded anteriorly by the posterior margins of the pericardium and great vessels and posteriorly by the thoracic vertebral bodies	Descending thoracic aorta Esophagus Thoracic duct Azygous or hemiazygous vein Autonomic nerves Lymph nodes Fat

Modified from Fraser RG, Paré JAP, Paré PD, et al (eds): Diagnosis of Diseases of the Chest, 3rd ed. Philadelphia, WB Saunders, 1998.

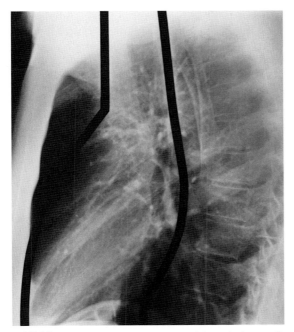

FIGURE 15-10. Mediastinal compartments. A lateral chest radiograph shows boundaries of the anterior, middle, and posterior compartments of the mediastinum.

TABLE 15-3 Differential Diagnosis of Mediastinal Masses

Location	Diagnoses
Anterior mediastinum	Thymoma* Lymphoma Germ cell neoplasms Thyroid abnormalities†
Middle mediastinum	Lymphadenopathy* Bronchogenic cyst Vascular abnormalities Pericardial cyst Tracheal tumor
Posterior mediastinum	Neurogenic tumors* Paravertebral abnormalities Vascular abnormalities Esophageal abnormalities Lymphadenopathy Neurenteric cyst Bochdalek hernia Extramedullary hematopoiesis

* Signifies the most common entity in each group.
† Thyroid abnormalities are the most common cause of a thoracic inlet mass in adults and also commonly extend into middle and posterior compartments of the mediastinum.

■ SUGGESTED READINGS

Felson, B., 1973. Chest Roentgenology. WB Saunders, Philadelphia.
Fraser, R.G., Coleman, N., Müller, N.L., Paré, P.D. (Eds.), Fraser and Paré's Diagnosis of Diseases of the Chest. fourth ed. WB Saunders, Philadelphia, 1999.
Heitzman, E.R., 1988. The Mediastinum: Radiologic Correlations with Anatomy and Pathology, third ed. Springer-Verlag, Berlin.
Martinez, S., McAdams, H.P., Erasmus, J.J., 2009, Mediastinum. In: Haaga, J.R., Dogra, V.S., Forsting, M., Gilkeson, R.C., Ha, H.K., Sundaram, M. (Eds.), CT and MRI of the whole body, 5th ed. Philadelphia, Mosby, pp. 969–1036.
McLoud, T.C., Ragozzino, M.W., 1990. MR imaging of the thorax. In: Edelman, R.R., Hesselink, J.R. (Eds.), Clinical Magnetic Resonance Imaging. WB Saunders, Philadelphia, pp. 731–744.
Naidich, D.P., Webb, W.R., Müller, N.L., et al. 1999. Computed Tomography and Magnetic Resonance of the Thorax. third ed. Raven Press, New York.
Müller, N.L., Silva, C.I. (Eds.), 2008. Imaging of the chest. Philadelphia, Saunders.
Reed, J.C., 2003. Chest radiology: plain film patterns and differential diagnoses. fifth ed. Mosby–Year Book, St. Louis.
Shaffer, K., Pugatch, R.D., 1992. Diseases of the mediastinum. In: Freundlich, I.M., Bragg, D.G. (Eds.), Radiologic Approach to Diseases of the Chest. Williams & Wilkins, Baltimore, pp. 171–185.
Vail, C.M., Ravin, C.E., 1992. Mediastinal masses. In: Freundlich, I.M., Bragg, D.G. (Eds.), Radiologic Approach to Diseases of the Chest. William & Wilkins, Baltimore, pp. 360–373.
Webb, W.R., 1994. Diseases of the mediastinum. In: Putman, C.E., Ravin, C.E. (Eds.), Textbook of Diagnostic Imaging. second ed. WB Saunders, Philadelphia, pp. 428–447.

CHAPTER 16
Mediastinal Masses

Phillip M. Boiselle

DIAGNOSTIC IMAGING WORKUP OF MEDIASTINAL MASSES

Radiologic examination of a mediastinal mass usually can narrow the differential diagnosis to two or three likely candidates. In some cases, imaging features enable the radiologist to make a specific diagnosis. The radiologic workup depends on the location of the mass (Fig. 16-1 and Box 16-1).

For masses localized within the anterior compartment of the mediastinum, computed tomography (CT) is a good diagnostic choice. It provides information about the precise location of a mass and its relation to adjacent mediastinal structures. CT can also determine whether a mass is cystic or solid and whether it contains calcium or fat. In many cases, non–contrast-enhanced CT is sufficient, but in others, contrast-enhanced CT can provide important information concerning enhancement of the mass and its relation to adjacent vascular structures. Correlative nuclear medicine studies may help in suspected cases of Hodgkin's lymphoma (i.e., gallium scan) and substernal goiter (i.e., radioiodine scan).

CT is the preferred imaging modality for further evaluation of a middle mediastinal mass. Contrast-enhanced CT is preferred for the evaluation of middle mediastinal masses, especially when you suspect a vascular abnormality. The development of multidetector-row spiral CT scanners has improved the ability to evaluate mediastinal vascular abnormalities. Compared with single-detector spiral CT scanners, multidetector-row CT scanners are associated with improved spatial resolution, faster scanning, improved vascular enhancement, and higher-quality multiplanar reformation images.

Magnetic resonance imaging (MRI) has historically been considered superior to contrast-enhanced CT in assessing relationships of masses and vascular structures and in determining vascular invasion. However, in the era of multidetector-row CT scanners, there is less of a distinction between these two modalities for assessing these parameters, especially when a CT study is specifically tailored to evaluate vascular structures. MRI should be the first cross-sectional imaging study for patients with a suspected vascular abnormality who have a contraindication to intravenous contrast. MRI also plays an important second-line role to CT by providing further tissue characterization in cases in which a mass is incompletely characterized by CT.

For masses localized within the posterior mediastinum, MRI is usually preferred because of its superior ability to assess the relationship of the mass to the adjacent spine. An exception occurs when a posterior mediastinal mass is suspected to be of esophageal origin. In this situation, a barium swallow should be obtained.

The algorithm presented in this chapter is a general guideline. The decision to obtain CT or MRI data depends on several factors, including the availability of MRI, patient factors (contraindication to intravenous contrast or MRI), and institutional practices. In some cases, CT and MRI provide complementary information, and both may be indicated.

ANTERIOR MEDIASTINAL MASSES

Thymic Abnormalities

The thymus is a bilobed structure that is normally located within the anterior mediastinum. The thymus reaches its maximum weight at puberty and subsequently undergoes fatty involution over a 5- to 15-year period. Many thymic abnormalities can manifest as an anterior mediastinal mass, but the most common are thymic hyperplasia and thymic epithelial tumors.

Thymic Epithelial Tumors

The most widely accepted classification scheme for thymic epithelial neoplasms is the World Health Organization (WHO) histologic classification that was published in 1999 and updated in 2004. It divides thymic epithelial neoplasms into three main groups: low-risk thymomas (types A, AB, and B1), high-risk thymomas (types B2 and B3), and thymic carcinomas, including neuroendocrine epithelial tumors (type C).

The most common thymic abnormality that manifests as an anterior mediastinal mass is *thymoma* (Box 16-2).

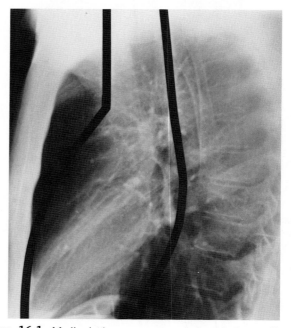

FIGURE 16-1. Mediastinal compartments. A lateral chest radiograph demonstrates the boundaries of the anterior, middle, and posterior mediastinal compartments.

Box 16-1. Algorithm for Imaging Evaluation of Mediastinal Masses

Mediastinal mass detected on chest radiograph

↓

Localize mass into anterior, middle, or posterior compartment

↙ ↓ ↘

Anterior mass — Middle mass — Posterior mass

↓

Chest CT

↓

Chest CT (I+)*

↓

MRI *or* Barium swallow if esophageal origin is suspected

Other studies:
Gallium scan if Hodgkin's lymphoma is suspected

Radioiodine scan if thyroid goiter is suspected

Other studies:
MRI if there is a contraindication to contrast and a vascular abnormality is suspected or if vascular invasion is suspected

*I+ refers to contrast-enhanced chest CT.

Box 16-2. Thymoma

DEMOGRAPHICS
Age: usually 40 to 60 years old; unusual in patients younger than 30 years old
Gender: men and women equally affected
Associations: myasthenia gravis, hypogammaglobulinemia, red cell aplasia, and stiff-person syndrome

DESCRIPTIVE FEATURES

Low-Risk Thymoma
Well-defined, round, soft tissue density mass with homogenous enhancement
Usually located anterior to the junction of the heart and great vessels

High-Risk Thymoma or Thymic Carcinoma
Irregularly marginated mass with necrotic components and heterogeneous enhancement
Additional findings of invasion of adjacent mediastinal vascular structures, chest wall invasion, or contiguous spread along pleural surfaces (usually unilaterally)

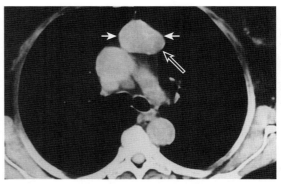

FIGURE 16-2. Thymoma. Axial CT shows an oval, homogeneous soft tissue mass *(short solid arrows)* in the anterior mediastinum, with a thin rim of peripheral calcification posteriorly *(open arrow)*. Calcification occurs in approximately 20% of thymomas.

Thymomas account for most anterior mediastinal masses in adults and typically occur as incidental findings in otherwise healthy individuals. However, thymomas may be associated with other abnormalities, including myasthenia gravis, red cell aplasia, hypogammaglobulinemia, and stiff-person syndrome. The association with myasthenia gravis is the most common of the three; about 15% of patients with myasthenia gravis have a thymoma, and about 50% of patients with thymomas have myasthenia gravis.

As with other midline anterior mediastinal masses, conventional radiographic findings are often limited to the lateral chest radiograph, which may demonstrate a well-defined mass in the normally clear retrosternal space. Small masses may not be detectable on plain radiographs, but CT can help to identify a thymoma in patients with myasthenia gravis. Characteristic CT imaging features include a well-defined, round, or oval mass, usually of homogeneous soft tissue density, that is located within the anterior mediastinum (Fig. 16-2). Although they are most commonly located anterior to the junction of the heart and great vessels, thymomas may occur at any level from the thoracic inlet to the diaphragm. In about 20% of cases, there is evidence of calcification, which is typically curvilinear.

Most thymomas are benign lesions confined within a fibrous capsule, but about 30% of thymomas are more aggressive and demonstrate invasion through the fibrous capsule. The WHO classification scheme correlates with the likelihood of invasiveness, a factor that has an important influence on treatment and prognosis. Types A and AB are usually encapsulated, type B (especially B3) has a greater likelihood of invasiveness, and type C is almost always invasive. Although CT and MRI findings are often of limited value in differentiating histologic subtypes of thymic epithelial neoplasms, certain findings have predictive value. For example, a small, smooth, round, homogeneous anterior mediastinal mass usually corresponds to a type A thymoma, whereas irregular contours and heterogeneous attenuation favor a type C thymic carcinoma (Fig. 16-3). Calcification is most commonly observed in type B thymomas and type C thymic carcinoma.

When interpreting CT scans or MRI studies of patients with suspected or proven thymic neoplasms, signs of capsular invasion or extracapsular extension should be carefully sought. They include irregular tumor margins; invasion of surrounding mediastinal fat, vascular structures, or chest wall; and irregular interface with the adjacent lung. Invasive thymomas typically spread locally (Fig. 16-4), and metastases outside of the thorax are rare. Pleural dissemination, also referred to as *drop metastases*, and pericardial involvement are common, whereas lung metastases are rare. The extent of involvement by thymic

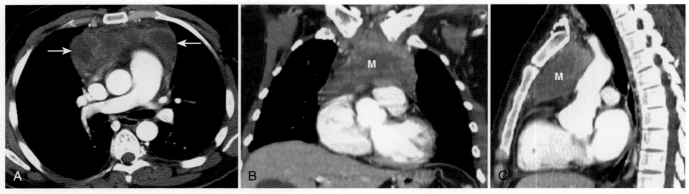

Figure 16-3. Thymic carcinoma. Axial, contrast-enhanced CT (**A**) at the level of main pulmonary artery shows a large, heterogeneously enhancing, anterior mediastinal mass with foci of low attenuation *(arrows)*, consistent with necrosis. Coronal (**B**) and sagittal (**C**) reformation images improve the assessment of the craniocaudal extent of the neoplastic mass (M) compared with axial images.

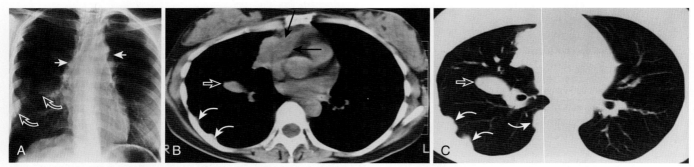

Figure 16-4. Invasive thymoma. **A,** The posteroanterior chest radiograph shows a lobulated, anterior mediastinal mass *(white arrows)* and multiple pleural masses in the right hemithorax *(open arrows)*. **B,** Axial CT image of the chest (filmed using soft tissue windows) shows an anterior mediastinal mass *(black arrows)* and multiple, unilateral pleural masses *(curved arrows)*. Notice that one of the pleural masses is located within the minor fissure *(open arrow)*. **C,** Axial CT image of the chest (filmed using lung windows) shows multiple pleural masses *(curved arrows)*, including a pleural mass within the minor fissure *(open arrow)*. The presence of an anterior mediastinal mass and unilateral pleural masses strongly suggests invasive thymoma.

neoplasms is often best determined by viewing CT or MRI data in axial, sagittal, and coronal planes rather than relying solely on axial images (see Fig. 16-3).

Thymic Hyperplasia

Thymic hyperplasia (Box 16-3) is associated with a wide variety of systemic abnormalities, including hyperthyroidism. Rebound thymic hyperplasia may be seen in patients who have been treated with chemotherapy.

Thymic hyperplasia is usually identified on CT as enlargement of the thymus gland, which maintains its normal bilobed, arrowhead configuration (Fig. 16-5). In contrast, most other thymic abnormalities appear as a discrete mass rather than as uniform glandular enlargement. ^{18}F-fluorodeoxyglucose positron emission tomography (FDG-PET) is of limited value in differentiating thymic

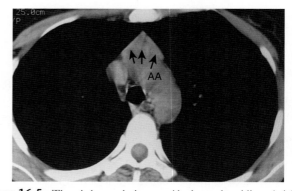

Figure 16-5. Thymic hyperplasia caused by hyperthyroidism. Axial CT image of the chest at the level of the aortic arch (AA) shows enlargement of the thymus gland *(arrows)*, which maintains its normal bilobed, arrowhead configuration.

Box 16-3. **Thymic Hyperplasia: Associated Systemic Abnormalities**

Hyperthyroidism
Acromegaly
Addison's disease
Myasthenia gravis
Systemic lupus erythematosus
Scleroderma
Rheumatoid arthritis

---

hyperplasia from thymic neoplasms because both may demonstrate FDG avidity. MRI imaging using a chemical shift technique can reliably differentiate thymic hyperplasia from thymic neoplasms. On chemical shift imaging, thymic hyperplasia is associated with a characteristic decrease in signal intensity within the thymus gland.

Thymic lymphoid hyperplasia is a distinct entity that is characterized by an increased number of lymphoid follicles, but the gland is usually not enlarged. Thymic lymphoid hyperplasia is most commonly associated with myasthenia gravis. On imaging studies, the thymus gland usually appears normal, but it may uncommonly may appear as a focal mass or diffuse glandular enlargement.

Thymic Carcinoid

Thymic carcinoid tumor is rare and is thought to arise from thymic cells of neural crest origin. It is now included in the same histologic category as thymic carcinomas in the 2004 WHO classification of thymic epithelial neoplasms.

Patients with thymic carcinoid tumors often present with endocrine abnormalities, including Cushing's syndrome, the syndrome of inappropriate antidiuretic hormone secretion (SIADH), hyperparathyroidism, and multiple endocrine neoplasia (MEN 1) syndrome.

No radiologic features differentiate thymic carcinoid from thymic carcinoma. The diagnosis is often suspected on the basis of endocrine abnormalities in a patient with an anterior mediastinal mass.

Thymic Cyst

Thymic cysts may be congenital or acquired. Acquired thymic cysts are most often associated with Hodgkin's disease after radiation therapy.

Radiographically, a thymic cyst usually appears as a well-defined, cystic mass with an imperceptible wall. The CT attenuation values are typically consistent with fluid; however, the appearance may vary if hemorrhage or infection complicates the cyst. Curvilinear calcification of the cyst wall occurs in a few cases.

Thymic Lymphoma

Thymic involvement may occur in up to one third of patients with Hodgkin's lymphoma. It is usually accompanied by involvement of mediastinal lymph nodes.

Thymic lymphoma usually manifests as a homogeneous, round mass with soft tissue density and without calcification. The presence of enlarged mediastinal lymph nodes may suggest the diagnosis.

Thymolipoma

Thymolipoma is a rare, benign thymic neoplasm composed primarily of fat, but it also contains strands of thymic tissue. Thymolipomas most often occur in younger patients and are usually identified on chest radiographs as incidental findings.

Because of their soft, pliable nature, thymolipomas commonly drape around the heart and other mediastinal structures. They are often quite large at the time of presentation, and they may mimic cardiac enlargement on chest radiographs. Identification of fat within the mass on CT or MRI suggests the diagnosis (Fig. 16-6).

Primary Mediastinal Lymphoma

Primary mediastinal lymphoma (Box 16-4) refers to malignant lymphoma that is exclusively or mostly limited to the mediastinum. The most common cell types to arise in the anterior mediastinum include the nodular sclerosing subtype of Hodgkin's lymphoma, primary mediastinal large B-cell lymphoma, and lymphoblastic lymphoma.

Approximately 40% of these patients present with enlargement of a single anterior mediastinal nodal group. Imaging features vary, ranging from a single, spherical soft

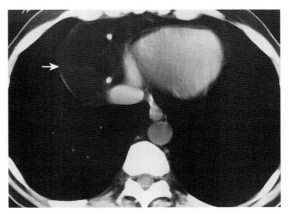

FIGURE 16-6. Thymolipoma. Axial CT image of the chest shows a right cardiophrenic angle mass, which is predominately fat attenuation. Notice the thin strands of soft tissue attenuation *(arrow)* within the mass, representing strands of thymic tissue, and the foci of calcification.

Box 16-4. Primary Mediastinal Lymphoma

DEMOGRAPHICS
Age: mostly young adults, but Hodgkin's lymphoma has a bimodal distribution, with initial peak in young adults and a second peak after age 50 years
Gender: female predominance, except for lymphoblastic lymphoma

DESCRIPTIVE FEATURES
Variable appearance, ranging from a single, spherical soft tissue mass to a large, lobulated mass
Margins may be well defined or irregular
Mass may have homogeneous or heterogeneous soft tissue attenuation
Calcification rare in untreated cases

---

tissue mass in the anterior mediastinum to a large, lobulated mass representing a conglomeration of lymph nodes. CT may show a mass with homogeneous soft tissue density, or it may appear heterogeneous, in which the low-attenuation areas represent necrosis. Whereas anterior mediastinal masses from lymphoma typically demonstrate well-defined margins, invasion of adjacent lung parenchyma may result in irregular margins. Invasion into the chest wall may also occur (Fig. 16-7).

Lymphoma that manifests as a solitary, spherical mass may be indistinguishable from thymoma. Correlative nuclear medicine gallium imaging may be helpful because most Hodgkin's lymphomas take up gallium avidly.

Associated lymphadenopathy in other compartments of the mediastinum and associated extrathoracic lymphadenopathy each suggest the diagnosis of lymphoma. An important discriminating feature is the absence of calcification in untreated lymphoma. Although the presence of calcification strongly suggests a diagnosis other than lymphoma, calcification frequently occurs in cases of treated lymphoma, but only rarely in untreated cases.

FDG-PET and FDG-PET/CT play important roles in staging lymphoma and in assessing the response to therapy. After treatment, patients often have residual mediastinal masses. PET is especially helpful in this setting because

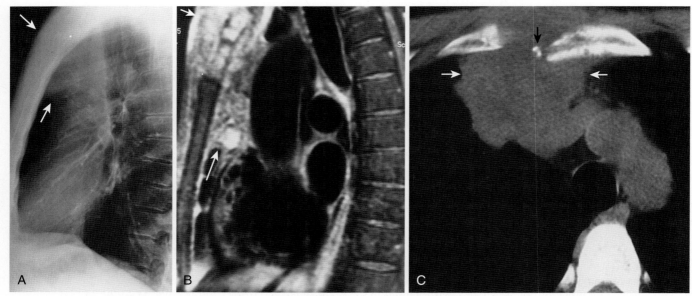

FIGURE 16-7. Lymphoma. **A,** The lateral chest radiograph reveals increased opacity in the normally clear retrosternal space *(lower arrow)* and a presternal soft tissue mass *(upper arrow)*. **B,** Sagittal MRI confirms the presence of a heterogeneous anterior mediastinal mass *(long arrow)* with invasion of the chest wall and extension into the presternal soft tissues *(short arrow)*. **C,** Axial noncontrast CT scan shows destruction of the sternum *(black arrow)* by the anterior mediastinal mass *(white arrows)*.

it can differentiate a residual, benign, fibrotic tissue mass from incompletely treated, viable tumor.

Germ Cell Neoplasms

Primary germ cell neoplasms (GCNs) arise from rests of primitive germ cells that were left within the mediastinum during their migration from the yolk sac to the urogenital ridge. The anterior mediastinum is the most common extragonadal site of GCNs.

There are a variety of benign and malignant GCNs (Box 16-5). Seventy percent of GCNs are benign, comprising mostly

---

Box 16-5. Germ Cell Neoplasms

DEMOGRAPHICS

Age: young patients, usually in third decade
Gender: malignant germ cell neoplasms have marked male predominance

DESCRIPTIVE FEATURES

Benign Forms (Teratoma, Dermoid Cyst)

Heterogeneous, predominately cystic mass with solid components
Well-defined margins
Calcification common
Presence of fat is suggestive; identification of a tooth, although rare, is diagnostic

Malignant Forms (Seminoma, Choriocarcinoma, Embryonal Cell Carcinoma, Yolk Sac Tumor)

Heterogeneous, solid mass
Irregular margins
Calcification uncommon

---

teratomas and dermoid cysts. Dermoid cysts contain only ectodermal layer elements, but teratomas contain elements of all three germinal layers. Several types of malignant GCNs occur within the anterior mediastinum, including pure seminomas and several nonseminomatous tumors (i.e., choriocarcinoma; embryonal cell carcinoma, yolk sac tumors, and mixed GCNs). Teratomas usually are benign, but carcinoma may rarely develop within one of the germinal layer elements.

Patients with GCNs may be asymptomatic or may have symptoms from compression or invasion of adjacent mediastinal structures. Because GCNs grow rapidly and have a propensity to invade mediastinal structures, patients with malignant GCNs are more likely to be symptomatic.

Dermoid cysts and teratomas have similar imaging features. They typically appear as heterogeneous, sharply marginated, multiloculated, cystic, anterior mediastinal masses. A combination of fluid, fat, and calcification is frequently observed. This unique combination of findings makes teratoma one of the few mediastinal tumors that can confidently be diagnosed by radiographic findings alone. A fat-fluid level is seen in 10% of cases and is highly specific for teratoma (Fig 16-8). The identification of dental tissue, such as a well-formed tooth, is rare, but it is also diagnostic of this entity. If a dominant, solid soft tissue component is observed within the mass, a malignant GCN or a teratoma with malignant components should be considered in the diagnosis.

Surgical excision of teratomas and dermoid cysts is usually curative. Thorough pathologic sampling is recommended to exclude small foci of immature tissue, other germ cell tumors, or carcinoma. In contrast, patients with malignant GCNs usually have a poor prognosis, with the exception of those with seminoma. Mediastinal seminomas are usually radiosensitive, and patients have an overall survival rate of about 75%.

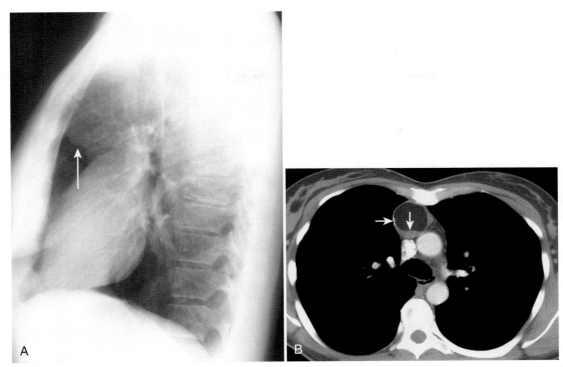

FIGURE 16-8. Teratoma. **A,** The lateral chest radiograph shows increased opacity in the normally clear retrosternal space, with a well-defined, round border inferiorly *(arrow)*. **B,** Axial, contrast-enhanced CT image reveals a round, anterior mediastinal mass with a partially calcified rim *(right arrow)* and a fat-fluid level *(down arrow)*. The latter finding is essentially diagnostic of a teratoma.

Thyroid Abnormalities

Thyroid abnormalities account for most thoracic inlet masses in adults (Box 16-6). They may extend inferiorly into the anterior, middle, and posterior compartments of the mediastinum. When located in the anterior mediastinum, thyroid masses are almost always located posterior to the great vessels, usually in a paratracheal location. However, most other anterior mediastinal masses are located anterior to the great vessels, and a mediastinal mass located anterior to the great vessels in a retrosternal location is unlikely to be of thyroid origin.

Most mediastinal masses of thyroid origin represent thyroid goiters, and they almost always extend inferiorly from the thyroid gland. A truly ectopic thyroid goiter is rare. Other thyroid abnormalities, such as thyroid adenomas and malignant thyroid neoplasms, infrequently extend into the mediastinum.

Because thyroid goiters account for most mediastinal masses of thyroid origin, the demographics of thyroid mediastinal masses are similar to those of thyroid goiter, with a tendency to occur predominately in middle-aged women. Most patients are asymptomatic, but symptoms may arise from compression of the trachea or esophagus.

CT imaging features of mediastinal thyroid goiters include continuity of the mass with the cervical thyroid gland; foci of high attenuation on non–contrast-enhanced examination (reflecting high iodine content of thyroid tissue); foci of heterogeneous attenuation (i.e., low attenuation cystic areas and high-attenuation foci of calcification); and intense and prolonged enhancement after administration of intravenous contrast. As on plain radiographs, deviation or compression of the trachea is frequently identified on CT. Large thyroid masses, especially posterior descending goiters, may compress the esophagus.

The most important of these features is demonstration of continuity of the mass with the cervical thyroid gland. A combined CT examination of the lower neck and chest is best (Fig. 16-9), although MRI can be used (Fig. 16-10). A radioiodine scan may be confirmatory, with demonstration of radioiodine uptake from foci of functioning thyroid tissue within the mass.

BOX 16-6. Thyroid Masses

DEMOGRAPHICS
Age: usually older than 30 years
Gender: female predominance

DESCRIPTIVE FEATURES

Chest Radiographic Features
Well-defined mass that extends from above the thoracic inlet
Displacement or compression of the trachea
Foci of calcification occasionally visible

Computed Tomography Features
Continuity with the cervical thyroid gland
Foci of high attenuation on noncontrast-enhanced images
Intense enhancement after intravenous contrast administration
Cystic areas and foci of calcification common

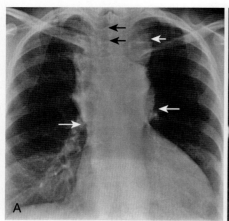
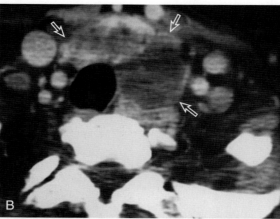
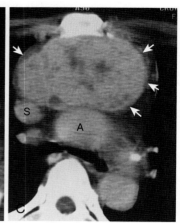

FIGURE 16-9. Thyroid goiter. **A,** The posteroanterior chest radiograph shows a large, anterior mediastinal mass. The superior extent of the mass *(upper white arrow)* extends above the thoracic inlet and is associated with rightward deviation of the trachea *(black arrows)*. The mass extends inferiorly to the level of the base of the heart *(lower white arrows)*. **B,** Axial, contrast-enhanced CT image of the lower neck shows a heterogeneous mass *(open arrows)* that is continuous with the isthmus and left lobe of the thyroid gland. The mass contains foci of thyroid tissue that demonstrate intense enhancement and foci of low attenuation consistent with cysts. **C,** Axial, contrast-enhanced CT image at the level of the aortic arch shows the large, substernal component of the mass *(arrows)*, which displaces the ascending aorta (A) and superior vena cava (S) posteriorly.

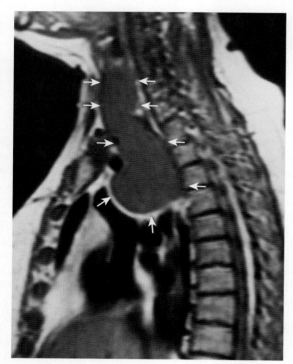

FIGURE 16-10. Thyroid goiter. Right parasagittal, T1-weighted MRI shows a homogeneous mass *(arrows)* that extends inferiorly from the right lobe of the thyroid gland to involve the middle and posterior mediastinal compartments.

▬ MIDDLE MEDIASTINAL MASSES

Lymphadenopathy

Neoplastic, inflammatory, or infectious lymphadenopathy (Box 16-7) is the most common cause of a middle mediastinal mass (Box 16-8). It is therefore no surprise that there are no distinguishing demographic features.

Lymphadenopathy should be considered in assessing a middle mediastinal mass when the mass is localized to a known anatomic lymph node site, such as the

---

Box 16-7. Lymphadenopathy

DEMOGRAPHICS
No general distinguishing demographic features

DESCRIPTIVE FEATURES
Single or multiple, round or elliptical masses located within known anatomic sites of lymph nodes
Often homogeneous, soft tissue density on CT but may have calcification, low-density centers, or vascular enhancement (see Box 16-9)

Box 16-8. Mediastinal Lymphadenopathy Differential Diagnosis

NEOPLASTIC CAUSES
Metastatic disease (bronchogenic carcinoma or extrathoracic primary*)
Lymphoma
Leukemia

INFECTIOUS CAUSES
Tuberculosis
Fungal infection (especially histoplasmosis)
Viral infection (measles, infectious mononucleosis)†
Bacterial infection†

DRUG REACTION
Diphenylhydantoin (Dilantin)

INFLAMMATORY CAUSES
Sarcoidosis
Castleman's disease
Angioimmunoblastic lymphadenopathy

---

*Extrathoracic primaries that commonly metastasize to mediastinal lymph nodes include genitourinary tumors, head and neck carcinomas, thyroid carcinomas, melanoma, and breast carcinoma.
† Lymphadenopathy is infrequently detected on chest radiography but often is seen on CT.

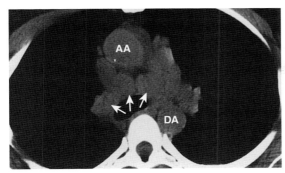

FIGURE 16-11. Sarcoidosis. Axial, non–contrast-enhanced CT image shows discrete, round, soft tissue masses *(arrows)* in the anterior subcarinal region, consistent with enlarged lymph nodes. Other images demonstrated lymphadenopathy in the right paratracheal region and both hila, a characteristic distribution of lymphadenopathy in sarcoidosis. AA, ascending aorta; DA, descending aorta.

azygous, subcarinal, or aortopulmonary window regions. Lymphadenopathy often manifests as multiple, discrete masses (Fig. 16-11), in contrast to most other causes of mediastinal masses, which usually manifest as a single mass. Multiple masses within known anatomic lymph node sites suggest lymphadenopathy.

CT plays a role in detecting and characterizing lymph nodes. Although lymph nodes often appear as homogeneous soft tissue density on CT, they may also demonstrate calcification, low-density centers, or vascular enhancement. Identification of these lymph node characteristics can shorten the lengthy differential diagnosis of mediastinal lymphadenopathy (Box 16-9).

Identification of low-density mediastinal lymph nodes is particularly helpful in narrowing the differential diagnosis of lymphadenopathy in patients with acquired immunodeficiency syndrome (AIDS) (Fig. 16-12) because low-density lymph nodes in an AIDS patient usually represent an infectious process, particularly tuberculosis, *Mycobacterium avium-intracellulare* (MAI), or a fungal infection. Low-density lymph nodes are not usually seen in neoplastic processes in AIDS patients.

Although calcified lymph nodes have many causes, the presence of peripheral calcification within a lymph node, referred to as *eggshell calcification,* suggests silicosis or coal worker's pneumoconiosis. However, eggshell calcification is not pathognomonic of these entities because it may be an unusual manifestation of sarcoidosis, granulomatous infection, treated lymphoma, scleroderma, or amyloidosis. Associated hilar lymphadenopathy and its distribution (i.e., unilateral or bilateral) also help to narrow the differential diagnosis of lymphadenopathy (Box 16-10).

Bronchogenic Cyst

Bronchogenic cysts (Box 16-11) are the result of an abnormality in primitive foregut development. Although they occur in all three mediastinal compartments, the middle mediastinum is the most common site. The cysts are lined by respiratory epithelium, and their walls contain cartilage, smooth muscle, or mucous glands.

Bronchogenic cysts usually are incidental findings in asymptomatic patients, but they occasionally cause symptoms because of compression of adjacent structures. They infrequently cause symptoms because of infection.

> *Box 16-9.* **Mediastinal Lymphadenopathy: Characteristic Features**
>
> **LOW-DENSITY LYMPH NODES**
>
> ***Infectious Causes***
> Tuberculosis*
> Mycobacterium avium-intracellulare (MAI)*
> Fungal*
>
> ***Neoplastic Causes***
> Metastases (seminoma, lung cancer)
> Lymphoma
>
> **CALCIFIED LYMPH NODES**
>
> ***Infectious Causes***
> Fungal (especially histoplasmosis)
> Tuberculosis
>
> ***Neoplastic Causes***
> Hodgkin's lymphoma after radiation therapy
> Metastases (especially mucinous adenocarcinoma)
>
> ***Inflammatory Causes***
> Sarcoidosis (5% of cases)
>
> ***Inhalational Causes***
> Silicosis (often eggshell appearance of calcification)
>
> **ENHANCING LYMPH NODES**
>
> ***Neoplastic Causes***
> Metastases (especially renal cell carcinoma, thyroid carcinoma, and small cell lung cancer)
>
> ***Inflammatory Causes***
> Castleman's disease (benign lymph node hyperplasia)
> Sarcoidosis (rare)

*May have a low-density center.

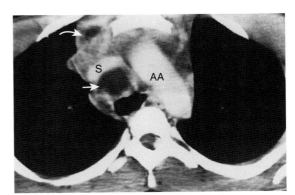

FIGURE 16-12. Mediastinal lymphadenopathy caused by tuberculosis infection in an AIDS patient. The axial, contrast-enhanced CT image shows pretracheal *(straight arrow)* and prevascular *(curved arrow)* enlarged lymph nodes. Notice the low attenuation of the lymph nodes and the peripheral enhancement, a characteristic appearance of tuberculosis lymphadenopathy in HIV-positive patients.

The most common location is subcarinal, and the presence of a well-defined subcarinal mass in an asymptomatic patient suggests a bronchogenic cyst (Fig. 16-13). The right paratracheal region is the second most common location (Fig. 16-14).

Box 16-10. **Hilar Lymphadenopathy: Differential Diagnosis**

UNILATERAL LYMPHADENOPATHY

Neoplastic Causes
Metastases (bronchogenic carcinoma, extrathoracic primary*)
Lymphoma

Infectious Causes
Tuberculosis
Fungal infections
Viral infections

BILATERAL, ASYMMETRIC LYMPHADENOPATHY

Neoplastic Causes
Lymphoma
Leukemia (chronic lymphocytic leukemia)
Metastases (bronchogenic carcinoma, extrathoracic primary*)

Infectious Causes
Fungal infections

BILATERAL, SYMMETRIC LYMPHADENOPATHY
Inflammatory conditions (sarcoidosis)

---

*Extrathoracic primaries that commonly metastasize to mediastinal lymph nodes include genitourinary tumors, head and neck carcinomas, thyroid carcinomas, melanoma, and breast carcinoma.

Imaging features include a well-defined, round or oval, homogeneous mass with a thin, often imperceptible wall. Air within the cyst is uncommon and suggests secondary infection and communication with the tracheobronchial tree. The CT and MRI characteristics depend on the contents. In a significant number of cases, bronchogenic cysts appear as soft tissue attenuation on CT and demonstrate bright signal on T1-weighted images (Fig. 16-15). These seemingly paradoxical imaging features of a cystic structure can be explained by the presence of proteinaceous, mucinous, or hemorrhagic contents within the cyst.

Box 16-11. **Bronchogenic Cyst**

DEMOGRAPHICS
Age: often occurs in younger patients but may be detected at any age
Gender: affects males and females equally

DESCRIPTIVE FEATURES
Subcarinal or right paratracheal location
Well-defined, homogeneous mass with imperceptible wall
Fluid or soft tissue attenuation on CT
MRI appearance depends on cyst contents: low signal intensity on T1 and bright on T2 or bright signal intensity on T1 and bright on T2-weighted images (if cyst contains mucin, protein, or hemorrhage)

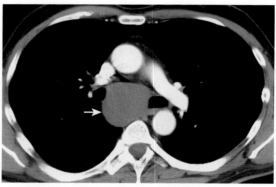

FIGURE 16-13. Bronchogenic cyst. The axial, contrast-enhanced CT image shows a well-defined, oval, simple fluid attenuation (0 HU) mass *(arrow)* in the subcarinal region that does not have a perceptible wall. The subcarinal region is the most common location of a bronchogenic cyst.

Calcification is uncommon, but it may occur in the wall or within the cyst contents.

Vascular Structures

Vascular structures, including anatomic variants and acquired abnormalities, are a common cause of middle

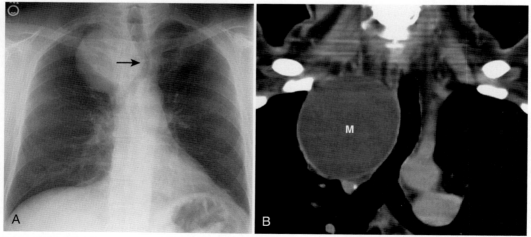

FIGURE 16-14. Bronchogenic cyst. **A,** The frontal chest radiograph shows a large, middle mediastinal mass that displaces the trachea to the left *(arrow)*. **B,** The coronal reformation CT image reveals simple fluid attenuation (0 HU) contents of the mass (M).

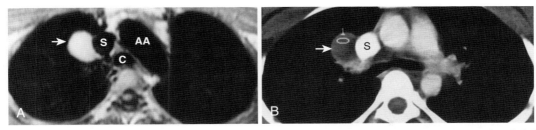

FIGURE 16-15. Bronchogenic cyst. **A,** Axial, T1-weighted MRI at the level of the carina (C) and aortic arch (AA) reveals an oval, well-defined mass *(arrow)* adjacent to the superior vena cava (S). The mass has homogenous, bright signal intensity. **B,** Axial, contrast-enhanced CT at the level of the main bronchi shows a homogeneous mass *(arrow)* adjacent to the superior vena cava (S). The mass measured 30 HU, consistent with soft tissue attenuation. When bronchogenic cysts contain mucin, protein, or hemorrhage, they appear as soft tissue attenuation on CT and as bright signal intensity on T1-weighted MRI.

mediastinal masses. It is extremely important to consider that a mediastinal mass may be vascular in origin, particularly when a biopsy is being considered.

Vascular Anatomic Variants

The demographics and descriptive features of vascular variants are summarized in Box 16-12.

Aberrant Right Subclavian Artery

An aberrant right subclavian artery is a relatively common normal variant, occurring in approximately 1% of the population. The anomalous right subclavian artery arises as the last branch of the aortic arch and courses obliquely from left to right behind the trachea and esophagus as it heads cephalad.

On chest radiographs, an aberrant right subclavian artery may appear as an oblique opacity coursing superiorly from left to right, beginning at the superior margin of the aortic arch (Fig. 16-16). On lateral chest radiographs, a posterior impression may be detected infrequently on the tracheal air column. Barium swallow examination can demonstrate an oblique indentation on the posterior wall of the esophagus (Fig. 16-17). An aberrant right subclavian artery is

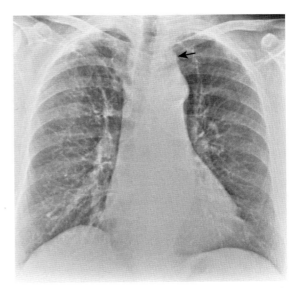

FIGURE 16-16. Aberrant right subclavian artery. The frontal radiograph of the chest reveals an oblique opacity *(arrow)* arising from the aortic arch and coursing superiorly from left to right.

Box 16-12. Vascular Variants

DEMOGRAPHICS

No distinguishing demographic features

DESCRIPTIVE FEATURES

Aberrant Right Subclavian Artery

Chest radiograph: oblique opacity coursing superiorly from left to right, beginning at the superior margin of the aortic arch.

Barium swallow: oblique indentation on the posterior wall of the esophagus

CT or MRI: vascular structure arising from the distal aortic arch and coursing obliquely behind the trachea and esophagus

Left-Sided Superior Vena Cava

CT or MRI: vascular structure located lateral to the left common carotid artery, which lies anterior to the left hilum as it courses caudally to drain into the right atrium through a dilated coronary sinus

Right-Sided Aortic Arch

Chest radiograph: right-sided, convex mediastinal contour with associated leftward deviation of the trachea; absent left-sided aortic arch

Barium swallow: right-sided, lateral impression on the esophagus; in the case of a right-sided aortic arch with an aberrant left subclavian artery, an oblique impression on the posterior wall of the esophagus is seen

CT or MRI: vascular arch located to the right of the trachea

Double Aortic Arch

Chest radiograph: convex mediastinal contours bilaterally, corresponding to two aortic arches; the right arch is usually larger and more cephalad than the left

Barium swallow: bilateral impressions on the esophagus on the anteroposterior projection; posterior compression of the esophagus on the lateral projection

CT or MRI: bilateral vascular arches join posterior to the trachea and esophagus to form a single descending aorta

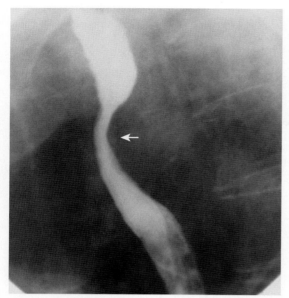

FIGURE 16-17. Aberrant right subclavian artery. The barium swallow shows a posterior impression on the barium column *(arrow)*, corresponding to an aberrant right subclavian artery.

readily identified on MRI and CT (Fig. 16-18). It is often dilated at its origin, and the adjacent esophagus may be slightly displaced or compressed by the dilated vessel.

Left-Sided Superior Vena Cava

A persistent left superior vena cava, which occurs in less than 0.5% of the population, is caused by failure of embryologic regression of a portion of the left common and anterior cardinal veins. A persistent left superior vena cava usually drains the left jugular and left subclavian veins, the latter of which may be small or absent in these patients. Most often, the right superior vena cava is present.

The persistent left superior vena cava, located lateral to the left common carotid artery, courses inferiorly in a position analogous to the right-sided superior vena cava (Fig.

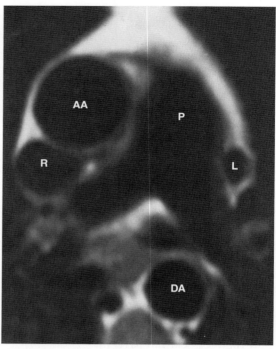

FIGURE 16-19. Left-sided superior vena cava. Axial, T1-weighted MRI shows a left-sided superior vena cava (L) located lateral to the main pulmonary artery (P) in a position analogous to the right-sided vena cava (R). More caudal images show that the left-sided superior vena cava drains into a dilated coronary sinus. AA, ascending aorta; DA, descending aorta.

16-19). As it courses caudally, the left superior vena cava lies anterior to the left hilum and usually drains into the right atrium by way of a dilated coronary sinus. Chest radiographs may show a widening of the left superior mediastinal contour and a well-defined vertical opacity lateral to the aortic arch contour. The diagnosis is easily confirmed on CT or MRI. The key to diagnosing this and other vascular anomalies on cross-sectional imaging is to carefully follow the course of the vessel on serial axial images. Two-dimensional coronal and sagittal reformatted images may be particularly helpful in determining the course of these vessels.

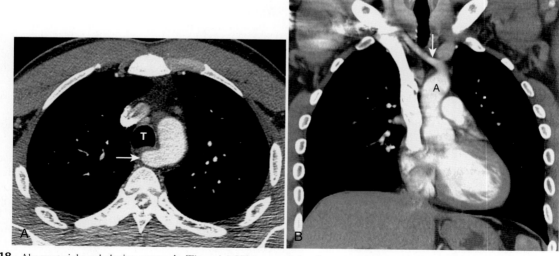

FIGURE 16-18. Aberrant right subclavian artery. **A,** The axial CT image of the chest reveals a vessel arising from the distal aortic arch and coursing posteriorly behind the trachea (T), corresponding to an aberrant right subclavian artery *(arrow)*. **B,** Coronal reformation CT image shows the origin of the aberrant vessel at the aortic arch (A) and its oblique course *(arrow)*.

Right-Sided Aortic Arch

Depending on the point of interruption of the aortic arch, at least five potential types of right-sided aortic arches are possible, although radiologists usually encounter only two. The most common type is a right-sided aortic arch with an aberrant left subclavian artery; this type of aortic arch is infrequently (10% incidence) associated with congenital heart disease. The second most common type is a right-sided aortic arch with mirror-image branching, an anomaly that has a very high (98%) incidence of associated congenital heart disease, especially tetralogy of Fallot.

Chest radiographs can identify a right-sided aortic arch in most affected patients as an abnormal convex mediastinal contour located to the right of the trachea, analogous to that produced by the left-sided aortic arch (Fig. 16-20). The trachea is frequently deviated to the left at the level of the right-sided arch, and the normal left-sided aortic arch contour is absent. In the case of a right-sided aortic arch with an anomalous left subclavian artery, the lateral radiograph may demonstrate an impression on the posterior wall of the tracheal air column. Barium swallow examination can demonstrate an impression on the right lateral wall of the esophagus from the right-sided aortic arch; in the case of a right-sided aortic arch with an aberrant left subclavian artery, it can also demonstrate an oblique impression along the posterior wall of the esophagus. CT or MRI easily confirms the presence of a right-sided aortic arch and the presence of an associated aberrant left subclavian artery.

Double Aortic Arch

A double aortic arch is an anomaly characterized by the presence of a left- and a right-sided aortic arch, each of which gives rise to its own subclavian and common carotid arteries. The two arches join posteriorly to form a single descending aorta, forming a vascular ring around the trachea and esophagus. The right-sided arch is usually larger and is located more cephalad than the left-sided arch. Most

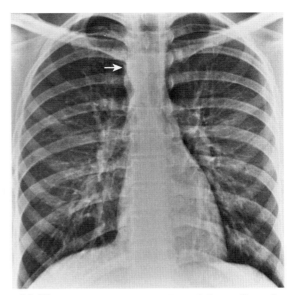

FIGURE 16-20. Right-sided aortic arch. Frontal chest radiograph reveals a convex contour to the right of the trachea *(arrow)*, corresponding to a right-sided aortic arch. Notice the leftward deviation of the trachea and the absence of the normal left-sided aortic arch contour.

often, both arches are patent and functioning; rarely, there is atresia of a portion of the left arch.

Because the two arches form a vascular ring, affected patients often have symptoms because of tracheal or esophageal compression, or both. The diagnosis of a double aortic arch may be suggested by chest radiography, which demonstrates right- and left-sided mediastinal convex contours corresponding to the two arches. Barium swallow can demonstrate bilateral impressions on the anteroposterior view, and posterior compression on the lateral projection. MRI (Fig. 16-21) or CT can confirm the diagnosis.

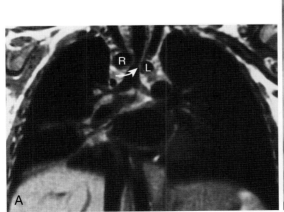
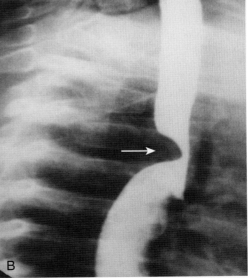

FIGURE 16-21. Double aortic arch in a male infant. **A,** Coronal, T1-weighted MRI of the chest shows bilateral aortic arches. The right-sided arch (R) is larger and is located more cephalad than the left-sided arch (L), a common appearance in patients with double aortic arches. The two arches form a vascular ring around the trachea and esophagus. Notice the narrowed coronal diameter of the trachea *(arrow)*. **B,** The lateral radiograph obtained during a barium swallow study in the same patient reveals a posterior impression on the barium column *(arrow)*, with pronounced narrowing of the anteroposterior diameter of the esophagus. On the anteroposterior view, there were bilateral impressions on the barium column from the two aortic arches.

Box 16-13. Aortic Aneurysms

DEMOGRAPHICS
Cause: atherosclerosis most common cause
Age: usually affects patients older than 40 years

DESCRIPTIVE FEATURES

Chest Radiography
Mass indistinguishable from the aortic contour
Curvilinear calcification (especially atherosclerotic
  aneurysms)

CT, MRI, and Angiography
Mass contiguous with the aorta
Mass demonstrates characteristics of a vascular
  structure (enhancement, flow void, contrast
  opacification), unless thrombosed

CLASSIFICATION
Integrity of Aortic Wall
True aneurysm has intact but dilated aortic wall.
False aneurysm has disrupted aortic wall, contained
  by surrounding tissues.

Shape
Fusiform aneurysm is characterized by cylindrical
  dilation of entire aortic circumference.
Saccular aneurysm is characterized by a focal area of
  outpouching of the aorta.
Location
Ascending
Transverse
Descending

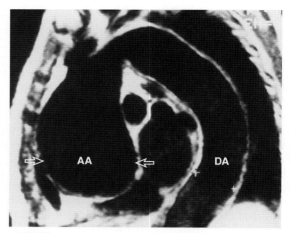

FIGURE 16-22. Ascending aortic aneurysm caused by cystic medial necrosis. Sagittal-oblique, T1-weighted MRI of the chest shows aneurysmal dilation *(arrows)* of the ascending aorta (AA), which does not extend into the descending aorta (DA).

Acquired Aortic Abnormalities
Aortic Aneurysm
A thoracic aortic aneurysm (Box 16-13) is an abnormal dilation of the aorta. The aortic lumen usually is larger than 4 cm in diameter.

Aneurysms may be classified based on several features, including integrity of the aortic wall, aneurysm shape, and aneurysm location. Based on the integrity of the aortic wall, aneurysms may be classified as *true aneurysms*, characterized by an intact aortic wall, and as *false aneurysms*, characterized by a disrupted aortic wall, in which case the aneurysm is contained by surrounding tissues.

Aneurysms may be further classified by their shape as *fusiform* or *saccular*. Fusiform aneurysms are characterized by cylindrical dilation of the entire aortic circumference, whereas saccular aneurysms are characterized by a focal area of outpouching of the aorta. By location, aneurysms may be classified as occurring within the ascending, transverse, and descending aorta.

Aneurysms that classically involve the ascending aorta include those related to cystic medial necrosis and syphilis. The latter, previously a common cause of ascending aortic aneurysms, is infrequently seen today. Aneurysms that commonly involve the descending thoracic aorta include atherosclerotic, posttraumatic, and mycotic aneurysms. The transverse aorta, usually involved by processes similar to those in the descending thoracic aorta, is uncommonly affected by cystic medial necrosis.

Most thoracic aortic aneurysms are atherosclerotic and are true aneurysms. Because atherosclerosis usually affects long segments of the aorta, atherosclerotic aneurysms are usually fusiform. They most commonly affect the aortic arch and descending thoracic aorta. Atherosclerotic aneurysms typically contain mural thrombus and calcification.

Aneurysms resulting from connective tissue disorders such as Marfan syndrome and Ehlers-Danlos syndrome most often affect the ascending aorta and are caused by cystic medial necrosis (Fig. 16-22). Complications of ascending aortic aneurysms include rupture, dissection, aortic insufficiency, and pericardial tamponade.

Posttraumatic aneurysms are usually the result of a rapid deceleration injury and often caused by a motor vehicle accident. Among patients who survive the initial injury, most aortic transections (80%) occur at the level of the ligamentous arteriosum, which is located just distal to the origin of the left subclavian artery. Posttraumatic aneurysms are classified as false aneurysms and are an acute surgical emergency, because the associated mortality rate is very high. Most patients who sustain a traumatic transection of the aorta do not survive the initial injury; for those who do survive, prompt diagnosis and treatment are critical. Uncommonly, a patient may present with a chronic false aneurysm from previous trauma; as in acute posttraumatic aneurysms, the most common location is at the level of the ligamentum arteriosum (see Chapter 6).

Infectious aneurysms are also known as mycotic aneurysms. They are classified as false aneurysms and are usually saccular. Mycotic aneurysms may be associated with periaortic inflammation and abscess formation.

On chest radiographs, an aortic aneurysm should be suspected whenever a mediastinal mass is immediately adjacent to the aorta, particularly if a border of the mass is indistinguishable from the aortic contour. Peripheral calcification within such a mass is supportive evidence of a vascular cause, particularly in atherosclerotic aneurysms. The diagnosis can be confirmed by contrast-enhanced CT, MRI, or angiography. Important information provided by these studies includes the precise location and size of the aneurysm, the relationship of the aneurysm to the great vessels, and the presence of complications, including aortic rupture and dissection. It is important to accurately measure the maximal diameter of an aortic aneurysm, because the incidence of rupture correlates with the size of the aneurysm and increases significantly for aneurysms greater than 5 cm in diameter. Aneurysms can dilate at a mean rate of 0.12 cm/year. For these reasons, elective surgical repair has been recommended for ascending aortic aneurysms of 5 to 5.5 cm and for descending thoracic aortic aneurysms of 5.5 to 6.5 cm in diameter.

Contrast-enhanced CT and MRI play an important role in imaging aortic aneurysms. The location of the abnormality and the expected cause should be considered when deciding which imaging modality to use for further evaluation. For abnormalities of the ascending aorta, MRI is usually preferred over CT, but MRI has less of an advantage in the current era of multidetector CT scanners. The direct multiplanar capability of MRI, including the ability to image in sagittal-oblique (LAO) and coronal projections, allows for precise measurement of an ascending aortic aneurysm; MRI can accurately identify associated effacement of the sinotubular junction by an aortic root aneurysm. Contrast-enhanced CT usually is sufficient for the evaluation of aneurysms of the aortic arch and descending thoracic aorta. CT can accurately demonstrate aortic dilation, intramural thrombus, and perianeurysmal hemorrhage or infection. However, a tortuous aorta occasionally courses obliquely on a transaxial CT image and may be difficult to measure accurately. Sagittal-oblique and coronal reformation images should be obtained to accurately measure and characterize aortic aneurysms using CT. Although catheter angiography was historically the method of choice for the evaluation of acute posttraumatic aortic transection (Fig. 16-23), CT angiography has largely replaced catheter angiography for this indication at most institutions. This topic is discussed further in Chapter 6.

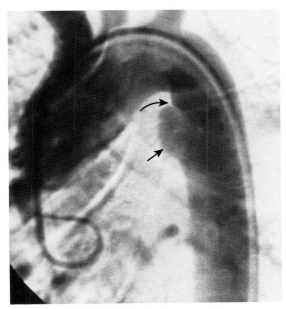

FIGURE 16-23. Acute aortic transection. Digital subtraction angiogram shows a posttraumatic pseudoaneurysm *(straight arrow)* of the proximal descending thoracic aorta at the level of the ligamentum arteriosum. Notice the presence of intimal disruption *(curved arrow).*

> **Box 16-14. Aortic Dissection**
>
> **DEMOGRAPHICS**
> Associated conditions: systemic hypertension (most common)
> Age: usually occurs in patients older than 40 years
>
> **DESCRIPTIVE FEATURES**
> **Chest Radiography**
> Widened mediastinum
> Inward displacement of intimal calcifications
> Diffuse aortic dilation
>
> **CT, MR, Transesophageal Echocardiography, and Angiography**
> Intimal flap
> Differential flow between the true and false lumens
> Pericardial effusion (suggests rupture)

Aortic Dissection

Aortic dissection (Box 16-14) is a life-threatening condition characterized by a tear in the intima of the aortic wall, followed by separation of the tunica media that creates two channels for the passage of blood: a true and false lumen. Aortic dissection is most commonly associated with systemic hypertension. It is also associated with a variety of other entities, including cystic medial necrosis, syphilitic aortitis, coarctation of the aorta, and pregnancy. Affected patients most often present with acute onset of chest and back pain, and they are usually hypertensive.

Chest radiograph findings suggesting aortic dissection include widening of the mediastinum, inward displacement of intimal calcifications, and diffuse aortic enlargement. The best way to appreciate these findings is by an interval change in appearance compared with previous chest radiographs (Box 16-15). The definitive diagnosis of dissection depends on identification of an intimal flap, for which contrast-enhanced CT, MRI, transesophageal echo, or angiography (Fig. 16-24) is useful. The decision of which imaging modality to choose is often based on several factors, including the stability of the patient and individual institutional practices.

Because management depends on the site of involvement, it is important to accurately localize the site of dissection. There are two main classification systems for aortic

> **Box 16-15. Aortic Dissection: Use of Imaging Studies**
>
> 1. Identification of an intimal flap
> 2. Determination of the site of involvement, particularly whether there is involvement of the ascending aorta
> 3. Visualization of differential flow between the true and false lumens
> 4. Determination of whether the dissection extends into the origin of the great vessels
> 5. Assessment for the presence of associated pericardial or pleural effusion in cases complicated by rupture
> 6. Assessment for the presence of aortic regurgitation

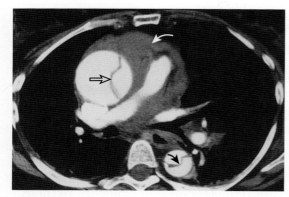

FIGURE 16-24. Stanford Type A aortic dissection with aortic rupture. Axial, contrast-enhanced CT image shows intimal flaps within the ascending aorta *(open arrow)* and descending aorta *(curved black arrow)*. Notice the presence of hemopericardium *(curved white arrow)* resulting from aortic rupture.

Box 16-16. Aortic Dissection: Classification Systems

DEBAKEY CLASSIFICATION
Type I: Dissection involves ascending and descending aorta
Type 2: Dissection involves ascending aorta only
Type 3: Dissection involves descending aorta only

STANFORD CLASSIFICATION
Type A: Dissection involves ascending aorta ± descending aorta
Type B: Dissection involves descending aorta only

---

dissections, the DeBakey and Stanford classification systems, both of which are based on the site of aortic dissection (Box 16-16). Because of their propensity to rupture across the coronary ostia and into the aortic valve and pericardium, dissections that involve the ascending aorta (i.e., DeBakey I, DeBakey II, and Stanford A) are treated surgically. Dissections that begin distal to the origin of the left subclavian artery (i.e., DeBakey III and Stanford B) are treated medically by controlling the patient's hypertension.

Intramural Hematoma
Intramural hematoma is a variant of aortic dissection in which hemorrhage is localized to the aortic media, without an intimal flap. Unenhanced CT shows a crescent-shaped area of high attenuation along the wall of the aorta that represents hemorrhage within the aortic media (Fig. 16-25A). After contrast administration, the hematoma does not enhance and appears hypodense compared with the aortic lumen (see Fig. 16-25B). Unlike an aortic dissection, an identifiable intimal flap or evidence of flowing blood within a false channel is not observed. Both CT and MRI are highly accurate for diagnosing intramural hematoma, but catheter angiography is insensitive for detecting this complication.

Intramural hematoma may be complicated by aneurysm formation, ulceration, rupture, or intimal disruption with dissection (see Fig. 16-25C). It is classified similar to aortic dissections. Similar to dissection, involvement of the ascending aorta usually is treated surgically. Patients with disease limited to the descending aorta are usually treated medically, with close follow-up imaging within the first 30 days after presentation. If progression or complications are detected, open surgical or endovascular stent repair may be indicated.

Penetrating Atherosclerotic Ulcer
Penetrating atherosclerotic ulcer is an ulcer that develops within an atherosclerotic portion of the aorta. The ulcer penetrates through the elastic lamina into the aortic media, with associated intramural hematoma.

Contrast-enhanced CT shows a localized ulceration penetrating through the aortic intima, most commonly involving the middle to distal third of the descending aorta. Coronal and sagittal reformation images aid accurate measurement of the craniocaudal length of the ulcer.

Complications include progression to aortic dissection, distal embolization, extensive intramural hematoma, and development of a pseudoaneurysm with possible rupture. Treatment decisions depend on patient factors and the extent of ulceration. Many patients are managed conservatively, but they require close follow-up within days of presentation to exclude progression or complications. Patients requiring surgery may undergo

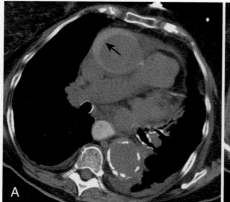
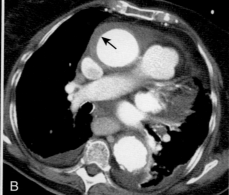
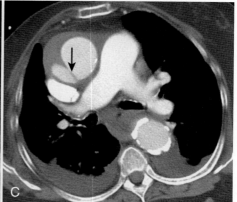

FIGURE 16-25. Intramural hematoma complicated by aortic dissection. **A,** Unenhanced, axial CT image at the level of the proximal ascending aorta shows a crescentic, hyperdense rim along the wall of the aorta *(arrow)*, consistent with an intramural hematoma. **B,** Contrast-enhanced, axial CT image at the same level shows the hematoma *(arrow)* to be hypodense compared with the contrast-enhanced aortic lumen. **C,** Contrast-enhanced, axial CT image performed 1 week later shows development of a frank aortic dissection, with a characteristic intimal flap *(arrow)*.

replacement of the diseased portion of the aorta with an interposition graft, but endovascular stent-graft repair is increasingly performed as an alternative to open surgical procedures.

Pericardial Cyst

Pericardial cysts are attached to the parietal pericardium and are lined by mesothelial cells. They usually contain clear fluid and do not communicate with the pericardial space.

Pericardial cysts often are detected as incidental findings in asymptomatic patients, usually after the age of 30 years. There is no sexual predilection.

Most pericardial cysts are in the anterior right cardiophrenic angle, but they may occur in other locations, including the left cardiophrenic angle, in up to one third of cases. On plain radiographs, they appear as well-defined, round or oval masses located in the normally clear cardiophrenic angle (Fig. 16-26). On CT, pericardial cysts typically demonstrate fluid attenuation; however, they may infrequently contain viscous fluid that measures soft tissue attenuation. Similarly, the MR signal characteristics are typically that of water (i.e., low signal intensity on T1-weighted images and bright signal intensity on T2-weighted images), they but may vary depending on the cyst's content.

Other Cardiophrenic Angle Masses

An important differential diagnosis is that of a cardiophrenic angle mass. Although most causes of cardiophrenic angle masses are benign entities (e.g., lipoma, pericardial fat pad, foramen of Morgagni hernia, pericardial cyst), enlarged epicardial lymph nodes due to lymphoma or metastases may also be identified in this location. It may be difficult to distinguish a mediastinal cardiophrenic angle mass from a pleural mass such as a fibrous tumor of the pleura. Sometimes, a well-defined lung mass in the right middle lobe may mimic a mediastinal cardiophrenic angle mass.

Pericardial Fat Pad and Lipoma

A prominent pericardial fat pad may simulate a cardiophrenic angle mass. Large pericardial fat pads are often seen in obese patients, in patients receiving exogenous steroid therapy, and in patients with Cushing's syndrome. In many cases, excess fat deposition in the pericardial region is associated with generalized excess fat deposition throughout the mediastinum (i.e., mediastinal lipomatosis). A focal fatty mass, a benign lipoma, may manifest as a cardiophrenic angle mass and may be indistinguishable from a prominent pericardial fat pad.

Previous radiographs are often helpful in the evaluation of patients with prominent pericardial fat pads, because they usually demonstrate a stable appearance over time. However, pericardial fat pads occasionally may increase in size in response to interval weight gain. CT can confirm that the mass demonstrates fat attenuation. It is helpful in differentiating a pericardial fat pad from epicardial lymph nodes, which demonstrate soft tissue attenuation, and from pericardial cysts, which usually demonstrate fluid attenuation.

Foramen of Morgagni Hernia

Herniation of abdominal contents through the anteromedial diaphragmatic foramen of Morgagni may result in a cardiophrenic angle mass, most often on the right side.

The imaging features depend on the contents that herniate through the foramen. Most often, herniated contents include omentum, liver, or colon. When the hernia contains only omentum, the CT appearance is similar to that of a lipoma. However, identification of fine linear densities representing omental vessels within the fat suggest the diagnosis of herniated omental fat rather than a lipoma. CT with multiplanar reformation images or a nuclear medicine hepatobiliary scan can confirm the presence of herniated liver. When a Morgagni hernia contains bowel, the diagnosis often can be made by identifying gas-filled loops of bowel within the mass on chest radiographs (Fig. 16-27).

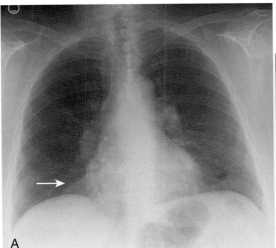
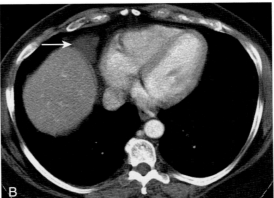

FIGURE 16-26. Pericardial cyst. **A,** The frontal chest radiograph shows a well-defined mass in the right cardiophrenic angle *(arrow).* **B,** The axial CT image shows fluid attenuation that is consistent with a pericardial cyst *(arrow).*

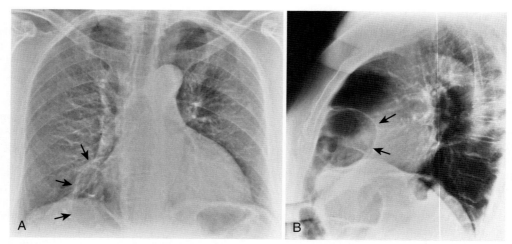

FIGURE 16-27. Foramen of Morgagni hernia. The frontal and lateral chest radiographs demonstrate a well-defined mass in the right cardiophrenic angle *(arrows)* that contains gas-filled loops of bowel, which is diagnostic of a Morgagni hernia. When the hernia contains omental fat or liver without bowel, additional imaging studies, such as CT, are required for the diagnosis.

Epicardial Lymph Nodes

Enlarged epicardial lymph nodes may manifest as a cardiophrenic angle mass. Because epicardial lymph nodes are rarely enlarged from benign processes, a neoplastic process, such as lymphoma or metastatic disease, should be suspected. Epicardial lymph nodes are a common site of recurrence in patients with Hodgkin's lymphoma after radiation therapy. On CT, epicardial lymph nodes appear as single or multiple masses with soft tissue attenuation.

Tracheal Neoplasms

Tracheal neoplasms should be considered in the differential diagnosis of a middle mediastinal mass, especially when a mass extends into or narrows the tracheal lumen. These tumors are discussed in Chapter 12.

▬ POSTERIOR MEDIASTINAL MASSES

Neurogenic Tumors

Neurogenic tumors (Box 16-17) are the most common cause of a posterior mediastinal mass. About 70% of neurogenic tumors are benign. There are three main groups: those arising from peripheral nerves (e.g., schwannoma, neurofibroma); those arising from the sympathetic chain (e.g., ganglioneuroma, ganglioneuroblastoma, neuroblastoma); and those arising from the paraganglia (e.g., pheochromocytoma, chemodectoma). The first group is the most common, and the third group is the least common.

Neurogenic tumors typically occur in younger patients. Although most patients are asymptomatic, these tumors may cause neurologic symptoms such as radicular pain and neuresthesias. Intravertebral extension may result in symptoms of cord compression.

Tumors arising from the peripheral nerves tend to be round, and those arising from the sympathetic chain are usually fusiform with a more vertical orientation. Neurogenic tumors usually occur in a paraspinal location. Benign neurogenic neoplasms typically appear homogeneous and have well-defined margins. Malignant neurogenic tumors are more likely to appear heterogeneous and have irregular margins. Associated bony abnormalities, including rib

---

Box 16-17. Neurogenic Tumors

DEMOGRAPHICS

Age: usually occur in younger patients, first 4 decades of life
Gender: males and females equally affected

DESCRIPTIVE FEATURES

Nerve Sheath Tumors

Round, homogeneous, paraspinal mass
May be associated with widening of the neural foramen
MRI: slightly brighter signal than muscle on T1-weighted and very bright on T2-weighted images; homogeneous enhancement after gadolinium administration

Sympathetic Chain Tumors

Fusiform, homogeneous, paraspinal mass
May be associated with vertebral body erosion
MRI characteristics similar to those of nerve sheath tumors

---

spreading and rib erosion, are commonly seen, but they do not imply malignancy (Fig. 16-28). Frank bone destruction, however, should raise the suspicion for malignancy.

MRI is the preferred cross-sectional imaging modality because of its superb ability to demonstrate intraspinal extension of tumor or an associated spinal cord abnormality. On MRI, neurogenic tumors are typically well-defined masses of homogeneous appearance, demonstrating signal intensity slightly greater than that of skeletal muscle on T1-weighted images and markedly increased signal on T2-weighted images (Fig. 16-29). Neurogenic tumors typically enhance homogeneously after gadolinium administration.

Associated abnormalities of the vertebral bodies are well demonstrated on CT. Because nerve sheath tumors arise posterolaterally, they are often associated with widening of the neural foramen. In contrast, tumors arising from the sympathetic ganglia are located anterolateral to the vertebral bodies and more often result in vertebral body erosion.

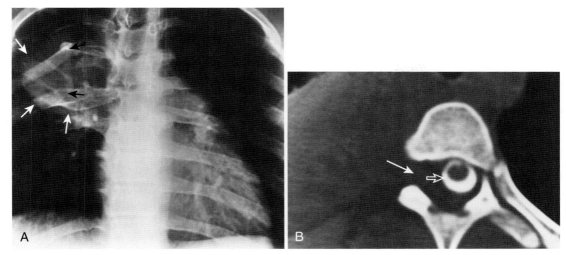

FIGURE 16-28. Ganglioneuroma. A, The frontal chest radiograph shows a large, posterior mediastinal mass *(white arrows)* with associated rib spreading and rib erosions *(black arrows).* B, An axial image from a CT-myelogram study shows extension of the right paraspinal mass into the neural foramen *(white arrow)*, with associated displacement of the thecal sac and spinal cord *(open arrow).*

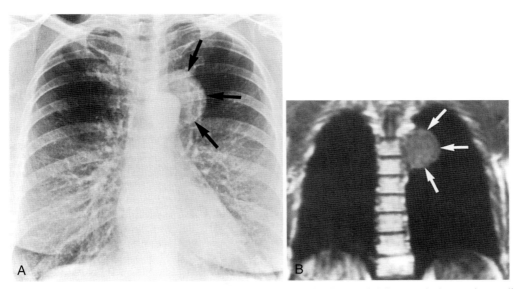

FIGURE 16-29. Schwannoma. A, The frontal chest radiograph reveals a well-defined, round, left paraspinal posterior mediastinal mass *(arrows).* B, Coronal, T1-weighted MRI shows homogeneous, intermediate signal intensity within the mass *(arrows)*, which is slightly brighter than skeletal muscle. T2-weighted images can demonstrate homogeneous bright signal within the mass. These MRI signal characteristics are typical of neurogenic tumors.

Paravertebral Abnormalities

Infectious, malignant, and traumatic abnormalities of the thoracic spine may result in a posterior mediastinal mass. Paravertebral abnormalities have many causes (Box 16-18). They may occur in patients of any age, and there is no sex predilection. Patients with paravertebral posterior mediastinal masses often present with back pain. Patients with infectious processes may have fever and leukocytosis. An important infectious cause is Pott's disease, a paraspinal abscess from tuberculous infection. Malignant causes include metastatic disease and myeloma. Traumatic causes include vertebral fracture with associated paraspinal hematoma.

On imaging studies, paravertebral posterior mediastinal masses are often bilateral and fusiform. Bilaterality may help distinguish paravertebral masses from neurogenic tumors, which are usually unilateral paraspinal masses. An important exception is neurofibromatosis, which may manifest with multiple, bilateral neurofibromas.

Associated abnormalities of the vertebral bodies or intervertebral disk spaces suggest a paravertebral origin. Disk space involvement can help differentiate infectious from malignant causes. Narrowing of the intervertebral disk spaces and abnormalities of the adjacent vertebral body end plates suggest an infectious cause. Malignant processes are associated with destruction of the vertebral body, but they usually spare the intervertebral disk spaces.

Posttraumatic paraspinal hematoma usually is associated with fracture of one or more thoracic vertebral bodies. MRI demonstrates signal characteristics of hemorrhage within the paraspinal mass, which vary according to the stage of hemorrhage.

Box 16-18. Paravertebral Abnormalities

DEMOGRAPHICS

No general distinguishing demographic features

DESCRIPTIVE FEATURES

Paravertebral masses are often bilateral and fusiform

Associated abnormalities of the vertebral bodies or intervertebral disk spaces are important features of paravertebral abnormalities.

Involvement of the intervertebral disk indicates an infectious cause, whereas involvement of the vertebral body with sparing of the disk space suggests a neoplastic process.

Posttraumatic paravertebral abnormalities are characterized by a vertebral body fracture and paraspinal hematoma.

Vascular Abnormalities

The descending thoracic aorta and the azygous vein are located within the posterior mediastinum, and abnormalities of these structures may result in a posterior mediastinal mass (Box 16-19). Abnormalities of the descending thoracic aorta include atherosclerotic, mycotic, and posttraumatic aneurysms. Azygous vein enlargement may result from increased flow (i.e., obstruction of the superior or inferior vena cava) or from increased pressure (i.e., tricuspid insufficiency or right-sided heart failure). The azygous vein may be enlarged in the congenital condition known as *azygous continuation of the inferior vena cava*. Esophageal varices also may result in a posterior mediastinal mass.

Most thoracic aortic aneurysms are atherosclerotic and therefore more common in older patients. Mycotic and posttraumatic aneurysms may be seen in any age group. Azygous continuation of the inferior vena cava is associated with polysplenia and asplenia, and it may also be an incidental finding. Esophageal and paraesophageal varices are associated with portal hypertension and cirrhosis and are often seen in patients with a history of alcohol abuse.

On chest radiographs, thoracic aortic aneurysms typically produce an abnormal contour of the descending thoracic aortic interface and often demonstrate curvilinear calcification (Fig. 16-30). The diagnosis may be confirmed with contrast-enhanced CT, MRI, or angiography.

Azygous continuation of the inferior vena cava may manifest with enlargement of the azygous arch and lateral displacement of the azygoesophageal interface (Fig. 16-31). The diagnosis can be confirmed by contrast-enhanced CT, which demonstrates enlargement of the azygous arch and the paraspinal and retrocrural portions of the azygous vein, as well as absence of the suprarenal portion of the inferior vena cava.

Esophageal and paraesophageal varices may manifest as a mass in the inferior aspect of the posterior mediastinum. Barium swallow typically demonstrates serpiginous filling defects in the barium column; these defects change in configuration with the Valsalva maneuver. Contrast-enhanced CT, MRI, or angiography can confirm the vascular origin of this abnormality. Associated findings on cross-sectional imaging include a cirrhotic liver and splenomegaly.

Box 16-19. Vascular Abnormalities of the Posterior Mediastinum

DEMOGRAPHICS

Aortic Aneurysms

Cause: atherosclerosis most common cause of thoracic aortic aneurysms

Age: usually occurs in patients older than 40 years

Azygous Continuation of the Inferior Vena Cava

Associations: polysplenia and asplenia

Age: may be detected in patients of any age

Esophageal Varices

Usually seen in adult patients with a history of alcohol abuse and cirrhosis

DESCRIPTIVE FEATURES

Thoracic Aortic Aneurysm

Chest radiograph: abnormal convex contour of the descending thoracic aortic interface; may contain peripheral calcification

CT, MRI, or angiography: confirms vascular cause; may detect complications, including rupture

Azygous Continuation of the Inferior Vena Cava

Chest radiograph: enlargement of the azygous arch and lateral displacement of the azygoesophageal interface; decrease in size after a Valsalva maneuver

CT or MRI: enlargement of the azygous arch and the paraspinal and retrocrural portions of the azygous vein; absence of the suprarenal portion of the inferior vena cava

Esophageal Varices

Chest radiograph: may present as a mass in the inferior aspect of the posterior mediastinum

Barium swallow: demonstrates serpiginous defects in the barium column that change in configuration after a Valsalva maneuver

CT or MRI, or angiography: confirms the vascular origin of the abnormality; CT or MRI may also demonstrate a cirrhotic liver and splenomegaly

Esophageal Abnormalities

A wide variety of esophageal abnormalities (Box 16-20) may result in a posterior mediastinal mass, such as benign and malignant neoplasms, achalasia, hiatal hernia, and duplication cyst. Because of the wide variety of causes, there are no general distinguishing demographic features, but there are some helpful guidelines.

Even though many esophageal abnormalities may occur in patients of any age group, malignant esophageal neoplasms are more common in older men and are associated with smoking and alcohol abuse. Leiomyoma, the most common benign tumor of the esophagus, occurs in patients between the ages of 20 and 60 years, and it has a male predominance. Achalasia usually occurs in patients 30 to 50 years old, with equal frequency among men and women.

Patients with malignant esophageal neoplasms tend to present with symptoms of dysphagia before they become large enough to result in a mediastinal mass. Obstructing esophageal malignancies may produce an air-fluid level

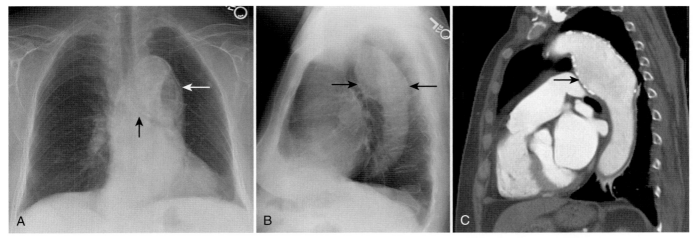

FIGURE 16-30. Descending thoracic aortic aneurysm. **A,** The frontal chest radiograph shows a mediastinal mass *(white arrow),* which is continuous with the proximal descending thoracic aortic contour and contains curvilinear calcifications *(black arrow).* **B,** Lateral chest radiograph confirms the presence of a posterior mediastinal mass with peripheral, curvilinear calcifications *(arrows)* that are continuous with the adjacent descending aorta. **C,** Sagittal-oblique CT reformation image confirms the presence of a descending thoracic aortic aneurysm *(arrow).*

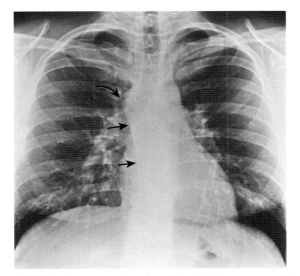

FIGURE 16-31. Azygous continuation of the inferior vena cava. Frontal chest radiograph reveals enlargement of the azygous arch contour *(curved arrow)* and lateral displacement of the azygoesophageal interface *(straight arrows),* corresponding to the presence of an enlarged azygous vein.

within the esophagus and thickening of the tracheoesophageal stripe (Fig. 16-32). In contrast, benign esophageal neoplasms are usually asymptomatic and larger than malignant neoplasms at diagnosis, although most benign esophageal neoplasms are not detectable on chest radiographs. Barium swallow is helpful for confirming the esophageal origin and in further characterizing the abnormality as mucosal or submucosal (Fig. 16-33).

Nonneoplastic esophageal abnormalities that may result in a posterior mediastinal mass include achalasia and hiatal hernia. Achalasia, a primary dysmotility disorder of the esophagus, results in aperistalsis of the esophagus below the level of the aortic arch, and subsequent diffuse esophageal dilation with retention of food and secretions. On chest radiographs, achalasia often appears as a longitudinal posterior mediastinal mass, extending the entire length of the mediastinum (Fig. 16-34). The azygoesophageal interface is typically

> **Box 16-20. Esophageal Abnormalities**
>
> **DEMOGRAPHICS**
> No general distinguishing demographic features
>
> **DESCRIPTIVE FEATURES**
>
> *Malignant Esophageal Neoplasm*
> Obstructing lesions may present as thickening of the tracheoesophageal stripe on the lateral chest radiograph; an air-fluid level may be identified within the esophagus.
> CT may demonstrate esophageal wall thickening and may show nodal spread or distant metastases.
>
> *Benign Esophageal Neoplasm*
> Neoplasm may manifest as a smooth mass that distorts the azygoesophageal interface.
>
> *Achalasia*
> Typically manifests as a longitudinal mass extending the length of the mediastinum with diffuse, rightward, lateral displacement of the azygoesophageal interface; an air-fluid level may be visible.
>
> *Hiatal Hernia*
> The hernia typically manifests as a round, retrocardiac mass that causes a focal, rightward, lateral displacement of the inferior aspect of the azygoesophageal interface; an air-fluid level is often visible.

laterally displaced and often demonstrates a rightward convexity. An air-fluid level within the mass strongly suggests achalasia. Barium swallow demonstrates aperistalsis below the level of the aortic arch and a characteristic bird's beak appearance of the distal esophagus.

A hiatal hernia results from the extension of the stomach into the chest through the esophageal hiatus. On chest radiographs, hiatal hernias typically appear as rounded, retrocardiac masses that often cause a focal rightward convexity in the inferior aspect of the azygoesophageal interface (Fig. 16-35). Air-fluid levels often are identified, and barium swallow is diagnostic.

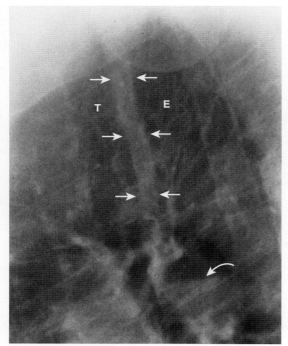

FIGURE 16-32. Esophageal carcinoma. Magnified image of a lateral chest radiograph shows thickening of the tracheoesophageal stripe *(straight arrows)* and an air-fluid level within the midthoracic esophagus *(curved arrow)* in a patient with esophageal obstruction caused by squamous cell carcinoma. E, esophagus; T, trachea.

Other Posterior Mediastinal Masses

Posterior Mediastinal Lymphadenopathy

Posterior mediastinal lymphadenopathy may be caused by neoplasms, especially lymphoma and bronchogenic carcinoma, and by inflammatory conditions, including sarcoidosis. However, involvement of this lymph node group is an uncommon manifestation of these disorders. Posterior mediastinal lymphadenopathy typically results in bilateral

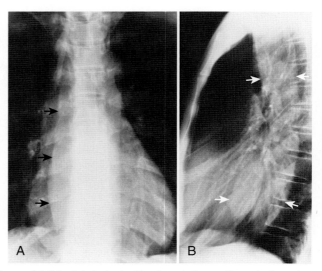

FIGURE 16-34. Achalasia. **A,** The frontal chest radiograph shows lateral displacement of the azygoesophageal interface *(arrows).* **B,** The lateral chest radiograph reveals a longitudinal, posterior mediastinal mass that extends the entire length of the thorax *(paired arrows).* **C,** The axial CT image of the chest obtained after administration of oral contrast shows pronounced dilation of the esophagus *(arrow),* which is characteristic of achalasia.

paraspinal masses and may be seen as widening of the paraspinal lines on chest radiographs.

Neurenteric Cyst

Neurenteric cysts are rare developmental anomalies that contain neural and gastrointestinal elements. They are often painful, and they usually develop at a young age.

Often associated with vertebral anomalies and scoliosis, they typically manifest as a well-defined, homogeneous cystic mass. They rarely fill with contrast after myelography.

Meningocele

Anterior and lateral meningoceles represent herniations of meninges through the neural foramina or

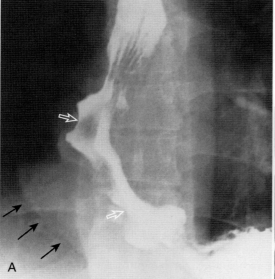

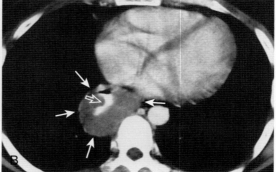

FIGURE 16-33. Leiomyoma. **A,** The coned-down image of the lower mediastinum from a barium esophagogram reveals a posterior mediastinal mass *(black arrows)* with an associated submucosal impression on the barium-filled esophagus *(open arrows).* **B,** The axial CT image obtained after administration of oral and intravenous contrast shows a circumferential mass *(white arrows)* arising from the esophageal wall. Notice the submucosal impression on the esophageal lumen *(open arrow).*

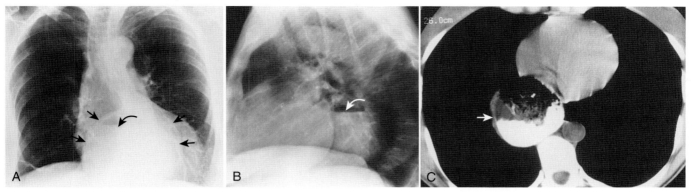

FIGURE 16-35. Hiatal hernia. Frontal and lateral chest radiographs reveal a large, round, retrocardiac mediastinal mass *(straight arrows)* that contains an air-fluid level *(curved arrow)*. Notice the lateral displacement of the azygoesophageal interface on the frontal radiograph.

through defects in the vertebral bodies. Meningoceles are usually asymptomatic and most often are diagnosed in adulthood. They are often associated with neurofibromatosis.

Meningoceles typically appear as well-defined, homogeneous, paraspinal masses. Like neurenteric cysts, they are often associated with vertebral anomalies and scoliosis. In contrast to neurenteric cysts, they frequently fill with contrast after myelography.

Bochdalek Hernia

Herniation of omental fat, kidney, or spleen through the foramen of Bochdalek may result in a posterior mediastinal mass. On chest radiographs, a Bochdalek hernia usually appears

as a smooth bulge in the posterior aspect of the left hemidiaphragm. The diagnosis can be confirmed by demonstration of a diaphragmatic defect on CT with herniated fat, kidney, or spleen.

Extramedullary Hematopoiesis

Extramedullary hematopoiesis is a rare compensatory response of marrow expansion. It is associated with severe anemias, particularly thalassemia intermedia.

Extramedullary hematopoiesis typically manifests as longitudinal, bilateral, lobulated paraspinal masses (Fig. 16-36). Associated osseous findings of marrow expansion, including expanded ribs with narrowed rib interspaces, suggest the diagnosis.

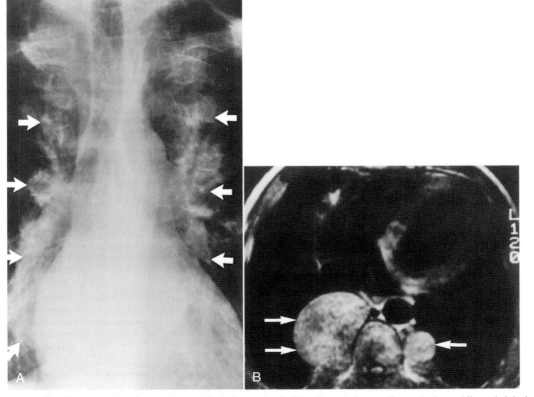

FIGURE 16-36. Extramedullary hematopoiesis in a patient with thalassemia. **A,** The frontal chest radiograph shows bilateral, lobulated paraspinal masses *(arrows)* that extend the entire length of the mediastinum. Notice the widening of the ribs, which is consistent with marrow expansion. **B,** Axial, T1-weighted MRI reveals bilateral, round, paraspinal masses of bright signal intensity *(arrows)*.

■ Suggested Readings

Davis, R.D., Oldham, H.N., Sabiston, D.C., 1987. Primary cysts and neoplasms of the mediastinum: recent changes in clinical presentation, methods of diagnosis, management and results. Ann. Thorac. Surg. 44, 229–237.

Duwe, B.V., Sterman, D.H., Musani, A.I., 2005. Tumors of the mediastinum. Chest 128, 2893–2909.

Felson, B., 1973. Chest Roentgenology. WB Saunders, Philadelphia.

Fraser, R.G., Colman, N., Müller, N., Paré, P.D., 1999. Fraser and Paré's Diagnosis of Diseases of the Chest. fourth ed. WB Saunders, Philadelphia.

Fujimoto, K., Müller, N., 2008. Anterior mediastinal masses. In: Müller, N., Silva, C.S. (Eds.), Imaging of the Chest, Saunders, Philadelphia.

Green, C.E., Klein, J.S., 2008. Multidetector row CT angiography of the thoracic aorta. In: Boiselle, P.M., White, C.S. (Eds.), New Techniques in Cardiothoracic Imaging. Informa, New York, pp. 105–126.

Grillo, H.C., Mathieson, D.J., 1990. Primary tracheal tumors: treatment and results. Ann. Thorac. Surg. 49, 69–77.

Halpert, R.D., Goodman, P., 1993. Gastrointestinal Radiology: The Requisites. Mosby–Year Book, St. Louis.

Heitzman, E.R., 1988. The Mediastinum, Radiologic, Correlations, Anatomy, and Pathology, second ed. Springer-Verlag, Berlin.

Hunsaker, A.R., 2004. MDCT in mediastinal imaging. In: Schoepf, U.J. (Ed.), Multidetector-Row CT of the Thorax. Springer-Verlag, Berlin, pp. 215–224.

Inaoka, T., Takahashi, K., Mineta, M., et al., 2007. Thymic hyperplasia and thymus gland tumors: differentiation with chemical shift MR imaging. Radiology 243, 869–876.

McCarthy, M.J., Rosado-de-Christenson, M.L., 1995. Tumors of the trachea. J. Thorac. Imaging 10, 180–198.

McLoud, T.C., Ragozzino, M.W., 1990. MR imaging of the thorax. In: Edelman, R.R., Hesselink, J.R. (Eds.), Clinical Magnetic Resonance Imaging. WB Saunders, Philadelphia, pp. 731–744.

Nadler, L.M., 1991. The malignant lymphomas. In: Wilson, J.D., Braunwald, E., Isselbacher, K.J., et al. (Eds.), Harrison's Principles and Practices of Internal Medicine, twelveth ed. vol. 2. McGraw-Hill, New York, pp. 1599–1612.

Naidich, D.P., Webb, W.R., Müller, N.L., et al., 1999. Computed Tomography and Magnetic Resonance of the Thorax, third ed. Raven Press, New York.

Nishino, M., Ashiku, S.K., Kocher, O.N., et al., 2006. The thymus: a comprehensive review. Radiographics 26, 335–348.

Palmer, E.L., Scott, J.A., Strauss, H.W., 1992. Practical Nuclear Medicine. WB Saunders, Philadelphia.

Pierson, D.J., 1991. Disorders of the pleura, mediastinum and diaphragm. In: Wilson, J.D., Braunwald, E., Isselbacher, K.J., et al. (Eds.), Harrison's Principles and Practices of Internal Medicine, twelfth ed. vol. 2. McGraw-Hill, New York, pp. 1111–1116.

Reed, J.C., 2003. Chest Radiology: Plain Film Patterns and Differential Diagnoses, fifth ed. Mosby–Year Book, St. Louis.

Shaffer, K., Pugatch, R.D., 1992. Diseases of the mediastinum. In: Freundlich, I.M., Bragg, D.G. (Eds.), Radiologic Approach to Diseases of the Chest. Williams & Wilkins, Baltimore, pp. 171–185.

Vail, C.M., Ravin, C.E., 1992. Mediastinal masses. In: Freundlich, I.M., Bragg, D.G. (Eds.), Radiologic Approach to Diseases of the Chest. Williams & Wilkins, Baltimore, pp. 360–373.

Webb, W.R., 1994. Diseases of the mediastinum. In: Putman, C.E., Ravin, C.E. (Eds.), Textbook of Diagnostic Imaging. second ed. WB Saunders, Philadelphia, pp. 428–447.

CHAPTER 17

Diffuse Mediastinal Abnormalities

Phillip M. Boiselle

Unlike focal mediastinal masses, which usually can be localized within a single mediastinal compartment, diffuse mediastinal abnormalities almost always involve more than one compartment of the mediastinum and therefore preclude classification by the traditional compartmentalization method. The common feature of these entities is that they all may present with *diffuse mediastinal widening* on chest radiographs.

RADIOLOGIC APPROACH TO DIFFUSE MEDIASTINAL WIDENING

Recognition and evaluation of diffuse mediastinal widening on plain radiographs can be challenging, even for experienced radiologists. The first challenge is recognizing the abnormality. Accurate recognition is particularly difficult on anteroposterior portable supine radiographs because they result in magnification of normal mediastinal structures. The mediastinum often must be assessed on portable radiographs, especially for trauma patients, even though posteroanterior and lateral chest radiographs are superior. Assessment of the mediastinum is also difficult in older patients with atherosclerotic vascular disease, because the mediastinum may appear wide because of tortuosity of the aorta and great vessels. Comparison with prior radiographs is particularly helpful in evaluating this population.

After recognizing diffuse mediastinal widening, its cause must be determined, which can be a difficult task based on chest radiographic findings alone. Assessment of the mediastinal contours and normal mediastinal landmarks is essential. Subtle alterations are often best appreciated as a change in appearance from previous radiographs. The identification of diffuse mediastinal widening on plain radiographs, particularly when accompanied by abnormalities of the normal mediastinal landmarks, usually requires further evaluation with computed tomography (CT) or magnetic resonance imaging (MRI).

DIFFUSE MEDIASTINAL ABNORMALITIES

Mediastinal Lipomatosis

Mediastinal lipomatosis is the diffuse accumulation of excess unencapsulated fat within the mediastinum. This benign condition is usually seen in adult patients and may be associated with Cushing's syndrome, exogenous steroid use, and obesity.

Fat accumulation is usually most prominent in the anterior and superior portions of the mediastinum, where it surrounds the great vessels and results in lateral displacement of the pleural reflections. It may be detected in other parts of the mediastinum, including the cardiophrenic angles, paravertebral regions, retrocrural, and subcostal regions.

The appearance on chest radiographs and CT depends on the distribution of excess fat deposition. Accumulation of fat in the anterior and superior portions of the mediastinum results in smooth widening of the anterior and superior mediastinal contours as seen on chest radiographs (Fig. 17-1). An important feature is the lack of mass effect on the trachea and esophagus, structures that are often displaced or compressed by other mediastinal abnormalities. Excess fat deposits within the cardiophrenic angles result in cardiophrenic angle "masses," and excess fat within the paravertebral regions may result in bilateral lateral displacement of the paraspinal lines.

A definitive diagnosis of mediastinal lipomatosis may be made on CT (Fig. 17-2). Fat is recognized on CT by its low CT numbers, which typically vary from –70 to –130 Hounsfield units (HU). Although CT is considered the imaging modality of choice, the diagnosis also can be made by MRI. On MRI, fat demonstrates bright signal intensity on T1-weighted images. Using a fat-suppression sequence results in suppression of the normally bright T1 signal from fat tissue and helps to differentiate it from other tissues with bright T1 signal. An important feature of mediastinal lipomatosis on CT or MRI is a homogeneous appearance of the mediastinal fat. An inhomogeneous appearance, such as the presence of high-attenuation foci within the fat, should raise the suspicion of a superimposed process, such as mediastinal hemorrhage or neoplastic infiltration.

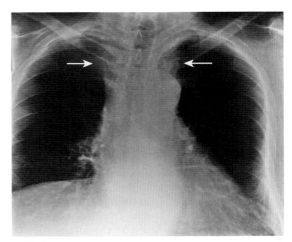

FIGURE 17-1. Mediastinal lipomatosis. The frontal chest radiograph reveals smooth widening of the superior mediastinum *(arrows)*. Notice the absence of a mass effect on the trachea, which has a midline position.

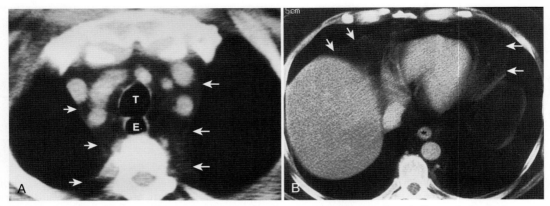

Figure 17-2. Mediastinal lipomatosis. **A,** Axial, noncontrast CT of the chest at the level of the brachiocephalic vessels shows a large amount of fat within the mediastinum that surrounds the vessels and results in lateral displacement of the pleural reflections *(arrows)*. Notice the normal midline position of the trachea (T) and esophagus (E). **B,** Axial CT of the chest at the level of the diaphragm reveals excess fat within the cardiophrenic angles *(paired arrows)*.

Mediastinitis

Diffuse mediastinitis may be acute or chronic. Both forms are most often caused by infections. Acute mediastinitis is often the result of a bacterial infection, and chronic mediastinitis is more often related to a granulomatous infection, such as histoplasmosis. Patients with acute mediastinitis usually present with an acute onset of symptoms, including fever and leukocytosis, whereas patients with chronic mediastinitis are often asymptomatic. If symptoms occur, they usually result from compression of mediastinal structures.

Acute Mediastinitis

Acute mediastinitis may occur after esophageal perforation, from extension of an infectious process from thoracic and extrathoracic structures (especially from the neck), and as an infrequent complication of cardiac surgery (Box 17-1). Most cases are caused by esophageal perforation.

Esophageal Perforation

Patients with esophageal perforation frequently present with fever, leukocytosis, dysphagia, and retrosternal chest pain, which often radiates into the neck. On physical examination, they may demonstrate subcutaneous emphysema and Hamman's sign, a crunching or rasping sound that is synchronous with the heartbeat and heard on auscultation over the cardiac apex and that is associated with pneumomediastinum.

Chest radiographic findings include diffuse widening of the mediastinum and pneumomediastinum (Fig. 17-3). Associated pleural abnormalities are usually left sided and include pneumothorax and empyema. When the diagnosis is delayed, complications may include mediastinal abscess formation and rupture of the abscess into the adjacent bronchus (i.e., esophagobronchial fistula) and pleura (i.e., esophagopleural fistula, often with subsequent development of empyema). The diagnosis of esophageal perforation can be confirmed by fluoroscopic examination after administration of water-soluble contrast, which demonstrates extravasation of contrast at the site of perforation (Fig. 17-4). In complicated cases that have progressed to mediastinal abscess formation, CT may be helpful in identifying the precise location and extent of fluid collections (Fig. 17-5).

Box 17-1. Causes of Acute Mediastinitis

ESOPHAGEAL PERFORATION
Iatrogenic (after esophagoscopy or esophageal dilation)
Impacted foreign body (chicken bone, sharp objects)
Obstructing esophageal neoplasm
Trauma (penetrating trauma more than blunt trauma)
Repeated episodes of vomiting (Boerhaave's syndrome)

EXTENSION OF INFECTION FROM ADJACENT SPACES
Pharynx (retropharyngeal or nasopharyngeal abscess)
Retroperitoneum (pancreatic pseudocyst)
Abdomen (subphrenic abscess)

EXTENSION OF INFECTION FROM ADJACENT THORACIC STRUCTURES
Lung
Lymph nodes
Pleura (empyema)
Pericardium

POSTOPERATIVE COMPLICATIONS
Cardiovascular surgery
Esophageal surgery

AIRWAY RUPTURE
Iatrogenic
Trauma
Foreign body
Erosion from adjacent malignancy

Prompt diagnosis and treatment of esophageal perforation are critical. Very high morbidity and mortality rates are associated with delay in diagnosis beyond 24 hours.

Other Causes of Acute Mediastinitis

Other causes of acute mediastinitis are less common. They include extension of infection from adjacent thoracic structures, including the lungs, pleura, pericardium and mediastinal lymph nodes; extension of infection from adjacent anatomic regions, especially from the neck; traumatic tra-

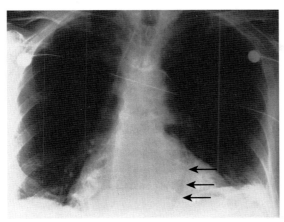

FIGURE 17-3. Acute mediastinitis caused by esophageal perforation (i.e., Boerhaave's syndrome). The frontal radiograph of the chest reveals an abnormal linear lucency *(arrows)* adjacent to the descending aortic interface, consistent with pneumomediastinum.

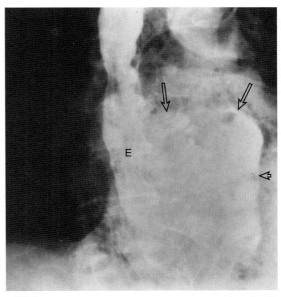

FIGURE 17-4. Acute mediastinitis caused by esophageal perforation (i.e., Boerhaave's syndrome). Coned-down image of the distal esophagus after administration of water-soluble contrast shows extravasation of contrast *(arrows)* from the distal esophagus, consistent with an esophageal perforation.

cheobronchial rupture; and cardiac surgery (an infrequent postoperative complication).

Chest radiographs may demonstrate diffuse mediastinal widening and findings associated with a mediastinal abscess, including gas bubbles or an air-fluid level. Pneumomediastinum and pneumothorax, findings frequently associated with esophageal perforation, are not usually seen with other causes of acute mediastinitis. An important exception is traumatic tracheobronchial rupture, which frequently manifests with pneumomediastinum and pneumothorax.

CT is helpful in diagnosing acute mediastinitis, because it is more sensitive than chest radiographs for detecting the presence and extent of mediastinal fluid collections and the presence of extraluminal gas. Because mediastinitis may result from extension of infection from adjacent thoracic

and extrathoracic structures, CT can determine the relationship of mediastinal fluid collections to these structures. CT may play a role in guiding drainage of mediastinal fluid collections.

Chronic Mediastinitis

Chronic mediastinitis is the result of chronic inflammation of the mediastinum, which may progress to diffuse mediastinal fibrosis. In patients with chronically enlarged inflammatory lymph nodes, the rupture of lymph nodes may incite an inflammatory response that results in diffuse

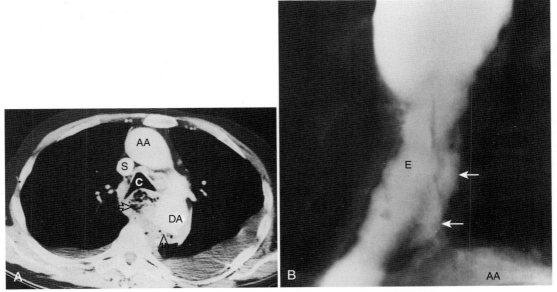

FIGURE 17-5. Mediastinal abscess after esophageal perforation from penetrating trauma. **A,** Axial contrast-enhanced CT of the chest at the level of the carina (C) reveals a large, subcarinal fluid collection *(arrows)* containing foci of gas, consistent with a mediastinal abscess. AA ascending aorta; DA, descending aorta; S, superior vena cava. **B,** Coned-down image of the upper thoracic esophagus after administration of water-soluble contrast media shows extravasation of contrast *(arrows)*, consistent with an esophageal perforation. AA, aortic arch; E, esophagus.

Box 17-2. Causes of Chronic Mediastinitis

INFECTION
Fungal (histoplasmosis, coccidiomycosis)
Tuberculosis

INFLAMMATION
Sarcoidosis

IMMUNOLOGIC
Systemic lupus erythematosus
Rheumatoid arthritis
Raynaud's phenomenon

DRUGS
Methysergide

TRAUMA
Mediastinal hemorrhage (rare)

IDIOPATHIC CAUSES
Sclerosing mediastinitis

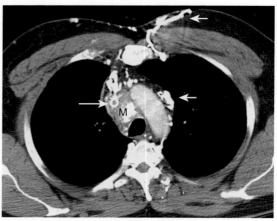

FIGURE 17-6. Mediastinal fibrosis resulting from histoplasmosis. Contrast-enhanced, axial CT shows obstruction of the superior vena cava caused by a large, calcified, right paratracheal mass (M). Notice the opacification of extensive venous collaterals throughout the chest *(short arrows)* and the obstructed stent *(long arrow)* in the superior vena cava. Histoplasmosis is a common benign cause of superior vena caval obstruction.

fibrosis. Over time, enlarged mediastinal lymph nodes and adjacent fibrous tissue may compress adjacent mediastinal and hilar structures, including arteries, veins, the trachea and bronchi, and the esophagus.

Chronic mediastinitis has many causes (Box 17-2). Most cases result from granulomatous processes, including infections such as histoplasmosis, coccidiomycosis, and tuberculosis, and less commonly, noninfectious granulomatous processes such as sarcoidosis. Sclerosing mediastinitis refers to a noninfectious, nongranulomatous cause of chronic mediastinitis, which is frequently associated with other sites of fibrosis, including the retroperitoneum (i.e., retroperitoneal fibrosis), thyroid gland (i.e., Riedel's struma), the orbit (i.e., orbital pseudotumor), and the cecum (i.e., ligneous perityphlitis). Chronic mediastinitis has been associated with immunologic abnormalities (e.g., systemic lupus, erythematosus rheumatoid arthritis, Raynaud's phenomenon), and drugs (e.g., methysergide).

Histoplasmosis is the most common cause of chronic mediastinitis and mediastinal fibrosis. Endemic areas in North America for the organism *Histoplasma capsulatum* include the Ohio, Mississippi, and St. Lawrence river valleys. Histoplasmosis can be acquired during even a brief stay in an endemic area. Individuals of all ages and both genders may be affected.

Patients with chronic mediastinitis are often asymptomatic. The diagnosis of chronic mediastinitis is frequently suggested after the incidental detection of characteristic abnormalities on chest radiographs. When present, symptoms usually arise as a result of compression of mediastinal structures, including vascular structures (e.g., superior vena cava, pulmonary arteries, pulmonary veins), the airway, and the esophagus. Mediastinal fibrosis, particularly from histoplasmosis, should be considered in the differential diagnosis of superior vena cava obstruction. The most common cause of superior vena caval obstruction is neoplastic (especially lung carcinoma), and mediastinal fibrosis is a common benign cause of superior vena caval obstruction (Fig. 17-6).

On chest radiographs, mediastinal fibrosis may manifest as diffuse widening of the mediastinal contours or as a localized mass. When it occurs as a localized mass, it is most commonly in the right paratracheal region (see Fig. 17-6). In cases resulting from granulomatous infections, such as histoplasmosis or tuberculosis, calcifications are frequently identified within enlarged mediastinal and hilar lymph nodes (Fig. 17-7). CT is more sensitive than chest radiographs for detecting enlarged mediastinal lymph nodes, fibrosis, and calcification. In addition to detecting mediastinal fibrosis, CT plays an important role in evaluating the effect of fibrosis on adjacent mediastinal structures. Contrast-enhanced CT is helpful in evaluating the presence of vascular compression, including obstruction of the superior vena cava, pulmonary arteries, and pulmonary veins (Fig. 17-8). CT also can detect airway narrowing and obstruction.

Lung abnormalities may be identified in patients with chronic mediastinitis and may result from the underlying granulomatous process (e.g., fungal or tuberculous infection, sarcoidosis) or from complications of mediastinal fibrosis. For example, pulmonary artery or vein compression may result in pulmonary infarcts, and bronchial obstruction may result in postobstructive pneumonitis and atelectasis.

Mediastinal fibrosis is often suggested on CT by the findings of abnormal fibrous tissue and multiple, calcified mediastinal lymph nodes. The diagnosis may be more difficult to make in patients who present with diffuse fibrosis without calcification. In these cases, the appearance of mediastinal fibrosis may be difficult to distinguish from diffuse mediastinal involvement by malignancy, including lymphoma and metastatic carcinoma. MRI plays an important diagnostic role in these cases, because benign mediastinal fibrosis has low signal intensity on T1- and T2-weighted images (Fig. 17-9), and malignant processes typically demonstrate bright signal intensity on T2-weighted images. Fibrosis, unlike malignancy, usually does not demonstrate enhancement after gadolinium contrast administration. MRI is also helpful for assessing vascular patency in cases of suspected

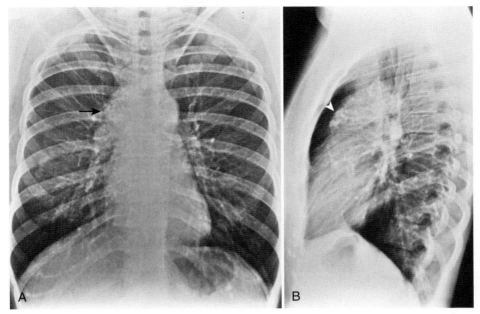

FIGURE 17-7. Mediastinal fibrosis caused by histoplasmosis. **A,** The frontal radiograph of the chest shows a large, calcified, right paratracheal mass *(arrow).* **B,** The lateral chest radiograph reveals calcified, anterior mediastinal lymph nodes *(arrowhead).*

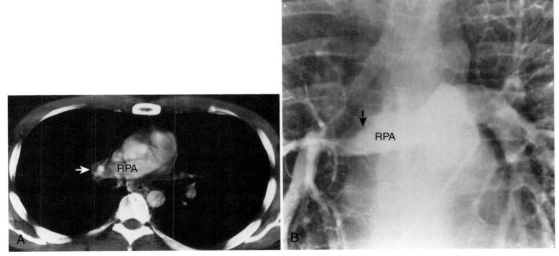

FIGURE 17-8. Mediastinal fibrosis caused by histoplasmosis. **A,** Axial, contrast-enhanced CT shows a calcified nodal mass *(arrow)* compressing the distal right pulmonary artery (RPA). **B,** The pulmonary artery angiogram reveals obstruction of the truncus anterior branch of the RPA. Notice the contour deformity of the distal right pulmonary artery *(arrow),* which results from extrinsic compression by the calcified nodal mass.

vascular obstruction, particularly in patients who have contraindications to intravenous contrast.

Diffuse Mediastinal Lymphadenopathy

When lymphadenopathy involves multiple lymph node sites, it may cause diffuse mediastinal widening. This is especially true of diffuse neoplastic mediastinal lymphadenopathy, particularly if it results from lymphoma (Fig. 17-10) or small cell lung cancer. Metastases from extrathoracic neoplasms that may present with diffuse mediastinal lymphadenopathy include poorly differentiated neoplasms; tumors arising in the head and neck, genitourinary tract, and breast; and melanoma or seminoma (Box 17-3).

Identification of enlarged lymph nodes on chest radiographs depends on recognition of characteristic alterations in the normal mediastinal landmarks. Table 17-1 reviews the typical radiographic findings associated with lymph node enlargement in various lymph node stations. Characteristic radiographic appearances of lymphadenopathy correlate with CT images (Figs. 17-10 to 17-16).

Multiple mediastinal contour abnormalities corresponding to known anatomic lymph node sites suggest the diagnosis of diffuse lymphadenopathy. CT usually shows multiple, discrete masses located in known lymph node sites, such as the azygous, subcarinal, and aortopulmonary window regions. CT is helpful for detecting

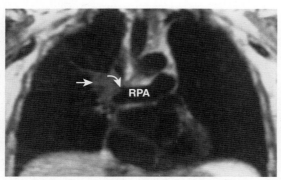

FIGURE 17-9. Mediastinal fibrosis caused by histoplasmosis. Coronal, T1-weighted MRI (same patient as in Fig. 17-7) shows a nodal mass *(straight arrow)* that is characterized by relatively low signal intensity. The truncus anterior *(curved arrow)* is obstructed just distal to its origin from the right pulmonary artery (RPA). The nodal mass also was seen as low signal intensity on T2-weighted images, a characteristic feature of mediastinal fibrosis.

Box 17-3. Diffuse Neoplastic Mediastinal Lymphadenopathy

Lymphoma (especially Hodgkin's lymphoma)

Bronchogenic carcinoma (especially small cell carcinoma)

Extrathoracic primary neoplasm (especially poorly differentiated neoplasms; neoplasms of the head and neck, genitourinary tract, and breast; and melanoma)

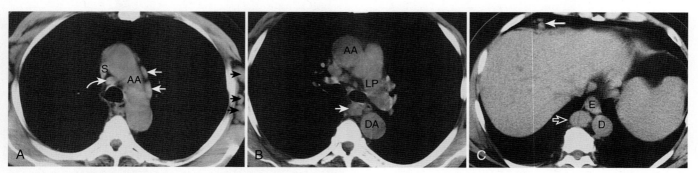

FIGURE 17-10. Diffuse lymphadenopathy caused by lymphoma. **A,** Axial, noncontrast CT of the chest at the level of the aortic arch (AA) shows prevascular *(white arrows),* pretracheal *(curved arrow),* and left axillary *(black arrows)* lymphadenopathy. S, superior vena cava. **B,** Axial CT of the chest at the level of the left pulmonary artery (LP) reveals an enlarged, posterior mediastinal lymph node *(arrow).* DA, descending aorta. **C,** Axial CT at the level of the diaphragm shows additional lymph nodes anterior to the liver *(arrow)* and in the para-aortic region *(open arrow).* D, descending aorta; E, esophagus.

TABLE 17-1 Mediastinal Lymphadenopathy: Radiographic Findings

Lymph Node Station	Radiographic Findings
ANTERIOR MEDIASTINAL	
Internal mammary	Lobulated upper retrosternal opacity on lateral CXR; parasternal mass on the posteroanterior CXR (see Fig. 17-11)
Prevascular	
Left prevascular	Partial or complete obscuration of the aortic knob (see Fig. 17-12)
Right prevascular	Usually not demonstrated on the CXR
Aorticopulmonary window	Convex bulge at junction of the descending aorta and left pulmonary artery (see Fig. 17-13)
MIDDLE MEDIASTINAL	
Paratracheal	
Right paratracheal	Thickened right paratracheal stripe (>3 mm) (see Fig.17-15)
Left paratracheal	Usually not demonstrated on the CXR
Azygous	Enlarged azygous diameter (>10 mm) (see Fig. 17-12)
Subcranial	Lateral convex bulge in the azygoesophageal interface; widened subcranial angle (see Fig. 17-15)
POSTERIOR MEDIASTINAL	
Paraesophageal	Usually not demonstrated on the CXR
Para-aortic	Usually not demonstrated on the CXR
Paravertebral	Lateral displacement of the paraspinal lines (see Fig. 15-2 in Chapter 15)

CXR, chest radiograph.

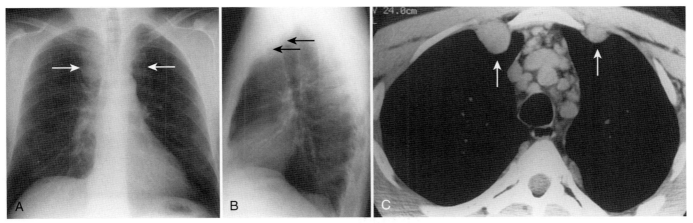

FIGURE 17-11. Internal mammary lymph node enlargement caused by lymphoma. **A,** The frontal radiograph of the chest reveals a large, right parasternal mass and a subtle, left parasternal mass *(arrows)*. Internal mammary nodes must be considerably enlarged before they are detectable on frontal radiographs. **B,** The lateral chest radiograph shows lobulated, upper retrosternal opacities *(arrows)*. Internal mammary node enlargement is usually easier to detect on the lateral projection. **C,** Axial, noncontrast CT at the level of the great vessels reveals bilateral, lobulated, soft tissue masses *(arrows)*, representing enlarged internal mammary lymph nodes. They are most commonly enlarged in patients with lymphoma and metastatic breast cancer. Notice the presence of extensive lymphadenopathy in the prevascular, paratracheal, and paravertebral regions.

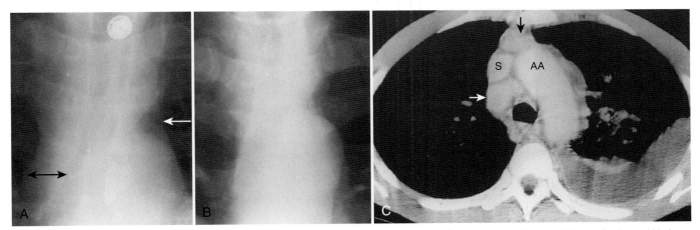

FIGURE 17-12. Diffuse mediastinal lymphadenopathy caused by metastatic carcinoma. **A** and **B,** Coned-down image of the mediastinum (A) shows widening of the left supra-aortic mediastinal contour *(white arrow)* and indistinctness of the superior aspect of the aortic arch, corresponding to the presence of enlarged, left, prevascular lymph nodes. **B,** These abnormalities are more apparent compared with a normal radiograph of the same patient obtained several years earlier. Notice the widening of the right paratracheal stripe and enlargement of the azygous contour in **A** *(black arrows)*. **C,** Contrast-enhanced axial CT at the level of the aortic arch (AA) shows enlarged, enhancing lymph nodes in the azygous *(white arrow)* and right prevascular *(black arrow)* regions. Enlarged, right, prevascular lymph nodes are not usually apparent on chest radiographs. S, superior vena cava.

enlarged lymph nodes and for further characterizing them (Fig. 17-16).

Mediastinal Hemorrhage

Mediastinal hemorrhage has a variety of causes, including traumatic, iatrogenic, and spontaneous events (Box 17-4). It often results form abnormalities of the thoracic aorta, including traumatic aortic transection and rupture of a tho-

racic aortic aneurysm. However, mediastinal hemorrhage may also result from abnormalities of other vascular structures in the thorax, including veins and arteries, or from trauma to the cervical and thoracic spine. Spontaneous mediastinal hemorrhage is an uncommon complication of coagulopathies. The most common chest radiographic finding of hemorrhage is diffuse mediastinal widening (Fig. 17-17). Mediastinal hemorrhage due to traumatic transection of the aorta is discussed in Chapter 6.

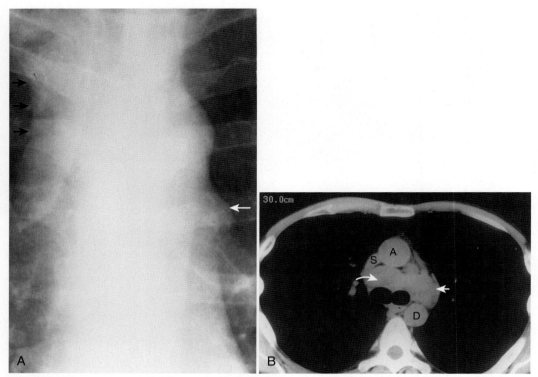

FIGURE 17-13. Diffuse mediastinal lymphadenopathy caused by metastatic carcinoma. **A,** Coned-down image of the mediastinum shows a convex bulge *(white arrow)* at the junction between the descending aorta and left pulmonary artery (i.e., aortic-pulmonary window). Notice the presence of thickening of the right paratracheal stripe *(black arrows)* and enlargement of the azygous contour. **B,** Axial, noncontrast CT at the level of the origin of the right and left mainstem bronchi reveals a large nodal mass *(straight arrow)* in the aorticopulmonary region. Also note the presence of an enlarged lymph node in the anterior subcarinal region *(curved arrow)*, located posterior to the superior vena cava (S) and ascending aorta (A). D, descending aorta.

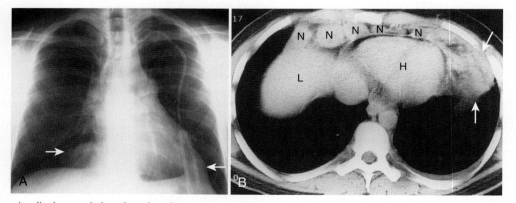

FIGURE 17-14. Anterior diaphragmatic lymph node enlargement caused by recurrent Hodgkin's lymphoma. **A,** The frontal chest radiograph reveals bilateral cardiophrenic angle masses *(arrows)*. **B,** Axial, contrast-enhanced CT at the level of the diaphragm shows multiple, discrete, enlarged lymph nodes (N) and a large nodal mass *(arrows)* along the superior surface of the diaphragm anterior to the heart (H) and liver (L). The most medial nodes are referred to as pericardiac lymph nodes. Anterior diaphragmatic lymph nodes are most frequently involved by lymphoma, and this is a frequent site of recurrence in patients with Hodgkin's disease.

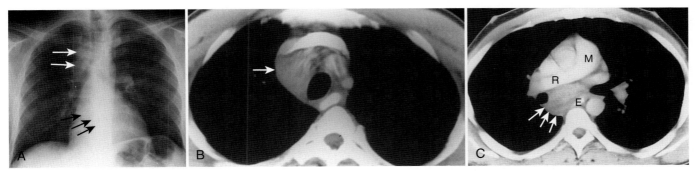

FIGURE 17-15. Diffuse mediastinal lymphadenopathy caused by lymphoma. **A,** The frontal chest radiograph shows widening of the right paratracheal stripe *(white arrows),* corresponding to the presence of enlarged right paratracheal lymph nodes. The abnormal lateral, convex bulge in the azygoesophageal interface *(black arrows)* corresponds to enlarged subcarinal lymph nodes. **B,** Contrast-enhanced CT at the level of the great vessels reveals an enlarged, right paratracheal lymph node *(arrow).* **C,** CT at the level of the main pulmonary artery (M) shows a large nodal mass in the subcarinal region *(arrows),* accounting for the laterally displaced azygoesophageal interface seen on the chest radiograph. E, esophagus; R, right pulmonary artery.

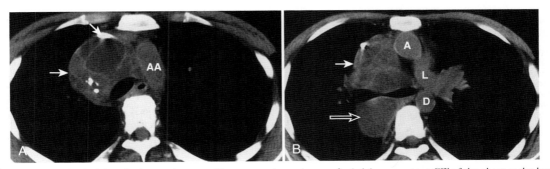

FIGURE 17-16. Diffuse mediastinal lymphadenopathy caused by metastatic seminoma. **A,** Axial, noncontrast CT of the chest at the level of the aortic arch (AA) shows a large, heterogeneous, right paratracheal mass *(right arrow),* which has central foci of low attenuation, which are consistent with necrosis, and several dense foci of calcification. A central venous catheter *(upper arrow)* is identified within the anteriorly displaced superior vena cava. **B,** Axial, noncontrast CT of the chest at the level of the left pulmonary artery (L) shows the inferior extent of the right paratracheal mass *(arrow)* and an additional low-attenuation lymph node mass *(open arrow)* posteriorly. Low-attenuation lymph nodes are a characteristic feature of metastatic seminoma. A, ascending aorta; D, descending aorta.

Box 17-4. **Causes of Mediastinal Hemorrhage**

TRAUMA
Aortic transection
Laceration of branch vessels of the aorta and thoracic
venous structures
Fracture of cervical or thoracic vertebral bodies

IATROGENIC CAUSES
Transection of subclavian artery or vein during central
venous catheter placement

Transection of adjacent vascular structures during sternal
marrow aspiration, pericardiocentesis, arteriography,
and cervical or thoracic surgical procedures

VASCULAR ABNORMALITIES
Aortic or aneurysmal rupture

SPONTANEOUS
Coagulopathy (rare)

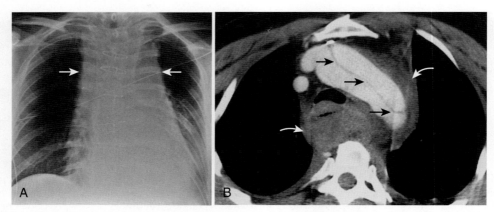

FIGURE 17-17. Mediastinal hemorrhage caused by aortic rupture. **A,** The frontal chest radiograph reveals diffuse widening of the mediastinum *(arrows)* and a left pleural effusion in a patient who underwent median sternotomy and aortic valve replacement. **B,** Axial, contrast-enhanced CT of the chest at the level of the aortic arch. The intimal flap within the aortic arch *(black arrows)* is consistent with aortic dissection. There is extensive, high-attenuation fluid throughout the mediastinum *(curved arrows)*, which is consistent with diffuse mediastinal hemorrhage.

■ SUGGESTED READINGS

Franquet, T., Mediastinitis. In: Müller, N.L., Silva, C.I. (eds.), 2008. Imaging of the chest. Philadelphia, Saunders pp. 1457–1472.

Fraser, R.S., Coleman, N., Müller, N.L., Paré, P.D., 1999. Fraser and Paré's Diagnosis of Diseases of the Chest, fourth ed. WB Saunders, Philadelphia.

Gavant, M.L., Menke, P.G., Fabian, T., et al., 1995. Blunt traumatic aortic rupture: detection with helical CT of the chest. Radiology 197, 125–133.

Halpert, R.D., Goodman, P., 1993. Gastrointestinal Radiology: The Requisites. Mosby–Year Book, St. Louis.

Heitzman, E.R., 1988. The Mediastinum: Radiologic Correlations with Anatomy and Pathology, second ed. Springer-Verlag, Berlin.

Libshitz, H.I., 1992. Intrathoracic lymph nodes. In: Freundlich, I.M., Bragg, D.G. (Eds.), A Radiologic Approach to Diseases of the Chest. Williams & Wilkins, Baltimore, pp. 100–114.

Martinez, S., McAdams, H.P., Erasmus, J.J., Mediastinum. In: Haaga, J.R., Dogra, V.S., Forsting, M., Gilkeson, R.C., Ha, H.K.,Sundaram, M. (eds.), 2009: CT and MRI of the whole body. 5th ed. Philadelphia, Mosby, pp. 969–1036.

Naidich, D.P., Webb, W.R., Müller, N.L., et al., 1999. Computed Tomography and Magnetic Resonance of the Thorax, third ed. Raven Press, New York.

Parker, M.S., Matheson, T.L., Rao, A.V., et al., 2001. Making the transition: the role of helical CT in the evaluation of potentially acute thoracic aortic injuries. AJR Am. J. Roentgenol. 176, 1267–1272.

Reed, J.C., 2003. Chest Radiology: Plain Film Patterns and Differential Diagnoses, fifth ed. Mosby–Year Book, St. Louis.

Rholl, K.S., Levitt, R.G., Glazer, H.S., 1985. Magnetic resonance imaging of fibrosing mediastinitis. AJR Am. J. Roentgenol. 145, 255–259.

Richardson, P., Mirvis, S.E., Scorpio, R., et al., 1991. Value of CT in determining the need for angiography when findings of mediastinal hemorrhage on chest radiographs are equivocal. AJR Am. J. Roentgenol. 156, 273–279.

Rivas, L.A., Fishman, J.E., Munera, F., Bajayo, D.E., 2003. Multislice CT in thoracic trauma. Radiol. Clin. North Am. 41, 599–616.

Shaffer, K., Pugatch, R.D., 1992. Diseases of the mediastinum. In: Freundlich, I.M., Bragg, D.G. (Eds.), A Radiologic Approach to Diseases of the Chest. Williams & Wilkins, Baltimore, pp. 171–185.

Webb, W.R., 1994. Diseases of the mediastinum. In: Putman, C.E., Ravin, C.E. (Eds.), Textbook of Diagnostic Imaging, second ed. WB Saunders, Philadelphia, pp. 428–447.

Woodring, J.H., Loh, F.K., Kryscio, R.J., 1984. Mediastinal hemorrhage: an evaluation of radiographic manifestations. Radiology 151, 15–21.

CHAPTER *18*

The Pleura

Theresa C. McLoud and Phillip M. Boiselle

Several imaging modalities are used to observe the pleural space. The most important is chest radiography, which remains the initial examination in the assessment of pleural disease. Other imaging techniques that may be used include computed tomography (CT) and ultrasound. Magnetic resonance imaging (MRI) plays a limited role in the assessment of pleural abnormalities. Positron emission tomography (PET) and integrated PET/CT scanning are increasingly used in the assessment of pleural malignancy.

ANATOMY AND PHYSIOLOGY OF THE PLEURAL SPACE

The pleura consists of a visceral and parietal layer that is composed of a continuous surface epithelium of mesothelial cells and underlying connective tissue. The visceral pleura covers the lungs and interlobar fissures, whereas the parietal pleura lines the ribs, diaphragm, and mediastinum. A double fold of pleura extends from the hilum to the diaphragm to form the inferior pulmonary ligament. There is no communication between the two pleural cavities. The pleural space is a potential space that contains 2 to 10 mL of pleural fluid in the normal individual. The pleura can produce up to 100 mL of fluid in an hour, and the absorption capacity of the pleural surface is approximately 300 mL per hour.

The parietal pleura is supplied by systemic capillary vessels and drains into the right atrium by way of the azygos, hemiazygos, and internal mammary veins. The visceral pleura is supplied by pulmonary arterioles and capillaries and drains mainly into the pulmonary veins. Fluid is usually produced at the level of the parietal pleura and is drained by the visceral pleura. Lymphatics also play a role in the clearance of pleural fluid in health and disease. Lymphatic drainage occurs through the parietal pleural lymphatics and ultimately reaches the thoracic duct. The lymphatic drainage of the pleural space begins within lymphatic stomas located mainly in the mediastinal, intercostal, and diaphragmatic portions of the parietal pleura. They eventually drain into larger lymphatic channels. The visceral subpleural space is in continuity with the interlobular septa of the pulmonary interstitium. Unlike the parietal pleura, there is no communication between lymphatic channels of the visceral pleura and the pleural space. Lymph from the visceral pleura flows centripetally toward the hila.

The main manifestations of disease in the pleura include pleural effusion, pleural thickening (which may or may not be calcified), pleural air (i.e., pneumothorax), and pleural neoplasms. Primary disease of the pleura is rare. Most pleural abnormalities result from disease processes in other organs.

PLEURAL EFFUSIONS

General Considerations and Clinical Features

Pleural effusions occur when the rates of entry and exit for pleural liquid and protein are no longer in equilibrium. Increased pleural fluid may result from one of six mechanisms (Box 18-1):

1. Increase in hydrostatic pressure in the microvascular circulation, for example, in congestive heart failure (CHF)
2. Decrease in osmotic pressure in the microvascular circulation, as seen in patients with hypoalbuminemia and cirrhosis
3. Decrease in pressure in the pleural space, as occurs in atelectasis
4. Increased permeability of the microvascular circulation, as seen in inflammatory and neoplastic processes in the pleura
5. Impaired lymphatic drainage from the pleural space due to blockage of the lymphatic system by tumor or fibrosis
6. Transport of fluid from the peritoneal space by way of diaphragmatic lymphatic vessels or through diaphragmatic defects, as may occur in patients with ascites

Pleural effusions may be transudates or exudates (Box 18-2). Transudates are usually caused by increased capillary hydrostatic pressure or decreased osmotic pressure, as in CHF, hypoalbuminemia, hepatic cirrhosis, and nephrotic syndrome. Management of transudates usually consists of treatment of the underlying cause, such as CHF. Exudates result from inflammatory and neoplastic processes involving the pleura. Other examples include pulmonary infarction and collagen vascular diseases.

The presence of an exudate requires a clinical investigation to determine the cause of the pleural effusion. Exudates are characterized by the following criteria: a pleural fluid protein concentration divided by the serum protein concentration that is greater than 0.5; a pleural fluid lactate dehydrogenase (LDH) level divided by the serum LDH level that is greater than 0.6; or a pleural fluid LDH level greater than two thirds of the upper limit of normal for the serum LDH level.

An exudative effusion with frank pus is referred to as an *empyema*. Hemothoraces may arise from traumatic laceration of vessels adjacent to the pleura. A pleural fluid hematocrit greater than 50% of the peripheral blood hematocrit establishes the diagnosis. Hemorrhagic effusions may also occur with neoplasms, tuberculosis, and infarction. Rupture or obstruction of major lymphatic channels, such as the thoracic duct, may result in a chylothorax, suggested by the presence of elevated triglyceride and cholesterol levels in the pleural fluid. Pleural effusions may also contain a high proportion of eosinophils. Causes include

379

Box 18-1. **Physiologic Mechanisms in the Development of Pleural Effusions**

Increase in hydrostatic pressure in microvascular circulation (congestive heart failure)
Decrease in osmotic pressure in microvascular circulation
    Hypoalbuminemia
    Cirrhosis
Decrease in pleural pressure
    Atelectasis
Increase in permeability of microvascular circulation
    Inflammatory conditions
    Neoplasms
Impaired lymphatic drainage
    Tumor
    Fibrosis
Transport of fluid from abdomen
    Ascites

Box 18-2. **Types of Effusions**

Transudates
Exudates
    Empyema
    Hemothorax
    Chylothorax

drug hypersensitivity, pneumonia, and pulmonary infarction. Intra-abdominal abnormalities may lead to pleural effusions such as ascites, benign ovarian fibroma (i.e., Meigs' syndrome), hydronephrosis, and pancreatitis.

Predominantly left-sided effusions may be caused by pancreatitis, distal thoracic duct obstruction, Dressler's syndrome, and postpericardiotomy syndrome. Predominantly right-sided effusions occur in proximal thoracic duct obstruction and ascites related to hepatic or ovarian disease and in endometriosis.

The leading causes of pleural effusion in the United States are CHF, pneumonia, malignancy, pulmonary embolism, viral infection, coronary artery bypass surgery, and cirrhosis. CHF and pneumonia account for more episodes of pleural effusion than the remaining five entities combined.

Radiologic Features

Standard Radiography

On an upright chest radiograph, a free pleural effusion demonstrates a meniscus sign, which is a concave, upward-sloping interface with the lung that causes sharp or indistinct blunting of the costophrenic angle (Figs. 18-1 and 18-2). Approximately 200 mL of fluid usually is necessary to blunt the lateral costophrenic angle, although smaller amounts (>75 mL) can

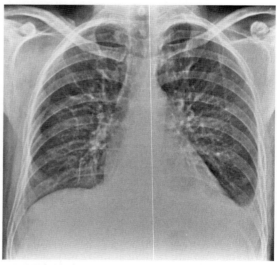

FIGURE 18-1. The frontal view shows a small pleural effusion on the left that causes blunting of the left costophrenic sulcus, producing a meniscus.

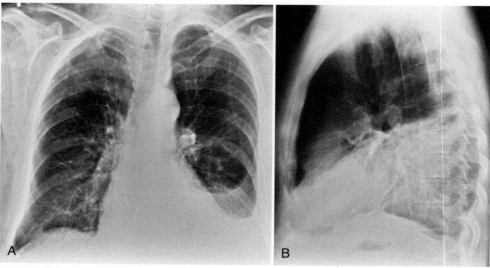

FIGURE 18-2. **A,** The frontal view shows a meniscus in the left costophrenic angle. The effusion extends upward along the left lateral chest wall. **B,** On the lateral view, the fluid extends anteriorly but reaches a higher level posteriorly than anteriorly.

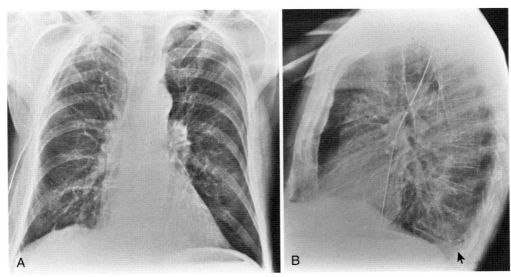

FIGURE 18-3. A small pleural effusion is seen only on the lateral view. **A,** On the frontal posteroanterior radiograph, the costophrenic angle on the right is sharp. **B,** The lateral view shows minimal blunting of the right costophrenic angle *(arrow)*.

produce a meniscus that blunts the posterior costophrenic angle on the lateral view (Fig. 18-3). A lateral decubitus view of the chest is much more sensitive than the upright view in the detection of pleural effusion, and as little as 5 mL of fluid can be demonstrated on decubitus views (Fig. 18-4).

In the upright position in the normal individual, a small amount of pleural fluid accumulates in a subpulmonic position. In certain individuals, a large amount of free-flowing pleural fluid may accumulate in this position before spilling into the costophrenic angles. On the frontal view, this produces a characteristic appearance with elevation of the apparent ipsilateral hemidiaphragm, flattening of the medial aspect, and displacement of the peak of the apparent diaphragm laterally. On the left side, this is easy to recognize because of separation of the stomach bubble from the apparent left hemidiaphragm (Fig. 18-5). A massive effusion produces a complete or nearly complete opacification of a hemithorax, with displacement of the mediastinum to

the opposite side (Fig. 18-6). This appearance contrasts with complete atelectasis of the lung, in which the shift of the mediastinum is toward the side of the opaque hemithorax. Moderate to large amounts of pleural effusion may be missed on supine radiographs. These effusions layer posteriorly and produce a generalized increase in opacity of the hemithorax, through which the pulmonary vessels can be visualized (Fig. 18-7). There may be blunting of the costophrenic angle, and the fluid occasionally tracks over the apex of the lung, producing an apical cap.

Fluid may occasionally accumulate within fissures, and these accumulations may produce the appearance of a mass or pseudotumor (Fig. 18-8). Differentiation from a mass can be easily made because the fluid is free and shifts on decubitus views.

Pleural effusions frequently loculate (Fig. 18-9); i.e., they do not shift freely in the pleural space because of adhesions between the visceral and parietal pleura. Loculation of

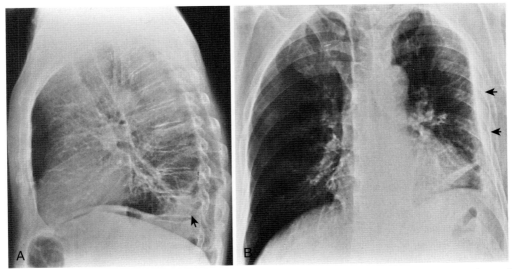

FIGURE 18-4. **A,** The lateral view shows blunting of the costophrenic angle posteriorly *(arrow)*. **B,** Left-side-down decubitus radiograph shows fluid layering along the left lateral chest wall *(arrows)*.

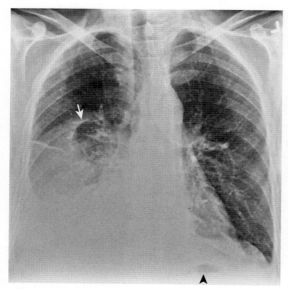

FIGURE 18-5. Subpulmonic effusion. On the left, there is separation of the apparent hemidiaphragm from the stomach bubble *(black arrow)*. There is also minimal blunting of the lateral costophrenic angle. On the right, a large effusion extends to the major fissure, subtending a lucent area that represents the superior segment of the right lower lobe *(white arrow)*.

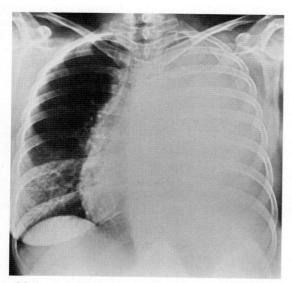

FIGURE 18-6. Massive effusion. There is a mediastinal shift to the opposite side and a completely opaque left hemithorax.

fluid occurs in exudative effusions, particularly in patients with empyema or hemothorax.

Ultrasound

Ultrasound may be used to detect pleural abnormalities and to differentiate solid pleural masses from pleural effusions. However, ultrasound is most frequently used for severely ill patients and for patients in the intensive care unit because of the ready availability for bedside imaging. Ultrasound is useful for detecting the presence of pleural fluid and as a guide to aspiration.

Pleural fluid collections may be anechoic or echoic, and they may change shape during respiration. Most collections are anechoic (Fig. 18-10) and are delineated by an echogenic

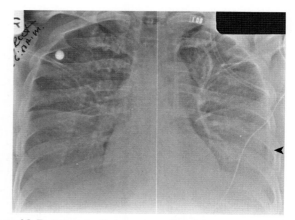

FIGURE 18-7. Bilateral effusions are seen with the patient in the supine position. Hazy opacification in both hemithoraces is caused by fluid layering posteriorly in the pleural spaces. The pulmonary vessels can be visualized through the fluid. Fluid is present laterally on the left *(arrow)* and in the minor fissure.

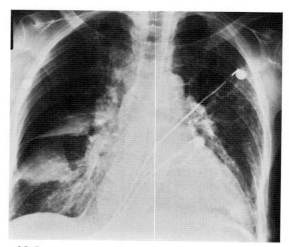

FIGURE 18-8. Pseudotumor. Fluid is seen in the upper and lower portions of the major fissure on the right, and it extends into the minor fissure. Fluid in the fissure may have a tapered or spindle-shaped configuration, as demonstrated in the more cephalad collection.

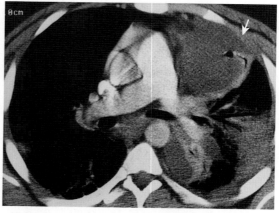

FIGURE 18-9. Loculated effusion. CT shows a large collection of pleural fluid in an anterior, nondependent location *(arrow)*. A lenticular collection of fluid lateral to the spine displaces the enhancing lung parenchyma of the left lower lobe.

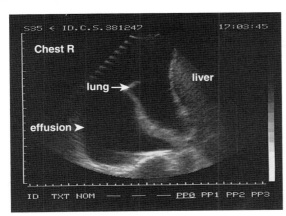

FIGURE 18-10. Anechoic pleural fluid collection. The sonogram shows a collapsed right lower lobe surrounded by a large pleural effusion. (From McLoud TC, Flower CD: Imaging of the pleura: sonography, CT and MR imaging. AJR Am J Roentgenol 156:1145-1153, 1991.)

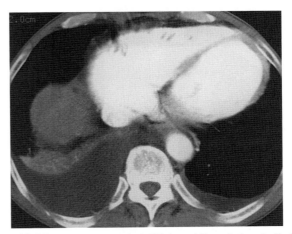

FIGURE 18-12. Contrast-enhanced CT shows bilateral pleural effusions; the right is greater than the left. Both have low attenuation and form sickle-shaped opacities posteriorly.

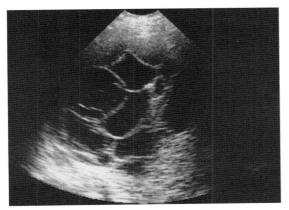

FIGURE 18-11. Empyema with multiple loculations. The transonic space is divided into multiple secondary loculations by curvilinear septa. (From McLoud TC, Flower CD: Imaging of the pleura: sonography, CT and MR imaging. AJR Am J Roentgenol 156:1145-1153, 1991.)

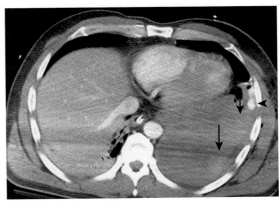

FIGURE 18-13. Hemothorax after a stab wound to left chest wall. Many areas of increased attenuation can be seen in the fluid collection *(arrow)*. Notice the area of active extravasation of contrast *(arrowhead)* due to injury to left intercostal vessel. (Case courtesy of Justin Kung, MD, Beth Israel Deaconess Medical Center, Boston, MA.)

line of visceral pleura and lung. Anechoic effusions are usually transudates, whereas effusions that contain septations represent exudates in approximately 80% of cases (Fig. 18-11).

Computed Tomography

Free-flowing pleural fluid produces a sickle-shaped opacity in the most dependent part of the thorax posteriorly on CT scanning (Fig. 18-12). CT allows very small amounts of pleural fluid to be detected. Loculated fluid collections are seen as lenticular opacities in fixed positions (see Fig. 18-9). CT is of limited value in differentiating transudates from exudates or in the diagnosis of chylous pleural effusions. Although most chylous effusions are indistinguishable from other causes of pleural effusion on CT, low attenuation consistent with fat or a fat-fluid level in the pleural collection is rarely seen. Acute pleural hemorrhage, however, can be identified by the presence of a fluid-fluid level or by increased attenuation of the pleural fluid collection (Fig. 18-13).

Pleural fluid can be distinguished from ascites by several CT features (Box 18-3), including the displaced crus sign, the interface sign, the diaphragm sign, and the bare area sign. If the diaphragmatic crus is displaced away from the spine by an abnormal fluid collection, the fluid is located in the pleural

Box 18-3. Computed Tomography: Pleural Fluid versus Ascites	
Pleural Fluid	**Ascites**
Displaced crus	
Ill-defined interface with liver and spleen	Sharp interface with liver or spleen
Fluid outside diaphragm contour	Fluid inside diaphragm contour
	Fluid excluded from bare area of liver

space (Fig. 18-14). The location of ascites is lateral and anterior to the crus. The interface sign describes a sharp interface that can be identified between fluid and the liver or spleen when ascites is present. In cases of ascites, the interface is sharp, whereas in cases of pleural effusion, the interface is ill defined (Fig. 18-15). If the diaphragm is identifiable adjacent to an abnormal fluid collection in the right upper quadrant, the diaphragm sign is probably the most reliable means of dif-

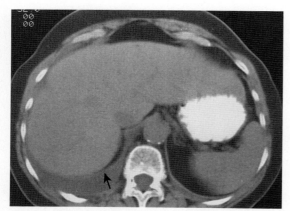

FIGURE 18-14. Displaced crus sign. The pleural fluid lies inside the crus of the diaphragm *(arrow)* and displaces it away from the spine. (From McLoud TC, Flower CD: Imaging of the pleura: sonography, CT and MR imaging. AJR Am J Roentgenol 156:1145-1153, 1991.)

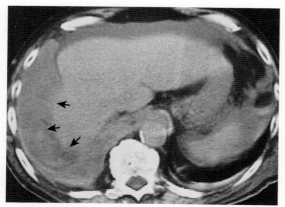

FIGURE 18-15. Interface sign. A hazy, indistinct interface is seen between the pleural effusion and liver laterally *(arrows)*, and ascites can be seen anteriorly. (From McLoud TC, Flower CD: Imaging of the pleura: sonography, CT and MR imaging. AJR Am J Roentgenol 156:1145-1153, 1991.)

ferentiating fluid from ascites (Fig. 18-16). The location of the diaphragm is readily visible in patients with ascites but may not be identified in patients with pleural effusions. Pleural effusion is visualized outside the hemidiaphragm, whereas ascites is seen within the hemidiaphragmatic contour. The

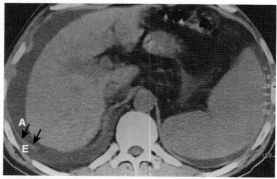

FIGURE 18-16. Diaphragm sign. Ascites (A) lies inside the diaphragm (arrows) and produces a sharp interface with the liver. The pleural effusion (E) is visualized outside the diaphragm. (From McLoud TC, Flower CD: Imaging of the pleura: sonography, CT and MR imaging. AJR Am J Roentgenol 156:1145-1153, 1991.)

bare area is the portion of the right lobe of the liver that lacks peritoneal covering. Restriction of peritoneal fluid by the coronary ligaments from that area is another useful distinguishing sign. To differentiate pleural effusions from intra-abdominal fluid collections, all four signs should be assessed in each case. The attempt to differentiate ascites from pleural effusion may have pitfalls. A large pleural effusion, particularly on the left side, may cause inversion of the diaphragm, resulting in the pleural fluid being located centrally rather than peripherally.

CT is helpful in the assessment and management of loculated pleural effusions (see Fig. 18-9). Accurate localization of loculated collections is useful before drainage. Loculated effusions have a lenticular configuration with smooth margins, and they displace the adjacent parenchyma. This typical appearance for any pleural process is a distinguishing feature that can help differentiate a pleural from parenchymal process.

Magnetic Resonance Imaging

The role of MRI in the evaluation of the pleura is somewhat limited. MRI does provide certain advantages because of its ability to image the thorax directly in the axial, sagittal, and coronal planes. MRI may be slightly superior to CT in the characterization of pleural fluid (Fig. 18-17). Typically, fluid collections in the pleural cavity have a low signal intensity

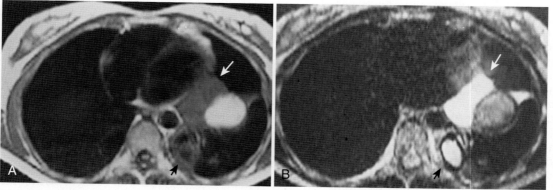

FIGURE 18-17. T1-weighted (**A**) and T2-weighted (**B**) MRI of a complex pleural effusion. The pleural fluid *(white arrows)* abuts the heart. The water content has low signal intensity on T1-weighted images and bright signal intensity on T2-weighted images. There is also a subacute hematoma *(black arrows)*, which on the T2-weighted image has bright internal signal characteristics and a dark concentric ring due to the hemosiderin content. The high signal intensity collection in the major fissure on the T1-weighted image represents fat (i.e., chylous effusion). There is T2 shortening, similar to that of subcutaneous fat. (From McLoud TC, Flower CD: Imaging of the pleura: sonography, CT and MR imaging. AJR Am J Roentgenol 156:1145-1153, 1991.)

on T1-weighted images and relatively high signal intensity on T2-weighted images because of the water content. It may be possible to differentiate transudates, simple exudates, and exudates with the use of a triple-echo pulse sequence. Complex exudates have greater signal intensity than simple exudates, which are brighter than transudates. Preliminary results also suggest chylothorax may have distinctive findings on MRI, with signal intensity characteristics similar to those of subcutaneous fat. Subacute or chronic hematomas demonstrate typical signal intensity on MRI with a concentric ring sign, consisting of an outer dark rim composed of hemosiderin and bright signal intensity in the center because of the T1 shortening effects of methemoglobin.

Positron Emission Tomography

PET and integrated PET/CT are playing an increasing role in the assessment of pleural malignancy, particularly in evaluating patients with non–small cell lung cancer (NSCLC) with suspected metastatic pleural effusions. For the diagnosis of pleural malignancy in patients with NSCLC, PET has reported sensitivities ranging from 92% to 100% and specificities of 67% to 94%. False-positive results may result from pleural infection or pleural inflammation after talc pleurodesis. Because integrated PET/CT scanners can accurately localize areas of increased FDG uptake to dense talc deposits in the pleura, this potential pitfall can be avoided by careful correlation between the CT and PET images.

A negative PET scan result can be useful for confirming the absence of pleural metastatic disease, particularly when the result of thoracentesis is also negative. However, false-negative PET studies may occur in the setting of small-volume pleural effusions.

■ EMPYEMA

Clinical Features

An empyema is an exudative effusion with pus in the pleural cavity. Several criteria are used for the diagnosis of empyema (Box 18-4): grossly purulent fluid; organisms identified on the basis of Gram stain or culture; a white blood cell count in the pleural fluid greater than 5×10^9 cells/L, and a pH below 7 or glucose level less than 40 mg/mL. The natural progression of an empyema consists of several phases: from an exudative to a fibropurulent phase to an organizing phase that results in the development of a thickened pleura, or *fibrin peel*. Early diagnosis and treatment is therefore imperative.

Most empyemas are the result of acute bacterial pneumonias or abscesses, but they may occur after thoracic surgery, as a result of trauma, or occasionally, from hematogenous dissemination from extrapulmonary sites or direct

---

Box 18-4. Fluid Characteristics of Empyema

Grossly purulent
Organisms identified by stain or culture
White blood cell count > 5×10^9 cells/L
pH < 7.0
Glucose level < 40 mg/mL

Box 18-5. Radiologic Features of Empyema

STANDARD RADIOGRAPHY
Loculation
Air-fluid level (bronchopleural fistula) varies in length on posteroanterior and lateral radiographs
COMPUTED TOMOGRAPHY
Lenticular shape
Compression of surrounding lung
Split pleura sign

---

spread through the diaphragm from a subphrenic abscess. Empyemas are frequently associated with a communication from the lung (i.e. bronchopleural fistula), which produces air in the pleural space. Empyemas may drain into the chest wall, producing an empyema necessitans.

Radiologic Features

The radiologic features of empyema are described in Box 18-5.

Standard Radiography

Most empyemas manifest as a classic pleural effusion. However, they tend to loculate early and, as a result, may not change with the patient's position, or they may not have a classic meniscus sign. Loculated collections have a lenticular shape that forms obtuse angles with the chest wall. If a bronchopleural fistula is present, an air-fluid level can be identified in the empyema space before thoracentesis (Fig. 18-18). On standard radiographs, the length of the air-fluid level varies on radiographs taken at 90 degrees to each other; there may be a short air-fluid level on the frontal radiograph and a long air-fluid level on the lateral radiograph. This finding contrasts with lung abscesses, in which the length of the air-fluid level is usually equal on both views.

Computed Tomography

CT is particularly helpful in establishing the diagnosis of empyema and in differentiating empyemas from lung abscesses. The most reliable sign is the split pleura sign, which is usually identified during the organizing phase of an empyema (Fig. 18-19). After intravenous administration of a bolus of contrast medium, the parietal and visceral pleura enhance vigorously, most likely due to the increased vascular supply in the inflamed pleura. In an empyema, the parietal and visceral pleura are thickened, and the extrapleural fat between the empyema space and the chest wall may be increased in size, particularly if the empyema is chronic, and attenuation of the fat may also be increased because of surrounding edema.

CT is the best method to differentiate empyemas from lung abscesses. Both may contain air-fluid levels. Characteristic features of empyema include a lenticular shape and compression of the surrounding lung by the empyema space, such that the pulmonary vessels and bronchi are displaced and draped around the pleural fluid collection (Fig. 18-20). Abscesses often have a rounded shape and lack a distinct boundary with the adjacent lung

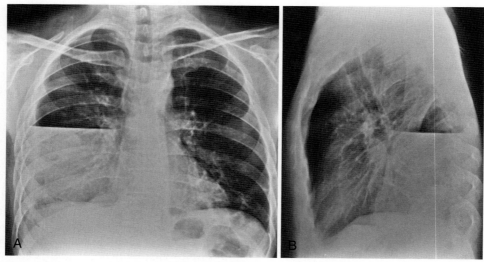

FIGURE 18-18. Empyema with bronchopleural fistula. **A,** The frontal radiograph shows an air-fluid level extending from the lateral chest wall to the mediastinum. **B,** On the lateral view, the air-fluid level is considerably shorter and located posteriorly.

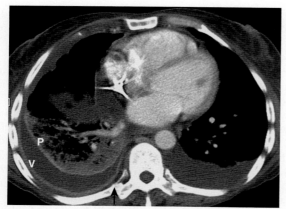

FIGURE 18-19. Split pleura sign. Enhancement and separation of the visceral (v) and parietal (p) pleura can be seen in a right-sided empyema. There is an increase in extrapleural fat *(arrow)*. Compare with the appearance of a simple pleural effusion on the left.

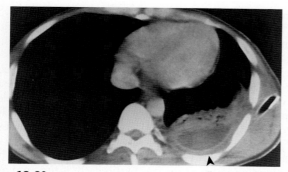

FIGURE 18-20. Empyema with a lenticular fluid collection posteriorly. Adjacent lung is compressed and displaced by the empyema space. There is an increase in extrapleural fat *(arrow)*. (From McLoud TC, Flower CD: Imaging of the pleura: sonography, CT and MR imaging. AJR Am J Roentgenol 156:1145-1153, 1991.)

parenchyma. The bronchi and vessels of the adjacent lung appear to end abruptly at the margins of the abscess. The split pleura sign also can be useful in differentiating empyemas from lung abscesses, although none of these criteria are absolutely reliable.

CT is a useful guide to the treatment and drainage of empyemas, particularly when the empyema contains multiple areas of loculation. Imaging-guided interventional methods for the treatment of empyema are discussed in Chapter 19.

▄ PNEUMOTHORAX

Pneumothorax (Box 18-6) may be defined as the presence of air or gas within the pleural space. A pneumothorax is considered to be under tension if pleural pressure exceeds alveolar pressure. In such situations, the pressure may reach atmospheric levels. Air may be combined with different types of fluid in the pleural space, producing a hydropneumothorax, hemopneumothorax, or pyothorax. Routes of entry of air into the pleural space include the lung and the mediastinum from pneumomediastinum. In the case of penetrating injury, the route may be from outside the chest.

Epidemiology and Etiology

Spontaneous pneumothorax is the most common cause, and it occurs predominantly in apparently healthy men during the third or fourth decade of life. It is associated with the presence of blebs, which are gas pockets within

---

Box 18-6. Causes of Pneumothorax

Spontaneous
    Associated with blebs
Chronic obstructive pulmonary disease
    Second peak in incidence
    Most patients 45 to 65 years old
Chronic infiltrative lung disease
    Langerhans cell histiocytosis
    Lymphangioleiomyomatosis
Metastatic sarcoma
Trauma
Catamenial pneumothorax
Iatrogenic cause
Barotrauma

the elastic fibers of the visceral pleura. This abnormality is localized and not necessarily associated with generalized pulmonary emphysema. Rupture of a bleb produces spontaneous pneumothorax.

In addition to apical blebs, many other causes of pneumothorax are related to underlying lung disease or trauma. Chronic obstructive pulmonary disease, especially chronic bronchitis and emphysema, accounts for a second peak in the incidence of pneumothorax that occurs between the ages of 45 and 65 years. In these conditions, the pneumothorax results from rupture of peripheral emphysematous areas. Recurrent pneumothorax may be associated with chronic infiltrative lung disease of any cause, but the prevalence is particularly high in two diseases: Langerhans cell histiocytosis (i.e., histiocytosis X) and lymphangioleiomyomatosis. However, pneumothorax may be seen as a complication of late stages of other types of infiltrative lung disease that are associated with fibrosis and honeycombing.

Malignant neoplasms, particularly metastatic sarcoma, are occasional causes of spontaneous pneumothorax. The most common tumor type is metastatic osteogenic sarcoma. Pneumothorax may be an occasional complication of septic infarcts and lung abscess. Catamenial pneumothorax is a rare but interesting manifestation of intrathoracic endometriosis.

A more common cause of pneumothorax is open or closed chest trauma. In blunt trauma, pneumothorax may occur without evidence of rib fracture, although rib fractures are commonly identified. In such cases, the lung may be lacerated by a rib fragment. Pneumothorax along with pneumomediastinum may occur in cases of tracheal, bronchial, and esophageal rupture. This is discussed in more detail in Chapter 6. Penetrating thoracic injuries from knife or bullet wounds also can produce pneumothorax. Iatrogenic pneumothorax may be produced as a result of subclavian line placement, liver biopsy, percutaneous needle aspiration biopsy of the lung, and renal biopsies. Pneumothorax is the most common form of barotrauma, occurring in patients maintained on mechanical ventilation and positive end-expiratory pressure. Pneumothorax associated with mechanical ventilation may be antedated by the development of interstitial or mediastinal emphysema. It is frequently bilateral and under tension.

Clinical Features

The clinical features of pneumothorax, particularly the spontaneous variety, are characterized by the development of dyspnea and chest pain, which is aggravated by deep breathing and body movement. Occasionally, asymptomatic pneumothorax is discovered incidentally. Bilateral pneumothorax is rare. In patients with chronic obstructive pulmonary disease, pneumothorax may potentially be lethal and lead to respiratory failure. Pneumothorax should always be suspected as a possible cause of sudden clinical deterioration in a patient with chronic obstructive pulmonary disease.

Radiologic Features

The radiologic findings of pneumothorax vary considerably, depending on the degree of pulmonary collapse, the presence of tension, and other associated conditions (Box 18-7).

Box 18-7. Radiologic Features of Pneumothorax

STANDARD RADIOGRAPHS
Visceral pleural line separated from chest wall by gas space devoid of vessels
Apex when upright
Lung opaque only with complete collapse
Tension
    Mediastinal shift
    Depression of hemidiaphragm
Supine
    Medial recess (juxtacardiac)
    Deep sulcus sign
    Subpulmonic
    Retrocardiac lucent triangle medially
Ancillary Views
Expiratory
Decubitus
Pitfalls
Skinfolds
Clothing
Tubing artifacts
Bullae
COMPUTED TOMOGRAPHY
More sensitive for detection of small pneumothoraces
More accurate for determining size

The basic observation consists of recognizing that the outer margin of the visceral pleura and lung is separated from the parietal pleura and chest wall by a lucent gas space devoid of pulmonary vessels (Fig. 18-21). Typically, the pneumothorax occurs at the lung apex in the upright patient. When a suspected pneumothorax is not definitely seen on an inspiration study, an expiration radiograph may be diagnostic. The constant volume of the pneumothorax gas is accentuated by an overall reduction in the size of the hemithorax on expiration. Similar accentuation of a small pneumothorax can be obtained with a lateral decubitus radiograph with the appropriate side up.

There are some pitfalls in the diagnosis of pneumothorax, including skinfolds, clothing, tubing artifacts, abnormalities of the chest wall, and cavitary and bullous lung disease. A skinfold can be particularly troublesome (Fig. 18-22). The density characteristics of a skinfold are different from those of the visceral pleural tangent. The lung opacity of a skinfold progressively increases until it reaches a maximum at its tangent, and it then abruptly becomes lucent. This is quite different from the uniform lucency of the pneumothorax lung and pleural space interrupted by a thin, visceral pleural line. Large, avascular bullae or thin-walled cysts have concave rather than convex inner margins and do not exactly conform to the normal shape of the costophrenic sulcus when they occur at the lung base (Fig. 18-23).

When lung collapse from pneumothorax is nearly complete, the lung hangs limply from the hilum, and the margins of the separate lobes can often be seen (Fig. 18-24). The collapsed lung is uniformly opaque. This contrasts with the pattern of a small pneumothorax, in which the lung, although partially collapsed, usually does not change

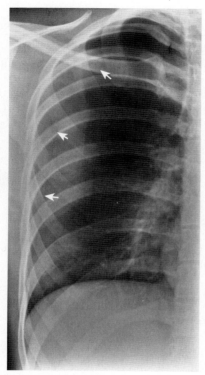

FIGURE 18-21. Pneumothorax in an upright patient. The extremely thin visceral pleural line can be seen extending along the lateral aspect of the lung to the apex *(arrows)*. Exterior to the line is a gas space devoid of vessels.

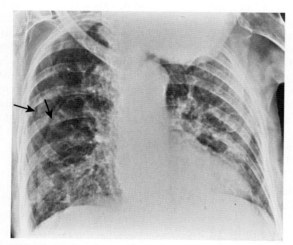

FIGURE 18-22. There are two skinfolds on the right *(arrows)*. Notice the increasing opacification that they produce, with an abrupt transition to lucency laterally. Skinfolds often produce an edge rather than the crisp visceral pleural line produced by a pneumothorax.

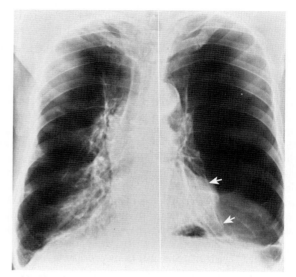

FIGURE 18-23. Large bullae simulating pneumothorax. The left lung is lucent, devoid of vessels, and almost completely replaced by bullae. The bullae have concave margins *(arrows)*, unlike pneumothorax, in which the lung margin is convex and parallels the chest wall.

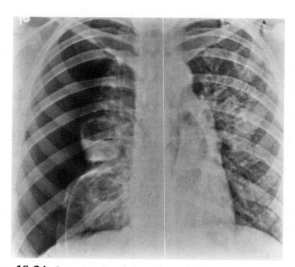

FIGURE 18-24. Large tension pneumothorax. The large pneumothorax on the right is associated with almost complete collapse of the right lung. The margins of the lobes can be seen. There is evidence of tension, with shift of the mediastinum to the left and depression of the right hemidiaphragm.

in density. When a flaplike pleural defect results in a tension pneumothorax, the pleural space becomes expanded. Manifestations of tension pneumothorax include mediastinal shift, diaphragmatic depression, and rib cage expansion at maximum inspiration (see Fig. 18-24). The degree of lung collapse is not a dependable sign for or against tension. Underlying lung disease may prevent total collapse even if tension is present. Little or no mediastinal shift occurs in patients maintained on positive airway pressure, despite the presence of a tension pneumothorax.

In the supine patient, identification of a pneumothorax is more difficult than in the erect patient, because air often accumulates along the long ventral surface of the lung rather than at the apex (Fig. 18-25). The medial pleural recess is a common site for pleural air to accumulate, and air can often be identified along the juxtacardiac area. Anteromedial air in the pleural space may produce a deep anterior costophrenic sulcus, often referred to as the deep sulcus sign, which outlines the medial hemidiaphragm under the heart. Air in this location often produces the appearance of a lucency projected in the right or left upper abdominal quadrants.

Pneumothorax may also accumulate in a subpulmonic location. This produces a sharply outlined hemidiaphragm that is well defined and a deep lateral costophrenic sulcus (see Fig. 18-25). Occasionally, pneumothorax accumulates posteromedially in supine patients and appears as a lucent

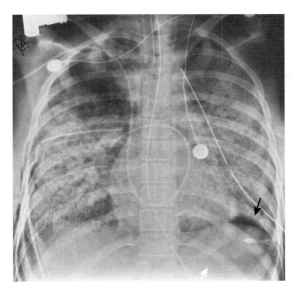

FIGURE 18-25. Pneumothorax in a supine patient. The portable antero-posterior radiograph shows a subpulmonic pneumothorax *(black arrow)* and a lucency projecting in the area of the left upper quadrant in the anterior costophrenic sulcus (i.e., deep sulcus sign) *(white arrow).*

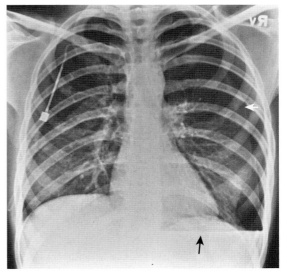

FIGURE 18-26. Hydropneumothorax. The erect frontal view shows an air-fluid level at the base of the left pleural space *(black arrow).* The pneumothorax can also be seen extending along the lateral chest wall and at the apex *(white arrow).*

triangle located medially at the lung base. This appearance was previously attributed to air in the pulmonary ligament. However, CT studies suggest that air at this location is usually posterior to the ligament and instead represents a pneumothorax. Occasionally, pneumothorax air may be identified in the major or minor fissures.

Subtle signs of pneumothorax should be searched for in intubated patients maintained on positive-pressure ventilation. Rapid increase in the size of a pneumothorax may occur with the development of tension and result in respiratory arrest. Heart-lung transplantation, bilateral lung transplantation, and lung volume reduction surgery for emphysema may create a communication between the right and left pleural spaces so that air or fluid can move from one side to the other.

The presence of fluid of any type in the pleural space accompanying a pneumothorax produces an air-fluid level if the radiograph is obtained with the patient in the erect position (Fig. 18-26). In the supine patient, the diagnosis of hydropneumothorax is more difficult. A hydrothorax or hemothorax frequently coexists with a pneumothorax. When the pneumothorax is small and pleural contact is maintained at the lung base, the fluid appears as a meniscus on the erect radiograph. When the pneumothorax is large, a typical air-fluid interface can be identified.

Other imaging studies are rarely used for the evaluation of pneumothorax. A ventilation scan may be helpful in distinguishing bullae from pneumothoraces because bullae will exhibit delayed wash-in and prolonged wash-out of xenon, and a pneumothorax fails to show evidence of ventilation. CT is much more sensitive than plain films in detecting small pneumothoraces, particularly in the supine patient. Unsuspected, small pneumothoraces are frequently detected at the bases of the lungs in patients who have sustained trauma and who undergo abdominal CT.

Accurately estimating the size of a pneumothorax is very difficult. It is not often realized that a pneumothorax that occupies the peripheral inch (2.5cm) of the hemithorax

amounts to about 30% of total lung volume. Percentage estimations usually are inaccurate and most often underestimate the true size of the pneumothorax.

■ FOCAL PLEURAL DISEASE

The most common focal pleural abnormalities include pleural plaques, localized pleural tumors, and local extension of bronchogenic carcinoma.

Pleural Plaques

Pleural plaques are discussed in the chapter dealing with pneumoconiosis (see Chapter 8).

Localized Pleural Tumors

Localized pleural tumors are relatively uncommon. They usually are one of two types: fibrous tumors of the pleura or lipomas. Liposarcomas are rare, but the pleura commonly may be invaded locally by adjacent bronchogenic carcinoma. CT is most commonly used for the assessment of localized pleural tumors because of its ability to determine the tissue composition (i.e., lipoma) and to determine extension into the lungs or chest wall.

Fibrous Tumors of the Pleura
Clinical Features

Fibrous tumors of the pleura (Box 18-8) were previously referred to as *benign fibrous mesotheliomas.* They account for less than 5% of all pleural tumors and have an equal sex incidence. The peak incidence occurs in the sixth to seventh decades. They are not related to asbestos exposure. Approximately 50% of individuals with fibrous tumors of the pleura are asymptomatic. These tumors occasionally reach extremely large sizes and produce symptoms that consist of cough, dyspnea, and chest pain. These tumors have a high incidence of associated hypertrophic osteoarthropathy, and episodic hypoglycemia may be present in 4% to 5% of cases.

Box 18-8. Fibrous Tumors of Pleura

CLINICAL FEATURES
Constitute < 5% of pleural tumors
Equal sex incidence
No symptoms in 50% of patients
Hypertrophic pulmonary osteoarthropathy
Episodic hypoglycemia (4% to 5%)

PATHOLOGIC FEATURES
Location: 80% in visceral pleura, 20% in parietal
   pleura
Encapsulated, pedunculated
60% benign, 40% malignant
Malignant tumors: invade chest wall, recur locally,
   produce pleural effusion

RADIOLOGIC FEATURES
Standard radiographs
   Round or lobulated
   Slow growth
   Variable size
   May be mobile

COMPUTED TOMOGRAPHY
Displace lung parenchyma
Enhancement after contrast
Acute angles with chest wall
Malignant tumors
   Large size
   Chest wall invasion
   Pleural effusion

Pathologic Features

Eighty percent of fibrous tumors of the pleura arise from the visceral pleura and 20% from the parietal pleura. They usually are encapsulated and frequently are pedunculated, with a broad-based pleural attachment. Vascular structures are present in the tumor pedicle. Microscopically, approximately 60% of the localized fibrous tumors of the pleura are benign, and 40% are malignant. They usually have a good prognosis; all benign tumors and 45% of malignant tumors are cured by means of surgical resection. The malignant tumors may invade the chest wall and then recur locally after surgical excision, but they do not metastasize widely. Some of the malignant lesions are associated with pleural effusion. These tumors may reach enormous sizes, and tumors larger than 10 cm in diameter are more likely to be malignant. Calcification is present in a minority of cases.

Radiologic Features

Fibrous tumors of the pleura usually appear as round or lobulated pleural masses of various sizes that show evidence of slow growth (Fig. 18-27). Those that are attached to the visceral pleura by a pedicle may be mobile and can change location over time on serial chest radiography or when the position of the patient is altered.

CT findings are similar to those observed on plain radiography (Fig. 18-28). When these tumors are large, it may be difficult to determine that they arise from the pleura, although they typically displace the lung parenchyma. Enhancement of tumor after contrast administration is a frequent finding. On CT scans, most of the tumors form acute angles with the chest wall. Lesions are frequently heterogeneous due to necrosis and hemorrhage. The malignant pleural fibrous tumors are usually larger than 10 cm in diameter, may invade the chest wall, and can be associated with pleural effusion. Central necrosis is common in the larger tumors. Calcification may be seen in roughly 25% of cases.

On MRI, these lesions often appear heterogeneous. Areas of relatively low signal intensity on T1-weighted and T2-weighted images may be observed because of the high fibrous content (Fig. 18-29).

Lipomas and Liposarcomas

Lipomas may occur in the pleural space or mediastinum. These lesions are asymptomatic and are usually discovered incidentally on chest radiographs. Some are purely intrathoracic, but others may be transmural and involve

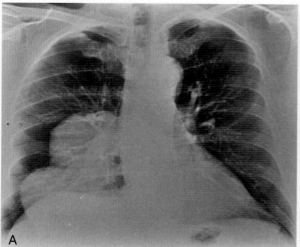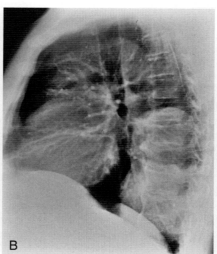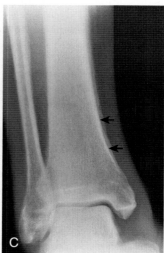

FIGURE 18-27. Fibrous tumor of the pleura. The posteroanterior (**A**) and lateral (**B**) views demonstrate a large, bulky mass medially and posteriorly in the right hemithorax. The origin from the pleura can be suspected, because the mass is longer than it is wide and conforms to the shape of the pleural space. In the right lower leg, there is periosteal reaction (**C**) along the medial surface of the distal, tibia indicating hypertrophic pulmonary osteoarthropathy *(arrows).*

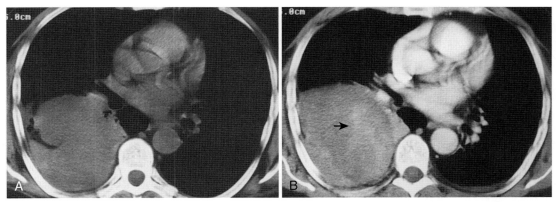

FIGURE 18-28. Fibrous tumor of the pleura. **A,** The precontrast CT scan shows a mass posteriorly of fairly uniform attenuation that makes an acute angle with the lateral chest wall. **B,** After the administration of contrast, focal areas of enhancement can be appreciated *(arrow)*.

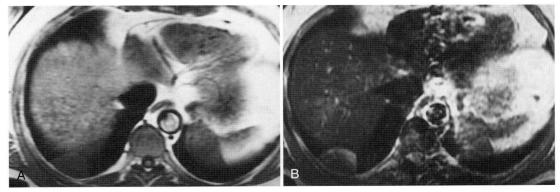

FIGURE 18-29. Fibrous tumor of the pleura. **A,** Spin-echo, T1-weighted MRI shows a mass posteriorly with signal intensity equal to that of muscle. **B,** On the T2-weighted image, most of the mass has low signal intensity with a slightly bright rim.

the chest wall. A definitive diagnosis is usually not possible on standard radiographs. However, CT clearly delineates the pleural origin of these lesions in most cases and their fatty composition (–50 to –150 Hounsfield units [HU]) (Fig. 18-30). Benign lipomas have a completely uniform fatty density, although linear soft tissue strands

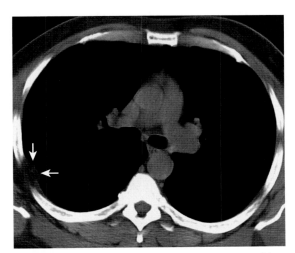

FIGURE 18-30. Lipoma. CT shows an intrapleural tumor of fatty composition (–90 HU).

due to fibrous stroma may be present. When the tumor is heterogeneous and has higher attenuation greater than –50 HU, a liposarcoma should be suspected. Liposarcomas usually contain a mixture of fat and soft tissue attenuation. These are rare tumors.

Pleural Extension of Lung Carcinoma

The features of pleural extension of bronchogenic carcinoma are discussed in Chapter 11.

■ DIFFUSE PLEURAL DISEASE

Benign and malignant diseases may cause diffuse pleural abnormalities. Causes include fibrothorax and malignant tumors such as malignant mesothelioma and metastatic carcinoma.

The radiographic definition of diffuse pleural thickening is somewhat arbitrary, and there is no general consensus on a definition. However, it has been suggested that diffuse pleural thickening consists of a smooth, uninterrupted pleural opacity extending over at least one fourth of the chest wall, with or without obliteration of the costophrenic angles. The CT definition that has been used in describing asbestos-related changes consists of thickening that extends more than 8 cm in the craniocaudal direction and 5 cm laterally and a pleural thickness more than 3 mm.

Fibrothorax

Causes and Clinical Features

Common causes of fibrothorax or diffuse pleural fibrosis (Box 18-9) include organized hemorrhagic effusions, tuberculous effusions, pyogenic empyema, and benign asbestos-related pleurisy. When it is bilateral, it may produce a restrictive defect leading to respiratory compromise and occasionally to respiratory failure.

One of the common causes of diffuse pleural thickening is asbestos exposure. This topic is discussed in Chapter 8.

Radiologic Features

Several radiologic features, particularly CT features, may permit determination of the cause of fibrothorax. Underlying parenchymal disease can be seen in patients who have had tuberculosis or empyema previously. Extensive calcification of the visceral pleura favors previous tuberculosis or empyema (Fig. 18-31). Calcification is seldom seen with asbestos-related pleurisy. When pleural thickening occurs as a sequela of a benign asbestos pleurisy, bilateral pleural abnormalities

usually are detected, whereas other causes of diffuse pleural thickening usually lead to unilateral pleural abnormalities (Fig. 18-32).

CT may help in differentiating benign from malignant pleural thickening (Box 18-10) (Figs. 18-33 and 18-34). Benign fibrothorax seldom involves the mediastinal pleura. Involvement of the mediastinal pleura is common with malignant mesothelioma and metastatic adenocarcinoma. Malignant thickening is more frequently nodular and masslike (see Fig. 18-34). CT is also helpful in the assessment of the underlying lung when extensive pleural thickening is present. The pleural thickening may interfere with the diagnosis of subtle parenchymal lung abnormalities, such as interstitial disease due to asbestosis.

Malignant Mesothelioma

Clinical Features

Diffuse malignant mesothelioma (Box 18-11) is a rare primary pleural neoplasm. Approximately 2000 to 3000 cases are reported each year in the United States. Approximately

---

Box 18-9. Fibrothorax

CAUSE
Hemorrhagic effusions
Tuberculous effusion
Pyogenic empyema
Benign asbestos pleurisy

RADIOLOGIC FEATURES
Standard Radiography
Length more than one fourth of chest wall
Computed Tomography
≥8 cm long
>5 cm laterally
>3 mm thick

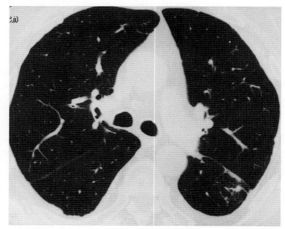

FIGURE 18-32. Asbestos-related pleural thickening. CT shows bilateral, diffuse thickening but no calcification.

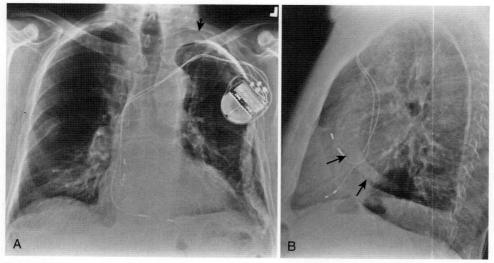

FIGURE 18-31. Calcified fibrothorax in a patient with pneumothorax treated many years ago for tuberculosis. There is extensive calcification surrounding the entire lung. **A,** On the frontal view the calcification can be easily localized to the visceral pleura *(arrow)*. **B,** On the lateral view, markedly thickened pleura can be seen anteriorly *(arrows)*.

Box 18-10. Benign versus Malignant Pleural Thickening

Benign	Malignant
<1 cm thick	>1 cm thick
Does not involve entire pleura	Circumferential
Spares mediastinal surface	Involves mediastinal surface
Smooth	Nodular

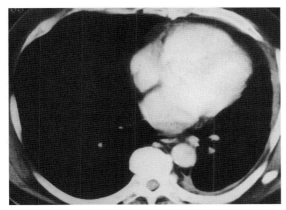

FIGURE 18-33. Benign, diffuse pleural thickening caused by empyema. CT shows smooth thickening without nodularity involving the lateral and posterior pleural surfaces but not the mediastinal pleural surfaces.

80% of these lesions occur in individuals exposed to asbestos. The amphibolic asbestos fibers are the most carcinogenic or tumorigenic type. There is usually a 30- to 40-year latency period between the time of initial exposure and the development of malignant mesothelioma. The prevalence is highest in cities with shipyards and asbestos plants. It usually occurs in the sixth to eighth decades of life, with a male-to-female predominance of approximately 4 to 1.

Box 18-11. Malignant Mesothelioma

CLINICAL FEATURES
Rare (2000 to 3000 cases/year)
80% of patients have a history of asbestos exposure
30- to 40-year latency period
Occurs in the 6th to 8th decade of life
Affects men more than women (4:1)
Symptoms
  Chest pain
  Dyspnea; weight loss

PATHOLOGIC FEATURES
Types
  Epithelial (50%)
  Sarcomatous
  Mixed
Gross features
  Encasement of lung
  Growth of tumor into lung, chest wall, mediastinum, diaphragm

RADIOLOGIC FEATURES
Standard radiography
  Diffuse pleural thickening
    Nodular
    Encases lung
  Pleural effusion
  Pleural mass
  Decrease in size of hemithorax, shift of mediastinum to affected side
  Plaques
Computed tomography
  Staging
  Extent
  Chest wall, mediastinal diaphragmatic invasion
Magnetic resonance imaging and PET/CT
  Improved staging

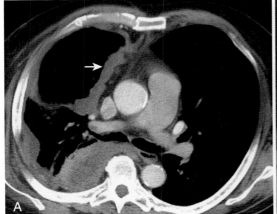
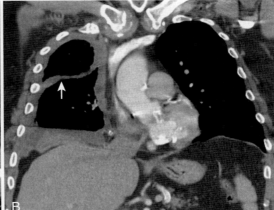

FIGURE 18-34. Malignant mesothelioma. **A,** The diffuse pleural thickening on the right is nodular and extends along the mediastinal pleural surface *(arrow)*. The volume of the right hemithorax is slightly reduced. **B,** Coronal reformation image shows the extent of pleural disease to greater detail and shows intrafissural extension *(arrow)*.

Clinical symptoms are frequently present 6 to 8 months before diagnosis and consist mainly of chest pain, although patients may also have dyspnea, cough, and weight loss. The prognosis for patients with this tumor is extremely poor, with a median survival of 10 months or less after diagnosis.

Pathologic Features

There are three major histologic types of malignant mesothelioma: epithelial, sarcomatous or mesenchymal, and mixed. The epithelial type is the most common and accounts for 50% of cases. The major differential diagnosis for the pathologist is metastatic adenocarcinoma, and a generous biopsy specimen that allows for immunohistochemistry and ultrastructural analysis is usually required to make the differentiation. The classic gross features include sheets, plaques, and masses of tumor that coat the pleural surface. There is involvement of the parietal and visceral pleura in most cases. The lung is encased, and tumor grows into the fissures and the interlobular septa, eventually producing parenchymal involvement. Crossover to the opposite pleural space and invasion of the mediastinum, chest wall, and diaphragm may occur.

Radiologic Features

The most common radiologic feature is diffuse pleural thickening that is irregular and nodular, with or without an associated pleural effusion (see Fig. 18-34). In a few cases, effusion alone or a pleural mass is detected. The irregular pleural surface progressively enlarges, producing multiple pleural masses. The diffuse pleural involvement often results in a decrease in the size of the hemithorax, with restriction of the underlying lung and a shift of the mediastinum toward the side of the disease (see Fig. 18-34). Other findings of asbestos-related pleural disease (e.g., plaques) occur in only 20% to 25% of cases. Occasionally, pleural effusions and mesothelioma may be associated with marked contralateral shift of the mediastinum.

CT is valuable in detecting and staging malignant mesothelioma. CT findings include pleural thickening (92%), thickening of the interlobular fissures (86%), pleural effusion (74%), loss of volume of the involved hemithorax (42%), pleural calcification (20%), and invasion of the chest wall 18% (Fig. 18-35). Malignant mesothelioma may metastasize to hilar and mediastinal nodes, but distant metastases are much less common. On CT, the pleu-

ral thickening is typically circumferential and involves the mediastinal pleural surface. It is nodular, and the thickness of the pleura usually exceeds 1 cm. However, malignant mesothelioma cannot be reliably differentiated from pleural metastases.

Extrapleural pneumonectomy is occasionally used in an attempt to produce a cure, but the results have been somewhat disappointing. Multimodality therapy consisting of surgery followed by chemotherapy and radiation therapy has been shown to prolong survival compared with surgery alone, but median survival is still less than 2 years.

Proper staging is necessary to assist treatment planning and to provide prognostic information. The most widely accepted staging system for mesothelioma is the International Mesothelioma Interest Group (IMIG) TNM staging system (Table 18-1). Accurate primary tumor (T) staging is important to distinguish patients who are potential surgical candidates from those who unlikely to benefit from surgery. It is important to distinguish locally advanced but potentially resectable T3 lesions (defined by involvement of endothoracic fascia, extension into mediastinal fat, nontransmural involvement of pericardium, or a solitary focus of chest wall invasion) from unresectable T4 lesions (defined by diffuse chest wall involvement or direct extension below the diaphragm to the contralateral pleura, mediastinal organs, the spine, or the inner surface of pericardium).

CT can be helpful in the preoperative staging of patients with this disease. CT may identify unresectable disease such as extensive chest wall and mediastinal invasion, spread to the contralateral thorax or mediastinal lymph nodes, or spread through the diaphragm to the abdomen (Fig. 18-36). CT is also useful for follow-up of patients who have undergone tumor resection, often suggesting the presence of tumor recurrence before there is other radiologic or clinical evidence.

MRI findings typically consist of tumor showing minimally increased signal on T1-weighted and moderately increased signal on T2-weighted images. MRI may be superior to CT in determining the extent of disease because it allows better evaluation of apical tumor, diaphragmatic and infradiaphragmatic extension, and the relation of tumors to mediastinal structures (Fig. 18-37, Fig. 18-38A).

On FDG-PET, mesotheliomas typically demonstrate high FDG avidity (Fig. 18-38B), with FDG uptake significantly

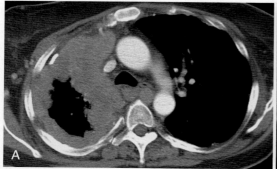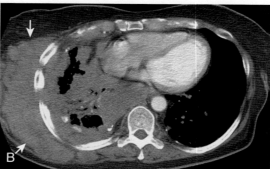

Figure 18-35. Malignant mesothelioma. **A** and **B**, There is diffuse, circumferential pleural thickening on the right, which is lobular. The tumor extends into the chest wall *(arrows)*. Notice the pleural plaques on the left.

TABLE **18-1** TNM International Staging System for Malignant Mesothelioma

Classification	Description of Involvement
TX	Primary tumor (T) cannot be assessed
T0	No evidence of primary tumor
T1	
T1a	Tumor limited to ipsilateral parietal, mediastinal, diaphragmatic pleura; no involvement of visceral pleura
T1b	Tumor involving ipsilateral parietal, mediastinal, diaphragmatic pleura, with focal involvement of viscera pleural surface
T2	Tumor involving any of the ipsilateral pleural surfaces with at least one of the following: confluent visceral pleural tumor, invasion of diaphragmatic muscle, or invasion of lung parenchyma
T3	Tumor involving any of the ipsilateral pleural surfaces with at least one of the following: invasion of the endothoracic fascia, invasion into mediastinal fat, solitary focus of tumor invading the soft tissues of the chest wall, or nontransmural involvement of the pericardium (locally advanced but resectable tumor)
T4	Tumor involving any of the ipsilateral pleural surfaces, with at least one of the following: diffuse or multifocal invasion of soft tissues of the chest wall, any involvement of rib, invasion through the diaphragm to the peritoneum, invasion of any mediastinal organ, direct extension to the contralateral pleura, invasion into the spine, extension to the internal surface of the pericardium, pericardial effusion with positive cytology, invasion of the myocardium, invasion of the brachial plexus (locally advanced, unresectable tumor)
NX	Regional lymph nodes (N) cannot be assessed
N0	No regional lymph node metastasis
N1	Metastases in the ipsilateral bronchopulmonary or hilar lymph nodes
N2	Metastases in the subcarinal or ipsilateral mediastinal lymph nodes
N3	Metastases in the contralateral mediastinal or internal mammary lymph nodes, or any supraclavicular node metastasis
MX	Presence of distant metastases (M) cannot be assessed
M0	No distant metastasis
M1	Distant metastasis present

Stage Grouping			
Stage I			
IA	T1a	N0	M0
IB	T1b	N0	M0
Stage II	T2	N0	M0
Stage III	T3	Any N	M0
	Any T	N1	M0
	Any T	N2	M0
Stage IV	T4	Any N	M0
	Any T	N3	M0
	Any T	Any N	M1

greater than that observed in most benign pleural diseases. Because patients with mesothelioma may have areas of pleural thickening that are not involved by malignancy, PET can help to direct biopsy procedures to areas of high FDG-avidity, thereby increasing the diagnostic yield and helping to avoid false-negative results.

Initial studies of FDG-PET for staging of mesothelioma were limited by the poor spatial resolution of PET images, which precluded accurate determination of the presence and extent of local tumor invasion. However, integrated PET/CT scanners have improved the accuracy of PET for staging mesothelioma due to improved anatomic localization of regions of FDG avidity. Integrated PET/CT typically detects more extensive involvement than shown by CT and MRI. It is also useful for identifying occult distant metastases. In addition to staging, integrated PET/ CT may play a role in determining prognosis and assessing response to therapy.

Pleural Metastases

Pleural metastases (Box 18-12) are the most common pleural neoplasm, accounting for 95% of cases. Metastases to the pleura are usually adenocarcinoma, with sites of origin including the lung, breast, ovary, and stomach. Lymphoma may also involve the pleural space. There are three major manifestations of pleural metastases, with pleural effusion being by far the most common. However, pleural metastases sometimes may produce diffuse pleural thickening with masses similar to malignant mesothelioma and involvement of the pleura occasionally may be caused by direct pleural seeding from tumors within the thorax, such as invasive thymoma.

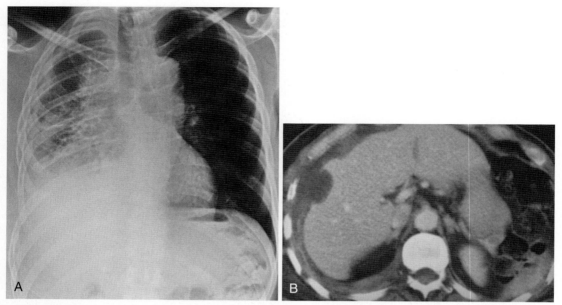

FIGURE 18-36. Malignant mesothelioma. **A,** Standard radiograph shows diffuse pleural thickening on the right and contracture of the right lung. **B,** CT shows involvement of the peritoneum and liver.

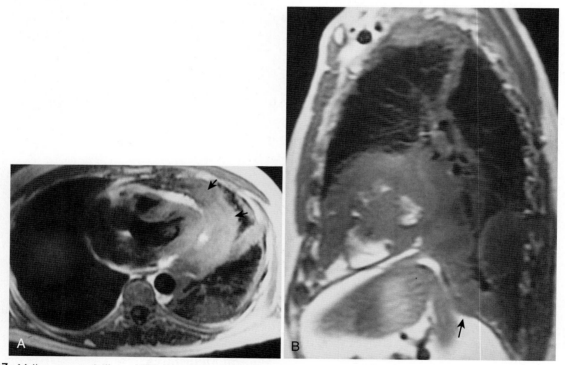

FIGURE 18-37. Malignant mesothelioma. MRI shows extensive left mesothelioma involving the pericardium (**A**) *(arrows)* and diaphragm (**B**) *(arrow)*.

Malignant Pleural Effusion

Malignant pleural effusion is the most common manifestation of metastatic involvement. Metastatic disease affecting the pleura is probably second only to CHF as a cause of pleural effusion in patients older than 50 years, and it is the most common cause of exudative effusion. The most common cause of a malignant pleural effusion is an underlying lung cancer. This is found in 15% of patients at initial evaluation and 50% of patients with disseminated disease. Breast cancer is the second most common cause of malignant effusion (25%), followed by lymphoma (10%) and ovarian and gastric carcinoma (≤5%). In approximately 10% of patients with malignant pleural effusion, the primary site is unknown (Fig. 18-38).

Diffuse Pleural Thickening

Diffuse pleural thickening due to solid pleural metastases may occur with peripheral lung adenocarcinoma,

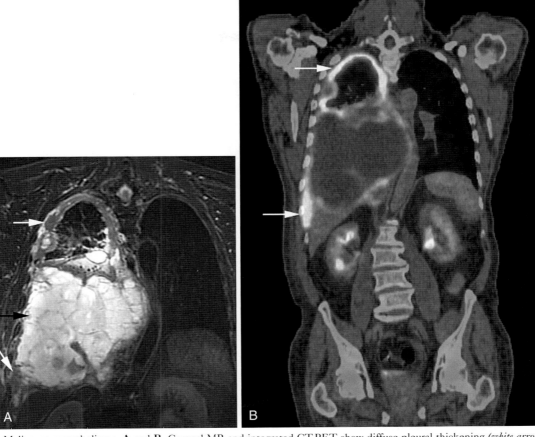

FIGURE 18-38. Malignant mesothelioma. A and B, Coronal MR and integrated CT-PET show diffuse pleural thickening *(white arrows)* that is FDG avid. There is an associated large multi-loculated pleural effusion *(black arrow)*. Note that tumor and fluid abut the diaphragm, which is caudally displaced. Laparoscopy revealed no evidence of transdiaphragmatic involvement. (Case courtesy of Dr. Jeremy Erasmus, M.D. Anderson hospital.)

Box 18-12. **Pleural Metastases**

Origins
  Lung
  Breast
  Ovary
  Stomach
  Lymphoma
Manifestations
  Malignant effusion
  Diffuse thickening
  Focal seeding

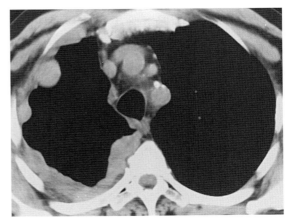

FIGURE 18-39. Metastatic disease to the right pleural space from renal cell carcinoma. Notice the nodular pleural thickening. (From McLoud TC, Flower CD: Imaging of the pleura: sonography, CT and MR imaging. AJR Am J Roentgenol 156:1145-1153, 1991.)

---

but it can also result from adenocarcinomas arising elsewhere. Lymphoma can manifest as a plaquelike or nodular thickening of the pleura or as large pleural masses. Extensive pleural thickening similar to that of malignant mesothelioma may occur with disease metastatic to the pleura (Fig. 18-39). Diffuse encasement of the underlying lung occurs with a shift of the mediastinum to the ipsilateral side.

Pleural Seeding
Solid pleural metastases may occur by means of direct seeding (Fig. 18-40), usually from primary intrathoracic tumors, and the most common source is invasive

thymoma. In patients in whom invasive thymoma has been resected, careful follow-up with CT is recommended to identify recurrence involving the pleura. It typically appears as small, plaquelike areas of pleural thickening.

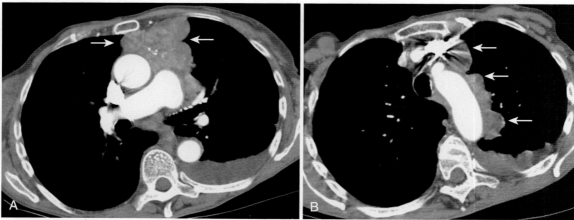

Figure 18-40. Invasive thymoma. **A,** Imaging shows a large, anterior mediastinal mass *(arrows)*. **B,** Nodular pleural thickening is present along the left mediastinal pleural surfaces *(arrows)*. Notice the left pleural effusion.

▄▄ SUGGESTED READINGS

Aberle, D.R., Gamsu, G., Ray, C.S., 1988. High-resolution CT of benign asbestos related diseases: clinical and radiographic correlation. AJR Am. J Roentgenol. 151, 883–891.

Antman, K.H., Corson, J.M., 1985. Benign and malignant pleural mesothelioma. Clin. Chest. Med. 6, 127–140.

Bressler, E.L., Francis, I.R., Glazer, G.M., Gross, B.H., 1987. Bolus contrast medium enhancement for distinguishing pleural from parenchymal lung disease: CT features. J. Comput. Assist. Tomogr. 11, 436–440.

Bruzzi, J.F., Munden, R.F., 2006. PET/CT imaging of lung cancer. J. Thorac. Imaging 21, 123–136.

Craighead, J.E., 1987. Current pathogenetic concepts of diffuse malignant mesothelioma. Hum. Pathol. 18, 544–557.

Dedrick, C.G., McLoud, T.C., Shepard, J.O., Shipley, R., 1985. Computed tomography of localized pleural mesothelioma. AJR Am. J. Roentgenol. 144, 275–280.

Dwyer, A., 1978. The displaced crus: a sign for distinguishing between pleural fluid and ascites on computed tomography. J. Comput. Assist. Tomogr. 2, 598–599.

England, D.M., Hochholzer, L., McCarthy, M.J., 1989. Localized benign and malignant fibrous tumors of the pleura: a clinicopathologic review of 223 cases. Am. J. Surg. Pathol. 13, 640–658.

Epler, G.R., McLoud, T.C., Munn, C.S., Colby, T.V., 1986. Pleural lipoma: diagnosis by computed tomography. Chest 90, 265–268.

Evans, A.R., Wolstenholte, R.J., Shettar, S.P., Yogish, H., 1985. Primary pleural liposarcoma. Thorax 40, 554–555.

Fleischner, F.G., 1963. Atypical arrangement of free pleural effusion. Radiol. Clin. North Am. 1, 347–362.

Fraser R.S., Muller N.L., Colman, N.C., Pare., P.D. 1999. Fraser and Pare's Diagnosis of Diseases of the Chest, 4th ed. Philadelphia. Elsevier,

Friedman, A.C., Fiel, S.B., Radecki, P.D., Lev-Toaff, A.S., 1990. Computed tomography of benign pleural and pulmonary parenchymal abnormalities related to asbestos exposure. Semin. Ultrasound CT MR 11, 393–408.

Friedman, P.J., Hellekant, C.A.G., 1977. Radiologic recognition of bronchopleural fistula. Radiology 124, 289–295.

Friedman, R.L., 1954. Infrapulmonary pleural effusions. Am. J. Roentgenol. Radium. Ther. Nucl. Med. 71, 613–623.

Greene, R., McLoud, T.C., Stark, P., 1977. Pneumothorax. Semin. Roentgenol. 12, 313–325.

Griffin, D.J., Gross, B.H., McCracken, S., Glazer, G.M., 1984. Observation on CT differentiation of pleural and peritoneal fluid. J. Comput. Assist. Tomogr. 8, 24–28.

Gupta N.C., Rogers J.S., Graeber G.M., et al., 2005. Clinical role of F 18 fluorodeoxyglucose positron emission tomography imaging in patients with lung cancer and suspected malignant pleural effusion. Chest 122, 1918–1924.

Halvorsen, R.A., Fedyshin, P.J., Korobkin, M., et al., 1986. Ascites or pleural effusion? Radiographics 6, 135–149.

Henschke, C.I., Davis, S.D., Romano, P.M., et al., 1989. Pleural effusions: pathogenesis, radiologic evaluation and therapy. J. Thorac. Imaging 4, 49–60.

Henschke, C.I., Yankelevitz, D.T., Davis, S.D., et al., 1992. Diseases of the pleura. In: Freundlich, I.M., Bragg, D.G. (Eds.), A Radiologic Approach to Diseases of the Chest. Williams & Wilkins, Baltimore, pp. 225–234.

Ismail-Khan, R., Robinson, L.A., Williams, C.C., et al., 2006. Malignant pleural mesothelioma: a comprehensive review. Cancer Control 13, 255–263.

Jones, R.N., McLoud, T., Rockoff, S.D., 1988. The radiographic pleural abnormalities in asbestos exposure: relationship to physiologic abnormalities. J. Thorac. Imaging 3, 56–66.

Kawashima, A., Libshitz, H.I., 1990. Malignant pleural mesothelioma: CT manifestations in 50 cases. AJR Am. J. Roentgenol. 155, 965–969.

Lee, K.S., Im, J.G., Choe, K.O., et al., 1992. CT findings in benign fibrous mesothelioma of the pleura: Pathologic correlation in nine patients. AJR Am. J. Roentgenol. 158, 983–986.

Leung, A.N., Müller, N.L., Miller, R.R., 1990. CT in differential diagnosis of diffuse pleural disease. AJR Am. J. Roentgenol. 154, 487–492.

Light, R.W., MacGregor, M.I., Luchsinger, P.C., et al., 1972. Pleural effusions: the diagnostic separation of transudates and exudates. Ann. Intern. Med. 77, 507–513.

Light, R.W., 2002. Clinical practice. Pleural effusion. N. Engl. J. Med. 346, 1971–1977.

Lipscomb, D.J., Flower, C.D.R., Hadfield, J.W., 1981. Ultrasound of the pleura: an assessment of its clinical value. Clin. Radiol. 32, 289–290.

Lorigan, J.G., Libshitz, H.I., 1989. MR imaging of malignant pleural mesothelioma. J. Comput. Assist. Tomogr. 13, 617–620.

Malatskey, A., Fields, S., Libson, E., 1989. CT appearance of primary pleural lymphoma. Comput. Med. Imaging Graph. 13, 165–167.

McLoud, T.C., Flower, C.D., 1991. Imaging the pleura: sonography, CT and MR imaging. AJR Am. J. Roentgenol. 156, 1145–1153.

McLoud, T.C., Woods, B.O., Carrington, C.B., et al., 1985. Diffuse pleural thickening in an asbestos-exposed population: prevalence and causes. AJR Am. J. Roentgenol. 144, 9–18.

McLoud, T.C., 1994. The pleura and chest wall. In: Haaga, J.R., Lanzieri, C.F., Sartoris, D.J., Zerhouni, E.A. (Eds.), Computed Tomography and Magnetic Resonance Imaging of the Whole Body. Mosby, St. Louis, pp. 772–787.

Mendelson, D.S., Meary, E., Buy, J.N., et al., 1991. Localized fibrous pleural mesothelioma: CT findings. Clin. Imaging 15, 105–108.

Mirvis, S., Dutcher, J.P., Haney, P.J., et al., 1983. CT of malignant pleural mesothelioma. AJR Am. J. Roentgenol. 140, 665–670.

Montalvo, B.M., Morillo, G., Sridhar, K., Christoph, C., 1991. MR imaging of malignant pleural mesotheliomas [abstract]. Radiology 181 (P), 109.

Moskowitz, H., Platt, R.T., Schachar, R., Mellins, H., 1973. Roentgen visualization of minute pleural effusion. Radiology 109, 33–35.

Müller, N.L., 1993. Imaging the pleura. Radiology 186, 297–309.

Munk, P.L., Müller, N.L., 1988. Pleural liposarcoma: CT diagnosis. J. Comput. Assist. Tomogr. 12, 709–710.

Naidich, D.P., Megibow, A.J., Hilton, S., et al., 1983. Computed tomography of the diaphragm: peridiaphragmatic fluid localization. J. Comput. Assist. Tomogr. 7, 641–649.

Naidich, D.P., Zerhouni, E.A., Siegelman, S.S., 1991. Pleura and chest wall. In: Naidich, D.P., Zerhouni, E.A., Siegelman, S.S. (Eds.), Computed Tomography and Magnetic Resonance of the Thorax, second ed. Raven-Lippincott, New York, pp. 407–471.

O'Moore, P.V., Mueller, P.R., Simeone, J.F., et al., 1987. Sonographic guidance in diagnostic and therapeutic interventions in the pleural space. AJR Am. J. Roentgenol. 149, 1–5.

Rigler, L.G., 1931. Roentgenologic observations on the movement of pleural effusions. AJR Am. J. Roentgenol. 25, 220–229.

Rosado-de-Christenson, M.L., Abbott, G.F., et al., 2003. Localized fibrous tumors of the pleura. Radiographics 23, 759–783.

Rusch, V.W., Godwin, J.D., Shuman, W.P., 1988. The role of computed tomography scanning in the initial assessment and the follow-up of malignant pleural mesothelioma. J. Thorac. Cardiovasc. Surg. 96, 171–177.

Ruskin, J.A., Gurney, J.W., Thorsen, M.K., Goodman, L.R., 1987. Detection of pleural effusions on supine chest radiographs. AJR Am. J. Roentgenol. 148, 681–683.

Saifuddin, A., Da Costa, P., Chalmers, A.G., et al., 1992. Primary malignant localized fibrous tumours of the pleura: clinical, radiological and pathological features. Clin. Radiol. 45, 13–17.

Schwartz, D.A., Fuortes, L.J., Galvin, J.R., et al., 1990. Asbestos-induced pleural fibrosis and impaired lung function. Am. Rev. Respir. Dis. 141, 321–325.

Shuman, L.S., Libshitz, H.I., 1984. Solid pleural manifestations of lymphoma. AJR Am. J. Roentgenol. 142, 269–273.

Silverman, S.G., Mueller, P.R., Saini, S., et al., 1988. Thoracic empyema: management with image-guided catheter drainage. Radiology 169, 5–9.

Sohn, S.A., 1988. The pleura. Am. Rev. Respir. Dis. 138, 184–234.

Stark, D.D., Federle, M.P., Goodman, P.C., et al., 1983. Differentiating lung abscess and empyema: radiography and computed tomography. AJR Am. J. Roentgenol. 141, 163–167.

Staub, N.C., Wiener-Kronish, J.P., Albertine, K.H., 1985. Transport through the pleura: physiology of normal liquid and solute exchange in the pleural space. In: Chretien, J., Bignon, J., Hirsch, A. (Eds.), The Pleura in Health and Disease. Marcel-Dekker, New York, pp. 169–193.

Teplick, J.G., Teplick, S.K., Goodman, L., Haskin, M.E., 1982. The interface sign: a computed tomographic sign for distinguishing pleural and intra-abdominal fluid. Radiology 144, 359–362.

Tocino, I., Miller, M.H., Frederick, P.R., et al., 1984. CT detection of acute pneumothorax in head trauma. AJR Am. J. Roentgenol. 143, 989–990.

Troung, M.T., Marom, E.M., Erasmus, J.J., 2006. Preoperative evaluation of patients with malignant pleural mesothelioma: role of integrated CT-PET imaging. J. Thorac. Imaging 21, 146–153.

van Sonnenberg, E., Nakamoto, S.K., Mueller, P.R., et al., 1984. CT- and ultrasound-guided catheter drainage of empyemas after chest-tube failure. Radiology 151, 349–353.

Vix, V.A., 1977. Roentgenographic manifestations of pleural disease. Semin. Roentgenol. 12, 277–286.

Yang, P.C., Luh, K.T., Chang, D.B., et al., Value of sonography in determining the nature of pleural effusion: analysis of 320 cases. AJR Am. J. Roentgenol. 159, 29–33.

Wang, Z.J., Reddy, G.P., Gotway, M.B., et al., 2004. Malignant pleural mesothelioma: evaluation with CT, MR imaging, and PET. Radiographics 24, 105–119.

Zerhouni, E.A., Scott, W.W., Baker, R.R., et al., 1982. Invasive thymomas: diagnosis and evaluation by computed tomography. J. Comput. Assist. Tomogr. 6, 92–100.

CHAPTER 19

Interventional Techniques

Theresa C. McLoud and Subba R. Digumarthy

Several interventional techniques are performed in thoracic radiology. The most important is percutaneous transthoracic needle biopsy (TNB) of lung and mediastinal lesions. Other interventional procedures that are mostly related to the pleura include drainage of fluid collections, catheter drainage of pneumothoraces, and sclerotherapy.

■ TRANSTHORACIC NEEDLE BIOPSY

Indications

Transthoracic needle biopsies (Box 19-1) are performed most commonly for the diagnosis of an indeterminate solitary pulmonary nodule. Not all solitary pulmonary nodules that are suspect for bronchogenic carcinoma require biopsy. If the pretest probability is very high for lung cancer or a biopsy is unlikely to have any impact on management, TNB should not be performed. For example, if a patient presents with a long history of smoking and a new, irregular, spiculated nodule in the lung, the likelihood is extremely high that this represents a lung cancer, and it is reasonable to proceed directly to staging and resection. Other indications for TNB include undiagnosed mediastinal masses, a hilar mass when the bronchoscopy result is negative, single or multiple pulmonary nodules in a patient with a known extrathoracic malignancy or a suspicion of metastatic disease, and suspected infectious lesions manifesting as solitary nodules, masses, or very focal areas of consolidation, particularly in the immunocompromised host.

There are several diagnostic alternatives to TNB. The most important is bronchoscopy. However, bronchoscopy is preferred for central lesions, particularly if a prebronchoscopy CT scan shows evidence of endobronchial involvement. Transthoracic biopsy may be used to diagnose hilar masses when the result of bronchoscopy is negative and extraluminal compression of the airway is identified. Transbronchial needle aspiration (i.e., Wang needle) is primarily used to establish metastatic malignancy in mediastinal nodes for the purposes of staging lung cancer. A needle is inserted using the bronchoscope through the tracheal wall or carina to facilitate the biopsy of the nodes. In the absence of a visible endobronchial lesion, the diagnostic yield for bronchoscopy in peripheral nodules is low (in the range of 58% to 80%) and is lowest for nodules less than 2 cm in diameter. Video-assisted thoracoscopy enables the diagnosis of peripheral subpleural pulmonary lesions. However, this is an operative procedure that requires an inpatient stay and general anesthesia, and it is more expensive than bronchoscopy or transthoracic needle aspiration biopsy.

Contraindications

Most contraindications to TNB are relative rather than absolute (Box 19-2). The most important are bleeding diatheses. A prebiopsy prothrombin time (PT), partial thromboplastin time (PTT), and platelet count are recommended. A careful history of coagulation abnormalities or the ingestion of drugs such as aspirin, which may lead to abnormal platelet function, should be obtained. Patients with low platelet counts who require an emergent biopsy, such as an immunocompromised patient with pulmonary infection, can receive platelet transfusions. Biopsy of lesions that have a marked vascular supply should be avoided.

Another relative contraindication is pulmonary hypertension. Needle biopsy can be safely attempted in patients with mild pulmonary hypertension if the nodule is peripheral. In the case of deep nodules or hilar masses, it is not recommended. Other relative contraindications include mechanical ventilation, bullae, or severe emphysema in the path of the lesion to be biopsied, severe chronic obstructive pulmonary disease (COPD, defined by a forced expiratory volume in 1 second [FEV_1] of less than 1 L), and intractable cough.

Patients should be cooperative and be able to maintain a certain position. Biopsies are performed with patients in the supine or prone position. The decubitus position is less preferable because it is difficult for the patients to maintain the position.

Local Anesthesia and Sedation

Lung biopsies can be performed under local anesthesia and breath-hold technique or under local anesthesia and intravenous conscious sedation with quiet breathing. Uncooperative patients need conscious sedation.

Box 19-1. **Indications for Transthoracic Needle Biopsy**

Indeterminate solitary pulmonary nodule
Undiagnosed mediastinal mass
Hilar mass when bronchoscopy is negative
Single or multiple nodules when metastases are
  suspect
Probable infectious lesions presenting as nodules or
  masses

Box 19-2. **Relative Contraindications to Transthoracic Needle Biopsy**

Bleeding diathesis
Pulmonary hypertension
Uncooperative patient
Mechanical ventilation
Bullae
Severe COPD (FEV$_1$ ≤ 1.0 L)
Intractable cough

COPD, chronic obstructive pulmonary disease; FEV$_1$, forced expiratory volume in 1 second.

Technique

Prebiopsy Imaging

Computed tomography (CT) is highly recommended before TNB. CT is useful in providing a specific benign diagnosis in certain instances, such as a calcified granuloma or hamartoma, and it can provide information concerning the optimal approach to the lesion (Figs. 19-1 and 19.2). Areas of necrosis within large masses can be identified. Such areas should be avoided because they often produce nondiagnostic samples. ^{18}F-fluorodeoxyglucose positron emission tomography (FDG-PET) is also useful for identifying the viable portion of the tumor (Fig 19-3). Vascular lesions such as aneurysms or arterial venous malformations can be easily recognized on contrast-enhanced CT.

Imaging Guidance

Fluoroscopy or CT can be used for imaging guidance. Ultrasound is occasionally used for chest wall or peripheral lesions abutting the pleura. Fluoroscopically guided biopsies are usually reserved for large masses (Fig. 19-4). Fluoroscopy allows real-time, moment-to-moment visualization and often enables the biopsy to be performed in less

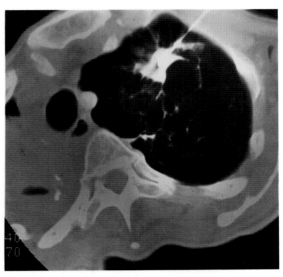

FIGURE 19-1. Anterior approach to a lesion in the left upper lobe. The patient was placed in a slightly oblique position, and an oblique anterior approach was chosen to avoid bullae surrounding the mass.

time than that required for a CT-guided biopsy. However, we prefer to use CT for imaging guidance in all transthoracic needle biopsies. It allows a more complex approach, and safe and accurate sampling of hilar or mediastinal masses is possible. CT also provides better visualization of severe emphysematous areas or bullae, which may lie within the path of a needle. Real-time, continuous CT fluoroscopy combines the advantages of standard fluoroscopy with CT guidance.

Needle Selection

A variety of needles can be used for TNB. Small-bore, 18- to 22-gauge needles are preferred because larger-bore needles have been associated with high complication

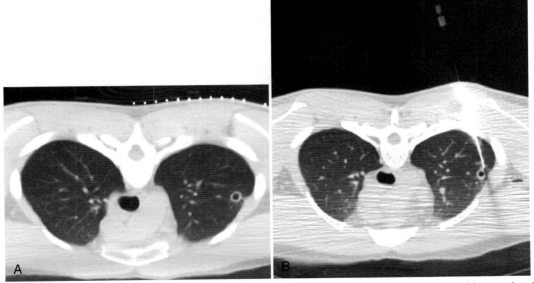

FIGURE 19-2. Prone biopsy of a cavitary lesion. **A,** New left upper lobe cavitary nodule was identified in a patient with treated nodular sclerosing Hodgkin's lymphoma. **B,** The biopsy specimen from the wall of the cavity showed coccidioidomycosis.

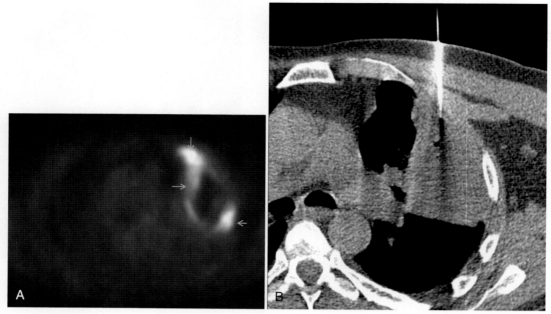

FIGURE 19-3. **A,** FDG-PET of a lung mass reveals viable metabolically active tumor only at the periphery. **B,** CT-guided biopsy, with a specimen obtained from the periphery, revealed non–small cell lung cancer.

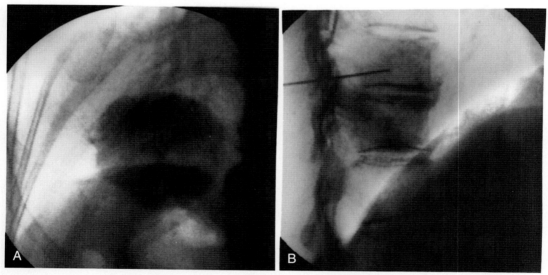

FIGURE 19-4. **A** and **B,** Fluoroscopically guided biopsy of a large right lower lobe mass. A C-arm or biplane fluoroscopic unit should be used for these procedures.

rates, particularly bleeding and pneumothorax. Aspirating needles commonly used include Chiba and Greene varieties. These needles provide only cytologic material from aspirates. Automatic biopsy devices that provide small cores of tissue, sometimes referred to as *biopsy guns,* are available. The length of the needle selected should be greater than the depth of the lesion from the skin and preferably 3 to 5 cm longer. If coaxial technique is used, the inner needle length should be 5 cm longer than the introducer needle.

On-Site Pathology

The high diagnostic accuracy of TNB can be attributed to improved radiologic techniques such as CT guidance and, even more importantly, to advances in cytologic techniques and interpretation. The TNB technique should be a cooperative effort between the cytologist and the radiologist. We prefer to have a cytologic technician available during the biopsy. Quick stains can be performed, and a cytologist can be called to provide a rapid interpretation of the specimen. This allows for repeat biopsy if the specimen is nondiagnostic or inadequate and permits the use of core-needle specimens as a supplement to the aspiration when the diagnosis cannot be obtained from the aspirated sample.

Technical Factors

The shortest, most vertical biopsy path should be chosen based on the prebiopsy CT scan (Fig. 19-5). Interlobar fissures, pulmonary vessels, bullae, and areas of severe emphysema should be avoided (see Fig. 19-1). Sometimes, this can be achieved by tilting the CT gantry (Fig. 19-6). Paraspinal and extrapleural saline injection creates safer access to paramediastinal lesions (Fig. 19-7). The patient is placed in a position that provides a safe approach—prone, supine, or occasionally, decubitus—as indicated. After a scanogram is performed, thin-section, 2- to 5-mm CT slices are obtained through the lesion with a localizing grid in place on the skin overlying the lesion. A desired skin

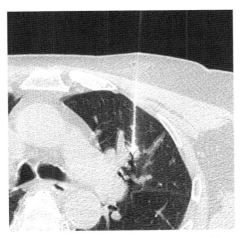

Figure 19-5. Biopsy of the left upper lobe nodule. The patient was placed in the supine position, and the most direct vertical path (avoiding the large vessels and bronchi) was used. The histologic diagnosis was metastatic adenocarcinoma from prostate cancer.

puncture site is identified using the grid, and the patient is prepared and draped in a sterile manner. After the injection of local anesthesia, a small puncture is made in the skin and subcutaneous tissues with a scalpel.

An introducer 19-gauge spinal needle is advanced through the chest wall using intermittent CT scans to verify the position of the needle. When performing TNB, the introducer needle must be perfectly aligned with the lesion before the pleural puncture. It is difficult to reposition or reorient the path of the needle after the lung is entered. Attempting to do so often produces a pleural tear.

Although the biopsy needle may be introduced alone, we prefer a coaxial technique. The 19-gauge introducer spinal needle is placed through the skin and chest wall and through the pleura just adjacent to or into the lesion to be biopsied. A 21- or 22-gauge aspirating needle is then used for the biopsy, and it is placed by way of the introducer needle. Ultrathin, 19-gauge introducer needles can accommodate 20-gauge automatic biopsy devices for core specimens. The coaxial technique allows several specimens to be obtained with only one pleural puncture.

After the introducer needle has been correctly positioned immediately adjacent to or in the lesion, the stylet is removed, and the 21- or 22-gauge aspirating needle is placed through the introducer needle into the lesion. A 10-mL syringe is then attached to the thin needle, and using a series of up and down and rotatory motions, an aspirate is obtained. The specimen should be immediately placed on glass slides and fixed with a number of available quick stains. If a core biopsy is used, the tissue can be rinsed with formalin or saline. A small amount of saline is placed in the introducer needle before withdrawing the stylet to reduce the risk of air embolism and reduce friction between the needles. If the cytologist thinks the original pass with the aspirating needle is nondiagnostic or negative, additional samples may be taken, as well as core samples, using the coaxial technique. If inflammatory changes are present or there is a suspicion of active infection, specimens should be sent to the bacteriology laboratory.

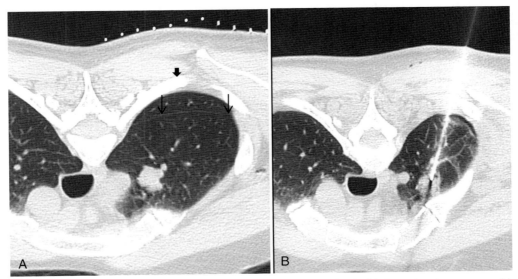

FIGURE 19-6. Biopsy with tilt of the CT gantry. **A,** CT of the left upper lobe nodule obtained with the patient in a prone position reveals ribs *(thick arrow)* and a left major fissure *(arrows)* in the path. **B,** CT obtained with 20 degrees of tilt of the gantry toward the head reveals a safe approach without intervening ribs or a fissure. The histologic diagnosis was hamartoma.

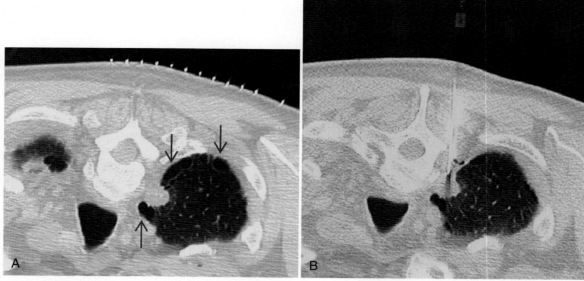

FIGURE 19-7. Biopsy after injection of paravertebral saline. **A,** CT of the left upper lobe with the patient in the prone position reveals a subpleural nodule surrounded by emphysematous bullae *(arrows)*. **B,** Needle placement through the paravertebral soft tissue was achieved after injecting saline to increase the soft tissue thickness and avoid the bullae. The biopsy specimen was positive for non–small cell lung cancer.

Postprocedural Management

We consider positional precautions to be the best postprocedural management option. Patients are removed from the CT table and immediately placed with the puncture side dependent. For example, if the needle has been introduced through the back with the patient in prone position, he or she is immediately turned into the supine position. The patient is then transferred to a holding area, where blood pressure and oxygen saturation (with a pulse oximeter) are monitored by the nursing staff. If the patient is asymptomatic, he or she is kept quiet on a stretcher, and a radiograph is obtained 1 hour later to determine if a pneumothorax is present. If no pneumothorax is identified, another film is obtained at 3 hours, and the patient can be discharged. If a small pneumothorax is present, it is followed for an additional 2 hours, and if there is no change in size, the patient can be discharged. However, symptomatic or enlarging pneumothoraces require treatment.

Most TNBs are performed on an outpatient basis. The patient should be instructed to come to the hospital with someone and be prepared to spend the evening of the biopsy in someone's company. Detailed instructions of signs and symptoms of pneumothorax are provided to the patients on discharge, with instructions to return to the nearest hospital if symptoms occur. However, discharge when there is no pneumothorax or a small, stable pneumothorax is considered to be extremely safe. Delayed pneumothorax developing after 3 hours is uncommon and is seen in about 3% of patients, predominantly in those with emphysema.

Complications

The most common complications of TNB (Box 19-3) are pneumothorax and hemoptysis (Fig 19-8). The incidence of pneumothorax has been reported to occur in 0% to 60% of patients, with most institutions reporting a rate of approximately 20% to

---

Box 19-3. Complications of Transthoracic Needle Biopsy

Pneumothorax (20% to 30%)
Chest tube (5% to 15%)
Hemoptysis (1% to 10%)
Seeding of biopsy track
Air embolism

30%. Risk factors for the development of pneumothorax include the size and depth of the lesion, the presence of emphysema and COPD, the use of multiple pleural punctures, and the transgression of a fissure. The percentage of biopsies requiring treatment (i.e., chest tube drainage) is much lower and ranges from about 5% to 15%.

Small pneumothoraces can be managed conservatively with monitoring of vital signs and follow-up radiographs to confirm stability. Large or symptomatic pneumothoraces require placement of a chest tube. Adequate treatment can usually be accomplished with small-bore, percutaneously inserted catheters. The catheters may be attached to suction or to a Heimlich valve. There is controversy about whether patients with small-bore chest catheters can be managed on an inpatient or outpatient basis. We prefer to admit all patients who require chest tubes. Many do have continuing air leaks that require suction. Most chest tubes, however, can be removed within 24 to 48 hours.

Hemoptysis occurs in 1% to 10% of cases. A large degree of hemoptysis or significant hemorrhage is unusual if no bleeding diathesis exists. The incidence of hemorrhage increases with the size and gauge of the needle used (see Fig. 19-8). Hemorrhage is almost always self-limiting. In cases with more severe hemorrhage, careful monitoring is required, and the patient with hemoptysis should be reassured and placed biopsy-side down to prevent transbronchial aspiration of blood.

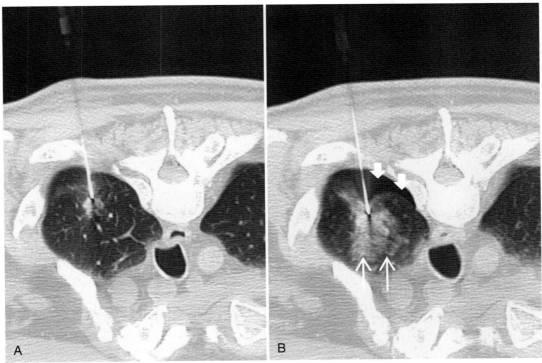

FIGURE 19-8. Biopsy complication. **A,** CT-guided biopsy of the right upper lobe nodule was done with the patient in the prone position. **B,** The procedure was complicated by hemorrhage *(thin arrows)* and a small pneumothorax *(thick arrows)*. The pneumothorax was aspirated during the needle removal, and the hemorrhage was asymptomatic. The biopsy specimen was positive for non–small cell lung cancer.

Malignant seeding of the biopsy track is a rare complication. The use of an introducer needle with a coaxial technique provides protection from seeding. Most cases of seeding have been reported in cases of malignant pleural tumors such as mesothelioma.

Systemic arterial air embolism is a rare but potentially fatal complication. It may produce myocardial infarction or stroke and occasionally can cause death. The mechanism is presumed to be air entry through a pulmonary vein into the left atrium and systemic circulation. Precipitating factors may include coughing and positive-pressure ventilation. We usually place saline in the introducer needle after the stylet is removed and before the aspirating needle is introduced into the lesion. This may prevent the sudden sucking of air through the needle and possibly lessen the danger of air embolism.

Diagnostic Value

TNB is extremely accurate in the diagnosis of cancer. Needle aspiration technique alone with excellent cytopathology has provided accurate diagnoses of more than 90% of lung cancers in most large series. However, despite the high sensitivity for the diagnosis of intrathoracic malignancy, TNB is somewhat limited in differentiating among different cell types of lung cancer. Several studies have shown approximately 80% accuracy in the typing of thoracic malignancies preoperatively. The accuracy usually is less in the diagnosis of thoracic malignancies that are not carcinomas. The diagnosis of lymphoma usually requires larger core-needle specimens to allow for the use of typing of lymphoma with immunoperoxidase staining.

A negative biopsy result for malignancy should not be considered diagnostic. Thirty percent of nonspecific negative biopsies are eventually proved to represent malignancy. It is therefore extremely important to establish a precise benign diagnosis for lesions that prove by biopsy to be nonmalignant. The inability of TNB to accurately diagnose benign disease has been cited as a major limitation of the technique. This limitation is primarily attributable to the aspiration technique with small-gauge needles. Active infections can be diagnosed using aspiration alone with a combination of cytologic analysis and appropriate stains or smears and cultures of aspirated material. However, the diagnosis of other benign, nonactive infections, such as well-established granulomas, hamartomas, and lipoid pneumonia, has been disappointingly low—in the range of 10% to 40% in most series.

The ability to obtain a specific benign diagnosis is greatly improved with the use of core-needle biopsies. These needles can provide histologic specimens in more than 80% of cases and can aid in the diagnosis of such lesions. The advent of small-gauge, spring-loaded, automatic cutting needles has allowed for reliable and safe retrieval of core tissue specimens from the lung, mediastinum, hila, and pleura. Small, 20-gauge core needles can be introduced through an ultrathin, 19-gauge introducing needle, permitting the use of the coaxial technique.

TNB may not be cost effective in adults with a high pretest likelihood of lung cancer who are candidates for curative surgical resection. However, there are several clinical situations in which needle biopsy may be extremely useful. It can establish the diagnosis in patients who are not operative candidates, and it may be useful in certain patient populations, such as when the prevalence of granulomatous disease is very high, as in river valleys in the United States, where most solitary pulmonary nodules are caused by histoplasmosis. In an unpublished report from our institution, we found that TNB had a major impact on clinical decision making in approximately 50% of the cases in which it was performed and resulted in marked cost savings compared with alternative diagnostic techniques, which included video-assisted thoracoscopic biopsy and thoracotomy.

TRANSTHORACIC HILAR AND MEDIASTINAL BIOPSY

Indications and Results

Most hilar lesions are biopsied by means of bronchoscopy. However, TNB may be useful in cases in which the bronchoscopy result is negative and the hilar mass is extrinsic to the airway. Most patients with mediastinal masses proceed directly to surgery without a preoperative diagnosis. Exceptions occur in the staging of lung cancer and when lymphoma is suspected. TNB has a high sensitivity and specificity for the diagnosis of metastatic carcinoma to the hilum and mediastinum. Sensitivities of more than 90% have been reported. TNB has advantages over mediastinoscopy for nodal evaluation. It is faster, is better tolerated, can be performed without general anesthesia, and is less costly. Other alternative procedures include transbronchial aspiration (i.e., Wang needle). This technique is useful when enlarged nodes are immediately adjacent to the trachea or are in the subcarinal location.

Fine-needle aspiration biopsy has a lower diagnostic accuracy for lymphoma than for carcinoma. Sensitivity for fine-needle aspiration has been reported in the range of 42% to 82%. However, the use of core biopsies has increased the yield, and patients can often be treated based on the results of core-needle biopsy alone.

In summary, the technique of TNB of the mediastinum is most useful for staging lung carcinoma, for which it is a less expensive and minimally invasive alternative to mediastinoscopy, and for the diagnosis of lymphoma when advances in immunohistochemistry are combined with core-needle biopsy techniques.

Technique

An anterior parasternal approach is preferred for most anterior mediastinal masses, and a posterior paravertebral approach is used for posterior mediastinal masses (Fig. 19-9). Often, a direct mediastinal approach can be used, and passing through the lung and pleura is avoided. This lessens the likelihood of pneumothorax because a transpulmonary approach often requires puncturing the pleural space in two locations. The pleural or extrapleural approach to the mediastinum can be enhanced by widening the tract with injections of saline or air.

The hilum is usually approached through the lung obliquely (Fig. 19-10). It is important to administer contrast before the biopsy to determine the exact location of the major pulmonary arteries and veins.

Complications

Serious complications from transthoracic biopsy of the mediastinum are rare. Occasionally, mediastinal bleeding occurs, but this is usually self-limited. However, at least one death due to pericardial tamponade has been reported. The incidence of hemoptysis and pneumothorax is similar to that for biopsy of lung lesions when the pulmonary parenchyma and pleura are traversed.

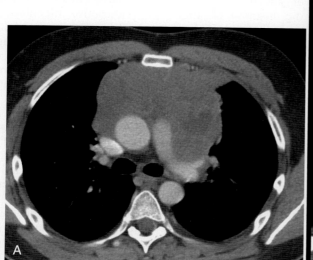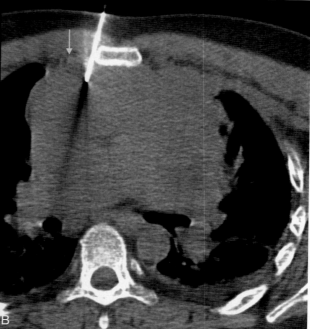

FIGURE 19-9. Anterior mediastinal biopsy. **A,** The large, partially necrotic anterior mediastinal mass displaces the mediastinal vessels. **B,** The biopsy used a parasternal approach medial to the internal mammary vessels *(arrow)*. The pathologic diagnosis was large B-cell lymphoma.

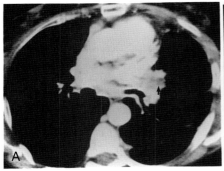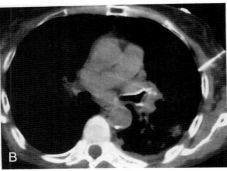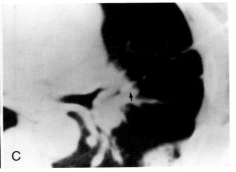

FIGURE 19-10. Transthoracic needle biopsy of a left hilar mass. **A,** A preliminary scan with contrast reveals a nonopacified lesion in the left hilum *(arrow)*. **B,** An oblique anterior approach was used. **C,** The needle has entered the lesion *(arrow)*, avoiding the pulmonary vessels. The biopsy specimen was positive for small cell carcinoma. Bronchoscopy showed extrinsic bronchial compression but no endobronchial lesion that could be biopsied.

■ RADIOFREQUENCY ABLATION OF MALIGNANT LUNG TUMORS

Radiofrequency ablation (RFA) is a minimally invasive technique for the treatment of malignant lung tumors. RFA has been an established technique in treatment of renal, hepatic, and bone tumors for several years. It has been applied to treatment of malignant lung tumors with encouraging results.

Indications

The ideal patients are those with small (<3 cm), localized, solitary primary lung cancers or metastasis from lung and other cancers. RFA is offered to patients who cannot undergo surgery, chemotherapy, or radiotherapy because of significant comorbidities or to those with disease recurrence after these treatments. It is also offered to patients who refuse these established treatments. Ongoing clinical trials are evaluating RFA as primary treatment. RFA is also used for palliation of symptoms in patients with advanced cancer typically for pain relief due to chest wall invasion (Box 19-4).

Contraindications

The absolute contraindications are bleeding diathesis and pulmonary arterial hypertension. Selected peripheral tumors in some patients with pulmonary arterial hypertension can be treated. The relative contraindications are severe emphysema with an FEV_1 value of less than 1.0 L and tumors close to a major blood vessels and central bronchi. Patients with pacemakers and intracardiac defibrillators can have malfunction due to radiofrequency (RF) interference (see Box 19-4).

Technique

Principle

The electromagnetic RF spectrum is between 3 KHz and 300 GHz. For tumor ablation, a frequency of less than 1 MHz is used. The basic principle is to cause thermal injury by converting RF energy into heat. The application of RF results in agitation of intracellular ions, which oscillate at high speed and generate frictional heat. The goal is to achieve a temperature beyond 60°C and cause cell death by irreversible protein denaturation and coagulation

---

Box 19-4. Radiofrequency Ablation

INDICATIONS
Localized solitary primary or metastatic lung cancer
Patients with comorbidities and not suitable for standard treatments
Palliation of symptoms in advanced lung cancer

RELATIVE CONTRAINDICATIONS
Bleeding diathesis
Pulmonary hypertension
Severe COPD ($FEV_1 \leq 1.0$ L)
Pacemaker and ICD

COMPLICATIONS
Postablation syndrome
Pneumothorax and potential chest tube requirement
Pleural effusion
Hemoptysis and pulmonary hemorrhage
Pneumonia
Hemothorax
Arrhythmias
ARDS
Air embolism
Transient nerve injury

ARDS, acute respiratory distress syndrome; COPD, chronic obstructive pulmonary disease; implantable cardioverter-defibrillator; FEV_1, forced expiratory volume in 1 second.

---

necrosis. An electrode that is connected to an RF generator is placed in the tumor to transmit the RF. The low-frequency RF results in an alternate current at the noninsulated tip of the electrode. The circuit is completed by grounding pads applied to the thighs of the patient that are connected to the RF generator.

The electrode is a 14- to 17-gauge, long, insulated needle with a short, noninsulated distal tip that is placed within the tumor. The needle tip can be straight (Valleylab) or multitined (RITA Medical Systems and Boston Scientific). The straight needles can be single or arrayed in a cluster, and they are internally cooled by circulating cold water. The flowing blood in the large vessels close to the tumor takes heat away from the tumor by a heat sink effect and results in inadequate treatment.

Preprocedural Workup

The preprocedural workup includes staging studies preferably with whole-body FDG-PET, CT, and blood tests for PT, PTT, and platelets. Patients with lung and airway infections are treated with antibiotics.

Patient Preparation, Sedation, and Anesthesia

Patients should be fasting overnight and stop all medications that interfere with coagulation and platelet function, similar to preparation for percutaneous needle biopsy. All procedures are done under conscious sedation or general anesthesia. Conscious sedation is adequate in most instances and is required to achieve patient immobility and analgesia. An adequate effect can be achieved with a combination of intravenous fentanyl, Versed, and Demerol administered in small doses during the procedure. General anesthesia is reserved for patients who have airway abnormalities, patients on home oxygen therapy, and those in whom severe chest wall pain is anticipated. Double-lumen tube intubation is used to reduce lung excursion for ablation of small tumors close to the diaphragm and in patients expected to have pulmonary hemorrhage.

Technical Factors

The steps involved in placement of an electrode are similar to those for needle placement for biopsy. The electrode should pass through the center of the tumor, and the tip should extend just beyond the far end of the tumor (Fig. 19-11). After satisfactory placement, treatment is started by switching on the RF generator. Typically, treatment lasts for 12 minutes. For irregularly shaped and large tumors, multiple treatments may be required after repositioning the electrode to cover the entire tumor. After successful treatment, a peripheral halo of ground-glass opacity is seen around the tumor, and the size of the treated tumor is larger the original tumor (see Fig. 19-11). After removal of the electrode, the patient is immediately placed with the treated area in a dependent position and transferred to observation room.

Postprocedural Care

Postprocedural chest radiographs are obtained at 1 and 3 hours to look for complications. Patients usually are admitted for overnight observations, although many medical centers send the patients home on the same day. Oral narcotic analgesics are prescribed for 2 weeks for treatment of potential pleuritic chest pain.

Complications

The patient may experience postablation syndrome with flulike symptoms such as fever, malaise, and fatigue. Most of the complications are minor and do not require treatment. The complications that may require chest tube are pneumothorax, pulmonary hemorrhage, hemoptysis, pleural effusion, persistent air leak, and infection. Burns can occur in the thighs at the site of grounding pads, mostly due to incorrect application techniques. Rare complications include hemothorax, acute respiratory distress syndrome (ARDS), cardiac arrhythmias, air embolus, transient mediastinal nerve injury, and rarely, death (see Box 19-4).

Follow-up

Postprocedural follow-up is done by periodic CT scans to detect complications and recurrence. The postablation lesion in the lung decreases in size during 1 to 3 months. An increase in size beyond 3 months or abnormal enhancement may indicate disease recurrence. After successful therapy, there is gradual retraction of treated lung lesion toward the pleura because of granulation tissue and scarring. Eventually, it develops into a subpleural, wedge-shaped opacity, similar to an infarct (see Fig. 19-11). Some medical centers perform magnetic resonance imaging (MRI) scans for follow-up. FDG-PET scans are also useful in detection of recurrence.

Alternative Methods of Ablation

Ablation of the tumors can be done using microwaves and laser and cryoablation.

▬ OTHER INTERVENTIONAL PROCEDURES IN THE THORAX

Radiologists may perform a spectrum of additional interventional procedures in the thorax. Many are done for pleural disease or processes. They include ultrasound-guided thoracenteses, drainage of empyemas or noninfected pleural collections, drainage of lung and mediastinal abscesses, and pleural sclerosis. Treatment of pneumothorax was discussed earlier.

Diagnosis and Treatment of Thoracic Fluid Collections

Thoracentesis

Most large pleural fluid collections can be tapped for diagnostic purposes by the attending clinician without the need for imaging guidance. Radiologic guidance increases the likelihood of obtaining pleural fluid and decreases the risk of pneumothorax. Ultrasound guidance is most useful when there are small amounts of fluid or when the fluid is loculated. Aspirated fluid can be sent for the usual diagnostic studies, including Gram stain, microbacteriologic culture, cytology, chemistry evaluations, and determinations of pH levels.

Small, 5- to 9-French (F) catheters may be inserted under ultrasound guidance along with the guiding localizing needle to permit therapeutic thoracentesis when the fluid is serous and noninfected. Ultrasound is the guidance procedure of choice for most thoracenteses; CT is reserved for loculated collections.

Empyema

If diagnostic aspiration reveals infection by Gram stain or culture, drainage is indicated. Large, free-flowing empyemas can be drained under ultrasound guidance. CT is usually reserved for loculated collections (Fig. 19-12). Radiologically guided catheters typically are used after large-bore thoracostomy tubes that have been introduced without imaging guidance have proved ineffective.

A needle is usually placed for localization, and then a catheter is introduced using a Seldinger or trocar technique. This technique is useful when collections are multiloculated or

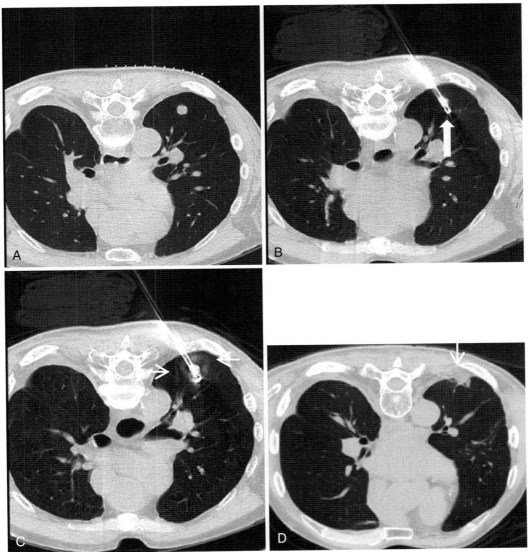

FIGURE 19-11. Radiofrequency ablation (RFA) of a left lower lobe metastasis. **A,** A new, 1.2-cm, metastatic nodule in the left lower lobe was determined to be from gastroesophageal cancer in a patient who previously underwent surgical metastasectomy. **B,** RFA was performed with the electrode placed through the center of nodule and the tip projecting just beyond the nodule *(arrow)*. **C,** Ground-glass halo *(arrows)* is seen around the nodule after completion of the treatment. **D,** Six months after the treatment, the lesion has retracted toward the pleura, forming a wedge-shaped opacity *(arrow)*.

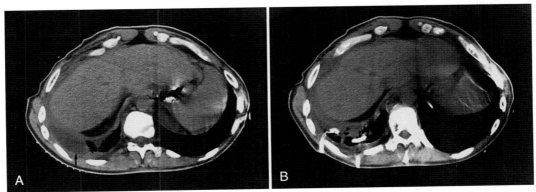

FIGURE 19-12. CT-guided empyema drainage. **A,** Preliminary CT shows a small, loculated fluid collection posteriorly *(arrow)*. **B,** Successful drainage has been achieved with a radiologically placed catheter.

multiple collections are present. Routinely, 12-F catheters are used, but larger catheters approaching the size of surgical chest tubes may be used. Most catheters contain several holes for better drainage. Multiple chest tubes can be paced for different fluid collections in cases of loculated empyema. Instillation of tissue plasminogen activator (tPA) through the chest tube helps to break up internal septations. Empyema drainage is effective in 80% to 90% of patients, and complications occur in less than 10% of cases.

Mediastinal Abscesses

Many mediastinal abscesses are drained surgically. However, radiologically guided percutaneous techniques used for drainage are particularly useful in extremely ill patients. Drainage is performed under CT guidance, and an anterior or posterior approach can be used. The pathway chosen to enter the collection should not traverse the pleura or the lung but cross only mediastinal structures.

Lung Abscesses

Most lung abscesses are treated effectively with antibiotics, and they drain spontaneously through the bronchial tree. However, lung abscesses occasionally fail to heal, particularly if there is bronchial obstruction, such as one caused by a primary lung carcinoma. Lung abscesses can also be successfully treated with percutaneous catheter drainage. The access route should be through the contiguous abnormal pleura so that the normal lung is not punctured.

Sclerotherapy

Sclerotherapy of the pleural cavity can be performed for recurrent malignant effusion. Although several agents, such as bleomycin and tetracycline, have been used, talc pleurodesis is preferred. Several sessions may be necessary for successful treatment, and the lung must be well expanded for the treatment to be effective.

▦ Suggested Readings

Austin, J.H., Cohen, M.B., 1993. Value of having a cytopathologist present during percutaneous fine-needle aspiration biopsy of lung: report of 55 cancer patients and metaanalysis of the literature. AJR Am. J. Roentgenol. 160, 175–177.

Beland, M.D., Wasser, E.J., Mayo-Smith, W.W., Dupuy, D.E., 2009. Primary non-small cell lung cancer: Review of frequency, location, and time of recurrence after radio frequency ablation. Radiology. Dec 17 (Epub ahead of print).

Cameron, E.W.J., Witton, I.D., 1977. Percutaneous drainage in the treatment of *Klebsiella pneumoniae* lung abscess. Thorax 32, 673–676.

Casola, G., vanSonnenberg, E., Keightley, A., et al., 1988. Pneumothorax: radiologic treatment with small catheters. Radiology 166, 89–91.

Choi, M.B., Um, S.W., Yoo, C.G., et al., 2004. Incidence and risk factors of delayed pneumothorax after transthoracic needle biopsy of the lung. Chest 126, 1516–1521.

Haramati, L.B., 1995. CT-guided automated needle biopsy of the chest. AJR Am. J. Roentgenol. 165, 53–55.

Khouri, N.F., Stitik, F.P., Erozan, Y.S., et al., 1985. Transthoracic needle aspiration biopsy of benign and malignant lung lesions. AJR Am. J. Roentgenol. 144, 281–288.

Klein, J.S., Salomon, G., Stewart, E.A., 1996. Transthoracic needle biopsy with a coaxially placed 20-gauge automated cutting needle: results in 122 patients. Radiology 198, 715–720.

Lee, S.I., Shepard, J.O., Boiselle, P.M., et al., 1996. Role of transthoracic needle biopsy in patient treatment decisions [abstract]. Radiology 201 (Suppl.), 269.

Lencioni, R., Crocetti, L., Cioni, R., et al., 2008. Response to radiofrequency ablation of pulmonary tumours: a prospective, intention-to-treat, multicentre clinical trial (the RAPTURE study). Lancet Oncol. 9, 621–628.

Moore, E.H., Shepard, J.O., McLoud, T.C., et al., 1990. Positional precautions in needle aspiration lung biopsy. Radiology 175, 733–735.

Morrissey, B., Adams, H., Gibbs, A.R., Crane, M.D., 1993. Percutaneous needle biopsy of the mediastinum: review of 94 procedures. Thorax 48, 632–637.

Naidich, D.P., Sussman, R., Kutcher, W.L., et al., 1988. Solitary pulmonary nodules: CT-bronchoscopic correlation. Chest 93, 595–598.

Pappa, V.I., Hussain, H.K., Reznek, R.H., et al., 1996. Role of image-guided core-needle biopsy in the management of patients with lymphoma. J. Clin. Oncol. 14, 2427–2430.

Parker, S.H., Hopper, K.D., Yakes, W.F., et al., 1989. Imaging-directed percutaneous biopsies with a biopsy gun. Radiology 171, 663–669.

Pennathur, A., Luketich, J.D., Abbas, G., et al., 2007. Radiofrequency ablation for the treatment of stage I non-small cell lung cancer in high-risk patients. J. Thorac. Cardiovasc. Surg. 134, 857–864.

Protopapas, Z., Westcott, J.L., 1996. Transthoracic needle biopsy of mediastinal lymph nodes for staging lung and other cancers. Radiology 199, 489–496.

Schenk, D.A., Bower, J.H., Bryan, C.L., et al., 1986. Transbronchial needle aspiration staging of bronchogenic carcinoma. Am. Rev. Respir. Dis. 134, 146–148.

Schenk, D.A., Bryan, C.L., Bower, J.H., Myers, D.L., 1987. Transbronchial needle aspiration in the diagnosis of bronchogenic carcinoma. Chest 92, 83–85.

Seyfer, A.E., Walsh, D.S., Graeber, G.M., et al., 1989. Chest wall implantation of lung cancer after thin-needle aspiration biopsy. Ann. Thorac. Surg. 48, 284–286.

Sider, L., Davis Jr., T.M., 1987. Hilar masses: evaluation with CT-guided biopsy after negative bronchoscopic examination. Radiology 164, 107–109.

Silverman, S.G., Mueller, P.R., Saini, S., et al., 1988. Thoracic empyema: management with image-guided catheter drainage. Radiology 169, 5–9.

Simon, C.J., Dupuy, D.E., DiPetrillo T.A., Safran H.P., Greico C.A., Mayo-Smith W.W., 2007. Pulmonary radiofrequency ablation:Long term safety and efficacy in 153 patients. Radiology 243(1) 268–275.

vanSonnenberg, E., D'Agostino, H., Casola, G., et al., 1991. Lung abscess: CT-guided drainage. Radiology 178, 347–351.

vanSonnenberg, E., Nakamoto, S.K., Mueller, P.R., et al., 1984. CT- and ultrasound-guided catheter drainage of empyema after chest tube failure. Radiology 151, 349–353.

Wang, K.P., Brower, R., Haponik, E.F., Siegelman, S., 1983. Flexible transbronchial needle aspiration for staging of bronchogenic carcinoma. Chest 84, 571–576.

Weisbrod, G.L., 1987. Percutaneous fine-needle aspiration biopsy of the mediastinum. Clin. Chest Med. 8, 27–41.

Weisbrod, G.L., 1991. Transthoracic percutaneous fine-needle aspiration biopsy in the chest and mediastinum. Semin. Interv. Radiol. 8, 1–14.

Westcott, J.L., 1980. Direct percutaneous needle aspiration of localized pulmonary lesions: results in 422 patients. Radiology 137, 31–35.

Westcott, J.L., 1981. Percutaneous needle aspiration of hilar and mediastinal masses. Radiology 141, 323–329.

Wholey, M.H., Machek, J.S., Rhinehart, E.R., et al., 1990. Automated, percutaneous biopsy device. Radiology 174, 567–568.

Zafar, N., Moinuddin, S., 1995. Mediastinal needle biopsy: a 15 year experience with 139 cases. Cancer 76, 1065–1068.

Index

Note:Page numbers followed by *b*, indicate boxes; *f*, figures; *t*, tables.